Multidisciplinary Management of Migraine

Pharmacological, Manual, and Other Therapies

Edited by

César Fernández-de-las-Peñas
Department of Physical Therapy, Occupational Therapy,
 Physical Medicine, and Rehabilitation
Esthesiology Laboratory
Universidad Rey Juan Carlos
Alcorcón, Madrid, Spain

Center for Sensory-Motor Interaction (SMI)
Department of Health Science and Technology
Aalborg University
Aalborg, Denmark

Leon Chaitow
Honorary Fellow, University of Westminster, London
Editor-in-Chief, *Journal of Bodywork and Movement Therapies*
United Kingdom

Jean Schoenen
Headache Research Unit
Department of Neurology and GIGA – Neurosciences
Liège University
Liège, Belgium

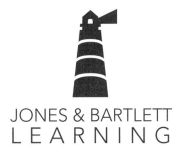

JONES & BARTLETT
LEARNING

World Headquarters
Jones & Bartlett Learning
5 Wall Street
Burlington, MA 01803
978-443-5000
info@jblearning.com
www.jblearning.com

Jones & Bartlett Learning books and products are available through most bookstores and online booksellers. To contact Jones & Bartlett Learning directly, call 800-832-0034, fax 978-443-8000, or visit our website, www.jblearning.com.

The authors, editors, and publisher have made every effort to provide accurate information. However, they are not responsible for errors, omissions, or for any outcomes related to the use of the contents of this book and take no responsibility for the use of the products and procedures described. Treatments and side effects described in this book may not be applicable to all people; likewise, some people may require a dose or experience a side effect that is not described herein. Drugs and medical devices are discussed that may have limited availability controlled by the Food and Drug Administration (FDA) for use only in a research study or clinical trial. Research, clinical practice, and government regulations often change the accepted standard in this field. When consideration is being given to use of any drug in the clinical setting, the health care provider or reader is responsible for determining FDA status of the drug, reading the package insert, and reviewing prescribing information for the most up-to-date recommendations on dose, precautions, and contraindications, and determining the appropriate usage for the product. This is especially important in the case of drugs that are new or seldom used.

Production Credits
Publisher: William Brottmiller
Acquisitions Editor: Joseph Morita
Editorial Assistant: Kayla Dos Santos
Production Manager: Julie Champagne Bolduc
Production Assistant: Emma Krosschell
Marketing Manager: Grace Richards
Manufacturing and Inventory Control Supervisor: Amy Bacus
Composition: Cenveo Publisher Services
Cover Design: Scott Moden
Permissions and Photo Research Assistant: Lian Bruno
Cover Image: © BioMedical/ShutterStock, Inc.
Printing and Binding: Malloy, Inc.
Cover Printing: Malloy, Inc.

Some images in this book feature models. These models do not necessarily endorse, represent, or participate in the activities represented in the images.

Library of Congress Cataloging-in-Publication Data
Fernández-de-las-Peñas, César.
 Multidisciplinary management of migraine : pharmacological, manual, and other therapies / by César Fernández-de-las-Peñas, Leon Chaitow, Jean Schoenen.
      p. ; cm.
 Includes bibliographical references and index.
 ISBN 978-1-4496-0050-1 -- ISBN 1-4496-0050-6
 I. Chaitow, Leon.   II. Schoenen, Jean.   III. Title.
 [DNLM: 1. Migraine Disorders--therapy. WL 344]

616.8'4912—dc23   2011045344

6048
Printed in the United States of America
16 15 14 13 12   10 9 8 7 6 5 4 3 2 1

In Memoriam

I am greatly saddened by the loss of my close friend and colleague Peter Huijbregts, who suddenly passed away on November 6, 2010. His death was a horrible tragedy and a great loss to his family and friends, the profession of physical therapy, and society in general. Peter was one of those individuals whom you never forgot once you were fortunate enough to have him cross your path.

I was aware of Peter's substantial contributions to the physical therapy profession well before I had an opportunity to meet and work personally with him. I first became friends with Peter during his tenure as Editor for the *Journal of Manual and Manipulative Therapy*. I was also extremely fortunate to work with him as Editor of *Contemporary Issues in Physical Therapy and Rehabilitation Medicine* for Jones & Bartlett Learning, as he entrusted me with editing the first textbook of the series, along with this book.

Peter was wonderfully articulate and never at a loss for words. I can recall some late-night evenings spent at national conferences enjoying conversations with Peter, who would frequently discuss his love for his wife, Rap, and his two children, Arun Joseph and Annika Dani. I will also never forget his sense of humor and can remember numerous occasions where Peter would entertain an entire room with his wit and comedy.

Peter has had a remarkable influence on many professionals who have had the fortunate opportunity to know him. His passing leaves a huge void in the manual therapy community around the entire world. Peter was a truly great gentleman, a wise scholar, and an inspiring man.

I will miss him greatly!

—César Fernández-de-las-Peñas

Contents

Foreword

Jes Olesen
Professor of Neurology, University of Copenhagen
Department of Neurology, Glostrup Hospital, Copenhagen, Denmark

The pharmacological treatment of migraine has progressed enormously over the last two decades. A wealth of randomized double-blind trials has documented the efficacy of the triptans and a huge number of post-marketing research studies have provided guidance on the practical use of these acute treatments. The combination of the triptans and nonsteroidal anti-inflammatory agents has delivered increased efficacy against migraine attacks as well. At the same time, a growing body of evidence has shown that overuse of triptans leads to deterioration and chronification in migraine patients. Although prophylactic treatment for migraine has also progressed, the gains realized have not matched those in acute treatment. Indeed, the gradually acquired knowledge of how to best use the different drugs, how to prioritize them, and when to stop prophylactic treatment, and a number of other clinical issues have been driving the agenda rather than the advent of new drugs.

All of these developments in pharmacotherapy have not obviated the need for a broader therapeutic approach to migraine. While patients with straightforward migraine as the only diagnosis are usually easy to treat, the patients seen at specialized clinics are increasingly being noted to suffer from a combination of problems that require a multidisciplinary therapeutic effort. Medication overuse, as already mentioned, is one problem observed in this setting, but comorbid depression and anxiety are also very important. Furthermore, it has become apparent that a relatively small segment of migraine patients experience deterioration of their condition over the years and may end up with the new diagnosis of chronic migraine. Chronic migraine is defined as suffering attacks for at least 8 days per month plus a total of at least 15 days of headache or more per month. Patients with this type of migraine are relatively resistant to existing prophylactic drugs and need multidisciplinary treatment. Although the efficacy of such regimens has not been proven in randomized controlled studies, the results of multidisciplinary treatment have been uniformly positive in a range of open studies in specialized centers in America, Europe, and elsewhere. These severely affected patients have often suffered with migraines for a decade or more, and so placebo effects are not likely to confound the clinical research picture.

This book is edited by an unusual combination of migraine experts—a physiotherapist, an osteopath, and a neurologist. They have recruited a number of international top-tier authors to write chapters on their areas of specialty. The result is a unique focus on the multidisciplinary aspects of migraine treatment, something to which no book has paid sufficient attention before. This book will undoubtedly be useful for those who specialize in the treatment of migraine and other headaches and, in fact, for all providers who care for headache patients.

Introduction

During the past decade, scientific research has improved our understanding of migraine pathogenesis, leading to more efficient pharmacological treatment protocols. Many migraineurs, however, remain dissatisfied with their anti-migraine medications because these agents are not sufficiently effective or have unpleasant side effects. It is not surprising, therefore, that in a recent survey by Wells et al. (2011), complementary and alternative medicine (CAM) was reportedly used more often among adults with migraines and severe headaches (49.5%) than by those persons without these diagnoses (33.9%). CAM therapies were grouped into four broad categories: alternative medical systems (e.g., acupuncture, homeopathy, naturopathy), manual therapies (e.g., massage, chiropractic care), biologically based therapies (e.g., herbs, food elimination), and mind–body therapies (e.g., biofeedback, hypnosis, meditation, relaxation).

Many—though by no means all—anti-migraine drugs have been studied in large, randomized, placebo-controlled trials and are the mainstay therapies cited in evidence-based international treatment guidelines. Such guidelines are chiefly focused on efficacy measures and seldom take into account side effects and tolerance. CAM therapies do not incorporate drugs and have relatively few adverse effects, but they also usually lack evidence-based data supporting their efficacy in treatment of migraine. Admittedly, this lack of research-based evidence is a major handicap according to modern scientific standards, and it is acknowledged that, whenever possible, adequate controlled trials should be performed. This standard can be problematic, however, as funding for such large trials is rarely available, and adequate, biologically nonactive placebos may not exist.

Meanwhile, the potential usefulness of CAM therapies is supported by the multifactorial pathophysiology of migraine and by its high comorbidity. Building on Kerr's principle (1961), Jes Olesen (1991) has conceptualized the *vascular–supraspinal–myogenic model* for headache where "the perceived pain is determined by the sum of nociception from cephalic arteries and pericranial myofascial tissues converging upon the same neurons and integrated with supraspinal effect." According to the author, this model provides "a rational explanation of empirically developed, internationally accepted, multimodal treatment strategies for migraine and tension-type headache." The majority of manual therapies described in this book are relevant to this multisensory convergent model of head pain.

Migraine, however, is also known to be comorbid with more than 20 somatic diseases (Le et al., 2011), among which musculoskeletal disorders, including fibromyalgia, are highly prevalent. Comorbidity with psychological disorders including generalized anxiety disorder, panic disorder, and depression is even more widespread (Radat et al., 2011).

Thus somatic and mental comorbidities are seen to contribute substantially to migraine disability. Both physical and mind–body strategies can beneficially modify such disability, thereby contributing to an increased quality of life for patients with migraine. Interestingly, only 4.5% of migraineurs who use CAM therapies (49.5%) declare that they use them specifically for migraines or severe headaches, suggesting that the majority use these therapies for comorbid symptoms (Wells et al., 2011).

To the best of our knowledge, this text is the first book that presents a comprehensive and cutting-edge overview of both the classical pharmacotherapies of migraine and the nondrug treatments, including the wide range of manual therapies and mind–body strategies. The chapter authors were asked to include illustrative clinical vignettes as well as therapeutic evidence scores based both on efficacy and tolerance whenever possible and appropriate. We are deeply indebted to them for their highly knowledgeable and well-balanced contributions.

Although this book's table of contents suggests that multidisciplinarity is the key to migraine therapy, the reader will not find a specific chapter on multidisciplinary treatment strategies here, because such an approach would vary with locally available expertise as well as the patient's clinical presentation and preferences. To conclude this introduction, we can do no better than to repeat David Peters' conclusion (Chapter 23) that "today . . . it is not merely a holistic notion of the patient that is needed, but a holistic notion of the medical context itself." We hope that this book will contribute to this model.

REFERENCES

Kerr FW. Structural relation of the trigeminal spinal tract to upper cervical roots and the solitary nucleus in the cat. *Exp Neurol* 1961;4:134–148.

Le H, Tfelt-Hansen P, Russell MB, et al. Co-morbidity of migraine with somatic disease in a large population-based study. *Cephalalgia* 2011;31:43–64.

Olesen J. Clinical and pathophysiological observations in migraine and tension-type headache explained by integration of vascular, supraspinal and myofascial inputs. *Pain* 1991;46:125–132.

Radat F, Kalaydjiana A, Merikangas KR. Psychiatric comorbidity in migraine. In: Schoenen J, Dodick DW, Sàndor P, eds. *Comorbidity in Migraine*. London: Wiley-Blackwell; 2011:1–13.

Wells RE, Bertisch SM, Buettner C, et al. Complementary and alternative medicine use among adults with migraines/severe headaches. *Headache* 2011;51:1087–1097.

Contributors

Nicole Elizabeth Acerra, PT, PhD
Rehabilitation Services, Vancouver General Hospital, Vancouver, Canada; Department of Physical Therapy, University of British Columbia, Vancouver, Canada; Physiotherapy Private Practice, Vancouver, Canada

Marta Allena, MD
University Consortium for Adaptive Disorders and Headache (UCADH) and Headache Science Centre (C. Mondino Foundation), Pavia, Italy

Frank Andrasik, PhD
Distinguished Professor and Chair, Department of Psychology, University of Memphis, United States

Fabio Antonaci, MD, PhD
University Consortium for Adaptive Disorders and Headache (UCADH) Pavia and Headache Medicine Centre, Policlinic of Monza, Italy

Lars Arendt-Nielsen, PhD, Dr. Med Sci
Center for Sensory-Motor Interaction (SMI), Laboratory for Musculoskeletal Pain and Motor Control, Aalborg University, Aalborg, Denmark

Thorsten Bartsch, MD
Department of Neurology, University Hospital of Schleswig Holstein, University of Kiel, Kiel, Germany

Michael H. Bennett, MBBS, MD, FANZCA, CertDHM
Associate Professor (Conjoint) of Anaesthesia and Hyperbaric Medicine, University of NSW, Sydney, Australia; Senior Staff Specialist, Prince of Wales Hospital, Sydney, Australia

Marcelo E. Bigal, MD, PhD
Head of the Merck Investigator Study Program and Scientific Education Division, Office of the Chief Medical Officer, Merck Department of Neurology, Albert Einstein College of Medicine, Bronx, New York, United States
Disclosure: Dr. Bigal is a full-time employee of Merck.

Mark Bovey, MSc, MBAcC
Acupuncture Research Resource Centre, Faculty of Health and Human Sciences, Thames Valley University, Brentford, Middlesex, United Kingdom

Dawn C. Buse, PhD
Assistant Professor, Department of Neurology, Albert Einstein College of Medicine of Yeshiva University, Bronx, New York, United States; Assistant Professor, Clinical Health Psychology Doctoral Program, Ferkauf

Graduate School of Psychology of Yeshiva University, New York, United States; Director of Psychology, Montefiore Headache Center, Bronx, New York, United States

Alessandro Capuano, MD, PhD
Division of Neurology, Headache Center, Bambino Gesù Pediatric Hospital, IRCCS, Rome, Italy

Leon Chaitow, ND, DO
Honorary Fellow, University of Westminster, London, United Kingdom; Editor-in-Chief, *Journal of Bodywork and Movement Therapies* (Elsevier), London, United Kingdom

Stefan Chmelik, MSc, MRCHM, MBAcC
Founder, New Medicine Group, Harley Street, London, United Kingdom; Senior Lecturer, London College of Traditional Acupuncture, London, United Kingdom

Bryan S. Dennison, PT, DPT, MPT, OCS, CSCS, FAAOMPT
Summit Physical Therapy, Mammoth Lakes, California, United States; Affiliate Faculty, Rueckert-Hartman College for Health Professions, Regis University, Denver, Colorado, United States

Ina Diener, PT, BAppSc (Physiology), PhD
Department of Physical Therapy, Stellenbosch University, Cape Town, South Africa

Jan Dommerholt, PT, DPT, MPS
President Myopain Seminars, LLC; Bethesda Physiocare, Inc., Bethesda, Maryland, United States

Anne Donnet, MD
Department of Neurology, Clinical Neuroscience Federation, La Timone Hospital, Marseille, France

Damien Downing, MBBS, MSB
New Medicine Group, Harley Street, London, United Kingdom

Marie-Elisabeth Faymonville, MD, PhD, Professor
Director of the Department of Algology and Palliative Care, University Hospital, University of Liège, Liège, Belgium

César Fernández-de-las-Peñas, PT, DO, PhD
Department of Physical Therapy, Occupational Therapy, Physical Medicine and Rehabilitation of Universidad

Rey Juan Carlos, Alcorcón, Madrid, Spain; Esthesiology Laboratory of Universidad Rey Juan Carlos, Alcorcón, Madrid, Spain; Centre for Sensory-Motor Interaction (SMI), Department of Health Science and Technology, Aalborg University, Aalborg, Denmark

Gary Fryer, PhD, BSc (Osteopathy), ND
Senior Lecturer, School of Biomedical and Clinical Sciences, Victoria University, Melbourne, Australia; Institute of Sport, Exercise and Active Living, Victoria University, Melbourne, Australia; Research Associate Professor, A.T. Still Research Institute, Kirksville, Missouri, United States

Andreas R. Gantenbein, MD
Department of Neurology, University Hospital Zurich, Zürich, Switzerland

Graham Gard, DO
Private Practice, Ware, Herts, United Kingdom; Independent Anatomically Based Osteopathic Research

Hong-You Ge, MD, PhD
Center for Sensory-Motor Interaction (SMI), Laboratory for Musculoskeletal Pain and Motor Control, Aalborg University, Aalborg, Denmark

Robert D. Gerwin, MD
Associate Professor of Neurology, Johns Hopkins University School of Medicine, Baltimore, Maryland, United States; Pain and Rehabilitation Medicine, Ltd., Bethesda, Maryland, United States

Paul Glynn, PT, DPT, OCS, FAAOMPT
Physical Therapy in Collaboration, Sudbury, Massachusetts, United States; Rehabilitation Manager, Newton-Wellesley Hospital, Newton, Massachusetts, United States

Peter J. Goadsby, MD, PhD
Headache Group, Department of Neurology, University of California, San Francisco, California, United States

Thomas Graven-Nielsen, PhD, Dr. Med Sci
Center for Sensory-Motor Interaction (SMI), Laboratory for Musculoskeletal Pain and Motor Control, Aalborg University, Aalborg, Denmark

Christian Gröbli, PT
President of the David G. Simons Academy, Winterthur, Switzerland

Javier González Iglesias, PT, DO, PhD
Centro de Fisioterapia Integral, Candás, Asturias

Peter Huijbregts, PT, MSc, MHSc, DPT, OCS, FAAOMPT, FCAMT (Deceased)
Shelbourne Physiotherapy, Victoria, British Columbia, Canada

John R. Krauss, PT, PhD, OCS, FAAOMPT
Program in Physical Therapy, School of Health Sciences, Oakland University, Rochester, Michigan, United States

Tarannum Lateef, MD, MPH
National Children's Medical Center and Staff Clinician, Genetic Epidemiology Research Branch, National Institute of Mental Health, Rockville, Maryland, United States

Meryl Latsko, MD, MPH
Research Instructor of Neurology, Thomas Jefferson University, Philadelphia, Pennsylvania, United States

Donald W. Lewis, MD, FAAP, FAAN
EVMS Foundation Professor and Chairman, Department of Pediatrics, Children's Hospital of The King's Daughters, Eastern Virginia Medical School, Norfolk, Virginia, United States

Adriaan Louw, PT, MAppSc (Physiology), GCRM, CSMT
International Spine and Pain Institute, Story City, Iowa, United States; Neuro Orthopaedic Institute, United States; Adjunct Faculty, Rockhurst University, Kansas City, Missouri, United States; Independent Anatomically Based Osteopathic Research

Nicole Malaise, MA
Department of Algology and Palliative Care, University Hospital, University of Liège, Liège, Belgium

Hélène Massiou, MD
Department of Neurology, Hospital Lariboisière, Paris, France

Johnson McEvoy, BSc, MSc, DPT, MISCP, MCSP, PT
United Physiotherapy Clinic, Unit 5c Whitethorns Castletroy, Limerick, Ireland

Kathleen R. Merikangas, PhD
Senior Investigator, Chief, Genetic Epidemiology Research Branch, National Institute of Mental Health, Rockville, Maryland, United States

Paul Mintken, PT, DPT, OCS, FAAOMPT
Assistant Professor, Department of Physical Therapy Education, University of Colorado, Denver, Colorado, United States

Koen Paemeleire, MD, PhD
Department of Neurology, Ghent University Hospital, Ghent, Belgium

Valérie Palmaricciotti, MA
Department of Algology and Palliative Care, University Hospital, University of Liège, Liège, Belgium

David Peters, MB, ChB, DRCOG, DMSMed, MFHom, FLCOM
Professor and Clinical Director, School of Life Sciences, University of Westminster, London, United Kingdom

Joseph Pizzorno, ND
President/CEO, Salugenecists Inc., Seattle, Washington, United States; President Emeritus, Bastyr University, Seattle, Washington, United States; Editor-in-Chief, *Integrative Medicine, A Clinician's Journal*; Chairman, Scientific Advisory Board, Bioclinic Naturals, Coquitlam, British Columbia, Canada

Geneviève Plu-Bureau, MD, PhD
Unit of Gynecology-Endocrinology, Hospital Hotel-Dieu, Paris, France; University Paris Descartes, Paris, France

Emilio J. Puentedura, PT, DPT, PhD, OCS, GDMT, CSMT, FAAOMPT
Assistant Professor, Department of Physical Therapy, University of Nevada, Las Vegas, Nevada, United States; International Spine and Pain Institute, Story City, Iowa, United States; Neuro Orthopaedic Institute, United States

Franz Riederer, MD
Department of Neurology, University Hospital Zurich, Zürich, Switzerland

Michael Bjørn Russell, MD, PhD, Dr. Med Sci
Professor of Neurology, Head and Neck Research Group, Research Centre, Akershus University Hospital,

Lørenskog, Oslo, Norway; Institute of Clinical Medicine, University of Oslo, Nordbyhagen, Oslo, Norway

Irène Salamun, MA
Department of Algology and Palliative Care, University Hospital, University of Liège, Liège, Belgium

Peter S. Sándor, MD
RehaClinic Zurzach and University Hospital Zurich, Zürich, Switzerland

Edgar Savidge, PT, DPT, OCS
Rehabilitation Supervisor, Newton-Wellesley Hospital, Newton, Massachusetts, United States

Jean Schoenen, MD, PhD
Department of Neurology and Neurobiology Research Centre, Liège University, Liège, Belgium

Stephen D. Silberstein, MD
Professor of Neurology, Jefferson Medical College, Thomas Jefferson University, Philadelphia, Pennsylvania, United States

Cristina Tassorelli, MD
University Consortium for Adaptive Disorders and Headache, Pavia, Italy; Headache Science Centre, IRCCS National Neurological Institute, C. Mondino Foundation, and University of Pavia, Pavia, Italy

Marina de Tommaso, MD, PhD
Neurological and Psychiatric Sciences Department, University of Bari, Aldo Moro, Bari, Italy

Michiel Trouw, PT, MT (OMT)
Physical-Manual Therapist, Private Practice, Hengelo, The Netherlands

Massimiliano Valeriani, MD, PhD
Division of Neurology, Headache Center, Bambino Gesù Pediatric Hospital, IRCCS, Rome, Italy; Center for Sensory-Motor Interaction, Aalborg University, Aalborg, Denmark

Harry Von Piekartz, PT, MSc, PhD
Department of Physical Therapy, Faculty of Business, Management and Social Science, University of Applied Science Osnabrück, Osnabrück, Germany; Clinic for Manual Therapy and Applied Neuro-Biomechanic Science, Ootmarsum, The Netherlands

Reviewers

Steve Agocs, DC
Clinician and Associate Professor, Cleveland
Chiropractic College, Overland Park, Kansas

Fernando Branco, MD, FAAPMR
Medical Director, Rosomoff Pain Center, Miami, Florida

Marni Capes, MS, DC, CCEP, CCSP
Associate Professor, Clinical Sciences Division, Life
University, Marietta, Georgia

Richard K. Compton, MS, CPAT, CH, CPH
Program Coordinator and Patient Care Coordinator,
Rosomoff Comprehensive Center, Miami, Florida

Thomas Denninger, DPT, CSCS
Clinic Director, Adjunct Faculty, and EIM Fellow in
Training, Proaxis Therapy Spine Center, Sports and
Orthopedic Physical Residencies, Greenville, South
Carolina

Deanna Dye, PT, PhD
Assistant Professor, Kasiska College of Allied Health
Professions, Idaho State University, Pocatello, Idaho

Matthew F. Funk, DC
Professor and Clinician, College of Chiropractic,
University of Bridgeport, Bridgeport, Connecticut

Connie Heflin, MSN, RN, CNE
Director of Online Learning, West Kentucky
Community and Technical College, Paducah,
Kentucky

Christopher P. Hurley, PT, DPT, DSc, OCS, SCS, ATC
Clinical Assistant Professor, Physical Therapy Program,
Carroll University, Waukesha, Wisconsin

Emmanuel B. John, BScPT, PhD
Assistant Professor and Director, Howard University,
Washington, District of Columbia

Gena E. Kadar, DC, CNS
Assistant Professor, Department of Diagnosis, Los
Angeles College of Chiropractic, Southern California
University of Sciences, Whittier, California

David Kujawa, PT, MBA, OCS
Assistant Professor and Doctor of Physical Therapy
Program, Department of Rehabilitation Science,
Judith Herb College of Education, Health Science
and Human Service University of Toledo,
Toledo, Ohio

John P. Mrozek, DC, MEd, FCCS
Dean of Academic Affairs, Texas Chiropractic College,
Pasadena, Texas

Shannon M. Petersen, PT, DScPT, OCS, FAAOMPT, COMT
Doctor of Physical Therapy Program, Des Moines University, Des Moines, Idaho

Stephen Ross, MD
Vice Chair for Clinical Affairs, Department of Neurology, Penn State College of Medicine, Hershey, Pennsylvania

Betty Sindelar, PT, PhD
Associate Professor, Ohio University, Athens, Ohio

H. Garrett Thompson, DC, PhD
Associate Professor and Chair, Evidence Based and Outcomes Focused Department, Department of Sciences, Los Angeles College of Chiropractic, University of Health Sciences, Whittier, California

Paul Wanlass, DC
Assistant Professor, Department of Principles and Practices, Southern California, University of Health Sciences, Whittier, California

INTRODUCTION

Epidemiology and Quality of Life with Migraine

Kathleen R. Merikangas, PhD, and Tarannum Lateef, MD, MPH

INTRODUCTION

Epidemiology is defined as the study of the distribution and determinants of diseases in human populations. Thus epidemiologic studies are concerned with the extent and types of illnesses in groups of people and with the factors that influence the distribution of those diseases (Gordis, 2000). Epidemiologists investigate the interactions that may occur among the host, the agent, and the environment (the classic epidemiologic triangle) to produce a disease state. An important goal of epidemiologic studies is to identify the *etiology* of a disease, thereby enabling health-care providers to prevent or intervene in the progression of the disorder. To achieve this goal, epidemiologic studies generally proceed from studies that specify the amount and distribution of a disease within a population by person, place, and time (that is, *descriptive* epidemiology), to more focused studies of the determinants of disease in specific groups (that is, *analytic* epidemiology) (Gordis, 2000). Whether descriptive or analytic, the ultimate goal of epidemiologic investigations is prevention.

Table 1.1 summarizes some contributions of epidemiology to our understanding of the magnitude, risk factors, and impact of migraine. The application of the tools of epidemiology to headache has generated substantial methodological developments designed to collect reliable and valid information on the prevalence of headaches in nonclinical samples. With these methodologies, the high prevalence of migraine in the general population has been consistently reported, and the sex- and age-specific patterns of onset and offset of migraine have been well established. Community-based studies have also demonstrated major biases in severity and comorbidity that characterize clinical samples, particularly those obtained at tertiary referral centers for headache. Finally, epidemiologic studies have provided data on the huge impact and the personal and societal costs of migraine and other headaches.

This chapter has two major goals: (1) to summarize the magnitude and sociodemographic correlates of headache subtypes in adults and children and (2) to present

Table 1.1 Goals of Epidemiologic Studies

- Develop standardized assessments of headache subtypes
- Establish validity of diagnostic nomenclature
- Estimate magnitude of headache subtypes in the general population
- Identify risk and protective factors for headache subgroups
- Collect information on patterns of use and adequacy of treatment

information on the individual and societal impact of migraine.

MAGNITUDE OF HEADACHE SYNDROMES IN THE GENERAL POPULATION

Adults

Table 1.2 summarizes recent international population-based studies of headache and specific headache subtypes in adults. Several community studies of European samples (Jensen & Stovner, 2008) have been undertaken, and a very large American study of 15,000 households representative of the U.S. population was conducted in 1989 (Stewart et al., 1992), followed by a 10-year replication with identical methodology (Lipton et al., 2001a).

Approximately 50% of persons in the general population suffer from headaches during any given year, and more than 90% report a lifetime history of headaches (Bigal et al., 2004; Stovner et al., 2007). The average lifetime prevalence of migraine is 18%, and the estimated average past-year prevalence is 13%. Tension-type headache is more common than migraine, with approximately 52% lifetime prevalence and 22% 12-month prevalence. Approximately half of those persons who report headaches suffer from tension-type headache. Only a small minority (3%) suffer from chronic headache (Jensen & Stovner, 2008).

Children

A recent systematic review of population-based studies reported the prevalence of headache and migraine among children and adolescents during the period between 1990 and 2007 (Abu-Arahef et al., 2010). It

has been difficult to summarize the rates in these studies because many studies focus on particular age subgroups, whereas few studies have examined prevalence of headache across all years of childhood and adolescence simultaneously. The prevalence of migraine in children and adolescents is 7.7% (95% confidence interval [CI]: 7.6–7.8), and that of headaches is 58.4% (95% CI: 58.1–58.8) over a range of prevalence periods between 1 month and lifetime. Variation in the prevalence rates of migraine can be attributed to sampling differences (age, sex, and ethnic composition of the sample); methodological differences, particularly related to the method of assessment of the diagnostic criteria for headache (e.g., structured diagnostic interview, questionnaire, symptom checklist); the mode of administration of headache assessments (i.e., direct interview, telephone interview, self-reported assessment); and variation in the time frame of prevalence estimates.

The variation in estimates of childhood migraine is in part due to methodological differences, but also to the inadequacy of the current diagnostic criteria in accurately capturing migraine among youth. As demonstrated in many studies, the *International Classification of Headache Disorders—I* (ICHD-I) does not adequately distinguish the primary headache syndromes in childhood. With the publication of the *International Classification of Headache Disorders—II* (ICHD-II) in 2004, the sensitivity of diagnosis of migraine without aura in children improved from 21% to 53%, yet continued to miss almost half of all pediatric migraine (Lima et al., 2007).

Headaches in early childhood are not only difficult to classify but also continuously evolve over time (Brna et al., 2005). The likelihood of migraine at puberty is practically equal among children who present with tension-type headache or migraine at 6 years of age (Virtanen et al., 2007).

Table 1.2 Twelve-Month and Lifetime Prevalence Rates of Headache in International Population Surveys of Adults

Headache Subtype	12 Month M	F	Total	Lifetime M	F	Total
Headaches	43 (19–69)	55 (40–83)	49 (29–77)	90 (90–93)	94 (94–99)	92 (71–96)
Migraine	8 (2–13)	16 (6–20)	13 (5–25)	13 (8–22)	23 (17–33)	18 (12–28)
Tension type	18 (13–21)	24 (23–25)	22 (18–25)	37 (32–69)	61 (37–88)	52 (35–78)

Prevalence Rates % [Median; (Range)]

RISK FACTORS AND CORRELATES

The evidence consistently indicates that migraine is far more common in women than in men, with one-year prevalence rates ranging from 1.5% to 18.3% among women and from 0.6% to 9.5% among males (Lipton & Bigal, 2005). The sex ratio for lifetime migraine remains stable at 2–3:1 and is generally consistent across countries. The female preponderance of headaches emerges in youth, with females having a 1.5-fold greater risk of headaches and 1.7-fold greater risk of migraine than male children and adolescents.

Numerous hypotheses have been proposed to explain the gender differences in migraines. However, few studies have systematically reviewed the evidence for both artifactual and true causes of women's increased risk for migraine. Potential sources of artifactual causes of the sex difference include biases associated with sampling (i.e., increased detection of females in clinical samples), reporting (i.e., a greater tendency for women to report or be aware of migraine), definitions (i.e., diagnostic criteria more likely to cover symptoms expressed by women than men), or confounding with other factors that are more common in women (i.e., depression, anxiety, gastrointestinal syndromes).

After exclusion of possible artifactual explanations for the excess number of cases of migraine noted in women, numerous hypotheses have been considered. These include hypotheses focusing on neurobiological factors (e.g., fluctuation of reproductive hormones, increased stress reactivity in women), greater exposure or sensitivity to environmental stressors (e.g., role stress, life events associated with certain sensory stimuli), and genetic factors (e.g., greater genetic loading for migraine in women) (Low et al., 2007).

With respect to specific headache subtypes, there is a twofold greater prevalence of migraine across the lifespan in women, whereas tension-type headache affects both sexes at approximately equal rates. Sex differences among migraineurs are by no means uniform across childhood and adolescence. Whereas post-pubertal rates of migraine are significantly higher among females in almost all studies, the rates of migraine are equivalent among boys and girls younger than 12 years of age; notably, some studies even suggest a higher prevalence of migraine among boys aged 3–5 years when compared with girls of the same age group (Winner & Rothner, 2001). The American Migraine study revealed that the female-to-male gender ratio of migraine increased steadily from age 12 to about age 42, after which it declined (Stewart et al., 1991). The decline in the sex-based ratio at mid-life may correspond with the decline in estrogen levels in women as menopause approaches. This pattern also suggests that hormonal events associated with menarche may contribute to the emerging relative increases in the migraine prevalence in females in early adolescence. Headache and migraine prevalence reliably increase across the pediatric age spectrum. In the United States, frequent or severe headaches, including migraine, were reported in 4% of 4- and 5-year-olds, with the prevalence increasing to 25% in the next 10 years of childhood (Lateef et al., 2009).

Aside from sex and age, a family history of migraine is one of the most potent and consistent risk factors for migraine. Findings from twin studies implicate genetic factors as underlying approximately one-third of familial clusters of migraine, but the mode of inheritance is clearly complex. Despite an increasing number of studies examining candidate genes' association with migraine, no replicated linkage or associations between specific genes and migraine have emerged as yet, except for hemiplegic migraine. To date, the application of genome-wide association studies in cases and controls has not yielded replicated associations between migraine and genetic markers.

Migraine is strongly associated with a variety of medical disorders, especially asthma, eczema, allergies, epilepsy, cardiovascular disease, cerebrovascular disease, and particularly ischemic stroke. Anxiety and mood disorders are also strongly associated with migraine. Prospective data from community studies of youth reveal that anxiety in childhood is associated with the subsequent development of headache in young adulthood.

INCIDENCE AND COURSE OF DISEASE

Despite the large body of cross-sectional studies on the prevalence and correlates of migraine, there is a dearth of prospective research from community samples that might provide information on the incidence, stability, and course of migraine in adults. Incidence data have been reported in three prospective community surveys of adults (Breslau & Davis, 1993; Swartz et al., 2000; Lyngberg et al., 2005a) and one such study of children (Anttila et al., 2006), but the longitudinal course of specific headache subtypes in adults has been studied in only two prospective studies of community samples (Lyngberg et al., 2005a; Merikangas et al., 2011). These studies revealed that there was substantial longitudinal overlap between migraine and tension-type headache and worse long-term outcome in terms of severity and recurrence among persons with coexisting migraine and tension-type headache (Lyngberg et al., 2005b; Merikangas et al., 2011). In contrast to the limited number of prospective studies of adults with migraine, several long-term follow-up studies of specific childhood headache subtypes have been conducted with school-based and clinical samples (Bille, 1997; Guidetti & Galli, 1998; Kienbacher et al., 2006).

The incidence of migraine is low before adolescence, but then rises rapidly until middle adulthood, and finally levels off in later life. The onset of migraine may occur in childhood, when boys and girls are equally likely to suffer from migraine. Migraine in childhood is more likely to be associated with gastrointestinal complaints, particularly episodic bouts of stomach pain, vomiting, or diarrhea, and its duration is shorter than that commonly observed in adults. In women, migraine is strongly associated with reproductive system function, with increased incidence during puberty and the first trimester of pregnancy, and is associated with exogenous hormone use. After menopause, the frequency of migraine attacks generally decreases dramatically, unless estrogen replacement therapy is administered.

The course of migraine is highly variable. Of the women in the United States who have migraine, 25% experience four or more severe attacks per month, 48% experience one to four severe attacks per month, and 38% experience one or fewer severe attacks per month. Similar frequency patterns have been observed in men (Lipton et al., 2001b). In general, both the frequency and the duration of migraine decrease at mid-life in both men and women, and the symptomatic manifestations may change substantially over time. Numerous precipitants of migraine attacks have been consistently implicated as precipitants of acute headache attacks (including hormonal changes, stress or its cessation, fasting fatigue, over-sleeping, particular foods and beverages, drug intake, chemical additives, bright light, weather changes, and exercise), but these agents/situations have been observed to vary dramatically within and between individuals in prospective research (see Chapter 4).

What happens to a child with migraine? Longitudinal population-based studies on pediatric migraine are relatively sparse. Bille (1997) reported the first extensive study of pediatric migraine epidemiology in 1962 and subsequently followed a group of children with severe migraine for 40 years. In this study, approximately 23% of these children became permanently migraine-free as adults (34% of the boys and 15% of the girls) (Bille, 1997). At the 40-year follow-up evaluation, of the initial group of migraineurs, 33% of those who had children

had offspring who developed their own headaches with migrainous features. The author also showed a considerable recall bias with regard to migraine with aura: 41% of middle-aged subjects could not remember that they had aura symptoms at younger ages. This finding highlights the need for prospective follow-up studies.

Other prospective studies, utilizing ICHD-II criteria, have shown that headaches remit in 17% to 34% of subjects, persist in 20% to 48%, and transform into other types of headache in 11% to 37% (Zebenholzer et al., 2000; Camarda et al., 2002). Studies that use detailed headache diagnostic criteria suggest that as many as one-fourth of patients may evolve from migraine to tension-type headache, and vice versa (Metsahonkala et al., 1997; Zebenholzer et al., 2000; Camarda et al., 2002). In terms of prognostic factors, early age at onset (Hernandez-Latorre & Roig, 2000), psychosocial stressors (Metsahonkala et al., 1997), and psychiatric comorbidity (Guidetti & Galli, 1998) may be linked to a less favorable outcome.

IMPACT OF MIGRAINE
Individual-Level Disability

Recent community studies have underscored the enormous personal and social burden imposed by migraine in terms of both direct and indirect costs. The severity of migraine ranges from mild inconvenience to nearly total disability. More than 80% of those persons with migraine report some degree of disability. For example, data from the American Migraine Study II (Lipton et al., 2001a) revealed that more than half (53%) of migraineurs reported severe impairment in activity or the requirement for bed rest with severe headaches. The same study revealed that 92% of women and 89% of men with severe migraine had some headache-related disability, and approximately half were severely disabled or required bed rest (Lipton et al., 2001a). In addition to attack-related disability, many patients with migraine live in fear, knowing that at any time an attack could disrupt their ability to work, care for themselves or their families, or meet social obligations. Abundant evidence indicates that migraine reduces the health-related quality of life (Dahlof et al., 1997; Santanello et al., 1997). Household and family or social activities are more likely than work or school activities to be disrupted by migraine.

Some of the disability among headache sufferers can be attributed to comorbid conditions that explain a substantial proportion of the disability associated with non-migraine severe headaches and approximately 65% of the disability associated with migraine headaches (Saunders et al., 2008). Despite the high magnitude of disability associated with migraine, only half of those individuals who suffer from debilitating migraine seek professional help.

Recurrent headaches have also been shown to have a negative impact on the quality of life in children. Children with migraine have more school absences, decreased academic performance, social stigma, and impaired ability to establish and maintain peer relationships. In a review of studies that examined the impact of headache on the functional status and quality of life of children with migraine, Kernick, Reinhold, and Campbell (2009) found substantial headache-related morbidity for a significant number of children, most notably in days lost and affected at school. On average, studies reflecting school settings found that 8% of children lost 6 days of school attendance per year. The impact of headache was directly related to headache frequency and severity of headaches. The same review also examined methodological factors in studies of headache effects in children, and recommended that future studies include control groups with standardized and validated measures of sleep impact. The quality of life in children with migraine is impaired to a degree similar to that in children with arthritis or cancer (Powers et al., 2003).

Impact of Migraine on Society

Severe headaches and migraine not only have substantial impact on the affected individual, but also have major economic implications in the form of medical expenses and employer costs (Dahlof & Solomon, 1998). The direct costs of migraine, including physician visits, emergency room visits, and prescribed and over-the-counter (OTC) medications, are estimated to exceed $17 billion to $19 billion per year (Andlin-Sobocki et al., 2005; Berg & Stovner, 2005). Indirect costs include the aggregate effects of migraine on productivity at work (paid employment), in performance of household work, and in other roles (Goldberg et al., 2005).

A recent European study of the impact of brain diseases revealed that migraine has the greatest health-care costs of all the neurologic disorders investigated, including epilepsy, multiple sclerosis, Parkinson disease, and stroke (Andlin-Sobocki et al., 2005). The bulk of the expenses attributable to migraine derive from its high population prevalence and indirect costs due to occupational disability rather than to direct health-care costs;

in fact, the latter costs are lower for migraine than for the other neurologic conditions. For example, the annual U.S. direct medical costs attributable to migraine totaled an estimated $1 billion in 1999 (Lipton et al., 2001a).

During the past few years, increasing attention has been directed to the enormous public health impact of migraine. In recognition of this condition's high prevalence and burden, as well as the limited amount of research resources devoted to migraine, the World Health Organization recently launched a global campaign—known as Lifting the Burden—to reduce the burden of headache (Osterhaus et al., 1992; Stang et al., 1996; Stewart et al., 1996; Hu et al., 1999; Holmes et al., 2001).

Migraine also has a marked impact on health-care utilization. The National Ambulatory Medical Care Survey in the United States, conducted from 1976 to 1977, found that 4% of all visits to physicians' offices (more than 10 million visits per year) were for headache (National Center for Health Statistics, 1979). Migraine also results in high utilization of emergency rooms and urgent care centers (Celentano et al., 1992; Fry, 1996; Bigal et al., 2000). Vast quantities of prescription and OTC medications are taken for headache-related disorders (Celentano et al., 1992). OTC sales of pain medication in the United States (for all conditions) were estimated to amount to $3.2 billion in 1999, and headache accounted for approximately one-third of OTC analgesic use (Lipton et al., 2001a). Gross sales for triptans total approximately $1 billion per year in the United States alone (Lipton et al., 2001a).

CONCLUSIONS

Approximately 50% of persons in the general population suffer from headaches during any given year, and more than 90% report a lifetime history of headache. The average lifetime prevalence of migraine is 18%, and the estimated average past-year prevalence is 13%. Tension-type headache is more common than migraine, with a lifetime prevalence of approximately 52%, and an average 12-month prevalence of 22%. About 58% of youth suffer from headache, and the prevalence of migraine in children and adolescents is about 8%. Approximately 20% of children and adults with headache continue to suffer from headache throughout their lives, whereas 50% experience remission over extended periods.

Recent community studies have underscored the enormous personal and social burden of migraine in terms of both direct and indirect costs. These findings strongly underscore the need for research that can elucidate targets for prevention of this serious condition.

REFERENCES

Abu-Arahef I, Razak S, Sivaraman B, Graham C. Prevalence of headache and migraine in children and adolescents: a systematic review of population-based studies. *Developmental Med and Child Neurology* 2010;1:1–10.

Andlin-Sobocki P, Jonsson B, Wittchen HU, Olesen J. Cost of disorders of the brain in Europe. *Eur J Neurol* 2005;12 (suppl 1):1–27.

Anttila P, Metsahonkalä L, Sillanpää M. Long-term trends in the incidence of headache in Finnish schoolchildren. *Pediatrics* 2006;117:1197–1201.

Berg J, Stovner LJ. Cost of migraine and other headaches in Europe. *Eur J Neurol* 2005;12(suppl 1):59–62.

Bigal ME, Bordini CA, Speciali JG. Headache in an emergency room. *São Paulo Med J* 2000;118:58–62.

Bigal M, Lipton R, Stewart W. The epidemiology and impact of migraine. *Curr Neurol Neurosci Rep* 2004;4:98–104.

Bille B. A 40-year follow-up of school children with migraine. *Cephalalgia* 1997;17:488–491.

Breslau N, Davis GC. Migraine, physical health and psychiatric disorder: a prospective epidemiologic study in young adults. *J Psychiatr Res* 1993;27:211–221.

Brna P, Dooley J, Gordon K, Dewan T. The prognosis of childhood headache: a 20-year follow-up. *Arch Pediatr Adolesc Med* 2005;159:1157–1160.

Camarda R, Monastero R, Santangelo G, et al. Migraine headaches in adolescents: a five-year follow-up study. *Headache* 2002;42:1000–1005.

Celentano DD, Stewart WF, Lipton RB, Reed ML. Medication use and disability among migraineurs: a national probability sample. *Headache* 1992;32:223–228.

Dahlof C, Bouchard J, Cortelli P, et al. A multinational investigation of the impact of subcutaneous sumatriptan. II. Health-related quality of life. *Pharmacoeconomics* 1997;1(suppl 1):24–34.

Dahlof CG, Solomon GD. The burden of migraine to the individual sufferer: a review. *Eur J Neurol* 1998;5:525–533.

Fry J. *Profiles of Disease.* Edinburgh: Churchill Livingstone; 1996:45–56.

Goldberg LD. The cost of migraine and its treatment. *Am J Manag Care* 2005;11:S62–S67.

Gordis E. *Epidemiology.* Philadelphia, PA: W.B. Saunders; 2000.

Guidetti V, Galli F. Evolution of headache in childhood and adolescence: an 8-year follow-up. *Cephalalgia* 1998;18:449–454.

Hernandez-Latorre MA, Roig M. National history of migraine in childhood. *Cephalalgia* 2000;20:573–579.

Holmes WF, MacGregor A, Dodick D, Holmes A. Migraine-related disability: impact and implications for sufferers' lives and clinical issues. *Neurology* 2001;56:S13–S19.

Hu XH, Markson LE, Lipton RB, Stewart WF, Berger ML. Burden of migraine in the United States: disability and economic costs. *Arch Intern Med* 1999;159:813–818.

Jensen R, Stovner LJ. Epidemiology and comorbidity of headache. *Lancet Neurol* 2008;7:354–361.

Kernick D, Reinhold D, Campbell JL. Impact of headache on young people in a school population. *Br J Gen Pract* 2009;59:678–681.

Kienbacher C, Wöber C, Zesch HE, et al. Clinical features, classification and prognosis of migraine and tension-type headache in children and adolescents: a long-term follow-up study. *Cephalalgia* 2006;26:820–830.

Lateef TL, Merikangas K, He J, et al. Headache in a national sample of American children: prevalence and comorbidity. *J Child Neurol* 2009;24:536–543.

Lima MM, Padula NA, Santos LC, Oliveira LD, Agapejev S, Padovani C. Critical analysis of the International classification of headache disorders diagnostic criteria (ICHD I–1988) and (ICHD II–2004), for migraine in children and adolescents. *Cephalalgia* 2007;25:1042–1047.

Lipton RB, Bigal ME. The epidemiology of migraine. *Am J Med* 2005;118:3S–10S.

Lipton R, Stewart W, Diamond S, Diamond M, Reed M. Prevalence and burden of migraine in the United States: data from the American Migraine Study II. *Headache* 2001a;41:646–657.

Lipton RB, Stewart WF, Scher AI. Epidemiology and economic impact of migraine. *Curr Med Res Opin* 2001b;17:4S–12S.

Low NC, Cui L, Merikangas KR. Sex differences in the transmission of migraine. *Cephalalgia* 2007;27:935–942.

Lyngberg AC, Rasmussen BK, Jorgensen T, Jensen R. Incidence of primary headache: a Danish epidemiologic follow-up study. *Am J Epidemiol* 2005a;161:1066–1073.

Lyngberg AC, Rasmussen BK, Jorgensen T, Jensen R. Prognosis of migraine and tension-type headache: a population-based follow-up study. *Neurology* 2005b;65:580–585.

Merikangas KR, Cui L, Richardson AK, et al. Magnitude, impact, and stability of primary headache subtypes: 30 year prospective Swiss cohort study. *BMJ* 2011;343:d507.

Metsahonkalä L, Sillanpää M, Tuominen J. Headache diary in the diagnosis of childhood migraine. *Headache* 1997;37: 240–244.

National Center for Health Statistics. *Vital and Health Statistics of the United States.* Department of Health, Education, and Welfare. Advance data. Hyattsville, MD: National Center for Health Statistics; 1979. PHS Publication No. 53. Available at: http://www.cdc.gov/nchs/products/pubs/pubd/nvsr/53/53-prehtm. Accessed February 7, 2005.

Osterhaus JT, Gutterman DL, Plachetka JR. Healthcare resource and lost labor costs of migraine headache in the US. *Pharmacoeconomics* 1992;2:67–76.

Powers SW, Patton SR, Hommel KA, Hershey AD. Quality of life in childhood migraines: clinical impact and comparison to other chronic illnesses. *Pediatrics* 2003;112:e1–e5.

Santanello NC, Polis AB, Hartmaier SL, Kramer MS, Block GA, Silberstein, SD. Improvement in migraine-specific quality of life in a clinical trial of rizatriptan. *Cephalalgia* 1997;17:867–872.

Saunders K, Merikangas K, Low NC, Von Korff M, Kessler RC. Impact of comorbidity on headache-related disability. *Neurology* 2008;70:538–547.

Stang PE, Sternfeld B, Sidney S. Migraine headache in a prepaid health plan: ascertainment, demographics, physiological and behavioral factors. *Headache* 1996; 36:69–76.

Stewart WF, Linet MS, Celentano DD, Van Natta M, Siegler D. Age and sex-specific incidence rates of migraine with and without visual aura. *Am J Epidemiol* 1991;34:1111–1120.

Stewart WF, Lipton RB, Celentano DD, Reed ML. Prevalence of migraine headache in the United States. *JAMA* 1992;267:64–69.

Stewart WF, Lipton RB, Liberman J. Variation in migraine prevalence by race. *Neurology* 1996;47:52–59.

Stovner L, Hagen K, Jensen R, Katsarava Z, Lipton R, Scher A, Steiner T, Zwart JA. The global burden of headache: a documentation of headache prevalence and disability worldwide. *Cephalalgia* 2007;27:193–210.

Swartz KL, Pratt LA, Armenian HK, Lee LC, Eaton WW. Mental disorders and the incidence of migraine headaches in a community sample: results from the Baltimore Epidemiologic Catchment area follow-up study. *Arch Gen Psychiatry* 2000;57:945–950.

Virtanen R, Aromaa M, Rautava P, Metsähonkala L, Anttila P, Helenius H, Sillanpää M. Changing headache from preschool age to puberty: a controlled study. *Cephalalgia* 2007;27:294–303.

Winner P, Rothner D. Headache in children and adolescents. *BC Decker* 2001;1:1–20.

Zebenholzer K, Wöber C, Kienbacher C, Wöber-Bingöl C. Migrainous disorder and headache of the tension-type not fulfilling the criteria: a follow-up study in children and adolescents. *Cephalalgia* 2000;20:611–616.

The Differential Diagnosis and Boundaries of Migraine

Michael Bjørn Russell, MD, PhD, Dr. Med Sci

INTRODUCTION

Migraine is the second most common pain condition, next to tension-type headache (Rasmussen et al., 1991; Russell et al., 1995). Its diagnosis relies exclusively on the patient's history and exclusion of secondary causes ruled out by a normal physical and neurologic examination or appropriate investigations (ICHD-II, 2004). The only objective marker in the most common types of migraine is the increased excretion of 5-hydroxyindoleacetic acid in urine after a migraine attack (Sicuteri et al., 1961), although some individuals with the rare sporadic or familial hemiplegic migraine might carry a point mutation in the *CACNA1A, ATP1A2,* or *SCN1A* genes (Ophoff et al., 1996; De Fusco et al., 2003; Dichgans et al., 2005). Thus the differential diagnosis and boundaries of migraine pose a real challenge.

DIFFERENTIAL DIAGNOSIS FOR MIGRAINE WITHOUT AURA

Migraine without aura is characterized by headache (symptoms) and accompanying symptoms (photophobia and phonophobia, nausea and vomiting). The most common differential diagnosis for migraine without aura is tension-type headache. The pain characteristics of migraine without aura and tension-type headache are complementary; that is, migraine without aura is usually a unilateral pulsating moderate/severe headache that is aggravated by physical activities, while tension-type headache is usually a bilateral pressing mild/moderate headache that is not aggravated by physical activities (ICHD-II, 2004). However, it is the usual lack of accompanying symptoms that makes the differential diagnosis of tension-type headache easy, although tension-type headache can also be accompanied by photophobia or phonophobia. The correct diagnosis of migraine without aura versus tension-type headache is important for correct management of the former condition, as triptans are not effective in tension-type headache (Tfelt-Hansen, 2007).

Cluster headache is another primary headache that is part of the differential diagnosis for migraine without aura. Usually it is easy to differentiate between cluster headache and migraine without aura owing to their different attack patterns—that is, attacks in clusters versus episodic attacks. Furthermore, cluster headache is characterized by one or more associated symptoms, such as lacrimation, conjunctival injection, miosis, eyelid edema, ptosis, nasal congestion, rhinorrhea, facial sweating, and a sense of restlessness or agitation that is not seen in migraine without aura (ICHD-II, 2004). At its onset, however, cluster headache might be mistaken for migraine without aura because the associated symptoms might be missed by the patient, may not be pronounced, or may not be present (Russell & Andersson, 1995; Sjöstrand et al., 2005). Similarly, chronic cluster headache might be difficult to differentiate from chronic migraine, given that chronic cluster headache is sometimes characterized by a milder headache between the more severe attacks of cluster headache.

The differential diagnoses for migraine without aura also include secondary migraine without aura. A major reason to suspect secondary migraine without aura is its onset in close temporal relation to another disorder. Migraine without aura is caused by a combination of genetic and environmental factors (Russell et al., 1995). First-degree relatives of probands with migraine without aura have a 1.9-fold (statistically significant) increased risk of migraine without aura compared to the general population (Russell & Olesen, 1995). Interestingly, first-degree relatives of probands with migraine without aura that occurred in relation to a head trauma have no increased risk of migraine without aura (Russell & Olesen, 1996b). Thus head trauma in a susceptible individual might cause migraine without aura. However, head trauma is very common, and not all people experience onset of migraine without aura after trauma. Other secondary causes include atriovenous malformation, MELAS (mitochondrial encephalomyopathy, lactic acidosis, and stroke), and antiphospholipid antibody disease (Pavalakis et al., 1984; Chabriat et al., 1995; Cervera et al., 2002).

Because migraine without aura is very common, co-occurrence of migraine without aura and other disorders is not rare. Thus, to establish a causal relationship, the occurrence of migraine without aura should be significantly increased as compared to the risk of migraine without aura in the general population (Weiss et al., 1982; Khoury et al., 1988). Suspicion of a secondary cause for migraine without aura should be raised if the symptoms are always located on the same side, attack frequency is dramatically changed, or age at onset is after age 40 years. This presentation requires a careful work-up that includes a physical and neurologic examination as well as magnetic resonance imaging (MRI) of the brain.

DIFFERENTIAL DIAGNOSIS FOR AURA

The migraine aura reflects reversible cerebral cortical dysfunction of vision, speech, sensory, and/or motor function. The gradual development and sequential march of the aura symptoms are caused by cortical spreading depression, in which a brief excitation of the occipital cortical neurons initiates a depolarization wave that moves across the cortex at a rate of 3–5 mm/min, and is followed by prolonged depression of the neurons (Leão, 1944a, 1944b). This event is followed by a reduction in the regional cerebral blood supply in persons with typical migraine with aura and hemiplegic migraine, which is not present in persons with migraine without aura (Olesen et al., 1981; Lauritzen & Olesen, 1984; Olesen et al., 1990).

The typical migraine with aura is characterized by visual aura followed by headache, with one-fourth and one-third of patients also experiencing dysphasic (speech) and sensory aura in some of their attacks (Russell & Olesen, 1996a). The sequence observed usually consists of first visual, then dysphasic, and finally sensory aura. If motor aura is present, the presentation is classified hemiplegic migraine (ICHD-II, 2004). Most persons with hemiplegic migraine experience all types of aura, including basilar-like aura, usually in the sequential order of visual, sensory, motor, aphasic, and basilar-like aura, although the order is different in approximately 30% of affected individuals (Thomsen et al., 2002, 2003). If the sequential order of the aura symptoms is not logical according to the locations of the different areas in the brain, the symptoms might be due to memory bias, and prospective recordings of the aura might illuminate this issue (Russell et al., 1994).

The gradual development and duration of the migraine aura over at least 20 minutes is unique for migraine with aura—that is, for typical migraine with aura and hemiplegic migraine. In contrast, an epileptic aura has a duration of a few seconds, transient ischemic attacks have a sudden onset with a duration of less than 24 hours, and stroke causes permanent neurologic signs. Thus a precise history of the aura will, in most cases, provide the crucial information necessary for a precise diagnosis.

DIFFERENTIAL DIAGNOSIS FOR TYPICAL MIGRAINE WITH AURA

The aura in typical migraine with aura can be followed by a migraine headache, a tension-type headache, or no headache. Onset may occur at all ages, though it usually takes place within the first four decades of life; by comparison, the typical migraine with aura without headache might have an onset later in life. Cautions should be taken with people in whom attack frequency is dramatically changed, as this alteration in pattern may be caused by reversible cerebral vasoconstriction (Ducros et al., 2007). The risk of typical migraine with aura is also increased in people with cerebral autosomal dominant arteriopathy with subcortical infarcts and leukoencephalopathy

(CADASIL) (Tournier-Lasserve, 1993). Other secondary causes could be similar to those causing hemiplegic migraine (discussed in the next section). Visual aura is nearly always present in typical migraine with aura (Russell & Olesen, 1996a). Thus a person without visual aura should be suspected to have a secondary cause.

DIFFERENTIAL DIAGNOSIS FOR HEMIPLEGIC MIGRAINE

Stroke is the first differential diagnosis considered for hemiplegic migraine, especially if the aura description is insufficient. A young age at onset points the diagnosis in the direction of a hemiplegic migraine attack. Although typical migraine with aura is a risk factor for stroke, particularly in young women, the risk of stroke in hemiplegic migraine is unknown (Tzourio et al., 1995).

Alternating hemiplegia of childhood (AHC) is characterized by paroxysmal episodes of hemiplegia, quadriplegia, choreoathetotic movements, and nystagmus that disappear immediately after sleep, along with progressive mental retardation and development of permanent neurologic deficits such as choreoathetosis, dystonia, and ataxia (Bourgeois et al., 1993). AHC is usually a sporadic disorder with onset prior to age 1 ½ year, whereas onset of hemiplegic migraine usually occurs at an older age. In addition, co-occurrence of mental retardation is rare in hemiplegic migraine.

Coma sometimes occurs in severe attacks of hemiplegic migraine. Its emergence requires an extensive work-up to exclude other symptomatic causes such as hypoglycemia, cerebral hemorrhages, mass lesion, and infections. Fever and meningismus can be observed during attacks of hemiplegic migraine, and their presence requires exclusion of bacterial and viral meningitis, sepsis, and inflammatory diseases from the diagnosis. Permanent cerebellar signs occur in 40% of the families with familial hemiplegic migraine caused by point mutations in the *CACNA1A* gene (Ducros et al., 2001).

A series of secondary causes of hemiplegic migraine have been reported. In one case reported in the literature, a parasagittal meningeoma in the left parietal-occipital region caused alternating attacks of typical migraine with aura and sporadic hemiplegic migraine for 17 years in a 42-year-old woman. The aura was strictly right-sided and spread in the sequential order of visual, aphasic, sensory and motor aura, including dysarthria, and then headache (Vetvik et al., 2005). Other secondary causes of hemiplegic migraine may include Sturge-Webers syndrome, Epstein-Barr virus infection, avascular necrosis associated with anticardiolipin antibodies, childhood lupus erythematosus, progressive facial hemiatrophy, ornithine transcarbamylase deficiency, MELAS, and CADASIL (Leavell et al., 1986; Montagna et al., 1988; de Grauw et al., 1990; Seleznick et al., 1991; Klapper, 1994; Parikh et al., 1995; Hutchinson et al., 1995; Woolfenden et al., 1998; Dora & Balkan, 2001). A secondary cause of hemiplegic migraine should be suspected if the aura symptoms always occur on the same side, as nonsymptomatic attacks of hemiplegic migraine usually change side from attack to attack. Other reasons to be suspicious for a symptomatic cause are atypical aura symptoms, increasing frequency of attacks, a change in the headache pain's character, a change in the efficacy of the usual medication, and occurrence of persistent neurologic symptoms or signs.

CONCLUSIONS

The paroxysmal nature of migraine and its reversible neurologic symptoms usually make the diagnosis of this condition straightforward, especially if a precise headache history and aura description are ascertained. The health-care provider should be suspicious of a secondary cause if the migraine headache and/or aura symptoms are always located on the same side, if the attack frequency increases significantly, if the efficacy of the usual medication changes, or if the neurologic symptoms or sign become permanent.

REFERENCES

Bourgeois M, Aicardi J, Goutieres F. Alternating hemiplegia of childhood. *J Pediatr* 1993;112:673–679.

Cervera R, Piette JC, Font J, Khamashta MA, et al. Antiphospholipid syndrome: clinical and immunologic manifestations and patterns of disease expression in a cohort of 1,000 patients. *Arthritis Rheum* 2002;46:1019–1027.

Chabriat H, Vahedi K, Iba-Zizen MT, Joutel A, Nibbio A, Nagy TG, Krebs MO, Julien J, Dubois B, Ducrocq X, et al. Clinical spectrum of CADASIL: a study of 7 families. Cerebral autosomal dominant arteriopathy with subcortical infarcts and leukoencephalopathy. *Lancet* 1995;346:934–939.

De Fusco M, Marconi R, Silvestri L, Atorino L, Rampoldi L, Morgante L, Ballabio A, Aridon P, Casari G. Haploinsufficiency of ATP1A2 encoding the Na$^+$/K$^+$ pump alpha$_2$ subunit associated with familial hemiplegic migraine type 2. *Nat Genet* 2003;33:192–196.

de Grauw TJ, Smit LM, Brockstedt M, Meijer Y, vd Klei-von Moorsel J, Jakobs C. Acute hemiparesis as the presenting sign in a heterozygote for ornithine transcarbamylase deficiency. *Neuropediatrics* 1990;21:133–135.

Dichgans M, Freilinger T, Eckstein G, Babini E, Lorenz-Depiereux B, Biskup S, Ferrari MD, Herzog J, van den Maagdenberg AM, Pusch M, Strom TM. Mutation in the neuronal voltage-gated sodium channel SCN1A in familial hemiplegic migraine. *Lancet* 2005;366:371–377.

Dora B, Balkan S. Sporadic hemiplegic migraine and Sturge-Weber syndrome. *Headache* 2001;41:209–210.

Ducros A, Denier C, Joutel A, Cecillon M, Lescoat C, Vahedi K, Darcel F, Vicaut E, Bousser MG, Tournier-Lasserve E. The clinical spectrum of familial hemiplegic migraine associated with mutations in a neuronal calcium channel. *N Engl J Med* 2001;345:17–24.

Ducros A, Boukobza M, Porcher R, Sarov M, Valade D, Bousser MG. The clinical and radiological spectrum of reversible cerebral vasoconstriction syndrome: a prospective series of 67 patients. *Brain* 2007;130:3091–3101.

Hutchinson M, O'Riordan J, Javed M, Quin E, Macerlaine D, Wilcox T, Parfrey N, Nagy TG, Tournier-Lasserve E. Familial hemiplegic migraine and autosomal dominant arteriopathy with leukoencephalopathy (CADASIL). *Ann Neurol* 1995;38:817–824.

ICHD-II: Headache Classification Committee of the International Headache Society. The International Classification of Headache Disorders (2nd edition). *Cephalalgia* 2004;24(suppl 1):1–160.

Khoury MJ, Beaty TH, Liang K-Y. Can familial aggregation of disease be explained by familial aggregation of environmental risk factors? *Am J Epidemiol* 1988;127:674–683.

Klapper J. Headache in Sturge-Weber syndrome. *Headache* 1994;34:521–522.

Lauritzen M, Olesen J. Regional cerebral blood flow during migraine attacks by xenon-133 inhalation and emission tomography. *Brain* 1984;107:447–461.

Leão AAP. Spreading depression of activity in the cerebral cortex. *J Neurophysiology* 1944a;7:359–390.

Leão AAP. Further observations on the spreading depression of activity in the cerebral cortex. *J Neurophysiology* 1944b;10:409–414.

Leavell R, Ray CG, Ferry PC, Minnich LL. Unusual acute neurologic presentations with Epstein-Barr virus infection. *Arch Neurol* 1986;43:186–188.

Montagna P, Gallassi R, Medori R, Govoni E, Zeviani M, Di Mauro S, Lugaresi E, Andermann F. MELAS syndrome: characteristic migrainous and epileptic features and maternal transmission. *Neurology* 1988;38:751–754.

Olesen J, Larsen B, Lauritzen M. Focal hyperemia followed by spreading oligemia and impaired activation of rCBF in classic migraine. *Ann Neurol* 1981;9:344–352.

Olesen J, Friberg L, Olsen TS, Iversen HK, Lassen NA, Andersen AR, Karle A. Timing and topography of cerebral blood flow, aura and headache during migraine attacks. *Ann Neurol* 1990;28:791–798.

Ophoff RA, Terwindt GM, Vergouwe MN, van Eijk R, Oefner PJ, Hoffman SM, Lamerdin JE, Mohrenweiser HW, Bulman DE, Ferrari M, Haan J, Lindhout D, van Ommen GJ, Hofker MH, Ferrari MD, Frants RR. Familial hemiplegic migraine and episodic ataxia type-2 are caused by mutations in the Ca^{2+} channel gene CACNL1A4. *Cell* 1996;87:543–552.

Parikh S, Swaiman KF, Kim Y. Neurologic characteristics of childhood lupus erythematosus. *Pediatr Neurol* 1995;13:198–201.

Pavlakis SG, Phillips PC, DiMauro S, De Vivo DC, Rowland LP. Mitochondrial myopathy, encephalopathy, lactic acidosis, and strokelike episodes: a distinctive clinical syndrome. *Ann Neurol* 1984;16:481–488.

Rasmussen BK, Jensen R, Schroll M, Olesen J. Epidemiology of headache in a general population: a prevalence study. *J Clin Epidemiol* 1991;44:1147–1157.

Russell MB, Andersson PG. Clinical intra- and interfamilial variation of cluster headache. *Eur J Neurol* 1995;1:253–257.

Russell MB, Olesen J. Increased familial risk and evidence of a genetic factor in migraine. *BMJ* 1995;311:541–544.

Russell MB, Olesen J. A nosographic analysis of the migraine aura in the general population. *Brain* 1996a;119:355–361.

Russell MB, Olesen J. Migraine associated with head trauma. *Eur J Neurol* 1996b;3:424–428.

Russell MB, Iversen HK, Olesen J. Improved description of the migraine aura by a diagnostic aura diary. *Cephalalgia* 1994;14:107–117.

Russell MB, Rasmussen BK, Thorvaldsen P, Olesen J. Prevalence and sex-ratio of the subtypes of migraine. *Int J Epidemiol* 1995;24:612–618.

Seleznick MJ, Silveira LH, Espinoza LR. Avascular necrosis associated with anticardiolipin antibodies. *J Rheumatol* 1991;18:1416–1417.

Sicuteri F, Testi A, Anselmi B. Biochemical investigations in headache: increase in the hydroxyindoleacetic acid excretion during migraine attacks. *Int Arch Allergy* 1961;19:55–58.

Sjöstrand C, Russell MB, Ekbom K, Hillert J, Waldenlind E. Atypical cluster headache: a variety of familial cluster headache. *Cephalalgia* 2005;25:1068–1077.

Tfelt-Hansen P. Acute pharmacotherapy of migraine, tension-type headache, and cluster headache. *J Headache Pain* 2007;8:127–134.

Thomsen LL, Eriksen MK, Roemer SF, Andersen I, Olesen J, Russell MB. A population-based study of familial hemiplegic migraine suggests revised diagnostic criteria. *Brain* 2002;125:1379–1391.

Thomsen LL, Østergaard E, Olesen J, Russell MB. Evidence for a separate type of migraine with aura: sporadic hemiplegic migraine. *Neurology* 2003;60:595–601.

Tournier-Lasserve E, Joutel A, Melki J, Weissenbach J, Lathrop GM, Chabriat H, Mas JL, Cabanis EA, Baudrimont M, Maciazek J, et al. Cerebral autosomal dominant arteriopathy with subcortical infarcts and leukoencephalopathy maps to chromosome 19q12. *Nat Genet* 1993;3:256–259.

Tzourio C, Tehindrazanarivelo A, Iglesias S, Alpérovitch A, Chedru F, d'Anglejan-Chatillon J, Bousser MG. Case-control study of migraine and risk of ischaemic stroke in young women. *BMJ* 1995;310:830–838.

Vetvik KR, Dahl M, Russell MB. Symptomatic sporadic hemiplegic migraine. *Cephalalgia* 2005;25:1093–1095.

Weiss KM, Chakraborty R, Majumder PP, Smouse PE. Problems in the assessment of relative risk of affected individuals. *J Chronic Dis* 1982;35:539–551.

Woolfenden AR, Tong DC, Norbash AM, Albers GW. Progressive facial hemiatrophy: abnormality of intracranial vasculature. *Neurology* 1998;50:1915–1917.

The Comorbidities of Migraine

Marcelo E. Bigal, MD, PhD

INTRODUCTION

The term *comorbidity*, which was coined by Feinstein in 1963, is now widely used to refer to the greater than coincidental association of two conditions in the same individual.

Epidemiological studies have identified a number of conditions that are comorbid with migraine headache (Breslau, 1998; Scher et al., 2006a). Failure to classify and analyze comorbid diseases can create misleading medical statistics and may cause spurious comparisons during the evaluation and treatment planning for patients (Merikangas & Stevens, 1997; Low & Merikangas, 2003). Comorbidity can alter the clinical course of patients with the same diagnosis by affecting the time of detection, prognosis, therapeutic selection, and post-therapeutic outcomes. In addition, it can affect the length of hospital stay, response to somatic treatment, and mortality (Lipton & Silberstein, 1994). Accordingly, comorbidity must be considered in formulating treatment plans and may provide insights into the mechanisms of disease (Solomon & Price, 1997).

Comorbidity does not mean random co-occurrence of two conditions, but rather occurrence at a rate that would be higher than what is expected by chance only. For example, assuming that migraine has a prevalence of 12% in the general population, and that the prevalence of obesity is approximately 30%, we can safely assume that 30% of the migraineurs are obese, and we can calculate expected confidence intervals for obesity in migraineurs. If a hypothetical study detected that the prevalence of obesity was 20% in migraineurs and determined that this rate fell below the lower limit of the confidence interval, then the researchers might conclude that suffering from one condition protected against the other (i.e., migraine protected against obesity, obesity protected against migraine, or an unidentified factor protected against both). Alternatively, if the prevalence of obesity was 40 % in migraineurs and this rate was also out of the confidence interval, both conditions would be called comorbid. The potential mechanisms of comorbidity are discussed later in the next section.

Studying comorbidities is not an easy task, and clinicians should be aware of spurious findings related to this issue (Bogenschutz & Nurnberg, 2000). For example, samples selected from clinical settings may not be representative of the general population. Assessment bias, in which the co-occurrence of two conditions is an artifact of overlap in the diagnostic criteria or in the assessments employed to ascertain the criteria, and the lack of an appropriate comparison (or control) group with which to account for factors that might potentially confound the association between the two conditions, must also be considered (Low & Merikangas, 2003).

In this chapter, we explore the comorbidities of migraine. We start by discussing the mechanisms of comorbidity. We then focus on the comorbidities of episodic migraine with psychiatric conditions, other forms of chronic pain, and cardiovascular disorders.

MECHANISMS OF COMORBIDITY

The mechanisms of comorbidity are multiple and non-mutually exclusive, and the readers are referred to other sources for a more detailed discussion (Lipton & Silberstein, 1994; Bigal & Lipton, 2008). **Figure 3.1** summarizes the possible reasons for migraine comorbidities, which are then briefly discussed in the remainder of this section. As you can see, Figure 3.1 uses the relationship between migraine and cardiovascular disease as an example (adapted from Bigal & Lipton, 2008).

Spurious Interaction

As mentioned previously, before claiming comorbidity, spurious association must be ruled out. For example, selection bias may exist. Additionally, if individuals with migraine and the comorbid disease are both more likely to be present in the health-care system, individuals with both disorders may be over-represented in clinic-based samples.

Unidirectional Causal Relationships

In a unidirectional causal relationship, one disease leads to the other. For example, aura seems to be a direct risk

A. Spurious

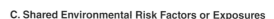

B. Undirectional Causal Relationship

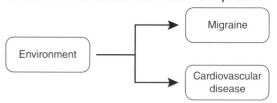

C. Shared Environmental Risk Factors or Exposures

D. Shared Genetic or Biological Risk Factors

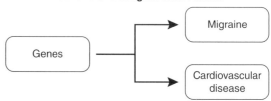

Figure 3.1 Conceptual Mechanisms of the Relationship Between Migraine with Aura and Cardiovascular Disease
Adapted from Lipton RD, Silberstein SD. Why study the comorbidity of migraine? *Neurology* 1994;44:S4–5.

factor for stroke (Kurth et al., 2005), meaning that both conditions are comorbid, but the first one (migraine) is a risk factor for the second one (stroke). As another example, among episodic migraineurs, obesity increases the risk of chronic migraine (Bigal & Lipton, 2006). Accordingly, although not comorbid with episodic migraine, obesity is comorbid with chronic migraine and, indeed, is a risk factor for it.

Shared Environmental Risk Factors

Comorbid relationships might be explained by shared environmental risks. For example, trauma may predispose individuals to both migraine and epilepsy (Haut et al., 2006). Likewise, chronic pain may predispose individuals to both depression and chronic migraine (Ratcliffe et al., 2008).

Shared Genetic Risk Factors

Migraine and comorbidities may share a common genetic underpinning. For example, specific genes have been reported to be linked to both migraine and stroke predisposition (Scher et al., 2006a). Serotoninergic dysfunction may explain both migraine and depression, for example.

THE COMORBIDITIES OF MIGRAINE

Migraine has been noted to be comorbid with a number of other illnesses in specialty care and in population samples (**Table 3.1**); for a review, see Breslau et al. (2003)

Table 3.1 Conditions Comorbid with Migraine

Psychiatric
- Depression
- Anxiety
- Panic disorder
- Bipolar

Neurologic
- Epilepsy
- Tourette syndrome*

Vascular
- Raynaud phenomenon
- Blood pressure (inconsistent)
- Ischemic stroke, subclinical stroke, white matter abnormalities

Heart
- Patent foramen ovale*
- Mitral valve prolapse*
- Atrial septal aneurysm*

Other
- Snoring/sleep apnea*
- Asthma/allergy
- Systemic lupus erythematosus*
- Non-headache pain

* Data from clinical samples only.

and Scher et al. (2005a). In this section, we discuss the comorbidity of migraine with psychiatric diseases, other forms of chronic pain, and vascular disorders.

Migraine and Psychiatric Disorders

Cross-sectional associations and bidirectional associations between migraine and a variety of psychiatric and somatic conditions have been reported in the literature (Hamelsky & Lipton, 2006; Holroyd, 2007). In an excellent review of the topic, Holroyd reports that, in large-scale population-based studies, individuals with migraine are 2.2 to 4.0 times more likely to have depression. In longitudinal studies, the evidence supports a bidirectional relationship between migraine and depression, with each disorder increasing the risk of the other disorder. Migraine is also comorbid with generalized anxiety disorder (odds ratio [OR]: 3.5 to 5.3), panic disorder (OR: 3.7), and bipolar disorder (OR: 2.9 to 7.3) (Holroyd, 2007).

Patel et al. (2004) assessed the prevalence of major depression in individuals with migraine, individuals with probable migraine (a subtype of migraine missing just one migraine feature), and healthy controls. Participants were identified from members of a mixed-model health maintenance organization. The overall prevalence of major depression was 28.1% for migraine, 19.5% for probable migraine, 23.9% for migraine and probable migraine polled together, and 10.3% for the controls. The prevalence of major depression was elevated in all migraine groups as compared to controls in terms of both crude and adjusted (by age, sex, and education) prevalence ratios.

Breslau et al. (2003) measured the bidirectional associations of migraine, severe non-migraine headache, and depression in a population-based cohort from the Detroit metropolitan area. A cross-sectional study involving more than 50,000 adults (the Nord-Trøndelag Health Study) measured the co-occurrence of headache and depression or anxiety disorders (Zwart et al., 2003). Participants were age 20 or older, with a headache diagnosis. On medical examination, they were administered the Hospital Anxiety and Depression scale. Overall, individuals with migraine were more likely to have depression (OR: 2.7; 95% CI: 2.3–3.2) or anxiety disorders (OR: 3.2; 95% CI: 2.8–3.6) than the non-headache controls. Similar associations were seen for non-migraine headache and depression (OR: 2.2; 95% CI: 2.0–2.5) or anxiety disorders (OR: 2.7; 95% CI: 2.4–3.0). There was a linear trend associated with headache frequency. Thus for migraine occurring on fewer than 7 days per month, 7 to 14 days per month, and 15 or more days per month, respectively, the associations with depression were (1) OR: 2.0; 95% CI: 1.6–2.5; (2) OR: 4.2; 95% CI: 3.2–5.6; and (3) OR: 6.4; 95% CI: 4.4–9.3. A similar trend was seen for anxiety disorders and for non-migraine headache with depression or anxiety disorders (Zwart et al., 2003).

Although most studies focused on the comorbidity of migraine and depression, recent evidence highlights the importance of anxiety as well. In a recent study, migraine risk was higher in participants with anxiety (OR: 2.30; 95% CI: 2.09–2.52), with depression (OR: 2.23; 95% CI: 1.93–2.58), who smoked (OR: 1.19; 95% CI: 1.09–1.30), or who consulted a mental health provider (OR: 1.45; 95% CI: 1.27–1.65) (Victor et al., 2010). Although migraine risk was increased in both women (OR: 1.93) and men (OR: 2.42), men with anxiety had a higher migraine risk than women with self-reported anxious symptoms (Victor et al., 2010).

Given that migraine is a form of chronic pain, it is of interest to what extent chronic pain conditions other than migraine are associated with depression and anxiety. A recent study (McWilliams et al., 2004) used data from an adult U.S. population (the Midlife Development in the United States Survey) to look at the cross-sectional associations between three pain conditions (migraine, arthritis, and back pain) and three psychiatric disorders (depression, generalized anxiety disorder, and panic attacks). The associations between the three psychiatric disorders were roughly similar for the three pain conditions; that is, the association between migraine and depression was roughly similar to the association between back pain and depression. However, the authors noted that the association between pain and anxiety was generally stronger than that between pain and depression (McWilliams et al., 2004).

Migraine and Comorbid Pain

Migraine has been reported to be comorbid with other chronic pain conditions in both cross-sectional and prospective studies of children or young adults (**Table 3.2**). In one study involving 1,756 third- and fifth-grade schoolchildren in Finland, children were examined for the presence of nontraumatic musculoskeletal pain symptoms and tested for hypermobility (El-Metwally et al., 2004). They were reevaluated after 1 and 4 years to determine factors related to the prognosis of musculoskeletal pain. Baseline headache once or more a week (not characterized by type) was found to be a negative prognostic

Table 3.2 Relationship Between Psychiatric Conditions and Chronic Pain

Depression and
- Arthritis: OR: 2.1, 95% CI: 1.6–2.7
- Migraine: OR: 2.4, 95% CI: 1.8–3.1
- Back pain: OR: 2.1, 95% CI: 1.6–2.6

Panic Attacks and
- Arthritis: OR: 2.5, 95% CI: 1.8–3.5
- Migraine: OR: 3.1, 95% CI: 2.2–4.3
- Back pain: OR: 2.7, 95% CI: 2.0–3.6

Generalized Anxiety Disorder and
- Arthritis: OR: 3.2, 95% CI: 2.0–5.2
- Migraine: OR: 3.1, 95% CI: 2.0–4.9
- Back pain: OR: 2.8, 95% CI: 1.8–4.3

Source: Data from McWilliams LA, Goodwin RD, Cox BJ. Depression and anxiety associated with three pain conditions: results from a nationally representative sample. *Pain* 2004;111:77–83.

factor; that is, children with comorbid headache were more likely to have persistent musculoskeletal pain at follow-up compared to the children without comorbid headache (El-Metwally et al., 2004).

Hestbaek et al. (2004, 2006) studied more than 9,000 adolescents and young adults in a cross-sectional, population-based study with the aim of describing conditions comorbid with low back pain (LBP). Headache (not characterized by type) was associated with both LBP experienced for fewer than 30 days per year (OR: 2.1; 95% CI: 1.8–2.5) and LBP lasting for more than 30 days per year (OR: 3.4; 95% CI: 2.3–5.0). Both LBP and headache were associated with asthma in this sample (Hestbaek et al., 2004, 2006).

The Nord-Trøndelag Health Study measured the co-occurrence of headache and musculoskeletal symptoms, defined as musculoskeletal pain and/or stiffness in muscles and joints lasting continuously for at least 3 months (Hagen et al., 2002). In this study, individuals with headache were roughly twice as likely to report musculoskeletal symptoms as those without headache. The elevated risk was similar in participants with non-migrainous (OR: 1.8; 95% CI: 1.8–1.9) and migrainous (OR: 1.9; 95% CI: 1.8–2.0) headaches. However, headache frequency was a stronger predictor of comorbid musculoskeletal symptoms than headache type. Thus, for headache experienced for fewer than 7 days per month, 7 to 14 days per month, and 15 or more days per month, respectively, the associations with musculoskeletal symptoms were as follows: (1) OR: 1.5; 95% CI: 1.4–1.6; (2) OR: 3.2; 95% CI: 2.9–3.5; and (3) OR: 5.3; 95% CI: 4.4–6.5 for women and (1) OR: 1.7; 95% CI: 1.6–1.8; (2) OR: 3.2; 95% CI: 2.8–3.8; and (3) OR: 3.6; 95% CI: 2.9–4.5 for men (Hagen et al., 2002).

A population-based study examined the comorbidity of chronic back and neck pain with other physical and mental disorders (Von Korff et al., 2005). These data came from the National Comorbidity Survey Replication (NCS-R), a nationally representative face-to-face household survey of adults 18 years of age and older. Chronic spinal pain was defined as self-reported "chronic back or neck problems." Comorbid mental disorders were based on DSM-IV criteria, and included mood disorders, anxiety disorders, and substance use disorders. Results showed that chronic spinal pain was associated with mood disorders (OR: 2.5; 95% CI: 1.9–3.2), anxiety disorders (OR: 2.3; 95% CI: 1.9–2.7), and substance use disorders, primarily alcohol abuse or dependence (OR: 1.6; 95% CI: 1.2–2.2). In addition, chronic spinal pain was associated with other chronic pain (OR: 4.8; 95% CI: 3.9–5.8), which included arthritis (OR: 3.9; 95% CI: 3.2–4.7), migraine (OR: 5.2; 95% CI: 4.1–6.4), other headache (OR: 4.0; 95% CI: 2.9–5.3), and other chronic pain (OR: 3.7; 95% CI: 2.9–4.7). Table 3.2 summarizes the associations between migraine and other forms of chronic pain and psychiatric conditions (McWilliams et al., 2004).

Migraine and Vascular Disorders

Migraine and Stroke

The association between migraine and ischemic stroke is well known and has been demonstrated in case-control studies as well as cross-sectional studies in patients selected from specialty care settings, from registries, and from the general population. A meta-analysis of 11 case-control studies and three cohort studies published before 2004 showed that, relative to individuals without migraine, the risk of stroke was increased in migraineurs [pooled relative risk (RR): 2.16; 95% CI: 1.9–2.5] (Etminan et al., 2005). This risk was nominally higher for individuals with migraine with aura (MA) (RR: 2.27; 95% CI: 1.61–3.19) but was also apparent in patients with migraine without aura (MO) (RR: 1.83; 95% CI: 1.06–3.15).

More recently, three large longitudinal studies added to the evidence base linking migraine and ischemic stroke. As a part of the Women's Health Study, the first of these studies, the relationship between migraine and stroke

was assessed using a large cohort and data prospectively gathered over an average of more than 10 years (Kurth et al., 2005). Compared with non-migraineurs, participants who reported any history of migraine or migraine without aura had no increased risk of any stroke type. Participants who reported MA had increased adjusted hazards ratios (HRs) of 1.53 (95% CI: 1.02–2.31) for total stroke and 1.71 (95% CI: 1.11–2.66) for ischemic stroke, but no increased risk for hemorrhagic stroke. The increased risk for ischemic stroke was further magnified (HR: 2.25; 95% CI: 1.30–3.91) for the youngest age group within this cohort (45–54 years). The associations remained statistically significant after adjusting for cardiovascular risk factors, and were not apparent for non-migraine headache (Kurth et al., 2005).

The second prospective study used data from the Atherosclerosis Risk in Communities Study and included more than 12,000 men and women aged 55 and older (Stang et al., 2005). Compared to participants without migraine or other headache, migraineurs had a 1.8-fold increased risk of ischemic stroke (RR: 1.84; 95% CI: 0.89–3.82). The fact that the risk estimates did not reach statistical significance may reflect the migraine classification used, as the category of "other headache with aura" showed a significant increased risk of ischemic stroke (RR: 2.91; 95% CI: 1.39–6.11). Similarly, in the stroke prevention in young women study, women with MA had 1.5 greater odds of experiencing ischemic stroke (MacClellan et al., 2006).

Finally, as part of the American Migraine Prevalence and Prevention study (AMPP), migraineurs (n = 6,102) and controls (n = 5,243) representative of the adult U.S. population were assessed (Bigal et al., 2010). Stroke occurred in 1.2% of the controls and 2.1% of the migraineurs (OR: 1.61; 95% CI: 1.2–2.2). Rates were 3.9% in MA (OR: 3.1; 95% CI: 2.2–4.4) and 1.12% in MO (OR: 0.9; 95% CI: 0.6–1.3). MA rates were elevated for both genders and in all ages older than 30. For MO, risk was not significantly different for either gender or any age group (Bigal et al., 2010) (**Table 3.4**).

Subclinical Brain Lesions

Deep brain lesions, found incidentally in neuroimaging exams, have long been reported as happening more frequently in migraineurs, although most studies lacked a contemporaneous control group (Porter et al., 2005). In a well-designed, population-based study from the Netherlands, Kruit et al. (2004) randomly selected approximately 150 individuals from each of three groups

Table 3.3 Cardiovascular Events as a Function of Migraine Type and of Demographics: Data from the American Migraine Prevalence and Prevention Study

	Control N (%)	Migraine Overall N (%)	OR (95% CI)	Migraine with Aura N (%)	OR (95% CI)	Migraine Without Aura N (%)	OR (95% CI)
Heart Attack							
Overall	100 (1.91)	249 (4.08)	2.19 (1.73–2.77)	110 (5.50)	2.99 (2.27–3.95)	139 (3.39)	1.80 (1.39–2.34)
Male	61 (2.47)	92 (7.65)	3.27 (2.35–4.55)	33 (8.59)	3.71 (2.39–5.74)	59 (7.21)	3.06 (2.12–4.42)
Female	39 (1.40)	157 (3.20)	2.32 (1.63–3.31)	77 (4.77)	3.52 (2.38–5.19)	80 (2.44)	1.75 (1.19–2.58)
18–29	5 (0.36)	1 (0.32)	0.88 (0.09–8.52)	1 (1.30)	3.67 (0.38–35.73)	0 (0.00)	Not available
30–39	3 (0.28)	10 (0.98)	3.55 (0.98–12.95)	7 (2.34)	8.59 (2.21–33.42)	3 (0.42)	1.50 (0.30–7.46)
40–49	6 (0.45)	30 (1.88)	4.25 (1.76–10.25)	10 (1.80)	4.07 (1.47–11.25)	20 (1.92)	4.35 (1.74–10.87)
50–59	24 (2.42)	96 (5.05)	2.15 (1.36–3.38)	51 (7.76)	3.40 (2.07–5.58)	45 (3.62)	1.52 (0.92–2.51)
60–69	64 (6.46)	112 (8.84)	1.40 (1.02–1.93)	41 (10.02)	1.61 (1.07–2.43)	71 (8.28)	1.31 (0.92–1.86)
White	85 (1.94)	214 (3.96)	2.09 (1.62–2.69)	88 (5.07)	2.70 (1.99–3.66)	126 (3.44)	1.80 (1.36–2.38)
Black	12 (1.97)	13 (3.44)	1.77 (0.80–3.93)	7 (4.90)	2.56 (0.99–6.62)	6 (2.55)	1.30 (0.48–3.51)
Other race	3 (1.20)	22 (6.79)	5.97 (1.77–20.19)	15 (12.61)	11.83 (3.35–41.72)	7 (3.41)	2.90 (0.74–11.36)
Stroke							
Overall	66 (1.26)	123 (2.02)	1.61 (1.19–2.18)	77 (3.85)	3.14 (2.25–4.38)	46 (1.12)	0.89 (0.61–1.30)
Male	27 (1.10)	25 (2.08)	1.92 (1.11–3.32)	16 (4.17)	3.93 (2.10–7.36)	9 (1.10)	1.00 (0.47–2.14)
Female	39 (1.40)	98 (2.00)	1.43 (0.99–2.08)	61 (3.78)	2.76 (1.84–4.14)	37 (1.13)	0.80 (0.51–1.26)
18–29	6 (0.71)	2 (0.63)	0.88 (0.18–4.40)	1 (1.30)	1.83 (0.22–15.39)	1 (0.42)	0.58 (0.07–4.85)
30–39	5 (0.46)	8 (0.79)	1.70 (0.55–5.21)	5 (1.67)	3.65 (1.05–12.69)	3 (0.42)	0.90 (0.21–3.77)
40–49	11 (0.82)	19 (1.19)	1.45 (0.69–3.06)	13 (2.33)	2.89 (1.29–6.49)	6 (0.58)	0.70 (0.26–1.90)
50–59	10 (1.01)	49 (2.58)	2.60 (1.31–5.16)	33 (5.02)	5.20 (2.54–10.62)	16 (1.29)	1.28 (0.58–2.84)
60–69	34 (3.43)	45 (3.55)	1.04 (0.66–1.63)	25 (6.11)	1.83 (1.08–3.11)	20 (2.33)	0.67 (0.38–1.18)
White	43 (0.98)	101 (1.87)	1.92 (1.34–2.76)	62 (3.57)	3.74 (2.52–5.54)	39 (1.06)	1.09 (0.70–1.68)
Black	19 (3.12)	10 (2.65)	0.84 (0.39–1.83)	6 (4.20)	1.36 (0.53–3.47)	4 (1.70)	0.54 (0.18–1.60)
Other race	4 (1.61)	12 (3.70)	2.36 (0.75–7.39)	9 (7.56)	5.01 (1.51–16.62)	3 (1.46)	0.91 (0.20–4.11)

OR; odds ratio; CI; confidence interval. All odds ratios are versus controls.

Table 3.4 Putative Mechanisms of the Relationship Between Migraine and Cardiovascular Disease

Mechanisms of Association	Putative Mechanisms	Comments
Causal association (migraine causes cardiovascular disease [CVD])	• Repetitive episodes of cortical spreading depression may predispose persons to ischemia, perfusion changes, and chronic inflammation.	• Justifies migraine with aura as a stronger risk factor. • Justifies the relationship with stroke but not with coronary problems.
Shared predisposition (environmental and/or biological factors predispose persons to both migraine and CVD)	• Migraineurs with aura are more likely to have a poor cholesterol profile, an elevated Framingham risk score for coronary heart disease, hypertension, and a history of heart attack in the family. • A polymorphism of the *C677T* gene was seen in one study and encodes high levels of homocysteine. This finding was not confirmed by a second study.	• Migraineurs with aura are more likely to present one or multiple risk factors for CVD.
Common comorbidities	• Obesity is associated with increased headache frequency in migraine both with and without aura. • Limited evidence suggests that metabolic syndrome predisposes individuals to increased headache frequency. • Clinic-based studies suggest that patent foramen ovale and other congenital heart problems are more common in persons with migraine with aura.	• Likely magnifies the relationship between migraine with aura and CVD, as the frequency of attacks is associated with number of deep brain lesions. However, in some studies, adjustments for body mass index were made.

for neuroimaging (MA, MO, and non-migraine controls). The researchers excluded individuals with a history of stroke or transient ischemic attack (TIA), or with an abnormal neurological exam. This study included blinded evaluation of MRI by a neuro-radiologist; aura classification was performed under the supervision of expert headache diagnosticians without knowledge of the patients' MRI results.

Overall, there were no differences in this study in the prevalence of clinically relevant infarcts between migraineurs and controls. This outcome might be explained by the exclusion of prior history of TIA and stroke (which would also exclude those patients with clinically relevant infarcts). However, those individuals with MA had a significant increase in the number of sub-clinical infarcts in the cerebellar region of the posterior circulation. The highest risk for these lesions was seen in those persons with MA and more than one headache attack per month (OR: 15.8; 95% CI: 1.8–14.0). In addition, women with migraine were roughly twice as likely to have deep white matter lesions as the non-migraineurs (OR: 2.1; 95% CI: 1.0–4.1) (Kruit et al., 2004). Consistent with the earlier studies on clinical stroke and white matter abnormalities, these findings were independent of the presence of some traditional cardiovascular risk factors (Kruit et al., 2006).

Migraine and Coronary Heart Disease

Due to the association between MA and ischemic stroke, it is of interest whether migraine is similarly associated with coronary heart disease as well. Although some studies have yielded negative or conflicting results for overall migraine (Rosamond, 2004), case reports and large-scale cohort studies have identified an association between migraine and chest pain; moreover, in some cases, migraine was associated with documented ischemic electrocardiographic changes (Etminan et al., 2005).

Several population studies have supported the relationship between migraine, especially MA, and coronary disease. In one study, Rose et al. (2004) looked at the association between headaches lasting 4 or more hours (including migraine and non-migraine headache) and Rose angina (i.e., identified through the Rose angina questionnaire). Participants, who were age 45–64 at baseline, were obtained from the Atherosclerosis Risk in Communities study. The headache group was roughly twice as likely to have a history of Rose angina, with the risk being most elevated in the group of patients with headache with aura (Rose et al., 2004).

In the Women's Health Study, MA (but not MO) approximately doubled the relative risk of major cardiovascular disease—that is, ischemic stroke, myocardial infarction, coronary revascularization procedures, and angina, as well as death related to ischemic cardiovascular events. These associations remained significant after adjusting for many cardiovascular risk factors (Kurth et al., 2006).

As part of the Physician's Health Study, men with migraine (with or without aura) were found to be at increased risk for major cardiovascular disease (HR: 1.24; 95% CI: 1.06–1.46), a finding that was driven by a 42% increased risk of myocardial infarction (Kurth et al., 2007).

In the AMPP study, migraine was associated with significantly increased risk of myocardial infarct relative to controls for participants of all ages older than 39 years (Bigal et al., 2010). Myocardial infarction occurred in 1.9% of controls and 4.1% of migraineurs (OR: 2.2; 95% CI: 1.7–2.7). The odds ratios were higher for both the 30–39 years and 40–49 years age groups (3.5 and 4.2, respectively) and decreased thereafter, although they remained significantly elevated. Rates were significantly increased in men (OR: 3.3; 95% CI: 2.4–4.6) compared to women (OR: 2.3; 95% CI: 1.6–3.3). Rates were significantly increased in white participants (OR: 2.1; 95% CI: 1.6–2.7) and nonsignificantly increased in black subjects. Ratios were further increased in MA relative to controls: men (OR: 3.7; 95% CI: 2.4–5.7) and women (OR: 3.5; 95% CI: 2.4–5.2). Risk was highest for those persons in the 30–39 years (OR: 8.6; 95% CI: 2.2–33.4) and 40–49 years (OR: 4.1; 95% CI: 1.5–11.2) groups. Risk was also elevated in patients with MO relative to controls: overall (OR: 1.8; 95% CI: 1.4–2.3), men (OR: 3.1; 95% CI: 2.1–4.4), and women (OR: 1.7; 95% CI: 1.2–2.6). The highest risk was observed in women aged 40–49 (OR: 4.4; 95% CI: 1.7–10.9) (**Figure 3.2**) (Bigal et al., 2010).

Migraine and Other Risk Factors for Cardiovascular Diseases

Specific disorders have been linked to migraine and cardiovascular diseases and may partially account for the relationships among them, although many studies have adjusted the findings based on these covariates. In this section, we consider some of these potential links, including obesity and metabolic syndrome.

Obesity   Obesity is a well-established risk factor for cardiovascular disease. In migraineurs, obesity has been associated with more frequent and severe headache attacks and with new onset of chronic migraine (Scher et al., 2003; Bigal et al., 2006; Bigal & Lipton, 2006), but

it is unrelated to MA (Winter, 2010). In a longitudinal study, the relative odds of chronic daily headaches were 5 times higher in individuals with a body mass index (BMI) greater than 30 compared to persons of normal weight (Scher et al., 2003). Overweight individuals had a 3-fold increased risk of developing chronic daily headache (CDH), suggesting a dose-response relationship between BMI and CDH.

Large cross-sectional studies confirm the longitudinal data. In one study, BMI was found to be a risk factor for high-frequency episodic migraine (OR: 2.9; 95% CI: 1.9–4.4 for obese persons; OR: 5.7; 95% CI: 3.6–8.8 for severely obese persons) (Bigal et al., 2006). Additionally, the prevalence of chronic migraine ranged from 0.9% of the normal weight cohort (reference group), to 1.2% of the overweight cohort (OR: 1.4; 95% CI: 1.1–1.8), 1.6% of the obese cohort (OR: 1.7; 95% CI: 1.2–2.4), and 2.5% of the severely obese cohort (OR: 2.2; 95% CI: 1.5–3.2) (Bigal et al., 2006).

Metabolic Syndrome and Its Components   Among the putative mechanisms to explain the obesity/cardiovascular disease relationship is metabolic syndrome, also known as the syndrome of insulin resistance (Bigal & Lipton, 2008). Metabolic syndrome has been associated with chronic pain in general. Women with fibromyalgia are 5 times more likely than healthy controls to have metabolic syndrome (Haffner, 2006). Elevated total and low-density lipoprotein (LDL) cholesterol levels have also been significantly associated with fibromyalgia among women (Haffner, 2006).

A recent study measured insulin and glucose levels in individuals with migraine, persons with other headaches, and controls (Cavestro et al., 2007). Tests were conducted at fasting and after administration of an oral glucose tolerance test. Compared to controls, migraineurs had significantly higher levels of glucose and of insulin, at fasting, and after glucose loading. After glucose loading, 65% of the migraineurs exhibited an insulin resistance pattern (19% in the control group).

Dyslipidemia, another component of metabolic syndrome, has also been associated with migraine. In the Genetic Epidemiology of Migraine study, compared to controls, migraineurs with aura were more likely to have an unfavorable cholesterol profile (Scher et al., 2006b). Risk for an elevated Framingham score for coronary heart disease, as well as reduced high-density lipoprotein (HDL) cholesterol levels, was doubled for persons with MA. This finding is of importance, because HDL cholesterol has anti-inflammatory properties that may

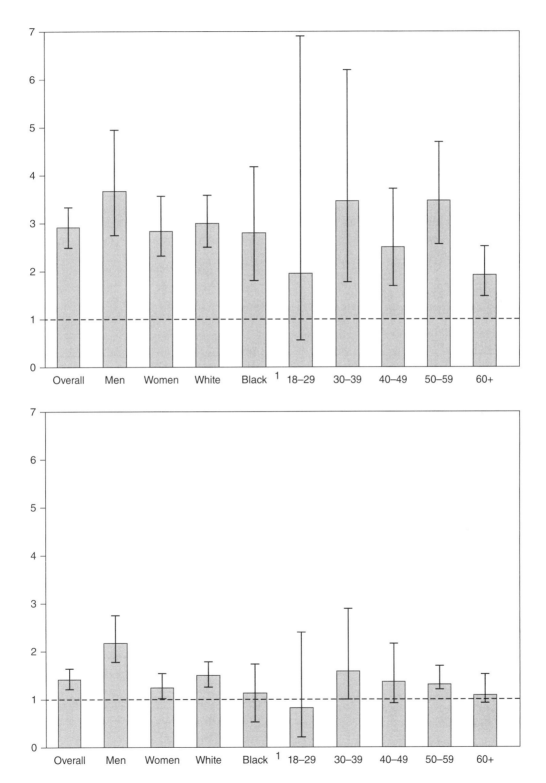

Figure 3.2 Odds Ratio of Reporting Any Cardiovascular Event in Individuals with Migraine with Aura (top) and Migraine Without Aura (bottom) / Footnote: Bars represent the odds ratio and whiskers represent the confidence intervals.

Adapted from Bigal ME, Kurth T, Santanello N et al. Migraine and cardiovascular disease: a population-based study. *Neurology* 2010;74:628-635.

diminish neurodegenerative processes and the perception of pain (Navab et al., 2007). Nonetheless, findings of the Women's Health Study showed that migraine was only weakly associated with elevated total cholesterol (OR: 1.09; 95% CI: 1.01–1.18) (Kurth et al., 2008).

Finally, a pro-inflammatory state has also been suggested to prevail in migraine. In the Women's Health Study, migraine was weakly associated with elevated levels of C-reactive protein (OR: 1.13; 95% CI: 1.05–1.22), although the magnitude of the effect was insufficient to support a strong biological link (Kurth et al., 2008). However, in a clinic-based sample, higher magnitudes of elevation were seen, suggesting that the levels of C-reactive protein are a function of severity of illness (Welch et al., 2006).

Migraine and Other Risk Factors for Cardiovascular Diseases in the AMPP Study

In the AMPP study, migraineurs were more likely than controls to have a medical diagnosis of diabetes (12.6% versus 9.4%; OR: 1.4; 95% CI: 1.2–1.6), hypertension (33.1% versus 27.5%; OR: 1.4; 95% CI: 1.3–1.6), and high cholesterol levels (32.7% versus 25.6%; OR: 1.4; 95% CI: 1.3–1.5) (**Figure 3.3**). Although migraineurs were significantly more likely to smoke, the differences found in this study were small, and the significance likely reflects the large sample size (Bigal et al., 2010).

MA was significantly associated with all risk factors. MO was significantly associated with diabetes, hypertension, and high cholesterol levels, but not with smoking (Bigal et al., 2010). Although the magnitude of the association was higher for MA than for MO, the differences were not as broad as seen for cardiovascular disease, as detailed in Table 3.1.

Figure 3.4 displays the odds of reporting at least two of the four assessed risk factors in persons with MA and MO relative to controls. Both individuals with MA and those with MO were significantly more likely to have more than one cardiovascular risk factor relative to controls for most demographic categories.

Assessment of Cardiovascular Risk: Framingham Scores

Figure 3.4 displays the Framingham risk scores for migraine overall, MA, and MO, as well as the scores by gender and age. Overall, risk scores were significantly higher for all migraineurs (mean: 10.7; standard deviation [SD]: 5.4), individuals with MA (mean ± SD: 11.0 ± 5.4),

and individuals with MO (mean ± SD: 10.6 ± 5.4) as compared to controls (mean ± SD: 8.5 ± 6.1) ($P < 0.001$ for all comparisons with controls). Scores were significantly higher in migraineurs of both genders (overall and for just MO and just MA). Scores were numerically higher for all age groups younger than 70 years. Scores were significantly higher for migraineurs in all age ranges from 30 to 59 years old.

Multivariate Analyses

Because migraine appears to be associated with both cardiovascular disease and risk factors for cardiovascular diseases, and because some medications used to treat migraine are vasoconstrictive, we tested main effects in our multivariate models after adjusting for gender, age, disability, triptan use, and the cardiovascular disease risk factors assessed in our study (diabetes, hypertension, smoking, and high cholesterol) (Bigal et al., 2010). Overall, migraine remained significantly associated with myocardial infarction (OR: 2.2; 95% CI: 1.7–2.8), stroke (OR: 1.5; 95% CI: 1.2–2.1), and claudication (OR: 2.69; 95% CI: 1.98–3.23). MA was significantly associated with the three outcomes, whereas MO remained associated with myocardial infarction and claudication but not stroke (Bigal et al., 2010). Table 3.4 shows the putative mechanisms that might explain the relationship between migraine and cardiovascular diseases.

Migraine and Patent Foramen Ovale

Initial studies indicate there is an increased prevalence of patent foramen ovale (PFO) in MA, as well as an increased prevalence of migraine and MA in persons with PFO (Diener et al., 2007a, 2007b). In a quantitative systematic review of articles on migraine and PFO, the estimated strength of association between PFO and migraine, reflected by the summary odds ratios, was 5.13 (95% CI: 4.67–5.59), and that between PFO and MA was 3.21 (95% CI: 2.38–4.17). The grade of evidence was low, however. The association between migraine and PFO was demonstrated by an OR of 2.54 (95% CI: 2.01–3.08); the grade of evidence was low to moderate (Schwedt et al., 2008).

CONCLUSIONS

Patients with comorbid medical or neurologic illness are often more difficult to treat. This understanding has particular significance in migraine, as several diseases

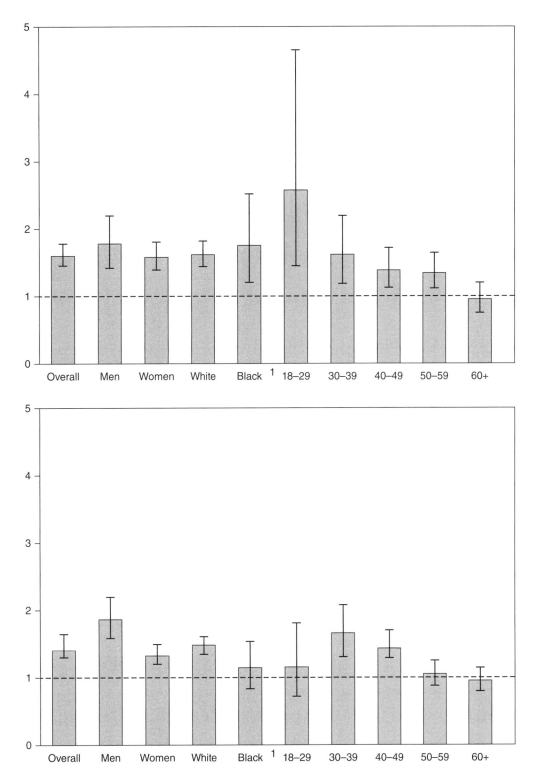

Figure 3.3 Odds Ratio of Reporting at Least Two Risk Factors for Cardiovascular Events in Individuals with Migraine with Aura (top) and Migraine Without Aura (bottom) / Footnote: Bars represent the odds ratio and whiskers represent the confidence intervals.

Adapted from Bigal ME, Kurth T, Santanello N et al. Migraine and cardiovascular disease: a population-based study. *Neurology* 2010;74:628-635.

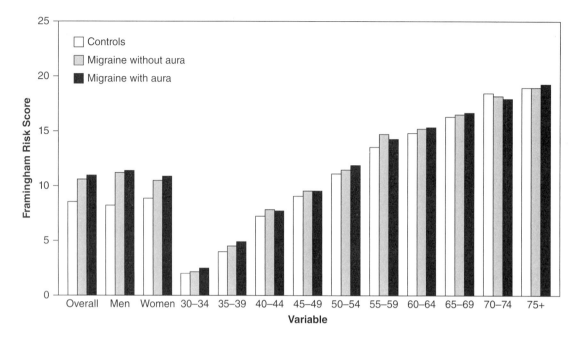

Figure 3.4 Mean Framingham Scores of Participants as a Function of Their Headache Status and of Demographics / Footnote: Stratification is by age in years.
Adapted from Bigal ME, Kurth T, Santanello N et al., 2010.

co-occur in migraineurs with a greater frequency than would be expected by chance. As discussed in this chapter, migraine is comorbid with depression, anxiety, affective disorders, stroke, and epilepsy, among other conditions. These disorders can pose therapeutic challenges and limit treatment options. A restricted therapeutic armamentarium can severely compromise treatment. Additionally, patients with major comorbid psychiatric disorders may require ongoing care from a mental health professional appropriate to the disorder.

REFERENCES

Bigal ME, Lipton RB. Obesity is a risk factor for transformed migraine but not chronic tension-type headache. *Neurology* 2006;67:252–257.

Bigal ME, Lipton RB. Putative mechanisms of the relationship between obesity and migraine progression. *Curr Pain Headache Rep* 2008;12:207–212.

Bigal ME, Liberman JN, Lipton RB. Obesity and migraine: a population study. *Neurology* 2006;66:545–550.

Bigal ME, Kurth T, Santanello N, et al. Migraine and cardiovascular disease: a population-based study. *Neurology* 2010;74:628–635.

Bogenschutz MP, Nurnberg HG. Theoretical and methodological issues in psychiatric comorbidity. *Harv Rev Psychiatry* 2000;8:18–24.

Breslau N. Psychiatric comorbidity in migraine. *Cephalalgia* 1998;22:56–61.

Breslau N, Lipton RB, Stewart W, et al. Comorbidity of migraine and depression: investigating potential etiology and prognosis. *Neurology* 2003;60:1308–1312.

Cavestro C, Rosatello A, Micca G, et al. Insulin metabolism is altered in migraineurs: a new pathogenic mechanism for migraine? *Headache* 2007;47:1436–1442.

Diener HC, Kurth T, Dodick D. Patent foramen ovale and migraine. *Curr Pain Headache Rep* 2007a;11: 236–240.

Diener HC, Kurth T, Dodick D. Patent foramen ovale, stroke, and cardiovascular disease in migraine. *Curr Opin Neurol* 2007b;20:310–319.

El-Metwally A, Salminen JJ, Auvinen A, et al. Prognosis of non-specific musculoskeletal pain in preadolescents: a prospective 4-year follow-up study till adolescence. *Pain* 2004;110:550–559.

Etminan M, Takkouche B, Isorna FC, et al. Risk of ischaemic stroke in people with migraine: systematic review and meta-analysis of observational studies. *BMJ* 2005;330:63.

Feinstein AR. The basic elements of clinical science. *J Chronic Dis* 1963;16:1125–1133.

Haffner SM. Risk constellations in patients with the metabolic syndrome: epidemiology, diagnosis, and treatment patterns. *Am J Med* 2006;119:S3–S9.

Hagen K, Einarsen C, Zwart JA, et al. The co-occurrence of headache and musculoskeletal symptoms amongst 51 050 adults in Norway. *Eur J Neurol* 2002;9:527–533.

Hamelsky SW, Lipton RB. Psychiatric comorbidity of migraine. *Headache* 2006;46:1327–1333.

Haut SR, Bigal ME, Lipton RB. Chronic disorders with episodic manifestations: focus on epilepsy and migraine. *Lancet Neurol* 2006;5:148–157.

Hestbaek L, Leboeuf-Yde C, Kyvik KO, et al. Comorbidity with low back pain: a cross-sectional population-based survey of 12- to 22-year-olds. *Spine* 2004;29:1483–1492.

Hestbaek L, Leboeuf-Yde C, Kyvik KO. Is comorbidity in adolescence a predictor for adult low back pain? A prospective study of a young population. *BMC Musculoskelet Disord* 2006;7:29.

Holroyd KA. Disentangling the Gordian knot of migraine comorbidity. *Headache* 2007;47:876–877.

Kruit MC, van Buchem MA, Hofman PA, et al. Migraine as a risk factor for subclinical brain lesions. *JAMA* 2004;291:427–434.

Kruit MC, Launer LJ, Ferrari MD, et al. Brain stem and cerebellar hyperintense lesions in migraine. *Stroke* 2006;37:1109–1112.

Kurth T, Slomke MA, Kase CS, et al. Migraine, headache, and the risk of stroke in women: a prospective study. *Neurology* 2005;64:1020–1026.

Kurth T, Gaziano JM, Cook NR, et al. Migraine and risk of cardiovascular disease in women. *JAMA* 2006;296:283–291.

Kurth T, Gaziano JM, Cook NR, et al. Migraine and risk of cardiovascular disease in men. *Arch Intern Med* 2007;167:795–801.

Kurth T, Ridker PM, Buring JE. Migraine and biomarkers of cardiovascular disease in women. *Cephalalgia* 2008;28:49–56.

Lipton RB, Silberstein SD. Why study the comorbidity of migraine? *Neurology* 1994;44:S4–S5.

Low NC, Merikangas KR. The comorbidity of migraine. *CNS Spectr* 2003;8:433–434, 437–444.

MacClellan LR, Mitchell BD, Cole JW, et al. Familial aggregation of ischemic stroke in young women: the Stroke Prevention in Young Women Study. *Genet Epidemiol* 2006;30:602–608.

McWilliams LA, Goodwin RD, Cox BJ. Depression and anxiety associated with three pain conditions: results from a nationally representative sample. *Pain* 2004;111:77–83.

Merikangas KR, Stevens DE. Comorbidity of migraine and psychiatric disorders. *Neurol Clin* 1997;15:115–123.

Navab M, Yu R, Gharavi N, et al. High-density lipoprotein: antioxidant and anti-inflammatory properties. *Curr Atheroscler Rep* 2007;9:244–248.

Patel NV, Bigal ME, Kolodner KB, et al. Prevalence and impact of migraine and probable migraine in a health plan. *Neurology* 2004;63:1432–1438.

Porter A, Gladstone JP, Dodick DW. Migraine and white matter hyper-intensities. *Curr Pain Headache Rep* 2005;9:289–293.

Ratcliffe GE, Enns MW, Belik SL, et al. Chronic pain conditions and suicidal ideation and suicide attempts: an epidemiologic perspective. *Clin J Pain* 2008;24:204–210.

Rosamond W. Are migraine and coronary heart disease associated? An epidemiologic review. *Headache* 2004;44:S5–S12.

Rose KM, Carson A, Sanford C, et al. Migraine and other headaches: associations with Rose angina and coronary heart disease. *Neurology* 2004;63:2233–2239.

Scher AI, Stewart WF, Ricci JA, et al. Factors associated with the onset and remission of chronic daily headache in a population-based study. *Pain* 2003;106:81–89.

Scher AI, Bigal ME, Lipton RB. Comorbidity of migraine. *Curr Opin Neurol* 2005a;18:305–310.

Scher AI, Terwindt GM, Picavet HS, et al. Cardiovascular risk factors and migraine: the GEM population-based study. *Neurology* 2005b;64:614–620.

Scher AI, Stewart WF, Lipton RB. The comorbidity of headache with other pain syndromes. *Headache* 2006a;46:1416–1423.

Scher AI, Terwindt GM, Verschuren WM, et al. Migraine and MTHFR C677T genotype in a population-based sample. *Ann Neurol* 2006b;59:372–375.

Schwedt TJ, Demaerschalk BM, Dodick DW. Patent foramen ovale and migraine: a quantitative systematic review. *Cephalalgia* 2008;28:531–540.

Solomon GD, Price KL. Burden of migraine. A review of its socioeconomic impact. *Pharmacoeconomics* 1997;11:1–10.

Stang PE, Carson AP, Rose KM, et al. Headache, cerebrovascular symptoms, and stroke: the Atherosclerosis Risk in Communities Study. *Neurology* 2005:64:1573–1577.

Victor TW, Hu X, Campbell J, et al. Association between migraine, anxiety and depression. *Cephalalgia* 2010;30:567–575.

Von Korff M, Crane P, Lane M, et al. Chronic spinal pain and physical–mental comorbidity in the United States: results from the national comorbidity survey replication. *Pain* 2005;113:331–339.

Welch KM, Brandes AW, Salerno L, et al. C-reactive protein may be increased in migraine patients who present with complex clinical features. *Headache* 2006;46:197–199.

Winter C, Buring J, Kurth T. Body mass index, migraine, migraine frequency, and migraine features in women. *Cephalalgia* 2009:29:269–278.

Zwart JA, Dyb G, Hagen K, et al. Depression and anxiety disorders associated with headache frequency: the Nord-Trøndelag Health Study. *Eur J Neurol* 2003;10:147–152.

Aggravating and Trigger Factors for Migraine

Anne Donnet, MD

INTRODUCTION

Triggers are factors that, alone or in combination, induce headache in predisposed individuals. The initiation of migraine headache is commonly associated with a wide variety of external and internal factors. Despite the progress made in elucidating the pathophysiology of migraine, only limited progress has been achieved in the study of trigger factors. Although many studies on these triggers have been published (Blau, 1992; Robbins, 1994; Peatfield, 1995; Scharff & Marcus, 1995; Silberstein, 1995; Evans, 1998; Chabriat et al., 1999; Spierings et al., 2001; Ierusalimschy & Filho, 2002; Zivadinov et al., 2003; Takeshima et al., 2004; Kelman, 2007; Wöber et al., 2007), some heterogeneity between studies persists. Better understanding of migraine triggers may lead to a better diagnostic approach, improved treatment strategies, and an understanding of the underlying pathophysiology of migraine.

PRECIPITATING FACTORS

Clinical evidence suggests that most migraine attacks are induced by a variety of endogenous and exogenous factors. The most commonly cited factors that could precipitate migraine attacks are endogenous triggers such as anxiety, irritation, and fatigue, and for women, menstruation (Chabriat et al., 1999; Henry et al., 2002). Migraine triggers are individual; thus they may differ from one migraine sufferer to another. They usually precede the attack by a short time interval. Triggers may vary between migraineurs, and the presence of a trigger does not always cause an attack in the same person. Furthermore, triggers may change during the lifetime of the migraineur or be modified by prophylactic treatment.

The fact that a precipitating factor is associated with headache does not prove causality or eliminate the need to consider etiology. Because common events happen commonly, the association between a headache and an exposure to a substance may be mere coincidence. Several trigger factors occurring within close proximity may be more likely to elicit a migraine than a single trigger factor. Moreover, triggers may sometimes be difficult to distinguish from the premonitory symptoms. Finally, triggers seem to be associated with a more florid acute migraine attack (Kelman, 2007).

Design of the Studies

Migraine attacks can be elicited by a variety of precipitants. Several designs have been used to study trigger factors. The realization of controlled clinical trials or prospective studies (Chabriat et al., 1999; Wöber et al., 2007) with high-level methodological conditions is difficult (Lipton, 2000). Controlled studies are rare and restricted to single trigger factors. The most common design is the patient survey. Migraine sufferers are asked to enumerate their headache triggers or asked whether they believe a specific factor triggers their headache (Hauge et al., 2011). This leads to subjective information. Thus, the validity of these data is reduced by recall bias, selective memory, and the patient's need for causal explanations (Wöber & Wöber-Bingöl, 2010).

Types of Triggers

All aspects of life have been suspected to trigger migraine, although scientific evidence supporting the validity of many of these triggers remains lacking.

Hormones

Menstruation has a prominent unfavorable role in migraine. Hormonal fluctuations occurring during the menstrual cycle also may trigger migraine. Menstrual migraine is defined as an attack that occurs as much as 1 day before and as long as 3 days after the onset of menses. Such attacks occur around menses in 60% of women with migraine, and exclusively during this period in 7% to 14% (Loder, 2006). Estrogen withdrawal is a trigger for headache in women who are susceptible to migraine. Women with an onset of migraine during the time of menarche seem to be affected more often by

menstrual migraine than women without an onset at that time. In prospective studies, evidence has not been found that ovulation initiates migraine attacks.

Migraine may worsen in the first trimester of pregnancy but often significantly improves during the latter half of the pregnancy. Notably, women with a history of menstrual migraine typically have an improvement of all types of migraine with pregnancy.

Although migraine prevalence typically decreases with advancing age, menopause may bring regression, worsening, or no change in migraine severity. Finally, the influence of oral contraception and hormone replacement therapy on the course of migraine varies. For more details, see Chapter 11.

Nutritional Triggers

Some foods (such as cheese, chocolate, or wine) are thought to be well-known triggers for migraine attacks. The proportion of patients reporting migraine related to intake of food or alcohol ranges between 12% and 58%. In the majority of studies, however, researchers have not reported data on the exact time between intake and onset of the migraine attack. Moreover, the role that food allergy plays in migraine remains controversial. Most food reactions are chemically mediated by one of the following substances: nitrites (hot dog headache; Henderson et al., 1972), glutamate (Chinese restaurant syndrome; Sauber, 1980), and possibly aspartame (Scharff & Marcus, 1995)

Chocolate is a "classical" migraine trigger, with as many as 20% of patients with migraine reporting that this food precipitates their headache. Nevertheless, the evidence supporting this link is inconsistent. In fact, Marcus et al. (1997) demonstrated that chocolate was no more likely to provoke headache than placebo, with these results being independent of subjects' beliefs regarding the role of chocolate in the instigation of headache. Precipitant agents may potentially include theobromine, caffeine, and biogenic amines such as phenylethylamine. In a review of intolerance to dietary biogenic amines in headache, two oral provocation studies found no effect of tyramine on migraine. In their study, Jansen et al. (2003) also failed to find any relationship between the amount of phenylethylamine in chocolate and headache attacks in migraineurs.

Cheese is another food that is frequently suspected of precipitating migraine attacks. The number of patients reporting migraine triggered by cheese consumption ranges between 0% and 19%, but no controlled study has been conducted to support the contention that cheese is a precipitant of migraine. If there is a link, biogenic amines contained in cheese may be at the origin of migraine attacks.

In terms of the relationship between caffeine and migraine, studies have produced contradictory results. Rasmussen (1993) failed to demonstrate that the intake of coffee was related to the prevalence of migraine. Nevertheless, headache attributed to the withdrawal of caffeine was included in the second edition of the *International Classification of Headache Disorders* (ICHD-II, 2004).

In a recent randomized, cross-over study in migraineurs, dietary restriction of IgG antibodies proved to be an effective strategy in reducing the frequency of migraine attack (Alpay et al., 2010). These results remain to be confirmed.

Patients should be advised that food plays a limited role as a precipitating factor of migraine. In particular, general dietary restrictions have not been proved to be useful in preventing attacks (Holzhammer & Wöber, 2006). Currently, scientific evidence is lacking to definitively prove that any other food or food additive plays a relevant role as a trigger factor of headaches (Wöber & Wöber-Bingöl, 2010).

In some retrospective studies, alcohol has been reported to be a migraine trigger; in contrast, the results from prospective studies limit considerably the importance of alcohol in this role. This risk factor is reported to be approximately 10% but ranges from less than 10% to 50%. Although red wine is frequently reported as the principal trigger of migraine (Holzhammer & Wöber, 2006), white wine and other alcoholic drinks also appear to have similar effects. Nevertheless, this influence greatly varies between the countries: in a study carried out in Japan, researchers found that wine never precipitated migraine with aura, and only 1.4% of patients experiencing migraine without aura reported wine as a trigger (Takeshima et al., 2004).

The mechanism underlying migraine precipitated by alcohol is unknown. The principal substances found in alcoholic drinks (histamine, tyramine, phenylethylamine, sulfites, flavonoid phenols, 5-hydroxytryptamine), dehydration, and vasodilatation are all thought to be involved in headache provoked by alcohol (Panconesi, 2008). Ethanol may lead to a vasodilatation of meningeal vessels by activation of TRPV1 and CGRP release (Nicoletti et al., 2008).

Skipping meals or fasting (Abu-Salameh et al., 2010), and dehydration (Blau, 2005) may also trigger migraine.

Weather

Among the most widely cited yet poorly documented triggers of headache are weather-related variables (Prince et al., 2004), such as temperature, humidity, and barometric pressure. Studies on barometric pressure have produced conflicting results in terms of their link with migraine. Spierings et al. (2001) found that weather changes were reported as a precipitating factor in 71% of migraineurs. The risk associated with this factor ranges from 8% to 86%. This variability may be explained by differences in patient recruitment, and by geographical, social, and cultural differences.

Two recent studies revealed a modest role of weather. In the first study, higher ambient temperature and, to a lesser degree, lower barometric pressure led to a transient increase in risk of headache (Mukamal et al., 2009). In the second study, both pre-Chinook and high-wind Chinook days increased the probability of migraine onset in a subset of migraineurs (Cooke et al., 2000). Most migraineurs who were influenced by the weather were sensitive to both temperature and humidity (Prince et al., 2004).

Stress, Tension, and Emotional Influences

Mental stressors are commonly perceived as important trigger factors by both patients and physicians, although solid evidence to back up this claim is lacking. In retrospective questionnaire studies, as many as 80% of migraine patients (Kelman, 2007) reported that stress was an important trigger factor for their attacks, but patients have a tendency to overestimate stress on retrospective measures. Chabriat et al. (1999) found that endogenous factors were the most common triggers for migraine attacks, with stress being the second most commonly reported trigger (after fatigue). The effect of stress as a trigger may be greater in migraine patients with a comorbid major depression (Sauro & Becker, 2009).

Only 15% of patients report pleasant experiences as trigger for headache, whereas negative feelings have been mentioned as triggers by as many as 58% (Hauge et al., 2011a). Various emotional subtypes—anxiety, irritation, worrying, distress, feeling depressed, and strong emotions—have been reported as being linked to migraine (Henry et al., 2002).

Stress-provocation studies, involving mental and physical stressors, have suggested that migraine patients demonstrate different sympathetic and parasympathetic changes compared to healthy volunteers (Avnon et al.,

2004). In a prospective longitudinal study, however, Schooman et al. (2007) failed to find any objective evidence for a temporal relationship between perceived stress, biological indicators for a stress response, and the onset of migraine attacks. Rarely, crying (Evans, 1998) or laughing has been described as a triggering factor.

Sensorial Triggers

Photophobia, phonophobia, and osmophobia are frequently associated with migraine attacks. Migraine attacks are often triggered by sensorial stimulation such as loud noise, bright light, strong odor, heat, or cold. Migraine patients reported odor to be a trigger factor for 36.5% to 70% of migraine attacks. The odors provoking migraine attacks most often in young women were perfume, followed by car exhaust, cigarette smoke, detergent, gasoline, vanilla, and fried or grilled food (Sjöstrand et al., 2010).

The relationship between migraine and smoking is controversial. In prospective studies, little or no evidence supported the role of smoke as a precipitating factor (Chabriat et al., 1999). Recent studies, by comparison, confirm that smoking cigarettes (Lopez-Mesonero et al., 2009) or passive smoking (Hauge et al., 2011) can be a precipitating factor for migraine attacks.

Lack of Sleep, Excess Sleep, and Fatigue

The relationship between sleep and migraine has been long recognized. Alteration in chronobiology, such as too much or too little sleep, may lead to a migraine attack. Under-sleeping (not sleeping enough or lack of sleep) is a more prevalent trigger than over-sleeping (Robbins, 1994). In Chabriat et al.'s (1999) study, fatigue and sleeping modifications were identified as triggers by 80% of patients with migraine. Fatigue was related to headache in 16% to 79% of migraineurs, but it remains an open question whether sleep disorders and fatigue are triggers of migraine or symptoms of migraine, or whether they are caused by a comorbid condition, such as a depressive disorder.

Weekends

Patients may experience migraine particularly or specifically during weekends. Such "weekend migraines" have been explained as deriving from relaxation and relief from stress after work. In particular, changes in lifestyle at weekends compared with working days, such as longer duration of sleep, skipping breakfast, caffeine

withdrawal, and use of alcohol and richer meals, have been discussed as headache triggers.

Physical Activity

Physical activities may trigger migraine, but they are also able to reduce the frequency and intensity of headache. In migraine patients, headache is also aggravated by physical activity. Primary exertional headache and primary headache associated with sexual activity are coded as separate entities in ICHD-II (2004), but are more frequently described in migraineurs.

Physical Musculoskeletal Factors

The body of knowledge has been increasing regarding how physical musculoskeletal triggers can initiate or precipitate a migraine attack. For instance, the referred pain from myofascial trigger points reproduces migraine attack (Fernández-de-las-Peñas et al., 2006) and is related to the presence of peripheral sensitization (Calandre et al., 2006). In addition, trigger point treatment is able to reduce central sensitization (Giambernardino et al., 2007). Different musculoskeletal factors related to migraine are covered in later chapters of this book.

Number of Triggers

Migraine attacks are initiated in many migraineurs by a variety of triggers; approximately three-fourths of patients report that their migraines are triggered by specific factors at least some of the time (Kelman, 2007). Sometimes multiple triggers may occur at the same time, such as stress, lack of sleep, and menses. Triggers may not operate independently. Occurrence of one trigger may increase the likelihood of exposure to one or more other triggers (Martin et al., 2009).

Precipitating Factors and the Type of Primary Headache

Several studies have identified a large number of trigger factors in migraine. Most of these studies have focused on migraine without aura. Few studies have analyzed trigger factors separately for patients with migraine with aura, patients without aura, and patients with tension-type headache (TTH). Stress, bright light, intense emotional influences, and sleep pattern changes are the trigger factors mentioned by most patients with migraine with aura (Hauge et al., 2010, 2011). Light, odors, or exercise may lead to an attack in less than

3 hours in 90% to 100% of patients with migraine with aura (Hauge et al., 2010).

Potential triggers have been examined most frequently in migraine and less often in TTH. Many of these factors are related to migraine as well as to TTH, but their prevalence may differ in the two types of headaches. The precipitating factors commonly acknowledged by both migraine and TTH patients include stress, not eating on time, fatigue, and lack of sleep (Spierings et al., 2001). Weather, odors, smoke, and light were the precipitating factors that differentiated migraine from TTH. Some precipitating factors differentiated migraine from TTH, but not vice versa (Spierings et al., 2001). No differences appear to exist between migraine and TTH patients in terms of the frequency with which alcohol acts as a trigger for headache (Panconesi, 2008).

Precipitating Factors and Age

Few studies in children and adolescents have addressed the subject of precipitating factors for headache. In a recent French study, precipitating factors were present in approximately 62% of children with headache. The most commonly reported precipitating factors were tantrums, school pressure, intense physical activity, heat, and lack of sleep (Cuvellier et al., 2008).

Physiopathology

Identifying triggers and the means by which they operate may help clarify the mechanisms of action underlying migraine. If genetics play an important role in migraine with and without aura, however, surely then environmental factors play an essential role. If trigger factors were better understood, it might be possible to modify factors in the environment, thereby reducing the frequency of migraine.

Excitability of the cell membranes of neurons in the occipital cortex appears fundamental to the brain's susceptibility to migraine attacks. Factors that increase or decrease neuronal excitability may, therefore, modulate the threshold for triggering attacks (Welch, 2003). Lambert and Zangami (2008) hypothesized that triggers may activate pathways in various parts of the cortex owing to variations in the susceptibility of neurons in different areas: according to these authors, migraine triggers activate multiple hypothalamic, limbic, and cortical areas, all of which contain neurons that project to the preganglionic parasympathetic neurons (Burstein & Jakubowski, 2005) in the superior salivatory nucleus. In fact, a trigger may cause a hypothalamic dysfunction, which can in turn activate the amygdala and trigeminal nuclei. Lambert and Zangami (2008) proposed a common downstream pathway, in which cortical activation by migraine triggers inhibits neuronal discharge in the brainstem—specifically, the periaqueductal gray matter and the nucleus raphe magnus—and facilitates trigeminovascular sensation.

Migraine triggers are likely to reflect a disturbance in overall balance of the circuits involved in the modulation of trigeminal afferent activity (Ho et al., 2010). Some authors suggest that a trigger, identifiable or not, must be present in all attacks of migraine headache and that these triggers induce the onset of cortical spreading depression in genetically predetermined individuals (Chakravarty, 2010).

Management of Triggers

Identification of trigger factors or precipitants is frequently recommended as a basic strategy in the treatment of migraine. In fact, patients are generally advised to avoid triggers. Keeping a detailed migraine calendar can help define which triggers are at play. At least some triggers, such as light, smoke, food, alcohol, and changes in sleep pattern, may be modified or avoided. In addition, hormonal triggers may respond to specific medications. Establishing proper sleep patterns, ensuring sufficient hydration, ceasing tobacco use, and avoiding excessive caffeine intake are some general practices that may help limit the outcome of migraine attack. Biofeedback, relaxation, and cognitive therapy may be helpful in patients whose most frequent trigger is stress. Of course, some environmental triggers are difficult to anticipate and to avoid.

If avoidance of triggers seems to be the logical solution to the problem, some authors suggest that advice to avoid triggers could result in maintaining the capacity of the trigger to precipitate headache or even inducing a process whereby existing tolerance diminishes to the trigger (Martin et al., 2009). In fact, another strategy advocates exposure to and focus on coping with triggers.

Finally, the effect of acute treatment on trigger factor–associated migraine is limited to menses-provoked attacks. Nevertheless, this approach may represent a springboard to treatments for migraine attacks induced by other specific trigger factors (Leone et al., 2010).

AGGRAVATING FACTORS

Factors that precipitate headache should be differentiated from those that exacerbate headache. According to the International Headache Society, migraine is aggravated by physical activity in adults, children (Cuvellier et al., 2008), and adolescents (Winner et al., 2003). Headache is aggravated by activity in 90.0% of patients at the following rates: occasionally in 13.5% of patients, frequently in 32.2% of patients, and very frequently in 44.3% of patients (Kelman, 2006). Patients with headache aggravated by activity have more headache-associated symptoms and triggers (Kelman, 2006). The most frequently described aggravating factors are physical activity, straining, bending over, stress, and tension (Spierings et al., 2001). In contrast to light and noise, which typically worsen headache, smell tends to aggravate nausea and vomiting.

CONCLUSIONS

All aspects of life have been suspected to trigger migraine, but scientific evidence supporting the validity of many of these triggers is lacking. Menses and alterations in chronobiology have prominent unfavorable roles in migraine.

The elucidation of factors that may trigger or precipitate headache can be diagnostically and therapeutically helpful. A better understanding of triggers is crucial for several reasons. In clinical practice, many migraine patients are interested in understanding what initiates their attacks. Identifying trigger factors can lead to preventive strategies such as trigger avoidance, stress management, and short-term prophylaxis of menstrual migraine.

Education of patients about trigger factors should be based on scientific evidence and should focus on those factors that can be modified. In addition, better understanding of trigger factors might enable researchers to identify those patients whose attacks can be precipitated, an approach used in the work conducted by Hadjikhani et al. (2001).

REFERENCES

Abu-Salameh I, Plakht Y, Ifergane G. Migraine exacerbation during Ramadan fasting. *J Headache Pain* 2010;11:513–517.

Alpay K, Orhan EK, Lieners C, Baykan B. Diet restriction in migraine, based on IgG against foods: a clinical double-blind, randomised cross-over trial. *Cephalalgia* 2010;30:829–837.

Avnon Y, Nitzan M, Sprecher E, Rogowski Z, Yarnitsky D. Autonomic asymmetry in migraine: augmented parasympathetic activation in left unilateral migraineurs. *Brain* 2004;127:2099–2108.

Blau JN. Migraine triggers: practice and theory. *Pathol Biol* 1992;40:367–372.

Blau JN. Water deprivation: a new migraine precipitant. *Headache* 2005;45:757–759.

Burstein R, Jakubowski M. Unitary hypothesis for multiple triggers of the pain and strain of migraine. *J Compar Neurol* 2005;493:9–14.

Calandre EP, Hidalgo J, Garcia-Leiva JM, Rico-Villademoros F. Trigger point evaluation in migraine patients: an indication of peripheral sensitization linked to migraine predisposition? *Eur J Neurol* 2006;13:244–249.

Chabriat H, Danchot J, Joire JE, Henry P. Precipitating factors of headache: a prospective study in a national control-matched survey in migraineurs and non-migraineurs. *Headache* 1999;39:335–338.

Chakravarty A. How triggers trigger acute migraine attacks: a hypothesis. *Med Hypotheses* 2010;74:750–751.

Cooke LJ, Rose MS, Becker WJ. Chinook winds and migraine headache. *Neurology* 2000;54:302–307.

Cuvellier JC, Donnet A, Guegan-Massardier E, et al. Clinical features of primary headache in children: a multicentre hospital-based study in France. *Cephalalgia* 2008;28:1145–1153.

Evans RW. Crying migraine. *Headache* 1998;38:799–800.

Fernández-de-las-Peñas C, Cuadrado ML, Pareja JA. Myofascial trigger points, neck mobility and forward head posture in unilateral migraine. *Cephalalgia* 2006;26:1061–1070.

Giamberardino MA, Tafuri E, Savini A, et al. Contribution of myofascial trigger points to migraine symptoms. *J Pain* 2007;8:869–878.

Hadjikhani N, Sanchez Del Rio M, Wu O, et al. Mechanisms of migraine aura revealed by functional MRI in human visual cortex. *Proc Natl Acad Sci USA* 2001;98:4687–4692.

Hauge AW, Kirchmann M, Olesen J. Trigger factors in migraine with aura. *Cephalalgia* 2010;30:346–353.

Hauge AW, Kirchmann M, Olesen J. Characterization of consistent triggers of migraine with aura. *Cephalalgia* 2011;31:416–438.

Henderson WR, Raskin NH. "Hot-dog" headache: individual susceptibility to nitrite. *Lancet* 1972;2:1162–1163.

Henry P, Auray JP, Gaudin AF, et al. Prevalence and clinical characterisics of migraine in France. *Neurology* 2002;59:232–237.

Ho TW, Edvinsson L, Goadsby PJ. CGRP and its receptors provide new insights into migraine pathophysiology. *Nat Rev Neurol* 2010;6:573–582.

Holzhammer J, Wöber C. Alimentäre triggerfaktoren bei migräne und kopfschmerz vom spannungstyp. *Schmerz* 2006;20:151–159.

Ierusalimschy R, Filho P. Fatores desencadeantes de crises de migranea em pacientes com migranea sem aura. *Arq Neuropsiquiatr* 2002;60:609–613.

ICHD-II: Headache Classification Subcommittee. The International Classification of Headache Disorders: 2nd edition. *Cephalalgia* 2004;24(suppl 1):9–160.

Jansen SC, van Dusselorp M, Bottema KC, Dubois AE. Intolerance to dietary biogenic amines: a review. *Ann Allergy Asthma Immunol* 2003;91:233–240.

Kelman L. Pain characteristics of the acute migraine attack. *Headache* 2006;46:942–953.

Kelman L. The triggers or precipitants of the acute migraine attack. *Cephalalgia* 2007;27:394–402.

Lambert GA, Zagami AS. The mode of action of migraine triggers: a hypothesis. *Headache* 2009;49:253–275.

Leone M, Vila C, McGown C. Influence of trigger factors on the efficacy of almotriptan as early intervention for the treatment of acute migraine in a primary care setting: the START study. *Expert Rev Neurother* 2010;10:1399–1408.

Lipton R. Fair winds and foul headaches. *Neurology* 2000;54:280–281.

Loder E. Menstrual migraine: pathophysiology, diagnosis and impact. *Headache* 2006;46:S55–S60.

Lopez-Mesonero L, Marquez S, Parra P, et al. Smoking as a precipitating factor for migraine: a survey in medical students. *J Headache Pain* 2009;10:101–103.

Marcus DA, Scharff L, Turk D, Gourley LM. A double-blind provocative study of chocolate as a trigger of headache. *Cephalalgia* 1997;17:855–862.

Martin PR, Mac Leod C. Behavioral management of headache triggers: avoidance of triggers is an inadequate strategy. *Clin Psychol Rev* 2009;29:483–495.

Mukamal KJ, Wellenius GA, Mittleman MA. Weather and air pollution as triggers of severe headaches. *Neurology* 2009;72:922–927.

Nicoletti P, Trevisani M, Manconi M, Gatti R, De Siena G, Zagli G, Benemei S, Capone JA, Geppetti P, Pini LA. Ethanol causes neurogenic vasodilatation by TRPV1 activation and CGRP release in the trigeminovascular system of the guinea pig. *Cephalalgia* 2008;28:9–17.

Panconesi A. Alcohol and migraine: trigger factor, consumption, mechanisms. A review. *J Headache Pain* 2008;9:19–27.

Peatfield RC. Relationship between food, wine, and beer-precipitated migrainous headaches. *Headache* 1995;35:355–357.

Prince PB, Rapoport A, Sheftell FD, et al. The effect of weather on headache. *Headache* 2004;44:596–602.

Rasmussen BK. Migraine and tension-type headache in a general population: precipitating factors, female

hormones, sleep pattern and relation to lifestyle. *Pain* 1993;53:65–72.

Robbins L. Precipitating factors in migraine: a retrospective review of 494 patients. *Headache* 1994;34:214–216.

Sauber WJ. What is Chinese restaurant syndrome? *Lancet* 1980;1:721–722.

Sauro KM, Becker WJ. The stress and migraine interaction. *Headache* 2009;1378–1386.

Scharff L, Marcus DA. Triggers of headache episodes and coping responses of headache diagnostic groups. *Headache* 1995;35:397–403.

Schooman GG, Evers DJ, Ballieux BE, et al. Is stress a trigger factor for migraine? *Psychoneuroendocrinology* 2007;32:532–538.

Silberstein S. Migraine symptoms: results of a survey of self-reported migraineurs. *Headache* 1995;35:387–396.

Sjöstrand C, Savic I, Laudon-Meyer E, et al. Migraine and olfactory stimuli. *Curr Pain Headache Rep* 2010;14:244–251.

Spierings ELH, Ranke AH, Honkoop PC. Precipitating and aggravating factors of migraine versus tension-type headache. *Headache* 2001;41:554–558.

Takeshima T, Ishizaki K, Fukuhara Y, et al. Population-based door to door survey of migraine in Japan: the Daisen study. *Headache* 2004;44:8–19.

Welch KMA. Contemporary concepts of migraine pathogenesis. *Neurology* 2003;61:S2–S8.

Winner P, Rothner AD, Putnam DG, Asgharnejad M. Demographic and migraine characteristics of adolescents with migraine: Glaxo Wellcome Clinical Trials' database. *Headache* 2003;43:451–457.

Wöber C, Brannath W, Schmidt K, Kapitan M, Rudel E, Wessely P, Wöber-Bingöl C, PAMINA Study Group. Prospective analysis of factors related to migraine attacks: the PAMINA study. *Cephalalgia* 2007;27:304–314.

Wöber C, Wöber-Bingöl C. Triggers of migraine and tension-type headache. *Handb Clin Neurol* 2010;97:161–172.

Zivadinov R, Willheim K, Sepic-Grahovac D, Jurjevic A, Bucuk M, Brnabic-Razmilic O, Relja G, Zorzon M. Migraine and tension-type headache in Croatia: a population-based survey of precipitating factors. *Cephalalgia* 2003;23:336–343.

The Trigeminocervical Complex and Migraine

Thorsten Bartsch, MD, and Peter J. Goadsby, MD, PhD

INTRODUCTION

Migraine is a common and debilitating disorder that is fundamentally episodic in nature. Its phenotype includes attacks of often severe headache involving the trigeminal and upper cervical dermatomes, sensory dysmodulation, and, in one-fifth of patients, an aura consisting of neurologic symptoms (Goadsby et al., 2002). Patients with primary headaches often report pain that involves the front of the head, in the cutaneous distribution of the first (ophthalmic) division of the trigeminal nerve. The trigeminocervical complex is the key structure processing cranial trigeminovascular nociceptive information. Its physiology and pharmacology provide insight into the processing of migraine pain and into acute and preventive medicine options (Goadsby et al., 2009).

THE NEURAL SUBSTRATE OF PAIN IN MIGRAINE: ANATOMY AND CONVERGENCE

Early neurosurgical studies in patients showed that stimulation of trigeminally innervated intracranial structures, such as the supratentorial dura mater and large cranial vessels, evoked painful sensations regardless of the stimuli applied and implied that the afferent input from dural structures is the neural substrate of head pain (Penfield & McNaughton, 1940; Ray & Wolff, 1940). Hence, afferent input, or at least perceived input, from dural structures is likely to be the neural substrate of pain in primary headaches, such as migraine or cluster headache.

The trigeminal nerve conveys sensory information, such as thermal, mechanical, and pain messages, to higher thalamic and neocortical centers (Malick & Burstein, 1998; Malick et al., 2000). The nociceptive input from the dura mater to the first synapse in the brainstem is transmitted via small-diameter A- and C-fiber afferents in the ophthalmic division of the trigeminal nerve via the trigeminal ganglia to nociceptive second-order neurons in the superficial and deep layers of the medullary dorsal horn of the trigeminocervical complex (Burstein et al., 1998; Schepelmann et al., 1999; Bartsch & Goadsby, 2002). Given that the trigeminal system constitutes the dominant sensory innervation of cranial vessels and the dura mater, this connection is termed the trigeminovascular system. The pseudo-unipolar cell bodies of the trigeminal nerve lie in the trigeminal ganglion in the Meckel cave and are analogous to the dorsal root ganglia of the spinal cord. All three divisions of the trigeminal nerve—ophthalmic (V1), maxillary (V2), and mandibular (V3)—innervate particular dermatomes of the head. The trigeminocervical complex is thus the key relay structure processing cranial trigeminovascular nociceptive pain information. Trigeminal fibers innervating cerebral vessels contain substance P and calcitonin gene-related peptide (CGRP). The trigeminocervical complex extends from the trigeminal nucleus caudalis to the segments of C_2 in the rat (Strassman et al., 1994), cat (Kaube et al., 1993b), and monkey (Goadsby & Hoskin, 1997).

Recent neuroimaging studies confirm the somatotopic representation of the trigeminal system to noxious stimulation (Borsook et al., 2004, 2006; Moulton et al., 2008). Dural-sensitive trigeminal neurons show a high degree of convergent input from other afferent sources, as they typically possess facial and corneal receptive fields as well (Burstein et al., 1998; Schepelmann et al., 1999).

With regard to the innervation of the head, the upper cervical spinal roots also contribute to the sensory innervation of cranial and cervical structures. Occipital and suboccipital structures, such as vessels and the dura mater of the posterior fossa, deep paraspinal neck muscles, and zygapophyseal joints and ligaments, are innervated by the upper cervical roots and are recognized sources of neck and head pain (Anthony, 1992; Bogduk & Bartsch, 2005; Bogduk & Govind, 2009). The nociceptive inflow from these suboccipital structures is also mediated by small-diameter afferent fibers in the upper cervical roots terminating in the dorsal horn of the cervical spine extending from the C_2 segment up to the medullary dorsal horn (Bakker et al., 1984; Pfister & Zenker, 1984; Neuhuber & Zenker, 1989). The major afferent contribution is mediated by the spinal root C_2, which is peripherally represented by the greater occipital nerve

(GON) (Vital et al., 1989; Becser et al., 1998). Similarly to the trigeminal sensory neurons, these cervical neurons show a high convergence of input from neck muscles and skin (Bartsch & Goadsby, 2002).

Experimentally, researchers have shown that spread and referral of pain can be induced by stimulation of structures in the neck that are innervated by the upper cervical roots. Posterior fossa tumors (Kerr, 1961), stimulation of infratentorial dura mater (Wolff, 1963), direct stimulation of cervical roots (Hunter & Mayfield, 1949), vertebral artery dissection (Hutchinson et al., 2000), and stimulation of subcutaneous tissue innervated by the greater occipital nerve (Piovesan et al., 2001, 2003) may all be perceived as frontal head pain. Similarly, direct stimulation of the supratentorial dura mater leads to pain that is mostly referred to the first (ophthalmic) division of the trigeminal nerve (Wolff, 1963), but may be also referred to dermatomes supplied by the upper cervical roots (Wirth & Van Buren, 1971).

Although an anatomic overlap of trigeminal and cervical afferents throughout the trigeminocervical complex from the level of the caudal trigeminal nucleus to at least the C_2 segment was first suggested by Kerr (1961), direct evidence for coupling between meningeal afferents and cervical afferents in the spinal dorsal horn was not described until recently (Bartsch & Goadsby, 2002). A population of neurons in the C_2 dorsal horn has been characterized that receives convergent input from the supratentorial dura mater and the greater occipital nerve (GON). These neurons demonstrate properties typical of dura-sensitive trigeminal neurons, with a convergent input from the facial skin corresponding to the dermatome of the ophthalmic division of the trigeminal nerve including the cornea; the same neurons also possess a receptive field corresponding to the cervical skin of the C_2/C_3 dermatomes and to deep paraspinal muscles innervated by the GON. Interestingly, these trigeminocervical neurons show convergent synaptic input not only from the supratentorial dura mater and from the ipsilateral GON, but also from the contralateral GON (**Figure 5.1**).

Taken together with the results of other studies that show similar contralateral projections of nociceptive afferents following labeling of the trigeminal and cervical dorsal root ganglia (Pfaller & Arvidsson, 1988) or after facial afferent or GON stimulation (Goadsby et al., 1997), these findings indicate that bilateral or contralateral endings of nociceptive afferents of visceral and deep-somatic tissues are more common than previously acknowledged. This anatomic arrangement may find its functional correlate in the dull and poorly localized quality of head and neck pain. A mechanism that

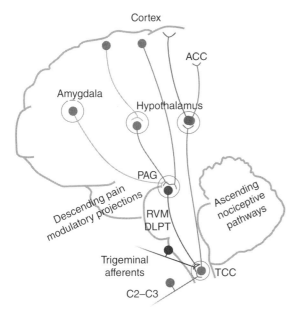

Figure 5.1 The Functional Anatomy of Pain-Modulatory Pathways in the Spinal Cord and Supraspinal Structures. Trigeminovascular nociceptive information is relayed in the trigeminocervical complex, where it is subject to segmental modulatory mechanisms, either intrinsic or extrinsic from descending projections. The convergent neuron in the dorsal horn may be sensitized due to an increased afferent inflow into the spinal cord by noxious stimuli. The nociceptive input is transmitted to supraspinal relay sites (e.g., the thalamus and cortex), and is subject to inhibitory anti-nociceptive projections by pain modulatory circuits in the brainstem.

Courtesy of Dr. Thorsten Bartsch.

PAG, periaqueductal gray; RV, rostral ventral medulla: DLPT, dorsal lateral pontine tegmentum.

explains these clinical and experimental findings posits the convergence of trigeminal and cervical afferents onto neurons in the trigeminocervical complex of the brainstem. Convergence taken together with sensitization of central trigeminal neurons provides a physiological basis for the clinical phenomenon of pain spread and referred pain, whereby pain originating from an affected tissue is perceived as originating from a distant receptive field (Mackenzie, 1909; Ruch, 1965).

PHARMACOLOGY OF TRIGEMINOVASCULAR NOCICEPTIVE TRANSMISSION IN THE TRIGEMINOCERVICAL COMPLEX

Considering that the trigeminocervical complex (TCC) is the major relay center processing nociceptive trigeminovascular input to higher central nervous system (CNS)

structures, elucidating its pharmacological mechanisms may provide insight into pathophysiological mechanisms and pharmacological treatment options of migraine. Indeed, the pharmacology of the nociceptive transmission has begun to be unraveled in recent years.

Recent experimental evidence has shown that anti-migraine drugs, including those with serotonergic action such as dihydroergotamine (Hoskin et al., 1996), sumatriptan (Kaube et al., 1993a; Storer & Goadsby, 1997), eletriptan (Goadsby & Hoskin, 1999), naratriptan (Cumberbatch, 1997; Goadsby & Knight, 1997b), rizatriptan (Cumberbatch et al., 1997), zolmitriptan (Goadsby & Hoskin, 1996), and NSAIDs such as acetylsalicylic acid (Kaube et al., 1993a), naproxen (Jakubowski et al., 2007), and ketorolac (Sokolov et al., 2010), have an effect on trigeminovascular nociception.

The trigeminal innervation of the cranial circulation contains a number of vasoactive neuropeptides; the most important for migraine seems to be calcitonin gene-related peptide (CGRP). With regard to the clinical effects of recently introduced CGRP receptor antagonists, micro-iontophoresis data indicate that non-presynaptic CGRP receptors in the TCC can be inhibited by CGRP-receptor blockers (Storer et al., 2004; Goadsby, 2005, 2008).

Serotonergic Targets

More recently, nonvascular serotonergic approaches involving 5-HT_{1F} receptors have been shown to have an anti-migraine effect in the TCC (Goldstein et al., 2001). These receptors are found in the trigeminal nucleus (Fugelli et al., 1997) and trigeminal ganglion (Bouchelet et al., 1996; Classey et al., 2010). 5-HT_{1F} receptor activation inhibits transmission in the trigeminal nucleus in the rat (Mitsikostas et al., 1999a) and the cat, although it seems less potent than 5-HT_{1B} or 5-HT_{1D} receptor activation in the cat (Goadsby & Classey, 2003). In a recent randomized proof-of-concept trial, the selective 5-HT_{1F} receptor agonist lasmiditan proved to be effective in the acute treatment of migraine (Ferrari et al., 2010).

Orexinergic Targets

Recently, two novel peptidergic neurotransmitters named orexin A (hypocretin) and orexin B, which are selectively synthesized in the lateral and posterior hypothalamus, have been described (De Lecea et al., 1998, 1999; De Lecea & Sutcliffe, 1999; Marcus et al., 2001). Orexin A and B are proteolytically derived from the same prepro-orexin precursor protein and bind to Gq-protein–coupled receptors named orexin A and B that act via PKC to phosphorylate voltage-activated calcium channels (Smart & Jerman, 2002). The orexins have been postulated to play a role in nociceptive processing, as application of orexin A elicits analgesic effects in behavioral pain assays, although the exact mechanisms by which this pain-modulating effect is mediated and the complete role of the orexins remain to be determined (Bingham et al., 2001; Yamamoto et al., 2002).

Anatomically, orexin A and B show widespread distribution throughout the brain and spinal cord, including sites that are involved in nociceptive processing such as the periaqueductal gray (PAG), raphe nuclei, and locus coeruleus (Trivedi et al., 1998; Hervieu et al., 2001). Orexinergic fibers have also been identified in the superficial and deep layers of the spinal and trigeminal dorsal horn (Van den Pol, 1999; Marcus et al., 2001; Van Den Pol et al., 2002). Orexins modulate synaptic transmission in the TCC. In studies, intravenous application of orexin A inhibited the A-fiber responses to dural electrical stimulation, an effect reversed by pretreatment with the OX1R antagonist SB-334867 (Holland et al., 2006; Holland & Goadsby, 2007; Holland & Bartsch, 2008). In contrast, orexin B administration had no significant effect on trigeminal neuronal firing. These data suggest that orexin A is able to inhibit A-fiber responses to dural electrical stimulation via activation of the OX1R. They are consistent with data showing a similar effect of inhibiting trigeminovascular activation in the dural circulation. Given that neurons in the hypothalamic area that is the source of CNS orexins can be activated with superior sagittal sinus stimulation, and also that these neurons contain orexin, CNS orexin mechanisms are a potential target for anti-migraine drugs (Benjamin et al., 2004; Holland et al., 2005).

Glutamatergic Targets

Glutamate is the major excitatory neurotransmitter in the CNS and plays a pivotal role in sensory and nociceptive transmission in both the brain and the spinal cord. Glutamatergic transmission acts through both ionotropic (ion channel type) and G-protein–coupled (metabotrophic) receptor classes. Glutamate-like immunoreactivity has been observed in neurons projecting to the trigeminal nucleus caudalis, whereas glutaminase immunoreactivity is most dense in the nucleus caudalis when compared with other parts of the trigeminal nucleus of the rat (Magnusson et al., 1986; Clements et al., 1991). Each of *N*-methyl-D-aspartate (NMDA), AMPA, kainate, and metabotropic glutamate receptors

have been identified in the superficial laminae of the trigeminal nucleus caudalis of the rat (Tallaksen-Greene et al., 1992). Ionotropic-receptor channel blockers, such as MK-801 acting at the NMDA receptor, and GYKI-52466, acting at the AMPA receptor, block trigeminovascular nociceptive transmission in the trigeminocervical nucleus (Storer & Goadsby, 1999; Classey et al., 2001). Similarly, both NMDA and non-NMDA ionotropic-receptor blockade reduces Fos protein expression in the trigeminal nucleus caudalis associated with intracisternal capsaicin injection (Mitsikostas, 1999a; Le Doare et al., 2006). Evidence suggests that group III metabotropic glutamate receptors are involved in trigeminovascular transmission, as their modulation decreases Fos expression in trigeminal nucleus caudalis in animal models of trigeminovascular nociceptive activation (Mitsikostas et al., 1999a, 1999b, 1999c). Moreover, it seems clear that the iGluR5 kainate subunit of the kainate receptor activation is important for trigeminocervical transmission after activation of durovascular afferents (Andreou et al., 2009). Clinical approaches to migraine treatment with the AMPA/kainate receptor antagonist LY293558 and the specific iGluR5 kainate receptor blocker LY466195 appear promising (Sang et al., 2004; Weiss et al., 2006).

Topiramate is an anticonvulsant that is known to have anti-migraine effects. Pharmacologically, this agent acts via inhibition of the carbonic anhydrase enzyme, blockage of voltage-dependent sodium channels, antagonism of AMPA/kainate receptors, and possibly amplification of gamma-aminobutyrate acid (GABA) activity. Besides its effects on a supraspinal level, topiramate inhibits neurovascular transmission in the trigeminocervical complex (Storer & Goadsby, 2004; Akerman & Goadsby, 2005a).

Cannabinoid Targets

Arachidonylethanolamide (AEA or anandamide) is one of the endogenous ligands to the cannabinoid CB1 and CB2 receptors (Devane et al., 1992). The known effects of anandamide are similar to those of Δ9-tetrahydrocannabinol, the active ingredient in cannabis—specifically, antinociception, catalepsy, hypothermia, and depression of motor activity (Adams et al., 1998). Blocking CB1 receptors in a model of intravital dural microscopy has been shown to affect neurogenic dural vasodilation, including CGRP-induced and nitric oxide (NO)–induced dural vessel dilation (Akerman et al., 2004). Moreover, anandamide-induced dural dilation was blocked by the TRPV1-receptor antagonist capsazepine (Akerman et al., 2004a). Anandamide is structurally related to capsaicin and olvanil (*N*-vanillyl-9-oleamide), two TRPV1 agonists that are known to have effects in the durovascular model (Akerman et al., 2003). From these data, one might predict that CB-receptor approaches in clinical trials might be effective against migraine (Akerman et al., 2007).

Dopamine Targets

Dopaminergic mechanisms have also been suggested to play a role in migraine head pain. Dopamine exerts antinociceptive effects when microiontophoresed directly into neurons in the TCC activated by trigeminovascular nociceptive inputs (Bergerot et al., 2007). Recently obtained experimental data suggest that dopamine binding to peripheral D1-like receptors may play a role in peripheral sensitization. Interestingly, the inhibitory or excitatory effects seen with administration of dopamine-receptor agonists are independent of blood vessel changes. In addition, central D2-like receptors inhibit trigeminocervical neurons and may provide insight into the role of dopamine and its receptors in migraine (Charbit et al., 2009a). Immunohistochemistry further demonstrates that both D1-like and D2-like dopamine receptors can be identified in the TCC (Bergerot et al., 2007).

One possible candidate for the supraspinal origin of this dopaminergic modulation is the hypothalamic A11 dopaminergic nucleus, which is distributed along the rostrocaudal axis, in the periventricular posterior region of the hypothalamus and the periventricular gray of the caudal thalamus (Fuxe et al., 2010). The A11 nucleus is known to send direct inhibitory projections to the spinal cord dorsal horn, and it is believed to be the sole source of dopamine in the spinal cord (Holstege et al., 1996). Stimulation of the A11 nucleus inhibits nociceptive trigeminocervical afferents (Goadsby et al., 2009). Furthermore, creating lesions in this area facilitates nociceptive and non-nociceptive trigeminocervical afferent activity (Charbit et al., 2010), indicating that the A11 nucleus provides a tonic inhibitory level of nociceptive neuronal firing, and suggesting that a dysfunction of A11 modulatory neurons would result in pain perception in the head without necessarily a change in peripheral signaling.

Calcium-Channel Targets

Selective large conductance calcium-activated potassium channels—that is, the BKCa or MaxiK channels—are thought to be involved in controlling neuronal excitability and transmitter release. A role for these calcium channels in the TCC was demonstrated through iontophoretic application of a BKCa analogue, which was also able to inhibit L-glutamate–induced firing in the TCC (Storer et al., 2009). Similarly, high-threshold VDCCs, including P/Q-, L-, and N-type VDCCs, have been shown to modulate nociceptive transmission in the TCC in vivo (Shields et al., 2005).

GABAergic Targets

Trigeminovascular nociceptive transmission in the TCC is also inhibited by GABA$_A$ receptor activation at the level of the TCC (Storer et al., 2001). Further, opioid agonists, potent analgesics with a certain role in the treatment of migraine, have been studied in the TCC showing that opiodergic receptors, in particular μ-receptors, modulate nociceptive input to the trigeminocervical complex (Silberstein & McCrory, 2000; Storer et al., 2003).

Figure 5.2 presents a schematic section of the trigeminocervical complex, indicating the intrinsic neuronal connections of afferent input, segmental interneurons, and ascending pathways.

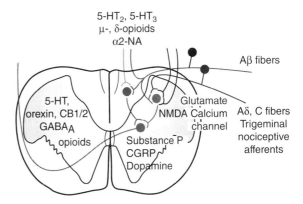

Figure 5.2 A Section of the Trigeminocervical Complex Indicating the Intrinsic Neuronal Connections of Afferent Input, Segmental Interneurons, and Ascending Pathways. Various neurotransmitter systems are involved in the processing of nociceptive trigeminovascular information and modulation by segmental and descending pathways.

Courtesy of Thorsten Bartsch.

CGRP: calcitonin gene-related peptide; GABA: gamma-aminobutyric acid; 5-HT: serotonin; NA: noradrenaline; NMDA: *N*-methyl-D-aspartic acid; cannabinoid CB1 and CB2 receptors.

CENTRAL MECHANISMS OF PAIN PROCESSING: CENTRAL SENSITIZATION AND DESCENDING INHIBITION

Nociceptive spinal cord neurons can become sensitized owing to a strong afferent stimulation by small-fiber afferents. This hyperexcitability is reflected in a reduction of the activation threshold, an increased responsiveness to afferent stimulation, an enlargement of receptive fields or the emergence of new receptive fields, and the recruitment of "silent" nociceptive afferents. The clinical correlates of this central hypersensitivity in migraine patients include the development of spontaneous pain, hyperalgesia, and allodynia (Burstein et al., 2000; Sandkuhler, 2009; Sokolov et al., 2010). The hypersensitivity of the afferent synaptic input in the spinal cord is thought to result from the stimulation-induced release of various neuropeptides, such as CGRP, or from augmented glutamate release and action at the NMDA receptor, but may also reflect a decrease of local segmental spinal inhibition in response to the afferent stimulation (Woolf & Salter, 2000; Sandkuhler, 2009).

These stimulation-induced neuroplastic changes may also be found in the neural population of the trigeminocervical complex, whose members receive convergent synaptic input from the dura mater and the greater occipital nerve (Bartsch & Goadsby, 2003). Noxious stimulation of the dura mater has been shown to elicit facilitated responses in the GON, and vice versa. These findings highlight the potential of dura-GON–sensitive neurons in the trigeminocervical complex to undergo a central sensitization, including increased excitability to converging synaptic inputs. This transformation indicates that dural afferents and GON afferents do not just represent an anatomic connection; rather, these connections are functionally relevant in terms of mutual changes of excitability. The previously described mechanisms of convergence and central sensitization are important to understand the clinical phenomena of spread and referral of pain, by which pain originating from an affected tissue is perceived as originating from a distant receptive field that does not necessarily involve a peripheral pathology in the cervical innervation territory (Ruch, 1965; Arendt-Nielsen et al., 2000).

It is now well established that the nociceptive inflow to second-order neurons in the spinal cord and the TCC is subject to a modulation by descending inhibitory projections from brainstem structures such as the periaqueductal gray (PAG), nucleus raphe magnus (NRM), and the rostroventral medulla (RVM), as stimulation of these regions produces profound anti-nociception (Sandkuhler et al., 1987; Behbehani, 1995; Fields, 2004; Heinricher & Ingram, 2008; Light, 2008; Ren & Dubner, 2008). In particular, recent findings suggest that the ventrolateral division of the PAG (vlPAG) plays a pivotal role in trigeminal nociception: stimulation of the vlPAG modulates dural nociception and selectively receives input from trigeminovascular afferents (Keay & Bandler, 1998; Hoskin et al., 2001; Knight & Goadsby, 2001; Knight et al., 2002; Bartsch et al., 2004). Injection of naratriptan, the $5-HT_{1B/1D}$ receptor agonist, into the vlPAG inhibits trigeminovascular nociceptive traffic in the TCC (Bartsch et al., 2004; Jeong et al., 2008). Injection of the P/Q-type calcium-channel blocker, omega-agatoxin IVA, into the periaqueductal gray (PAG) facilitates meningeal dural stimulation–evoked trigeminal nociceptive processing, whereas the $GABA_A$ antagonist bicuculline inhibits neuronal firing in the TCC (Knight & Goadsby, 2001; Knight et al., 2002). Trigeminal anti-nociception induced by bicuculline in the PAG is not affected by PAG P/Q-type calcium-channel blockade in the rat, however (Knight et al., 2003).

Dura-sensitive neurons in the trigeminal nucleus are also subject to modulation by hypothalamic projections. Stimulation of nociceptive trigeminovascular afferents leads to activation of neurons in the posterior hypothalamus (Benjamin et al., 2004). The posterior hypothalamus is embedded in a descending pain-modulating network system; this relationship was demonstrated by injection of orexin A into the posterior hypothalamus, which decreased the A- and C-fiber responses to dural electrical stimulation as well as spontaneous activity in trigeminal nucleus caudalis neurons (Bartsch et al., 2004). Injection of orexin B into the posterior hypothalamus, however, elicited increased responses to dural stimulation in A- and C-fiber input neurons studied and resulted in increased spontaneous activity. Similarly, somatostatinergic projections seem to be involved in this modulation of trigeminovascular pain (Bartsch et al., 2005). Stimulation of the dopaminergic/calcitonin gene-related peptide A11 cell group located in the posterior hypothalamus also has been shown to modulate nociceptive neurons in the TCC (Charbit et al., 2009b).

Functional neuroimaging has proved an important complementary technology in providing deeper understanding of the central modulation of the trigeminal system in migraine headache pathophysiology. Neuroimaging results suggest that brainstem descending modulatory centers appear to be dysfunctional in migraineurs, indicating an altered descending modulation in migraine.

This dysfunction may lead to a loss of inhibition or enhanced facilitation, resulting in episodic hyperexcitability of trigeminovascular neurons in the TCC (Weiller et al., 1995; Bahra et al., 2001; Afridi ct al., 2005a, 2005b; Denuelle et al., 2007; Moulton et al., 2008).

CONCLUSIONS

This chapter described the anatomic substrate of migraine headache, with a focus on basic mechanisms of pain processing in the trigeminocervical complex. The studies reviewed here provide evidence of anatomic and functional coupling between nociceptive dural afferents and cervical afferents in the greater occipital nerve on to neurons in the trigeminocervical complex. These convergent neurons may be sensitized during headache and may be involved in the clinical phenomenon of hypersensitivity, which is characterized by spread and referred pain to trigeminal and cervical dermatomes, whereby pain originating from an affected tissue is perceived as originating from a distant receptive field. An understanding of the physiology and pharmacology of the trigeminocervical complex has fundamental implications for the treatment of migraine.

ACKNOWLEDGMENTS

This work was supported by the Sandler Family Trust.

REFERENCES

Adams IB, Compton DR, Martin BR. Assessment of anandamide interaction with the cannabinoid brain receptor: SR 141716A antagonism studies in mice and autoradiographic analysis of receptor binding in rat brain. *J Pharmacol Exp Ther* 1998;284:1209–1217.

Afridi SK, Giffin NJ, Kaube H, et al. A positron emission tomography study in spontaneous migraine. *Arch Neurol* 2005a;62:1270–1275.

Afridi SK, Matharu MS, Lee L, et al. A PET study exploring the laterality of brainstem activation in migraine using glyceryl trinitrate. *Brain* 2005b;128:932–939.

Akerman S, Goadsby PJ. Topiramate inhibits cortical spreading depression in rat and cat: impact in migraine aura. *Neuroreport* 2005a;16:1383–13837.

Akerman S, Goadsby PJ. Topiramate inhibits trigeminovascular activation: an intravital microscopy study. *Br J Pharmacol* 2005b;146:7–14.

Akerman S, Kaube H, Goadsby PJ. Vanilloid type 1 receptors (VR1) on trigeminal sensory nerve fibres play a minor role in neurogenic dural vasodilatation, and are involved in capsaicin-induced dural dilation. *Br J Pharmacol* 2003;140:718–724.

Akerman S, Kaube H, Goadsby PJ. Anandamide acts as a vasodilator of dural blood vessels in vivo by activating TRPV1 receptors. *Br J Pharmacol* 2004a;142:1354–1360.

Akerman S, Kaube H, Goadsby PJ. Anandamide is able to inhibit trigeminal neurons using an in vivo model of trigeminovascular-mediated nociception. *J Pharmacol Exp Ther* 2004b;309:56–63.

Akerman S, Holland PR, Goadsby PJ. Cannabinoid (CB1) receptor activation inhibits trigeminovascular neurons. *J Pharmacol Exp Ther* 2007;320:64–71.

Andreou AP, Holland PR, Goadsby PJ. Activation of iGluR5 kainate receptors inhibits neurogenic dural vasodilatation in an animal model of trigeminovascular activation. *Br J Pharmacol* 2009;157:464–473.

Anthony M. Headache and the greater occipital nerve. *Clin Neurol Neurosurg* 1992;94:297–301.

Arendt-Nielsen L, Laursen RJ, Drewes AM. Referred pain as an indicator for neural plasticity. *Prog Brain Res* 2000;129:343–356.

Bahra A, Matharu MS, Buchel C, et al. Brainstem activation specific to migraine headache. *Lancet* 2001;357:1016–1017.

Bakker DA, Richmond FJ, Abrahams VC. Central projections from cat suboccipital muscles: a study using transganglionic transport of horseradish peroxidase. *J Comp Neurol* 1984;228:409–421.

Bartsch T, Goadsby PJ. Stimulation of the greater occipital nerve induces increased central excitability of dural afferent input. *Brain* 2002;125:1496–1509.

Bartsch T, Goadsby PJ. Increased responses in trigeminocervical nociceptive neurons to cervical input after stimulation of the dura mater. *Brain* 2003;126:1801–1813.

Bartsch T, Knight YE, Goadsby PJ. Activation of 5-HT$_{1B/1D}$ receptors in the periaqueductal grey inhibits meningeal nociception. *Ann Neurol* 2004;56:371–381.

Bartsch T, Levy MJ, Knight YE, Goadsby PJ. Inhibition of nociceptive dural input in the trigeminal nucleus caudalis by somatostatin receptor blockade in the posterior hypothalamus. *Pain* 2005;117:30–39.

Becser N, Bovim G, Sjaastad O. Extracranial nerves in the posterior part of the head: anatomic variations and their possible clinical significance. *Spine* 1998;23:1435–1441.

Behbehani MM. Functional characteristics of the midbrain periaqueductal gray. *Prog Neurobiol* 1995;46:575–605.

Benjamin L, Levy MJ, Lasalandra MP, et al. Hypothalamic activation after stimulation of the superior sagittal sinus in the cat: a Fos study. *Neurobiol Dis* 2004;16:500–505.

Bergerot A, Storer RJ, Goadsby PJ. Dopamine inhibits trigeminovascular transmission in the rat. *Ann Neurol* 2007;61:251–262.

Bingham S, Davey PT, Babbs AJ, et al. Orexin-A, an hypothalamic peptide with analgesic properties. *Pain* 2001;92:81–90.

Bogduk N, Bartsch T. Headache of cervical origin: focus on anatomy and physiology. In: Goadsby P, Dodick D,

Silberstein S, eds. *Chronic Daily Headache for Clinicians.* Philadelphia: Decker; 2005.

Bogduk N, Govind J. Cervicogenic headache: an assessment of the evidence on clinical diagnosis, invasive tests, and treatment. *Lancet Neurol* 2009;8:959–968.

Borsook D, Burstein R, Becerra L. Functional imaging of the human trigeminal system: opportunities for new insights into pain processing in health and disease. *J Neurobiol* 2004;61:107–125.

Borsook D, Burstein R, Moulton E, Becerra L. Functional imaging of the trigeminal system: applications to migraine pathophysiology. *Headache* 2006;46:S32–S38.

Bouchelet I, Cohen Z, Case B, et al. Differential expression of sumatriptan-sensitive 5-hydroxytryptamine receptors in human trigeminal ganglia and cerebral blood vessels. *Mol Pharmacol* 1996;50:219–223.

Burstein R, Yamamura H, Malick A, Strassman AM. Chemical stimulation of the intracranial dura induces enhanced responses to facial stimulation in brain stem trigeminal neurons. *J Neurophysiol* 1998;79:964–982.

Burstein R, Cutrer MF, Yarnitsky D. The development of cutaneous allodynia during a migraine attack clinical evidence for the sequential recruitment of spinal and supraspinal nociceptive neurons in migraine. *Brain* 2000;123:1703–1709.

Charbit AR, Akerman S, Goadsby PJ. Comparison of the effects of central and peripheral dopamine receptor activation on evoked firing in the trigeminocervical complex. *J Pharmacol Exp Ther* 2009a;331:752–763.

Charbit AR, Akerman S, Holland PR, Goadsby PJ. Neurons of the dopaminergic/calcitonin gene-related peptide A11 cell group modulate neuronal firing in the trigeminocervical complex: an electrophysiological and immunohistochemical study. *J Neurosci* 2009b;29:12532–12541.

Charbit AR, Akerman S, Goadsby PJ. Dopamine: what's new in migraine? *Curr Opin Neurol* 2010;23:275–281.

Classey JD, Knight YE, Goadsby PJ. The NMDA receptor antagonist MK-801 reduces Fos-like immunoreactivity within the trigeminocervical complex following superior sagittal sinus stimulation in the cat. *Brain Res* 2001;907:117–124.

Classey JD, Bartsch T, Goadsby PJ. Distribution of 5-HT$_{1B}$, 5-HT$_{1D}$ and 5-HT$_{1F}$ receptor expression in rat trigeminal and dorsal root ganglia neurons: relevance to the selective anti-migraine effect of triptans. *Brain Res* 2010;1361:76–85.

Clements JR, Magnusson KR, Hautman J, Beitz AJ. Rat tooth pulp projections to spinal trigeminal subnucleus caudalis are glutamate-like immunoreactive. *J Comp Neurol* 1991;309(8):281–288.

Cumberbatch MJ, Hill RG, Hargreaves RJ. Rizatriptan has central antinociceptive effects against durally evoked responses. *Eur J Pharmacol* 1997;328:37–40.

Date Y, Ueta Y, Yamashita H, et al. Orexins, orexigenic hypothalamic peptides, interact with autonomic, neuroendocrine and neuroregulatory systems. *Proc Natl Acad Sci USA* 1999;96:748–753.

De Lecea L, Kilduff TS, Peyron C, et al. The hypocretins: hypothalamus-specific peptides with neuroexcitatory activity. *Proc Natl Acad Sci USA* 1998;95:322–327.

De Lecea L, Sutcliffe JG. The hypocretins/orexins: novel hypothalamic neuropeptides involved in different physiological systems. *Cell Mol Life Sci* 1999;56:473–480.

Denuelle M, Fabre N, Payoux P, et al. Hypothalamic activation in spontaneous migraine attacks. *Headache* 2007;47:1418–1426.

Devane WA, Hanus L, Breuer A, et al. Isolation and structure of a brain constituent that binds to the cannabinoid receptor. *Science* 1992;258:1946–1949.

Ferrari MD, Farkkila M, Reuter U, et al. Acute treatment of migraine with the selective 5-HT$_{1F}$ receptor agonist lasmiditan: a randomised proof-of-concept trial. *Cephalalgia* 2010;30:1170–1178.

Fields H. State-dependent opioid control of pain. *Nat Rev Neurosci* 2004;5:565–575.

Fugelli A, Moret C, Fillion G. Autoradiographic localization of 5-HT$_{1E}$ and 5-HT$_{1F}$ binding sites in rat brain: effect of serotonergic lesioning. *J Recept Signal Transduct Res* 1997;17:631–645.

Fuxe K, Dahlstrom AB, Jonsson G, et al. The discovery of central monoamine neurons gave volume transmission to the wired brain. *Prog Neurobiol* 2010;90:82–100.

Goadsby PJ. Calcitonin gene-related peptide antagonists as treatments of migraine and other primary headaches. *Drugs* 2005;65:2557–2567.

Goadsby PJ. Calcitonin gene-related peptide (CGRP) antagonists and migraine: is this a new era? *Neurology* 2008;70:1300–1301.

Goadsby PJ, Classey JD. Evidence for serotonin (5-HT)$_{1B}$, 5-HT$_{1D}$ and 5-HT$_{1F}$ receptor inhibitory effects on trigeminal neurons with craniovascular input. *Neuroscience* 2003;122:491–498.

Goadsby PJ, Hoskin KL. Inhibition of trigeminal neurons by intravenous administration of the serotonin (5HT)$_{1B/D}$ receptor agonist zolmitriptan (311C90): are brain stem sites therapeutic target in migraine? *Pain* 1996;67:355–359.

Goadsby PJ, Hoskin KL. The distribution of trigeminovascular afferents in the nonhuman primate brain *Macaca nemestrina*: a c-fos immunocytochemical study. *J Anat* 1997;190:367–375.

Goadsby PJ, Hoskin KL. Differential effects of low dose CP122,288 and eletriptan on fos expression due to stimulation of the superior sagittal sinus in cat. *Pain* 1999;82:15–22.

Goadsby PJ, Knight YE. Direct evidence for central sites of action of zolmitriptan (311C90): an autoradiographic study in cat. *Cephalalgia* 1997a;17:153–158.

Goadsby PJ, Knight Y. Inhibition of trigeminal neurons after intravenous administration of naratriptan through an action at 5-hydroxy-tryptamine (5-HT$_{(1B/1D)}$) receptors. *Br J Pharmacol* 1997b;122:918–922.

Goadsby PJ, Charbit AR, Andreou AP, et al. Neurobiology of migraine. *Neuroscience* 2009;161:327–341.

Goadsby PJ, Knight YE, Hoskin KL. Stimulation of the greater occipital nerve increases metabolic activity in the trigeminal nucleus caudalis and cervical dorsal horn of the cat. *Pain* 1997;73:23–28.

Goadsby PJ, Lipton RB, Ferrari MD. Migraine: current understanding and treatment. *N Engl J Med* 2002;346:257–270.

Goldstein DJ, Roon KI, Offen WW, et al. Selective serotonin 1F (5-HT$_{(1F)}$) receptor agonist LY334370 for acute migraine: a randomised controlled trial. *Lancet* 2001;358:1230–1234.

Heinricher MM, Ingram SL. The brainstem and nociceptive modulation. In: Basbaum A, Bushnell A., eds. *Science of Pain*. New York: Academic Press; 2008.

Hervieu GJ, Cluderay JE, Harrison DC, et al. Gene expression and protein distribution of the orexin-1 receptor in the rat brain and spinal cord. *Neuroscience* 2001;103:777–797.

Holland PR, Bartsch T. Involvement of corticotrophin-releasing factor and orexin-A in chronic migraine and medication overuse headache: findings from cerebrospinal fluid. *Cephalalgia* 2008;28:681–682.

Holland P, Goadsby PJ. The hypothalamic orexinergic system: pain and primary headaches. *Headache* 2007;47:951–962.

Holland PR, Akerman S, Goadsby PJ. Orexin 1 receptor activation attenuates neurogenic dural vasodilation in an animal model of trigeminovascular nociception. *J Pharmacol Exp Ther* 2005;315:1380–1385.

Holland PR, Akerman S, Goadsby PJ. Modulation of nociceptive dural input to the trigeminal nucleus caudalis via activation of the orexin 1 receptor in the rat. *Eur J Neurosci* 2006;24:2825–2833.

Holstege JC, Van Dijken H, Buijs RM, et al. Distribution of dopamine immunoreactivity in the rat, cat and monkey spinal cord. *J Comp Neurol* 1996;376:631–652.

Hoskin KL, Kaube H, Goadsby PJ. Central activation of the trigeminovascular pathway in the cat is inhibited by dihydroergotamine: a c-Fos and electrophysiological study. *Brain* 1996;119:249–256.

Hoskin KL, Bulmer DC, Lasalandra M, et al. Fos expression in the midbrain periaqueductal grey after trigeminovascular stimulation. *J Anat* 2001;198:29–35.

Hunter C, Mayfield F. Role of the upper cervical roots in the production of pain in the head. *Am J Surg* 1949;78:743–751.

Hutchinson PJ, Pickard JD, Higgins JN. Neurological picture: vertebral artery dissection presenting as cerebellar infarction. *J Neurol Neurosurg Psychiatry* 2000;68:98–99.

Jakubowski M, Levy D, Kainz V, et al. Sensitization of central trigeminovascular neurons: blockade by intravenous naproxen infusion. *Neuroscience* 2007;148:573–583.

Jeong HJ, Chenu D, Johnson EE, et al. Sumatriptan inhibits synaptic transmission in the rat midbrain periaqueductal grey. *Mol Pain* 2008;4:54.

Kaube H, Hoskin KL, Goadsby PJ. Inhibition by sumatriptan of central trigeminal neurons only after blood–brain barrier disruption. *Br J Pharmacol* 1993a;109:788–792.

Kaube H, Keay KA, Hoskin KL, et al. Expression of c-Fos-like immunoreactivity in the caudal medulla and upper cervical spinal cord following stimulation of the superior sagittal sinus in the cat. *Brain Res* 1993b;629:95–102.

Keay KA, Bandler R. Vascular head pain selectively activates ventrolateral periaqueductal grey in the cat. *Neurosci Lett* 1998;245:58–60.

Kerr FWL, Olafson RA. Trigeminal and cervical volleys. *Arch Neurol* 1961;5:69–76.

Knight YE, Goadsby PJ. The periaqueductal grey matter modulates trigeminovascular input: a role in migraine? *Neuroscience* 2001;106:793–800.

Knight YE, Bartsch T, Kaube H, Goadsby PJ. P/Q-type calcium-channel blockade in the periaqueductal gray facilitates trigeminal nociception: a functional genetic link for migraine? *J Neurosci* 2002;22:1–6.

Knight YE, Bartsch T, Goadsby PJ. Trigeminal antinociception induced by bicuculline in the periaqueductal gray (PAG) is not affected by PAG P/Q-type calcium channel blockade in rat. *Neurosci Lett* 2003;336:113–116.

Le Doare K, Akerman S, Holland PR, et al. Occipital afferent activation of second order neurons in the trigeminocervical complex in rat. *Neurosci Lett* 2006;403:73–77.

Light AR, Lee S. Spinal cord physiology of nociception. In: Basbaum A, Bushnell A, eds. *Science of Pain*. New York: Academic Press; 2008:311–330.

Mackenzie J. *Symptoms and Their Interpretation*. London: Shaw and Sons; 1909.

Magnusson KR, Larson AA, Madl JE, et al. Co-localization of fixative-modified glutamate and glutaminase in neurons of the spinal trigeminal nucleus of the rat: an immunohistochemical and immunoradiochemical analysis. *J Comp Neurol* 1986;247:477–490.

Malick A, Burstein R. Cells of origin of the trigeminohypothalamic tract in the rat. *J Comp Neurol* 1998;400:125–144.

Malick A, Strassman RM, Burstein R. Trigeminohypothalamic and reticulohypothalamic tract neurons in the upper cervical spinal cord and caudal medulla of the rat. *J Neurophysiol* 2000;84:2078–2112.

Marcus JN, Aschkenasi CJ, Lee CE, et al. Differential expression of orexin receptors 1 and 2 in the rat brain. *J Comp Neurol* 2001;435:6–25.

Mitsikostas DD, Sanchez del Rio M, Moskowitz MA, Waeber C. Both 5-HT1B and 5-HT1F receptors modulate c-fos expression within rat trigeminal nucleus caudalis. *Eur J Pharmacol* 1999a;369:271–277.

Mitsikostas DD, Sanchez del Rio MS, Waeber C, et al. The NMDA receptor antagonist MK-801 reduces capsaicin-induced c-fos expression within rat trigeminal nucleus caudalis. *Pain* 1999b;76:239–248.

Mitsikostas DD, Sanchez del Rio M, Waeber C, et al. Non-NMDA glutamate receptors modulate capsaicin induced c-fos expression within trigeminal nucleus caudalis. *Br J Pharmacol* 1999c;127:623–630.

Moulton EA, Burstein R, Tully S, et al. Interictal dysfunction of a brainstem descending modulatory center in migraine patients. *PLoS One* 2008;3:e3799.

Neuhuber WL, Zenker W. Central distribution of cervical primary afferents in the rat, with emphasis on proprioceptive projections to vestibular, perihypoglossal, and upper thoracic spinal nuclei. *J Comp Neurol* 1989;280:231–253.

Penfield W, McNaughton F. Dural headache and innervation of the dura mater. *Arch Neurol Psychiatry* 1940;44:43–75.

Pfaller K, Arvidsson J. Central distribution of trigeminal and upper cervical primary afferents in the rat studied by anterograde transport of horseradish peroxidase conjugated to wheat germ agglutinin. *J Comp Neurol* 1988;268:91–108.

Pfister J, Zenker W. The splenius capitis muscle of the rat, architecture and histochemistry, afferent and efferent innervation as compared with that of the quadriceps muscle. *Anat Embryol (Berl)* 1984;169:79–89.

Piovesan EJ, Kowacs PA, Tatsui CE, et al. Referred pain after painful stimulation of the greater occipital nerve in humans: evidence of convergence of cervical afferences on trigeminal nuclei. *Cephalalgia* 2001;21:107–109.

Piovesan EJ, Kowacs PA, Oshinsky ML. Convergence of cervical and trigeminal sensory afferents. *Curr Pain Headache Rep* 2003;7:377–383.

Ray BS, Wolff HG. Experimental studies on headache: pain sensitive structures of the head and their significance in headache. *Arch Surg* 1940;41:813–856.

Ren K, Dubner R. Descending control mechanisms. In: Basbaum A, Bushnell A, eds. *Science of Pain*. New York: Academic Press; 2008:723–767.

Ruch TC. Pathophysiology of pain. In: Ruch TC, Patton HD, eds. *Physiology and Biophysics*. Philadelphia: Saunders; 1965:345–363.

Sandkuhler J. Models and mechanisms of hyperalgesia and allodynia. *Physiol Rev* 2009;89:707–758.

Sandkuhler J, Fu QG, Zimmermann M. Spinal pathways mediating tonic or stimulation-produced descending inhibition from the periaqueductal gray or nucleus raphe magnus are separate in the cat. *J Neurophysiol* 1987;58:327–341.

Sang CN, Ramadan NM, Wallihan RG, et al. LY293558, a novel AMPA/GluR5 antagonist, is efficacious and well-tolerated in acute migraine. *Cephalalgia* 2004;24:596–602.

Schepelmann K, Ebersberger A, Pawlack M, et al. Response properties of trigeminal brain stem neurons with input from dura mater encephali in the rat. *Neuroscience* 1999;90:543–554.

Shields KG, Storer RJ, Akerman S, Goadsby PJ. Calcium channels modulate nociceptive transmission in the trigeminal nucleus of the cat. *Neuroscience* 2005;135:203–212.

Silberstein SD, McCrory DC. Opioids. *Cephalalgia* 2000;20:854–864.

Smart D, Jerman J. The physiology and pharmacology of the orexins. *Pharmacol Ther* 2002;94:51.

Sokolov AY, Lyubashina OA, Panteleev SS, Chizh BA. Neurophysiological markers of central sensitisation in the trigeminal pathway and their modulation by the cyclooxygenase inhibitor ketorolac. *Cephalalgia* 2010;30:1241–1249.

Storer RJ, Goadsby PJ. Microiontophoretic application of serotonin (5HT)$_{1B/1D}$ agonists inhibits trigeminal cell firing in the cat. *Brain* 1997;120:2171–2177.

Storer RJ, Goadsby PJ. Trigeminovascular nociceptive transmission involves *N*-methyl-D-aspartate and non-*N*-methyl-D-aspartate glutamate receptors. *Neuroscience* 1999;90:1371–1376.

Storer RJ, Goadsby PJ. Topiramate inhibits trigeminovascular neurons in the cat. *Cephalalgia* 2004;24:1049–1056.

Storer RJ, Akerman S, Goadsby PJ. GABA receptors modulate trigeminovascular nociceptive neurotransmission in the trigeminocervical complex. *Br J Pharmacol* 2001;134:896–904.

Storer RJ, Akerman S, Goadsby PJ. Characterization of opioid receptors that modulate nociceptive neurotransmission in the trigeminocervical complex. *Br J Pharmacol* 2003;138:317–324.

Storer RJ, Akerman S, Goadsby PH. Calcitonin gene-related peptide (CGRP) modulates nociceptive trigeminovascular transmission in the cat. *Br J Pharmacol* 2004;142:1171–1181.

Storer RJ, Immke DC, Goadsby PJ. Large conductance calcium-activated potassium channels (BKCa) modulate trigeminovascular nociceptive transmission. *Cephalalgia* 2009;29:1242–1258.

Strassman AM, Potrebic S, Maciewick RJ. Anatomical properties of brainstem trigeminal neurons that respond to electrical stimulation of dural blood vessels. *J Comp Neurol* 1994;346:349–365.

Tallaksen-Greene SJ, Young AB, Penney JB, Beitz AJ. Excitatory amino acid binding sites in the trigeminal principal sensory and spinal trigeminal nuclei of the rat. *Neurosci Lett* 1992;141:79–83.

Trivedi P, Yu H, MacNeil DJ, et al. Distribution of orexin receptor mRNA in the rat brain. *FEBS Lett* 1998;438:71–75.

Van den Pol AN. Hypothalamic hypocretin (orexin): robust innervation of the spinal cord. *J Neurosci* 1999;19:3171–3182.

Van Den Pol AN, Ghosh PK, Liu RJ, et al. Hypocretin (orexin) enhances neuron activity and cell synchrony in developing mouse GFP-expressing locus coeruleus. *J Physiol* 2002;541:169–185.

Vital JM, Grenier F, Dautheeibwe M, et al. An anatomic and dynamic study of the greater occipital nerve (n. of Arnold). Applications to the treatment of Arnold's neuralgia. *Surg Radiol Anat* 1989;11:205–210.

Weiller C, May A, Limmroth V, et al. Brain stem activation in spontaneous human migraine attacks. *Nat Med* 1995;1:658–660.

Weiss B, Alt A, Ogden AM, et al. Pharmacological characterization of the competitive GLUK5 receptor antagonist decahydroisoquinoline LY466195 in vitro and in vivo. *J Pharmacol Exp Ther* 2006;318:772–781.

Wirth FP, Van Buren JM. Referral of pain from dural stimulation in man. *J Neurosurg* 1971;34:630–642.

Wolff H. *Headache and Other Head Pain*. New York: Oxford University Press; 1963

Woolf CJ, Salter MW. Neuronal plasticity: increasing the gain in pain. *Science* 2000;288:1765–1769.

Yamamoto T, Nozaki-Taguchi N, Chiba T. Analgesic effect of intrathecally administered orexin-A in the rat formalin test and in the rat hot plate test. *Br J Pharmacol* 2002;137:170–176.

Peripheral and Central Sensitization Mechanisms in Migraine

Marina de Tommaso, MD, PhD, Alessandro Capuano, MD, PhD,
and Massimiliano Valeriani, MD, PhD

INTRODUCTION

Our understanding of the neural correlates of nociceptive pain perception in humans has recently significantly increased. Today, pain is recognized as being a conscious experience, an interpretation of the nociceptive input influenced by memories and emotional, pathological, genetic, and cognitive factors. The resultant pain is not necessarily linearly related to the nociceptive drive or input, or to the extent of neurogen lesions, especially in the chronic pain state. Several cortical areas interact with the brainstem and the descending pain modulatory system in affecting the resultant pain experienced (Tracey & Mantyh, 2007). Whatever the type of pain, nociceptive or neuropathic, it has to produce memory and synaptic readaptation, so as to defend the animal from potentially dangerous elements and to maintain a high vigilance level toward any de-afferentated part of the body. As a consequence, a nociceptive stimulus that is able to recruit the C- and A-delta sensory fibers reduces, in only a short time, the pain threshold in the primarily involved areas, a phenomenon known as hyperalgesia; meanwhile, in the adjacent zones, any mechanical input becomes painful, as an effect of the so-called allodynia (Treede et al., 1992).

Migraine is a complex disorder characterized by (usually) throbbing headache and by (invariably) accompanying symptoms—namely, nausea, vomiting, phonophobia, or photophobia. The neuroanatomic and functional basis of migraine is constituted by episodic activation of the so called trigeminocervical complex. Indeed, although the brain is thought to be insensitive, other cranial structures are densely innervated by the trigeminal nerves, which are responsible for pain in the cranial district as well as in referred territories. Surrounding the large cerebral vessels, pial vessels, large venous sinuses, and dura mater is a plexus of largely unmyelinated fibers that arises from the ophthalmic division of the trigeminal ganglion and in the posterior fossa from the upper cervical dorsal roots. Trigeminal fibers innervating cerebral vessels arise from neurons located in the trigeminal ganglion; they contain a variety of neuropeptides involved in mediating pain processing in migraine headache, such as substance P and, particularly, calcitonin gene-related peptide (CGRP). The transient phenomenon of altered cortical excitability, termed *cortical spreading depression*, subtends the migraine aura and probably the initiation of migraine without aura (Ayata, 2010), and activates both meningeal and vessels' trigeminal nociceptors (Zhang et al., 2009). Stimulation of the trigeminal ganglion results in plasma protein extravasation (PPE) in the dura mater (Markowitz et al., 1988), cerebral vasodilation (Goadsby & Duckworth, 1987), and local nerve stimulation in dural vasodilation (Williamson et al., 1997).

Despite great efforts directed toward classification of chronic pain according to its main pathophysiological mechanism in the last few years (Treede et al., 2008), migraine pain has never been specifically interpreted as a nociceptive, neuropathic, or "sine materia" pain. (Readers are referred to Chapter 5 of this textbook for a better description of the trigeminocervical complex.) Nevertheless, the anatomic integrity of pain pathways and the occurrence of sterile neurogenic inflammation (Moskowitz, 1990) may account for self-generated nociceptive trigeminal pain. Although PPE seems to be a key event in migraine pathophysiology, several studies indicate that PPE alone is not sufficient to explain all characteristics of pain in migraine. Indeed, both peripheral and central sensitization phenomena, which are commonly noted in nociceptive pain, play roles that are particularly evident in migraine. Indeed, a recent theory attempted to unify migraine, nociceptive, and neuropathic pain on the basis of common peripheral and central sensitization mechanisms (Chakravarty & Sen, 2010).

WHAT IS "SPECIAL" IN MIGRAINE SENSITIZATION?

Sensory neurons in vertebrates connect peripheral tissues with the central nervous system, occupying a particularly prominent position in acute information reception, transduction, and integration. They may also undergo potentially long-lasting plastic changes. This plasticity, which may take the form of sensitization, memory for prior injury, or desensitization, can be beneficial in the case of avoidance of physical stimulation of injured tissue. In contrast, in cases of chronic inflammatory or neuropathic pain, these changes place an often disabling burden on the organism.

In mammals, the early-warning protective pain that occurs in response to noxious stimuli (nociceptive pain) is mediated by specialized high-threshold primary sensory neurons, the nociceptors. Activation of transduction molecules generates inward currents in the nociceptor peripheral terminal. If these currents exceed a threshold value, they cause action potentials in the nociceptor axon; following conduction and transmission to projection neurons in the spinal cord or brainstem, and transfer via the thalamus to the cortex, this phenomenon leads to pain sensation. Although nociceptive pain is characterized by a high threshold and is typically transient ("ouch" pain), clinical pain associated either with peripheral tissue damage and inflammation (inflammatory pain) or with lesions to the nervous system (neuropathic pain) is characterized by persistent hypersensitivity. This type of pain includes spontaneous pain (pain experienced in the absence of any obvious peripheral stimulus), hyperalgesia (an increased responsiveness to noxious stimuli), and allodynia (pain in response to normally innocuous stimuli). Two major mechanisms contribute to pain hypersensitivity—peripheral and central sensitization.

In their fundamental study, Burstein et al. (2004) reported that the typical throbbing pain of migraine, and its worsening after coughing or other innocuous activities that increase intracranial pressure, may be due to increased responsiveness (sensitization) of trigeminovascular afferents to mechanical stimuli. Indeed, chemical stimuli such as potassium ions (K^+), protons, or other inflammatory agents applied to rat dura mater have the capacity to activate the trigeminovascular afferents and sensitize them to mechanical stimuli. Interestingly, cortical spreading depression leads to an increased extracellular concentration of many of these sensitizing substances. Evidence of sensitization of second-order neurons during migraine attacks comes from recordings of wide dynamic sensory neurons within the trigeminal caudal nucleus and from the presence of cutaneous allodynia in most migraine patients. Cutaneous allodynia, as a sign of sensitization, entails a progressive enlargement of the allodynic area to the contralateral face and ipsilateral and contralateral arms, representing an effect of sensitization of third-order thalamic sensory neurons (Burstein et al., 2000). Sensitization of second- and of third-order neurons (allodynia in areas outside pain perception areas) is referred to as central sensitization.

Peripheral and central sensitization may occur in any type of acute pain (Treede et al., 1994). Nevertheless, neurophysiological methods able to explore the function of nociceptive afferents have shown that the trigeminal reflex activity is enhanced during migraine compared with typical nociceptive pain (Katsarava et al., 2002).

The peculiarity of migraine pain seems to be linked with its self-generation and its tendency toward persistence. Current theories propose that during a migraine attack, release of endogenous substances ("migraine mediators") can sensitize the trigeminal neurons (peripheral sensitization) to normally subthreshold stimuli and increase the nociceptive signal flow to the brainstem, leading to central sensitization of second order neurons (Giniatullin et al., 2008).

NEUROBIOLOGY OF PERIPHERAL AND CENTRAL SENSITIZATION IN MIGRAINE

Peripheral Sensitization

Intense mechanical and thermal stimuli as well as diverse chemical irritants act on the peripheral terminals of nociceptor sensory neurons to initiate nociceptive pain—the acute pain that accompanies noxious stimuli and warns of impending tissue damage. In the same manner, C fibers' activation within the dura mater plays a similar role in cranial structures. Nociceptor activators—the external stimuli that drive this pain—act on specific high-threshold chemical-sensitive ion-channel transducers expressed by the nociceptors, producing inward currents in their peripheral terminals. These inward currents create generator potentials that activate voltage-gated sodium currents; if the threshold is exceeded, they lead to a flow of action potentials from the periphery to the central nervous system, thereby signaling the presence, location, and intensity of noxious stimuli (Basbaum et al., 2009).

Normally, nociceptors are silent and there is no pain. When inflammation occurs, it results in spontaneous pain in the absence of any external stimulus, along with hypersensitivity to painful stimuli. Pain hypersensitivity at the site of inflammation (primary hyperalgesia) is largely the consequence of the sensitization of the peripheral terminals of nociceptors due to a reduction in their threshold and an increase in their excitability. Electrophysiologically, this sensitization is characterized by increased background firing, increased responses to supra-threshold (noxious) stimuli, and a decreased threshold for recognition of thermal and mechanical stimuli. These electrophysiological phenomena

may underlie corresponding behavioral phenomena—specifically, spontaneous pain, hyperalgesia (increased responses to noxious stimuli), and allodynia (nociceptive response to previously innocuous stimuli) (Basbaum et al., 2009).

During neurogenic inflammation in migraine, different inflammatory mediators are released and non-neural cells (e.g., fibroblasts, mast cells, and platelets) are recruited by inflammation in the environment. Activation of the nociceptor not only transmits afferent messages to the second-order neurons (and from there to the brain), but also initiates the process of neurogenic inflammation. In this efferent function of the nociceptors, release of neurotransmitters—notably substance P and, particularly, CGRP from the peripheral terminal—induces vasodilatation and plasma extravasation (leakage of proteins and fluid from post-capillary venules), as well as activation of many non-neuronal cells, including mast cells and neutrophils. These cells, in turn, contribute additional elements to the "inflammatory soup" (Levy, 2009) (**Figure 6.1**).

Pain hypersensitivity arises from the production and release of inflammatory mediators such as prostaglandin E_2 (PGE_2), bradykinin, ATP, protons, nerve growth factor (NGF), and pro-inflammatory cytokines such as tumor necrosis factor alpha (TNF-α) and interleukin-1-beta (IL-1β) from non-neuronal cells as well as from primary sensory terminals. The soma and axons of trigeminal sensory neurons contain receptors for these inflammatory mediators, such as G-protein–coupled receptors for PGE_2 and bradykinin, ionotropic receptors for ATP and protons, and tyrosine kinase receptors for NGF and cytokines. Importantly, these inflammatory mediators have been implicated in pain sensitization, and molecular mechanisms underlying the actions of these mediators have been intensively investigated.

Primary sensory neurons in the trigeminal ganglion (TG) may be divided into peptidergic neurons that express the neuropeptide CGRP and the NGF receptor TrkA, and non-peptidergic neurons that express isolectin B4 (IB4) and glia-derived neurotrophic factor (GDNF) receptor c-ret. Based on this neurochemical characterization, the majority of TG neurons are nociceptors, including (1) peripheral terminals (C fibers or nociceptors); (2) cell bodies in the TG; and (3) central axons in the trigeminal nucleus. Although peripheral sensitization is better studied in the peripheral terminals and cell bodies, it can occur at all sites within the trigeminal sensory system.

At the peripheral level, sensitization can occur rapidly (in a matter of minutes) by post-translational regulation via phosphorylation, as ion channels possess different

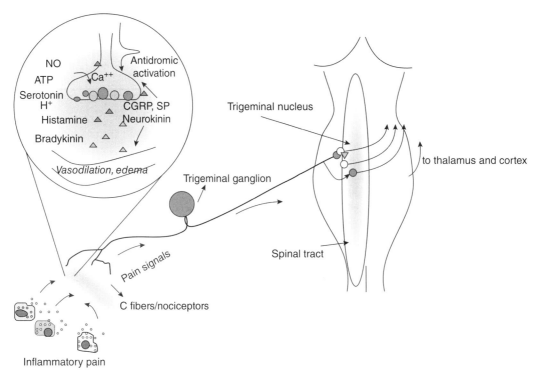

Figure 6.1 The Trigeminovascular System and Sensitizing Mediators in the Periphery

Courtesy of Alessandro Capuano, MD, PhD.

phosphorylation sites for several protein kinases. By comparison, transcriptional regulation often takes hours to days to manifest, leading to increased expression of pro-nociceptive molecules that then maintain peripheral sensitization and enhanced pain states. Tissue injury and persistent inflammation are known to induce the expression of multiple pro-nociceptive genes in nociceptors, such as genes encoding for substance P, CGRP, brain-derived neurotrophic factor (BDNF), TRPV1, and Nav1.8. Importantly, both rapid post-translational and slow transcriptional regulations in sensory neurons require the activation of multiple protein kinases via intracellular signaling transductions. The most important pathway comprises cAMP-PKA and the cAMP-epsilon isoform of protein kinase C (PKCε) (Strassman & Levy, 2006).

Nitric Oxide in Migraine Pain Sensitization

The bioactive free radical nitric oxide (NO) is an important messenger involved in the development and maintenance of inflammation and pain. NO is generated by the activity of NO synthases (NOS) during the enzymatic conversion of L-arginine to L-citruliline. The primary NO-producing enzymes in mammalian tissues are neuronal NOS (nNOS), endothelial NOS (eNOS), and inducible NOS (iNOS). The constitutive NOS isoforms—eNOS and nNOS—rapidly produce small amounts of NO that exert direct, short-acting effects on target cells. In contrast, iNOS produces large quantities of NO over a period lasting from hours to days, sustaining high levels of this free radical which may then cause tissue damage and cell death.

An important role for NO in migraine has been indicated by the finding that intravenous infusion of glyceryl trinitrate (GTN; an exogenous NO donor) produces a delayed headache in migraineurs that is indistinguishable from a spontaneous migraine attack (Thomsen & Olesen, 2001). Moreover, NOS inhibitors improve headache pain scores in spontaneous attacks of migraine. Animal experiments with either an exogenous NO donor or NOS inhibitors have provided evidence of NO's roles in mediating activation/sensitization of the trigeminovascular system after dural stimulation, and in mediating central sensitization of trigeminal nucleus neurons receiving dural input (Akerman et al., 2002; Lambert et al., 2002).

Within the meninges, a pro-inflammatory response to GTN, including up-regulation of cytokines (IL-1β and IL-6), iNOS, and defense proteins governed by the transcription factor NF-κB. Targeting the inflammatory response by selectively inhibiting NF-κB–driven transcription or downstream pro-inflammatory gene expression represents a promising therapeutic approach to the treatment of headache (Reuter et al., 2002). Indeed, GTN infusion causes a prototypical induction of migraine headache in susceptible humans, and the cellular and molecular features of this response in rodents resemble the well-known sensitizing agents found in other experimental migraine models—namely, delayed plasma protein extravasation, mast cell degranulation, and cytokine release. In addition, GTN increases electrophysiologically recorded neuronal responses to facial cutaneous stimuli in the trigeminal nucleus caudalis and increases early immediate gene response within this nucleus.

The Role of "Trigeminal Ganglion" Events in Peripheral Sensitization

As described earlier in this chapter, CGRP plays a pivotal role in migraine pain mechanisms. Recent evidence suggests that CGRP might be a sensitizing agent itself. The neuroanatomic basis of these findings lies within the trigeminal ganglion structure. Indeed, within the trigeminal ganglia, trigeminal sensory neurons are unsheathed by several glial cells, which together constitute a morphological and functional unit (Hanani, 2005). Glial cells not only provide a mechanical support to neurons, but also directly modulate their activity by controlling the ganglion microenvironment. Several findings demonstrate that glial cells modulate neuronal excitability, and profound changes in their functional state have been described in inflammatory pain as well as neuropathic pain. Interestingly, CGRP receptors have been detected within the trigeminal ganglion, both on neurons and glial cells, thus suggesting another site of CGRP release and action possibly relevant for migraine (Zhang et al., 2007). An intraganglionic release of CGRP has been suggested. Thus, CGRP released by trigeminal neurons might act (1) on trigeminal neurons themselves and (2) on satellite glial cells.

The CGRP binding site is located on a seven-transmembrane-spanning protein, named the calcitonin receptor-like receptor (CLR). This protein interacts with the receptor activity-modifying protein 1 (RAMP-1), a flanking protein that confers specificity for CGRP. Finally, the intracellular protein, receptor component protein (RCP), is necessary for signal transduction. CGRP binding to and activation of this receptor cause increased levels of intracellular cAMP, due to the recruitment of a Gs protein. Researchers have recently shown that CGRP can induce its own expression in trigeminal ganglia neurons by acting on CGRP gene promoter via a PKA-mediated pathway (Zhang et al., 2007). In this regard, a growing body of data indicates that the RAMP-1 component of the CGRP receptor constitutes a rate-limiting agent for CGRP action. In animal studies, over-expression of RAMP-1 enhances the expression of CGRP content within trigeminal neurons and mediates CGRP-induced mechanical allodynia, conferring sensitizing properties upon CGRP (Russo et al., 2009).

Although the role of the CGRP receptor in trigeminal satellite glial cells has only recently been investigated, reports indicate that CGRP can increase the production in trigeminal glial cells of known sensitizing substances, such as NO, and cytokines, such as IL-1β, that directly enhance the production and the release of neuronal CGRP. Finally, pro-inflammatory activation of satellite glial cells sensitizes trigeminal neurons to common depolarizing stimuli, thereby facilitating CGRP secretion (Capuano et al., 2009). Thus, taken together, these data depict a well-defined neuronal–glial loop inside the trigeminal ganglion, which might be a novel site of peripheral sensitization in migraine.

Central Sensitization

Several symptomatic features of migraine headache reflect central sensitization produced in trigeminal nuclei within the brainstem (Hu et al., 1992; Burstein et al., 2000). The original descriptions of central sensitization referred to an immediate-onset, activity- or use-dependent increase in the excitability of nociceptive neurons (neurons responsive to nociceptor inputs) in the spinal cord or in the trigeminal nucleus caudalis. This activity-dependent central sensitization is normally initiated only by nociceptor sensory inflow and is characterized by reductions in threshold and increases in the responsiveness of second-order neurons, as well as by enlargement of their receptive fields.

At cellular and molecular levels, central sensitization is explained by the synaptic efficacy phenomenon occurring during the activity-dependent phenomenon involving second-order neurons. A striking feature of the increase in synaptic efficacy characteristic of central sensitization is that it is also associated with synapses made by low-threshold, mechano-sensitive Aβ fibers

(Cook et al., 1987). During migraine attack, low-threshold sensory fibers activated by innocuous stimuli such as light touch become able to activate normally high-threshold nociceptive neurons, thereby contributing to a reduction in the pain threshold (tactile allodynia) that is the consequence of an increased excitability of central nervous system neurons. Although this pain is referred to the periphery, it arises from within the central nervous system. This activity-dependent central facilitation manifests within seconds of an appropriate nociceptive conditioning stimulus and can outlast the stimulus by several hours. If the stimulus is maintained, even at low levels, the central sensitization persists.

Activity-dependent sensitization is extremely robust and has been reported in rodent, cat, and primate dorsal horn neurons, including spinothalamic neurons. A central sensitization-like phenomenon can also be generated in neurons in other parts of the pain system, such as the rostro-ventral medulla, anterior cingular cortex, and amygdala. Furthermore, in addition to the immediate-onset activity-dependent form of central sensitization already described (often referred to as classical central sensitization), several other types of synaptic plasticity occur in response to noxious stimuli that modify nociceptive transmission by altering synaptic efficacy. These changes can be considered components of a more global phenomenon. They include other immediate-onset, transcription-independent phenomena, such as wind-up and long-term potentiation, as well as a late-onset, transcription-dependent, long-lasting facilitation. Invariably, glutamate neurotransmission is deeply involved in mediating these phenomena in migraine. Indeed, unmyelinated C-fiber nociceptor afferents co-express glutamate and CGRP, and glutamate immunoreactivity is most dense in the trigeminal nucleus caudalis. Glutamate can act through both ionotropic (NMDA) and G-protein–coupled receptor (metabotropic receptors) families. Thus activity of nociceptors normally produces a depolarization in the second-order neurons, mediated by glutamate metabotropic receptors.

An increasing activity of nociceptors (peripheral sensitization), in turn, leads to removal of the voltage-dependent Mg^{2++} channel blockade in NMDA receptors. By increasing glutamate sensitivity, this process progressively increases the action potential response to each stimulus in a train of inputs (wind-up). Glutamate-dependent activity induces an increased intracellular calcium influx, which first activates a calcium-dependent kinase cascade and finally leads to transcriptional (gene) modifications (Ji et al., 2003).

MECHANISMS OF SENSITIZATION IN MIGRAINE: A NEUROPHYSIOLOGICAL APPROACH

Much neurophysiological evidence favors the occurrence of trigeminal sensitization during and even between migraine attacks. For example, the threshold of a nociceptive trigemino-facial reflex—the corneal reflex—is reduced on the side of headache in the interictal phase of unilateral migraine (Sandrini et al., 2002). The same reflex, obtained by a stimulation method specific to Aδ afferents, was found to be increased in amplitude during migraine attack, as an effect of trigeminal sensitization (Kaube et al., 2002). Curiously, the reduced habituation of the same reflex seemed to rebound during migraine attack, a phenomenon scarcely compatible with its amplitude increase (Katsarava et al., 2003).

The amplitude increase of the trigeminal reflex may be partly mediated by the direct effect of endogenous substances causing migraine, as with NO (Di Clemente et al., 2009). In our opinion, it is more likely that the dysfunction of descending control pain systems plays a central role in extending and aggravating trigeminal pain and in favoring chronic migraine. The diffuse control system named DNIC, devoted to the inhibition of any pain sensation occurring after a painful stimulation in a remote part of the body, is unable to reduce the trigemino-facial and the nociceptive flexion reflexes in both episodic and chronic migraine (De Tommaso et al., 2007b; Perrotta et al., 2010). In addition, the remote somatic pain does not reduce those cortical potentials by trigeminal painful stimulation (De Tommaso et al., 2007a), which seems to originate from the associative zones elaborating the cognitive and emotive compounds of pain (Garcia-Larrea et al., 2003) and activating the descending system in an inhibitory versus excitatory modality (Valet et al., 2004; Tracey & Mantyh, 2007).

It is conceivable that the same neuronal dysfunctions that seem to subtend the onset of migraine attack might also cause its persistence, favoring central sensitization. In fact, it has been shown that the phenomenon of reduced habituation to repetitive sensory stimuli (Coppola et al., 2009) involves cortical responses to nociceptive stimuli (Valeriani et al., 2003; De Tommaso et al., 2005). This relationship is similar to that found with other forms of chronic pain, such as fibromyalgia (De Tommaso et al., 2011), whose pathogenesis has been attributed to an enhanced expression of central sensitization (Staud & Rodriguez, 2006). The reduced habituation to repetitive painful stimuli may be related to cortical and subcortical mechanisms. At the cortical level, reduced habituation may be a correlate of hyper-attention to pain, a pattern often observed in migraine patients (De Tommaso, 2008; De Tommaso et al., 2008). Moreover, during migraine attack, the pattern of reduced habituation recovers for most of the sensory modalities of stimulation (Ambrosini et al., 2003) except for the painful one, probably as a direct effect of central sensitization (De Tommaso et al., 2005). The increased amplitude of nociceptive cortical potentials observed during the migraine attack (De Tommaso et al., 2002) may be the result of cortical hyper-vigilance to pain during the acute phase with the persistence of reduced habituation. The abnormal cortical pain processing may induce a dysfunction of the descending modulatory system in the brainstem, along with a tendency toward an increase in (instead of a reduction of) pain transmission (Tracey & Mantyh, 2007).

According to many authors, the dysfunction of neuromodulatory structures in the brainstem, such as the locus coeruleus or the periaqueductal gray matter, may be a primary phenomenon in migraine, causing attack onset and maintenance. In positron emission tomography (PET) studies investigating acute migraine attacks, researchers observed activation of an area of the dorso-lateral brainstem that included the locus coeruleus and PAG (Weiller et al., 1995; Afridi et al., 2005). These findings have inspired the theory of a brainstem generator of migraine, although the PAG is generally activated during pain modulation and influenced by the cortical control (Valet et al., 2004). The dysfunction of descending modulating pain systems may play a key role in promoting sensitization of trigeminal nociceptive neurons, as also suggested by the finding of abnormal iron levels in the PAG of patients with chronic migraine (Welch et al., 2001).

FROM THE MECHANISMS TO CLINICAL PRACTICE: FEATURES OF CENTRAL SENSITIZATION IN PRIMARY HEADACHE PATIENTS

The clinical symptoms of central sensitization confirm that this effect may be promoted by an altered central control on trigeminal pain, leading to increased headache frequency and pain diffusion. In the presence of predisposing factors to headache generation, migraine severity is linked with expression of central sensitization phenomena, which causes hyperalgesia and allodynia, whose effects often spread beyond the sites of headache origin. These signs of sensitization are expressed as reduced pain threshold and increased peri-cranial tenderness, which may be present without headache episodes, especially in chronic forms (Buchgreitz et al., 2006).

A failure of pain modulation, favoring central sensitization phenomena, has been proposed to occur in chronic migraine (Goadsby, 2006) as well as in tension-type headache (Fumal & Schoenen, 2008). Cutaneous allodynia seems to prevail in patients presenting with symptoms of anxiety and depression (D'Agostino et al., 2010) confirming that enhanced expression of central sensitization during migraine attack may be induced by the same factors facilitating the evolution from the episodic to the chronic form of migraine (Juang et al., 2000).

Migraine with aura may represent an exception to this theory. This variant is characterized by clear allodynic symptoms (Lovati et al., 2007), such that one could expect to see an evolution in chronic migraine from migraine with aura. The new diagnostic criteria for chronic migraine (Headache Classification Committee, 2006), however, confirm that it occurs "in a patient who has had at least five attacks fulfilling criteria for 1.1 Migraine without aura," thereby excluding an evolution from migraine with aura. Moreover, few studies support the contention that the presence of aura conditions a reduced migraine frequency (Kelman, 2004). The reason why migraine does not become chronic in the form preceded by aura, despite the clear presence of central sensitization phenomena and the concomitance of potentially facilitating factors (Lovati et al., 2008; Tietjen et al., 2009), remains unclear and is worthy of further study.

The presence and the gravity of allodynia are accompanied by increased headache frequency, anxiety, depression, and various causes of comorbidity, such as irritable bowel, chronic fatigue, and fibromyalgia syndromes (Tietjen et al., 2009). These syndromes have been hypothesized to be primarily generated by enhanced expression of central sensitization (Yunus, 2007). In a recent study assessing fibromyalgia comorbidity in primary headaches, allodynia at the trigeminal and cervical levels was present in both migraine and tension-type patients (De Tommaso et al., 2009), according to previous findings (Lovati et al., 2008). In patients suffering from tension-type headache or migraine, the signs of central sensitization were linked with chronic pain and fibromyalgia comorbidity (De Tommaso et al., 2009).

Psychiatric comorbidity and sleep disorders are common factors facilitating central sensitization, and they are largely expressed in chronic headaches (Tietjen et al., 2009). Psychiatric comorbidity has been observed in both tension-type headache and migraine (Beghi et al., 2007), with a maximal expression in chronic headache populations (Juang et al., 2000; Wang et al., 2007; Tietjen et al., 2007a, 2007b), as a reflection of the burden of the disease rather than as a hallmark of a specific headache category. The marked expression of chronic pain in headache patients with symptoms of anxiety and depression may reflect a disturbed pain modulation with a facilitation of central sensitization (Tracey & Mantyh, 2007).

Sleep disorders are a frequent symptom in headache; they prevail in chronic forms and in patients with psychiatric comorbidity (Rains & Poceta, 2006). Although chronic pain may be per se a cause of poor sleep quality, and mediated by the same psychiatric comorbidities, an attractive hypothesis suggests that sleep deprivation is a factor inducing hyperalgesic change (Lautenbacher et al., 2006). Both psychiatric comorbidity and sleep disturbances were found to be pronounced in patients with primary headaches reporting allodynia and peri-cranial tenderness and presenting with fibromyalgia comorbidity (De Tommaso et al., 2009).

WHY EVALUATE CENTRAL SENSITIZATION SIGNS IN MIGRAINE?

The development of allodynia seems to reduce the efficacy of acute treatment of migraine with triptans (Burstein et al., 2004), despite results from a placebo-controlled, double-blind study suggesting that sensitivity to cutaneous inputs is not predictive of headache relief by a triptan in acute migraine (Cady et al., 2007). In fact, sumatriptan and its licensed successors reduce neuronal activity via $5HT_{1B/D}$ receptors at the trigeminocervical complex (Hoskin et al., 1996) and thalamic level (Shields & Goadsby, 2006) and, therefore, may have a potential role in preventing action on central sensitization development. Conceivably, the earlier the acute treatment, the

lesser the entity and extension of central sensitization, and the lower the risk for migraine persistence toward the chronic form.

The individuation of patients exhibiting serious symptoms of ictal allodynia and persistent phenomena of central sensitization, as peri-cranial muscle tenderness, should further support the necessity of an early intervention on acute symptoms. Moreover, clinical management should include education of patients about symptoms requiring early intervention, so as to prevent administration of useless therapies and avoid a tendency toward drug abuse. Most drugs used to prevent migraine have been studied for their efficacy in reducing migraine severity, with less attention being paid to their efficacy related to factors facilitating central sensitization, such as psychiatric comorbidity and sleep disturbances, and symptoms such as ictal and interictal allodynia and peri-cranial tenderness (De Tommaso et al., 2008). In our experience, patients with chronic migraine who exhibit enhanced expression of central sensitization phenomena and related comorbidities, such as diffuse muscle–skeletal pain and fibromyalgia syndrome, appear less responsive to both pharmacological and nonpharmacological approaches aiming to reduce headache severity (De Tommaso et al., 2008).

CONCLUSIONS

A growing body of evidence supports the idea that routine examination of migraine patients should include ictal and interictal allodynia, peri-cranial tenderness, and factors aggravating central sensitization, such as sleep disturbance, anxiety, depression, and comorbidity with those diseases sharing common mechanisms of chronic pain. If this type of evaluation could possibly imply a more appropriate acute and preventive approach, the time consumed would be fully rewarded.

REFERENCES

Afridi SK, Matharu MS, Lee L, Kaube H, Friston KJ, Frackowiak RS, Goadsby PJ. A PET study exploring the laterality of brainstem activation in migraine using glyceryl trinitrate. *Brain* 2005;128:932–939.

Akerman S, Williamson DJ, Kaube H, Goadsby PJ. Nitric oxide synthase inhibitors can antagonize neurogenic and calcitonin gene-related peptide induced dilation of dural meningeal vessels. *Br J Pharmacol* 2002;137:62–68.

Ambrosini A, de Noordhout AM, Sándor PS, Schoenen J. Electrophysiological studies in migraine: a comprehensive review of their interest and limitations. *Cephalalgia* 2003;23:13–31.

Ayata C. Cortical spreading depression triggers migraine attack: pro. *Headache* 2010;4:725–730.

Basbaum AI, Bautista DM, Scherrer G, Julius D. Cellular and molecular mechanisms of pain. *Cell* 2009;139:267–284.

Beghi E, Allais G, Cortelli P, et al. Headache and anxiety–depressive disorder co-morbidity: the HADAS study. *J Neurol Sci* 2007;28:S217–S219.

Buchgreitz L, Lyngberg AC, Bendtsen L, Jensen R. Frequency of headache is related to sensitization: a population study. *Pain* 2006;123:19–27.

Burstein R, Yarnitsky D, Goor-Aryeh I, Ransil BJ, Bajwa ZH. An association between migraine and cutaneous allodynia. *Ann Neurol* 2000;47:614–624.

Burstein R, Collins B, Jakubowski M. Defeating migraine pain with triptans: a race against the development of cutaneous allodynia. *Ann Neurol* 2004;55:19–26.

Cady R, Martin V, Mauskop A, Rodgers A, Hustad CM, Ramsey KE, Skobieranda F. Symptoms of cutaneous sensitivity pre-treatment and post-treatment: results from the rizatriptan TAME study. *Cephalalgia* 2007;27:1055–1060.

Capuano A, De Corato A, Lisi L, Tringali G, Navarra P, Dello Russo C. Proinflammatory-activated trigeminal satellite cells promote neuronal sensitization: relevance for migraine pathology. *Mol Pain* 2009;5:43

Chakravarty A, Sen A. Migraine, neuropathic pain and noci-ceptive pain: towards a unifying concept. *Med Hypotheses* 2010;74:225–231.

Cook AJ, Woolf CJ, Wall PD, McMahon SB. Dynamic recep-tive field plasticity in rat spinal cord dorsal horn following C-primary afferent input. *Nature* 1987;325:151–153.

Coppola G, Pierelli F, Schoenen J. Habituation and migraine. *Neurobiol Learn Mem* 2009;92:249–259.

D'Agostino VC, Francia E, Licursi V, Cerbo R. Clinical and personality features of allodynic migraine. *Neurol Sci* 2010;31:S159–S161.

De Tommaso M. Laser-evoked potentials in primary head-aches and cranial neuralgias. *Expert Rev Neurother* 2008;8:1339–1345.

De Tommaso M, Guido M, Libro G, Losito L, Sciruicchio V, Monetti C, Puca F. Abnormal brain processing of cutaneous pain in migraine patients during the attack. *Neurosci Lett* 2002;333:29–32.

De Tommaso M, Lo Sito L, Di Fruscolo O, Sardaro M, Pia Prudenzano M, Lamberti P, Livrea P. Lack of habituation of nociceptive evoked responses and pain sensitivity during migraine attack. *Clin Neurophysiol* 2005;116: 1254–1264.

De Tommaso M, Difruscolo O, Sardaro M, Libro G, Pecoraro C, Serpino C, Lamberti P, Livrea P. Effects of remote cutane-ous pain on trigeminal laser-evoked potentials in migraine patients. *J Headache Pain* 2007a;8:167–174.

De Tommaso M, Sardaro M, Pecoraro C, Di Fruscolo O, Serpino C, Lamberti P, Livrea P. Effects of the remote C fibres stimulation induced by capsaicin on the blink reflex in chronic migraine. *Cephalalgia* 2007b;27:881–890.

De Tommaso M, Sardaro M, Vecchio E, Serpino C, Stasi M, Ranieri M. Central sensitisation phenomena in primary headaches: overview of a preventive therapeutic approach. *CNS Neurol Disord Drug Targets* 2008;7:524–535.

De Tommaso M, Sardaro M, Serpino C, et al. Fibromyalgia comorbidity in primary headaches. *Cephalalgia* 2009; 29:453–464.

De Tommaso M, Federici A, Santostasi R, Calabrese R, Vecchio E, Lapadula G, Iannone F, Lamberti P, Livrea P. Laser-evoked potentials habituation in fibromyalgia. *J Pain.* 2011;12: 116–124.

Di Clemente L, Coppola G, Magis D, Gérardy PY, Fumal A, De Pasqua V, Di Piero V, Schoenen J. Nitroglycerin sensitises in healthy subjects CNS structures involved in migraine pathophysiology: evidence from a study of nociceptive blink reflexes and visual evoked potentials. *Pain* 2009;144: 156–161.

Fumal A, Schoenen J. Tension-type headache: current research and clinical management. *Lancet Neurol* 2008;7:70–83.

Garcia-Larrea L, Frot M, Valeriani M. Brain generators of laser-evoked potentials: from dipoles to functional significance. *Neurophysiol Clin* 2003;33:279–292.

Giniatullin R, Nistri A, Fabbretti E. Molecular mechanisms of sensitization of pain-transducing P2X3 receptors by the migraine mediators CGRP and NGF. *Mol Neurobiol* 2008;37:83–90.

Goadsby P. Recent advances in understanding migraine mechanisms, molecules and therapeutics. *Trends Mol Med* 2006;13:39–44.

Goadsby PJ, Duckworth JW. Effect of stimulation of trigemi-nal ganglion on regional cerebral blood flow in cats. *Am J Physiol* 1987;253:R270–R274.

Hanani M. Satellite glial cells in sensory ganglia: from form to function. *Brain Res Rev* 2005;48:457–476.

Headache Classification Committee (ICHD-II). New appendix criteria open for a broader concept of chronic migraine. *Cephalalgia* 2006;26:742–746.

Hoskin KL, Kaube H, Goadsby PJ. Sumatriptan can inhibit trigeminal afferents by an exclusively neural mechanism. *Brain* 1996;119:1419–1428.

Hu JW, Sessle BJ, Raboisson P, Dallel R, Woda A. Stimulation of craniofacial muscle afferents induces prolonged facili-tatory effects in trigeminal nociceptive brain-stem neurons. *Pain* 1992;48:53–60.

Ji RR, Kohno T, Moore KA, Woolf CJ. Central sensitization and LTP: do pain and memory share similar mechanisms? *Trends Neurosci* 2003;26:696–705.

Juang KD, Wang SJ, Fuh JL, Lu SR, Su TP. Co-morbidity of depressive and anxiety disorders in chronic daily headache and its subtypes. *Headache* 2000;40:818–823.

Katsarava Z, Lehnerdt G, Duda B, Ellrich J, Diener HC, Kaube H. Sensitization of trigeminal nociception specific for migraine but not pain of sinusitis. *Neurology* 2002;59:1450–1453.

Katsarava Z, Giffin N, Diener HC, Kaube H. Abnormal habitu-ation of "nociceptive" blink reflex in migraine: evidence for increased excitability of trigeminal nociception. *Cephalalgia* 2003;23:814–819.

Kaube H, Katsarava Z, Prywara S, Drepper J, Ellrich J, Diener HC. Acute migraine headache: possible sensitization of neurons in the spinal trigeminal nucleus? *Neurology* 2002;58:1234–1238.

Kelman L. The aura: a tertiary care study of 952 migraine patients. *Cephalalgia* 2004;24:728–734.

Lambert GA, Boers PM, Hoskin KL, Donaldson C, Zagami AS. Suppression by eletriptan of the activation of trigemino-vascular sensory neurons by glyceryltrinitrate. *Brain Res* 2002;953:181–188.

Lautenbacher S, Kundermann B, Krieg JC. Sleep deprivation and pain perception. *Med Rev* 2006;10:357–369.

Levy D. Migraine pain, meningeal inflammation, and mast cells. *Curr Pain Headache Rep* 2009;13:237–240.

Lovati C, D'Amico D, Rosa S, Suardelli M, Mailland E, Bertora P, Pomati S, Mariani C, Bussone G. Allodynia in different forms of migraine. *Neurol Sci* 2007;28:S220–S221.

Lovati C, D'Amico D, Bertora P, et al. Acute and interictal allo-dynia in patients with different headache forms: an Italian pilot study. *Headache* 2008;48:272–277.

Markowitz S, Saito K, Moskowitz MA. Neurogenically medi-ated plasma extravasation in dura mater: effect of ergot alkaloids. A possible mechanism of action in vascular head-ache. *Cephalalgia* 1988;8:83–91.

Moskowitz MA. Basic mechanisms in vascular headache. *Neurol Clin* 1990;8:801–815.

Perrotta A, Serrao M, Sandrini G, et al. Sensitisation of spinal cord pain processing in medication overuse headache involves supraspinal pain control. *Cephalalgia* 2010;30:272–284.

Rains JC, Poceta JS. Headache and sleep disorders: review and clinical implications for headache management. *Headache* 2006;46:1344–1363.

Reuter U, Chiarugi A, Bolay H, Moskowitz MA. Nuclear factor-kappaB as a molecular target for migraine therapy. *Ann Neurol* 2002;51:507–516.

Russo AF, Kuburas A, Kaiser EA, Raddant AC, Recober A. A potential preclinical migraine model: CGRP-sensitized mice. *Mol Cell Pharmacol* 2009;1:264–270.

Sandrini G, Proietti Cecchini A, Milanov I, Tassorelli C, Buzzi MG, Nappi G. Electrophysiological evidence for trigeminal neuron sensitization in patients with migraine. *Neurosci Lett* 2002;317:135–138.

Shields KG, Goadsby PJ. Serotonin receptors modulate trigeminovascular responses in ventroposteromedial nucleus of thalamus: a migraine target? *Neurobiol Dis* 2006;23:491–501.

Staud R, Rodriguez ME. Mechanisms of disease: pain in fibro-myalgia syndrome. *Nat Clin Pract Rheumatol* 2006;2:90–98.

Strassman AM, Levy D. Response properties of dural nociceptors in relation to headache. *J Neurophysiol* 2006;95:1298–1306.

Tietjen GE, Brandes JL, Digre KB, et al. High prevalence of somatic symptoms and depression in women with disabling chronic headache. *Neurology* 2007a;68:134–140.

Tietjen GE, Herial NA, Hardgrove J, Utley C, White L. Migraine co-morbidity constellations. *Headache* 2007b;47:857–865.

Tietjen GE, Brandes JL, Peterlin BL, et al. Allodynia in migraine: association with comorbid pain conditions. *Headache* 2009;49:1333–1344.

Thomsen LL, Olesen J. Nitric oxide in primary headaches. *Curr Opin Neurol* 2001;14:315–321.

Tracey I, Mantyh PW. The cerebral signature for pain percep-tion and its modulation. *Neuron* 2007;55:377–391.

Treede RD, Meyer RA, Raja SN, Campbell JN. Peripheral and central mechanisms of cutaneous hyperalgesia. *Prog Neurobiol* 1992;38:397–421.

Treede RD, Jensen TS, Campbell JN, et al. Neuropathic pain: redefinition and a grading system for clinical and research purposes. *Neurology* 2008;70:1630–1635.

Valeriani M, de Tommaso M, Restuccia D, et al. Reduced habituation to experimental pain in migraine patients: a CO_2 laser evoked potential study. *Pain* 2003;105:57–64.

Valet M, Sprenger T, Boecker H, Willoch F, Rummeny E, Conrad B, Erhard P, Tolle TR. Distraction modulates connec-tivity of the cingulo-frontal cortex and the midbrain during pain: an fMRI analysis. *Pain* 2004;109:399–408.

Wang SJ, Juang KD, Fuh JL, Lu SR. Psychiatric co-morbidity and suicide risk in adolescents with chronic daily headache. *Neurology* 2007;68:1468–1473.

Weiller C, May A, Limmroth V, et al. Brain stem activa-tion in spontaneous human migraine attacks. *Nat Med* 1995;1:658–660.

Welch KM, Nagesh V, Aurora SK, Gelman N. Periaqueductal gray matter dysfunction in migraine: cause or the burden of illness? *Headache* 2001;41:629–637.

Williamson DJ, Hargreaves RJ, Hill RG, Shepheard SL. Intravital microscope studies on the effects of neurokinin agonists and calcitonin gene-related peptide on dural blood vessel diameter in the anaesthetized rat. *Cephalalgia* 1997;17:518–524.

Yunus MB. Fibromyalgia and overlapping disorders: the unify-ing concept of central sensitivity syndromes. *Semin Arthritis Rheum* 2007;36:339–356.

Zhang X, Levy D, Kainz V, et al. Activation of meningeal nociceptor by cortical spreading depression. In: *Society for Neuroscience Annual Meeting*. Vol. 339.5. Chicago, IL: Society for Neuroscience; 2009.

Zhang Z, Winborn CS, Marquez de Prado B, Russo AF. Sensitization of calcitonin gene-related peptide receptors by receptor activity-modifying protein-1 in the trigeminal ganglion. *J Neurosci* 2007;27:2693–2703.

Neurophysiological Basis of Muscle-Referred Pain to the Head

Thomas Graven-Nielsen, PhD, Dr. Med Sci, Hong-You Ge, MD, PhD,
and Lars Arendt-Nielsen, PhD, Dr. Med Sci

INTRODUCTION

Headache symptoms are well known for being referred to the head, neck, and shoulder muscles. Likewise, in musculoskeletal pain conditions, pain from an arthritic hip joint may be referred to the thigh or knee joint, or vice versa, and in myofascial pain patients, trigger points typically produce referred pain to distant somatic structures (Simons et al., 1999). Evident manifestation of referred pain is often reported in visceral pain conditions, where pain is frequently felt in remote somatic structures from the affected visceral organs.

Referred pain has been formally recognized for more than a century, yet no strict definition for it exists. Originally the term "referred tenderness and pain" was used by Head (1893); it describes pain perceived remotely from the site of origin or pain locus. This definition does, however, not allow a distinction between the spread of pain and the actual referred pain. In this chapter, "referred pain" is defined as pain occurring predominately outside and remote from the local pain area.

This chapter outlines manifestations and mechanisms of referred pain to the head. The evidence for manifestations and mechanisms of referred pain is, however, mainly based on investigations of referred pain from extremity muscles. Consequently, this material will be presented in line with specific examples on referred pain to the head.

REFERRED HEAD PAIN FROM MYOFASCIAL TRIGGER POINTS

Pain patterns in headache can be composed of referred pain patterns from myofascial trigger points (TrPs) located in the neck, shoulder, and orofacial muscles. Active TrPs can induce spontaneous headache pain patterns or reproduce headache symptoms upon mechanical stimulation. Usually, multiple active TrPs in different muscles contribute to headache pain symptoms. Based on thorough pain mapping studies, it is clear that most of the muscles in the neck, shoulder, and orofacial regions can contribute to headache pain patterns (Simons et al., 1999). Muscles commonly involved in headache in the neck shoulder region are the upper trapezius, supraspinatus, levator scapulae, sternocleidomastoid, sub-occipital, and splenius capitis muscles (Fernández-de-las-Peñas et al., 2006; Giamberardino et al., 2007). Headaches with origin in the orofacial muscles typically derive from the temporalis, masseter, and pterygoid muscles (Fernández-de-las-Peñas et al., 2006; Calandre et al., 2006). The referred pain patterns are often muscle specific. For example, referred pain from the upper trapezius usually moves along the posterior-lateral aspect of the neck, behind the ear, and to the temple, in addition to the posterior aspect of the arm (**Figure 7.1**). Pain in the temporal region, eyebrow, and the maxilla areas can also be referred from active TrPs in the temporalis muscle. Mapping studies of the specific referred pain pattern have enhanced researchers' ability to localize those active myofascial TrPs responsible for the pain in a specific area related to headache. Chapter 15 of this book also provides more information on TrPs.

The common manifestations of active myofascial TrPs can be clinically identified and treated, whereas understanding the complex and esoteric presentations requires detailed knowledge of functional anatomy and factors that perpetuate the condition. A further challenge to this process is the fact that in some patients with chronic musculoskeletal pain, the pain complaints or referred pain pattern may mimic neuropathic pain symptoms (Giske et al., 2009).

EXPERIMENTAL REFERRED MUSCULOSKELETAL PAIN

Referred pain from muscle has been widely explored in studies involving injections of hypertonic saline (Graven-Nielsen, 2006), including injections made in the areas shown in **Figure 7.2**. Other deep structures, such as

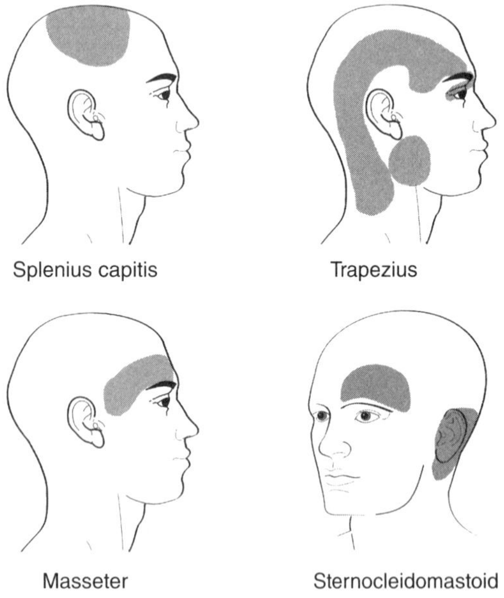

Splenius capitis

Trapezius

Masseter

Sternocleidomastoid

Figure 7.1 Examples of Referred Pain Following Manual Stimulation of Active Myofascial Trigger Points in the Splenius Capitis, Upper Trapezius, Masseter, and Sternocleidomastoid Muscles

Modified from Simons DG, Travell J, Simons L. *Travell and Simons' Myofascial Pain and Dysfunction: The Trigger Point Manual: Vol. 1.* 2nd ed. Baltimore: Williams & Wilkins; 1999.

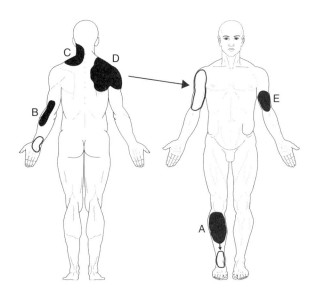

Figure 7.2 Typical Pain Distribution After Intramuscular Injection of Hypertonic Saline into the Tibialis Anterior (A), Brachioradialis (B), Trapezius (C), Infraspinatus (D), and Biceps Brachii Muscles (E). Distinct referred pain areas are shown by open shapes, whereas local and enlarged pain areas are illustrated by solid shapes. Arrows indicate which muscle is linked to a specific referred pain area.

tendons, interspinous ligaments, intervertebral discs, periostium, and joint-related components, may also evoke referred pain. Muscle or deep-tissue pain often evokes referred pain perceived in deep structures (Kellgren, 1938; Graven-Nielsen et al., 2002), in contrast to visceral referred pain, which is often experienced as a superficial and deep pain sensation (Ness & Gebhart, 1990).

Experimental deep-tissue pain studies have resulted in the development of pain models for localized pain as well as models with referred pain (Figure 7.2). The tibialis anterior and infraspinatus muscles typically give referred pain to distinct areas not included in the local pain area, whereas saline-induced biceps brachii muscle pain, for example, is only localized (Graven-Nielsen, 2006). Peri-cranial muscles have also been subjected to experimental investigations. Early pioneer studies showed that injections of hypertonic saline into the sub-occipital muscles evoked deep pain comparable to headache (Kellgren, 1938). Feinstein et al. (1954) presented examples of hypertonic saline injections into para-vertebral muscles at the cervical level, which evoked pain in the occipital and posterior neck areas and also in the forehead. Injections into the atlanto-occipital joint (C4–C5) frequently resulted in parieto-frontal pain areas (Campbell & Parsons, 1944). Hypertonic saline–induced pain in the sternocleidomastoid muscle gives rise to pain in the oculo-fronto-temporal region, whereas experimental pain induced in the splenius capitis induces pain in the occipito-parietal region (Falla et al., 2007).

Schmidt-Hansen et al. (2007) made a systematic map of the pain areas evoked by hypertonic saline injections in trigeminally and cervically innervated muscles (masseter, anterior and posterior parts of temporalis, trapezius, splenius capitis, and sternocleidomastoid). Among the different muscles, clear differences in the spread and location of pain were observed (**Figure 7.3**). The masseter and anterior temporalis muscles were extensively associated with a spread and referral of pain to the trigeminal territories, whereas pain in the posterior temporalis muscle more frequently spread to the cervical territories. Further, pain in the trapezius muscle was rarely associated with pain in the trigeminal territories. Pain within the splenius and sternocleidomastoid muscles frequently was reported in the ophthalmic division. Pain in the trigeminal area after induced pain in the trapezius muscle was found only after a low to moderate number of injections, in line with the observation of predominately local pain after induced pain in the anterior temporalis muscle.

Similar findings were previously reported in other studies involving experimental pain induced in the trapezius, masseter, and temporalis muscles (Jensen & Norup, 1992; Svensson & Graven-Nielsen, 2001; Mørk et al., 2003). Thus there appears to be a distinct difference between muscles innervated by the trigeminal and cervical systems, suggesting that there is only a limited functional overlap between upper cervical and trigeminal afferents, although extensive convergence has been reported in animal studies (Sessle et al., 1986; Bartsch & Goadsby, 2002).

The patterns of referred muscle pain from various skeletal muscles after activation of TrPs (discussed in the previous section) generally fit with the experimental referred pain pattern. In early reports, Kellgren (1938) concluded that referred pain followed a segmental pattern. Updated findings suggest, however, that the distributions of referred pain do not always follow a strict segmental pattern; that is, referred pain is not exclusively constricted to the myotome, sclerotome, or dermatome related to the spinal segment with afferent input from the painful muscle. Actually, referred pain to electrically stimulated areas three segments rostral to the dorsal root has been reported (Bogduk, 1980). As a consequence, both the tibialis anterior muscle and the typical referred pain areas (ankle) are included in myotomes/sclerotomes related to the L5 and L4 vertebral levels. A similar segmental relation has been reported for referred pain from myofascial TrPs in the trigeminal system, where an active TrP within the temporalis muscle (mandibular division, V3) induces referred pain to the maxillary teeth (maxillary branch, V2). Such segmental relation are even more evident in the trigeminocervical complex, where active TrPs in both the sub-occipital (C1) and splenius capitis (C2–C4) muscles refer pain to the temple regions supplied by trigeminal nerves (Simons et al., 1999). Therefore, referred muscle pain most likely extends to segmental areas neighboring the segment supplying the painful deep structures.

A feature of referred pain is the semi-directionality of occurrence. For example, experimental pain induced in the tibialis anterior muscle typically evokes referred pain to the ankle, but strong painful pressure stimulation on the ankle does not cause pain in the tibialis anterior muscle (Graven-Nielsen, 2006). Similar findings have been reported for other muscles, although other examples (Feinstein et al., 1954) suggest that the mechanisms for referred pain also can be bidirectional. Accordingly, experimental jaw-muscle pain can cause referred pain to the teeth (Svensson et al., 1998) and odontogenic pain may mimic jaw-muscle and facial pain (Wolff, 1963; Falace et al., 1996) illustrating the potential for a bidirectional mechanism for referred pain in the trigeminal system.

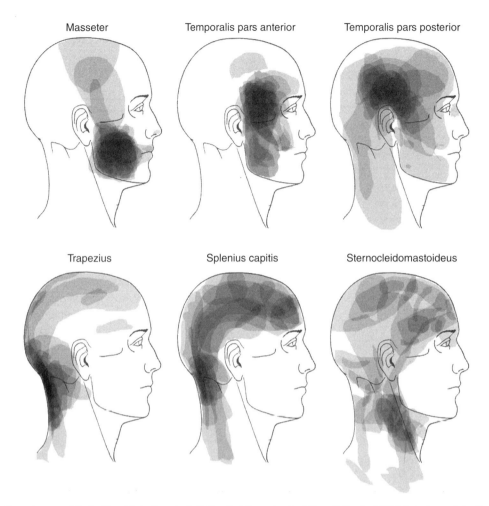

Masseter

Temporalis pars anterior

Temporalis pars posterior

Trapezius

Splenius capitis

Sternocleidomastoideus

Figure 7.3 Superimposed Body Chart Pain Drawings Following Hypertonic Saline (0.2 mL, 5.8%) Injections into the Masseter, Anterior, and Posterior Parts of the Temporalis, Trapezius, Splenius Capitis, and Sternocleidomastoid Muscles in 20 Subjects. The different stimulation sites were all accompanied by pain referral.

Adapted from Schmidt-Hansen PT, Svensson P, Jensen TS, Graven-Nielsen T, Bach FW. Patterns of experimentally induced pain in peri-cranial muscles. *Cephalalgia* 2006;26:568–577.

Temporal and Spatial Characteristics of Referred Pain

Saline-induced referred pain is delayed approximately 20 seconds compared with the appearance of local pain (Graven-Nielsen et al., 1997). In referred pain induced by continuous intramuscular electrical stimulation, the local nociceptive activity is instantaneous and constant. In addition, in this model, referred pain is delayed compared with local pain (Laursen et al., 1997), indicating involvement of a time-dependent process in evoking referred pain. Perhaps not surprisingly, then, more subjects in one study developed referred pain after 15 minutes with experimental muscle pain compared

with the initial phase of pain (Graven-Nielsen et al., 1998), and the frequency of referred pain from prolonged painful stimulation of the muscle is significantly higher than for brief painful stimulation, again indicating the time dependency of referred pain (Gibson et al., 2006).

The distribution of local and referred pain after noxious muscle stimulation can be categorized in three groups: (1) subjects with local and referred pain, (2) subjects with only referred pain, and (3) subjects with only local pain. For subjects developing both local and referred pain, there is a clear correlation between the local and referred pain intensity (Graven-Nielsen, 2006). Similar correlations between the overall pain intensity and the areas of pain (Graven-Nielsen, 2006) or the occurrence of referred pain (Jensen & Norup, 1992) have been reported as well. The size of the pain areas is correlated with pain intensity, and the local pain area may expand to the referred pain area; in such cases, the referred pain area will, by definition, be included in the local pain area, resulting in underestimates of the number of subjects with referred pain. In previous studies on extremity muscles, fewer than 50% of all hypertonic saline injections provoked true referred pain (i.e., pain not enclosed in the local pain area). However, more than 60% of subjects developed referred pain far away from the stimulation site or pain that expanded from the stimulation site to the typical area for referred pain (Graven-Nielsen, 2006).

It is not clear why some muscles have stronger abilities for evoking referred pain, whereas only local pain can be evoked in other muscles. Nonetheless, similar observations have been found in patients with myofascial pain—namely, TrP stimulation for some muscles gives referred pain in close vicinity of the TrP, but in other cases produces referred pain a long distance away from the myofascial TrP (Simons et al., 1999). Of particular interest are those subjects who develop only referred pain and not local pain. This situation conforms with the finding of referred pain from viscera where local pain in some situations is absent (Ness & Gebhart, 1990). Whether some groups of subjects may experience only referred pain or local pain due to the excitation of different subgroups of intramuscular nociceptors, perhaps dependent on anatomic variations, or different endogenous inhibitory systems, is not clear. Injections of hypertonic saline in the motor endplate zone were found to evoke higher pain intensities and larger referred pain areas compared with a control site (Qerama et al., 2004), suggesting that specific muscle structures are more susceptible to provoking referred pain. Conversely, a similar difference in the referred pain areas between the endplate zone and control site was not found with capsaicin-induced muscle pain (Qerama et al., 2004). Capsaicin and hypertonic saline injected in the endplate region and capsaicin injected in the control point induced more pain than hypertonic saline in the control point (Qerama et al., 2004)—a finding indicating that critical pain intensity is the main determinant for induction of referred muscle pain.

The Need for Somatosensory Afferent Information from the Referred Pain Area

In early studies of referred pain, this phenomenon was induced in structures with sensory loss due to spinal injury or nerve lesion, in phantom limbs, and in anesthetic limbs with unchanged or slightly decreased intensity (Kellgren, 1938; Harman, 1948; Feinstein et al., 1954; Whitty & Willison, 1958). Later, referred pain was induced in an anesthetic limb, albeit with a 40% reduction in the referred pain intensity (Laursen et al., 1999). This finding suggests that sensory input from the periphery is partly needed for the induction of referred pain.

A differential nerve block of the afferent fibers from the referred pain area showed that the referred pain intensity decreased when blocking the myelinated fibers, and no further reduction was found when blocking unmyelinated fibers (Laursen et al., 1999). Furthermore, the proprioceptive afferent fibers became inefficient when the referred pain intensity decreased during the differential nerve block, suggesting that these fibers might act as the peripheral component of referred pain (Laursen et al., 1999). Articular receptors generally do not show any resting activity, but some examples from joint afferent recordings have demonstrated irregular resting activity especially for units sensitive to non-noxious movements (Schaible & Schmidt, 1984). Thus referred pain to areas including the joints (Laursen et al., 1999; Graven-Nielsen et al., 2002; Graven-Nielsen et al., 2003) might be due to the facilitation of spontaneous sensory input from the joint. Additional afferent activity from the referred pain area might also be facilitated. This hypothesis meshes with the finding that deep-tissue hyperalgesia to pressure occurs in areas innervated by a branch of the afferent fibers also innervating the referred pain area (Graven-Nielsen et al., 2002). The degree of peripheral sensory input involved in referred pain may vary among various sites of referred pain (e.g., muscle versus joint), explaining the inconsistency in the effects of anesthetizing the referred pain area.

Experimental Pain Referral in Headache and Musculoskeletal Pain Patients

The distribution of experimentally induced, referred muscle pain seems to be changed in chronic musculoskeletal pain conditions. In patients with chronic or episodic tension-type headache, experimental pain induced in the anterior temporalis, masseter (**Figure 7.4**), and tibialis anterior (**Figure 7.5**) muscles resulted in larger pain areas as compared with controls, although such pain was mainly expressed for the anterior temporalis muscle (Schmidt-Hansen et al., 2007). This result suggests that these patients are experiencing a condition of generalized sensitization, as muscles both adjacent to and distant from the head showed facilitated mechanisms of referred pain.

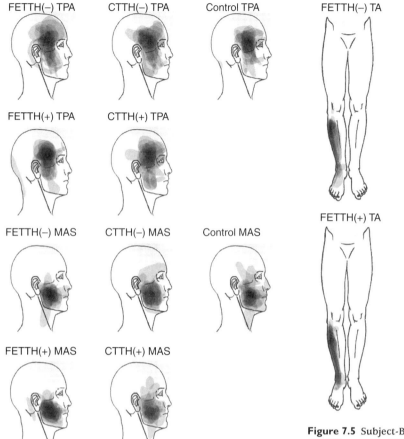

FETTH(–) TPA CTTH(–) TPA Control TPA

FETTH(+) TPA CTTH(+) TPA

FETTH(–) MAS CTTH(–) MAS Control MAS

FETTH(+) MAS CTTH(+) MAS

Figure 7.4 Subject-Based and Superimposed Drawings (FETTH: n = 24, CTTH: n = 22, Controls: n = 26) of the Extension of Perceived Pain Following Infusion of 0.5 mL Hypertonic Saline into the Anterior Part of the Temporalis (TPA) and Masseter (MAS) Muscles. Larger pain areas were found in chronic (CTTH) and frequent episodic (FETTH) tension-type headache patients compared with sex- and age-matched control subjects, especially for the anterior temporalis muscle. The patients were assessed on days with (FETTH + , CTTH +) and without (FETTH–, CTTH–) ongoing headache.

Figure provided courtesy of Schmidt-Hansen PT. *A Controlled Study on Muscle Pain Sensitivity in Tension-Type Headache Patients: Experimentally Induced Pain in Peri-cranial Muscles* [PhD thesis].

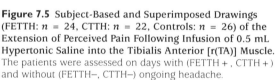

FETTH(–) TA CTTH(–) TA Control TA

FETTH(+) TA CTTH(+) TA

Figure 7.5 Subject-Based and Superimposed Drawings (FETTH: n = 24, CTTH: n = 22, Controls: n = 26) of the Extension of Perceived Pain Following Infusion of 0.5 mL Hypertonic Saline into the Tibialis Anterior [r(TA)] Muscle. The patients were assessed on days with (FETTH + , CTTH +) and without (FETTH–, CTTH–) ongoing headache.

Figure provided courtesy of Schmidt-Hansen PT. *A Controlled Study on Muscle Pain Sensitivity in Tension-Type Headache Patients: Experimentally Induced Pain in Peri-cranial Muscles* [PhD thesis].

In a study examining the condition of widespread pain, fibromyalgia patients were found to experience stronger pain and larger referred areas after saline-induced muscle pain as compared with matched controls (Arendt-Nielsen & Graven-Nielsen, 2003). Interestingly, these manifestations were present in muscles where the

patients typically did not experience ongoing pain. In patients, substantial proximal spread of the experimentally induced referred pain areas was found, unlike in healthy control subjects.

Furthermore, extended referred pain areas from the tibialis anterior muscle have been shown to exist in patients suffering from chronic whiplash pain; the extended areas of referred pain were also found in the neck/shoulder region (Johansen et al., 1999). Similarly, in patients with temporomandibular pain disorders, enlarged pain areas were found after masseter muscle pain was experimentally induced (Svensson et al., 2001).

Extended referred pain areas from the tibialis anterior muscle, indicating central sensitization, have also been identified in patients with low back pain (O'Neill et al., 2007). In patients suffering from chronic osteoarthritic knee pain, extended areas of saline-induced referred pain have been found (Bajaj et al., 2001). This finding indicates that noxious joint input to the central nervous system facilitates the mechanisms of referred pain from muscle, possibly due to the plasticity of the involved neural components.

Enlarged referred pain areas in pain patients suggest that the efficacy of central processing is increased (central sensitization). Moreover, the expansion of referred-pain areas in fibromyalgia patients was partly inhibited by an NMDA receptor antagonist (ketamine); this treatment inhibited central sensitization (Graven-Nielsen et al., 2000).

MECHANISMS FOR REFERRED PAIN

In the literature, several neuroanatomic and neurophysiological models of referred pain have been proposed. Most models explain why higher brain centers cannot identify correctly the actual afferent input source. Single-neuron recordings in experimental animals have, indeed, shown an extensive convergence between trigeminal and cervical afferent input into the caudal part of the trigeminal sensory nucleus complex (Amano et al., 1986; Sessle et al., 1986). Referred pain is probably a combination of central processing and peripheral input, given that it is possible to induce referred pain in limbs with complete sensory loss resulting from an anesthetic block. Central sensitization may also be involved in the generation of referred pain.

Animal studies have shown that noxious muscle stimuli can provoke the expansion and development of new receptive fields (Hu et al., 1992; Hoheisel et al., 1993). A complex network of extensive collateral synaptic connections for each muscle afferent fiber onto multiple dorsal horn neurons is assumed to exist (Mense & Simons, 2001). Under normal conditions, the afferent fibers have fully functional synaptic connections with dorsal horn neurons, as well as latent synaptic connections to other neurons within the same region of the spinal cord. Following ongoing strong noxious input, latent synaptic connections become operational, thereby allowing for the convergence of input from more than one source. Recordings from dorsal horn neurones with receptive fields located in the biceps femoris muscle reveal that this process leads to new receptive fields in the tibialis anterior muscle and at the foot after intramuscular injection of bradykinin into the tibialis anterior muscle (Hoheisel et al., 1993). In the context of referred pain, the unmasking of new receptive fields due to central sensitization could mediate this phenomenon (Neugebauer & Schaible, 1990; Sessle et al., 1993; Mense & Simons, 2001; Graven-Nielsen, 2006).

OTHER HEADACHE MODELS

Intradermal injection of capsaicin into the forehead provokes large pain areas that may mimic pain patterns following headache attacks in some cases (Gazerani et al., 2007). This model has been used to evaluate the effect of botulinum toxin (Botox; Gazerani et al, 2009), as craniofacial administration of Botox has been suggested as a method of migraine prophylaxis (Burstein et al., 2009). Migraine is more common in women than in men, and in an experimental pain study, intradermal delivery of capsaicin to the forehead also induced stronger hyperalgesic responses in females compared with males (Gazerani et al., 2005). This finding suggests that human experimental craniofacial pain models may mimic similar manifestations seen clinically in patients with headache. Glutamate has also been injected intradermally into the foreheads of males and females, and it has been demonstrated that sex-related differences also occur in some of the glutamate-evoked craniofacial responses (Gazerani et al., 2006).

More than 40 years ago, it was suggested that experimental tonic craniofacial pain created via pressure around the skull could evoke headache-like symptoms (Wolff, 1963). Recently, this model was revisited and elaborated, with researchers noting that standardized skull compression causes very well-defined headache-like symptoms (Sowman et al., 2011). With this technique, a head compression device is mounted with four compression points above the top of the ears bilaterally and above both the occiput and the nasion posteriorly and anteriorly, respectively (**Figure 7.6**). Compression forces are monitored for each compression point so that all clamping screws are pressed into the head with equal force. Adjusting the compression force targeting an initial pain intensity of 3 cm out of 10 cm on a visual analogue scale (VAS) evoked a mean pain intensity of approximately 8 cm on the VAS after 15 minutes of compression (Sowman et al., 2011). The pain area typically spread to larger areas than the area of compression points, and the pain quality was described as "intense," "pressing," "heavy," "exhausting," and "taut."

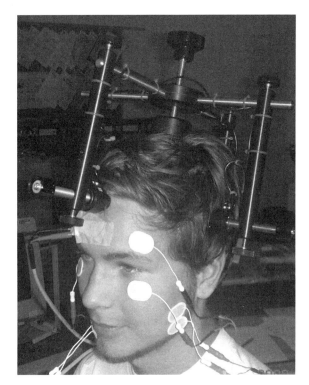

Figure 7.6 An Experimental, Pressure-Induced Head Pain Model. A head compression device is mounted with four compression points approximately 4 cm above the top of the ears bilaterally and 4 cm above both the occiput and the nasion posteriorly and anteriorly, respectively. Compression forces are monitored for each compression point so that all clamping screws are pressed into the head with equal force.

HEADACHE AND DESCENDING PAIN MODULATION

The perception of pain in response to a given painful stimulus can be reduced by the application of another painful stimulus to an extra-segmental body location. This phenomenon, which is known as counter-irritation analgesia, is the product of the endogenous pain modulation mechanism defined as diffuse noxious inhibitory control (DNIC), more recently redefined as conditioning pain modulation (CPM) (Yarnitsky et al., 2010). Conditioning pain modulation results from the activation of brainstem inhibitory projections, which in turn act to post-synaptically inhibit spinal and trigeminal wide-dynamic-range neurons (Le Bars et al., 1975). CPM can be evoked and studied experimentally in humans by

applying a tonic nociceptive conditioning stimulus prior to or during a segmentally distinct acute nociceptive test stimulus. The extent of the CPM response can be quantified as an increase in the threshold to a phasic, applied painful test stimulus. Depending on the relative intensities of the conditioning and test stimuli, experimentally evoked CPM can create a potent inhibition of nociception that lasts for several minutes beyond the application of the conditioning stimulus.

Some scientific evidence suggests that dysfunctional modulatory mechanisms are involved in craniofacial muscle pain conditions (Olesen, 1991; Tommaso et al., 2007) such as myofascial temporomandibular pain (Maixner et al., 1995) and chronic tension-type headache (Bragdon et al., 2002; Pielsticker et al., 2005; Sandrini et al., 2006). Alteration in descending modulation is likely to be a common characteristic of a variety of craniofacial pain syndromes and may contribute to the magnitude of chronic pain symptoms.

The role of the craniofacial nociceptive system in driving CPM has largely been overlooked to date. While a number of reports have demonstrated that spinal nociceptive systems can exert CPM over the craniofacial nociceptive system, the reverse case has been investigated to only a minimal extent (Wang et al., 2010; Sowman et al., 2011). In one study, a CPM effect, demonstrated as increased pressure pain thresholds on the masseter and tibialis anterior muscles, was induced by compression-induced head pain (Sowman et al., 2011). Substantial evidence exists to support the contention that there is convergence between trigeminal and spinal regions (Morch et al., 2007) and hence that CPM mechanisms also exist between trigeminal and spinal systems (Wang et al., 2010).

CONCLUSIONS

Relevant human pain models acting as proxies for headache are available, allowing pain referral from shoulder, neck, and peri-cranial muscles to be assessed experimentally. Through such research, distinct pain distribution patterns have been identified for specific muscles that may be relevant for the perception of pain in the head. In addition, TrPs may form the clinical basis for certain headache conditions. Finally, sensitization of pain referral mechanisms is found in patients with tension-type headache as well as those with chronic musculoskeletal pain, indicating the involvement of central sensitization; this mechanism represents a promising target for further development of rational treatment strategies.

REFERENCES

Amano N, Hu JW, Sessle BJ. Responses of neurons in feline trigeminal subnucleus caudalis (medullary dorsal horn) to cutaneous, intraoral, and muscle afferent stimuli. *J Neurophysiol* 1986;55:227–243.

Arendt-Nielsen L, Graven-Nielsen T. Central sensitization in fibromyalgia and other musculoskeletal disorders. *Curr Pain Headache Rep* 2003;7:355–361.

Bajaj P, Bajaj P, Graven-Nielsen T, Arendt-Nielsen L. Osteoarthritis and its association with muscle hyperalgesia: an experimental controlled study. *Pain* 2001;93:107–114.

Bartsch T, Goadsby PJ. Stimulation of the greater occipital nerve induces increased central excitability of dural afferent input. *Brain* 2002;125:1496–1509.

Bogduk N. Lumbar dorsal ramus syndrome. *Med J Aust* 1980;2:537–541.

Bragdon EE, Light KC, Costello NL, Sigurdsson A, Bunting S, Bhalang K, Maixner W. Group differences in pain modulation: pain-free women compared to pain-free men and to women with TMD. *Pain* 2002;96:227–237.

Burstein R, Dodick D, Silberstein S. Migraine prophylaxis with botulinum toxin A is associated with perception of headache. *Toxicon* 2009;54:624–627.

Calandre EP, Hidalgo J, Garcia-Leiva JM, Rico-Villademoros F. Trigger point evaluation in migraine patients: an indication of peripheral sensitization linked to migraine predisposition? *Eur J Neurol* 2006;13:244–249.

Campbell DG, Parsons CM. Referred head pain and its concomitants. *J Nerv Mental Dis* 1944;99:544–551.

Falace DA, Reid K, Rayens MK. The influence of deep (odontogenic) pain intensity, quality, and duration on the incidence and characteristics of referred orofacial pain. *J Orofac Pain* 1996;10:232–239.

Falla D, Farina D, Dahl MK, Graven-Nielsen T. Muscle pain induces task-dependent changes in cervical agonist/antagonist activity. *J Appl Physiol* 2007;102:601–609.

Feinstein B, Langton JNK, Jameson RM, Schiller F. Experiments on pain referred from deep somatic tissues. *J Bone Joint Surg Am* 1954;36A:981–997.

Fernández-de-las-Peñas C, Cuadrado ML, Pareja JA. Myofascial trigger points, neck mobility and forward head posture in unilateral migraine. *Cephalalgia* 2006;26:1061–1070.

Gazerani P, Andersen OK, Arendt-Nielsen L. A human experimental capsaicin model for trigeminal sensitization: gender-specific differences. *Pain* 2005;118:155–163.

Gazerani P, Wang K, Cairns BE, Svensson P, Arendt-Nielsen L. Effects of subcutaneous administration of glutamate on pain, sensitization and vasomotor responses in healthy men and women. *Pain* 2006;124:338–348.

Gazerani P, Andersen OK, Arendt-Nielsen L. Site-specific, dose-dependent, and sex-related responses to the experimental pain model induced by intradermal injection of capsaicin to the foreheads and forearms of healthy humans. *J Orofac Pain* 2007;21:289–302.

Gazerani P, Pedersen NS, Staahl C, Drewes AM, Arendt-Nielsen L. Subcutaneous botulinum toxin type A reduces capsaicin-induced trigeminal pain and vasomotor reactions in human skin. *Pain* 2009;141:60–69.

Giamberardino MA, Tafuri E, Savini A, Fabrizio A, Affaitati G, Lerza R, Di IL, Lapenna D, Mezzetti A. Contribution of myofascial trigger points to migraine symptoms. *J Pain* 2007;8:869–878.

Gibson W, Arendt-Nielsen L, Graven-Nielsen T. Referred pain and hyperalgesia in human tendon and muscle belly tissue. *Pain* 2006;120:113–123.

Giske L, Bautz-Holter E, Sandvik L, Roe C. Relationship between pain and neuropathic symptoms in chronic musculoskeletal pain. *Pain Med* 2009;10:910–917.

Graven-Nielsen T. Fundamentals of muscle pain, referred pain, and deep tissue hyperalgesia. *Scand J Rheumatol* 2006;35(suppl 122):1–43.

Graven-Nielsen T, Arendt-Nielsen L, Svensson P, Jensen TS. Stimulus-response functions in areas with experimentally induced referred muscle pain: a psychophysical study. *Brain Res* 1997;744:121–128.

Graven-Nielsen T, Babenko V, Svensson P, Arendt-Nielsen L. Experimentally induced muscle pain induces hypoalgesia in heterotopic deep tissues, but not in homotopic deep tissues. *Brain Res* 1998;787:203–210.

Graven-Nielsen T, Kendall SA, Henriksson KG, Bengtsson M, Sörensen J, Johnson A, Gerdle B, Arendt-Nielsen L. Ketamine reduces muscle pain, temporal summation, and referred pain in fibromyalgia patients. *Pain* 2000;85:483–491.

Graven-Nielsen T, Gibson SJ, Laursen RJ, Svensson P, Arendt-Nielsen L. Opioid-insensitive hypoalgesia to mechanical stimuli at sites ipsilateral and contralateral to experimental muscle pain in human volunteers. *Exp Brain Res* 2002;146:213–222.

Graven-Nielsen T, Jansson Y, Segerdahl M, Kristensen JD, Mense S, Arendt-Nielsen L. Experimental pain by ischaemic contractions compared with pain by intramuscular infusions of adenosine and hypertonic saline. *Eur J Pain* 2003;7:93–102.

Harman JB. The localization of deep pain. *Br Med J* 1948;188–192.

Head H. On disturbances of sensation with especial reference to the pain of visceral disease. *Brain* 1893;16:1–133.

Hoheisel U, Mense S, Simons DG, Yu X-M. Appearance of new receptive fields in rat dorsal horn neurons following noxious stimulation of skeletal muscle: a model for referral of muscle pain? *Neurosci Lett* 1993;153:9–12.

Hu JW, Sessle BJ, Raboisson P, Dallel R, Woda A. Stimulation of craniofacial muscle afferents induces prolonged facilitatory effects in trigeminal nociceptive brain-stem neurones. *Pain* 1992;48:53–60.

Jensen K, Norup M. Experimental pain in human temporal muscle induced by hypertonic saline, potassium and acidity. *Cephalalgia* 1992;12:101–106.

Johansen MK, Graven-Nielsen T, Olesen AS, Arendt-Nielsen L. Generalised muscular hyperalgesia in chronic whiplash syndrome. *Pain* 1999;83:229–234.

Kellgren JH. Observations on referred pain arising from muscle. *Clin Sci* 1938;3:175–190.

Laursen RJ, Graven-Nielsen T, Jensen TS, Arendt-Nielsen L. Quantification of local and referred pain in humans induced by intramuscular electrical stimulation. *Eur J Pain* 1997;1:105–113.

Laursen RJ, Graven-Nielsen T, Jensen TS, Arendt-Nielsen L. The effect of compression and regional anaesthetic block on referred pain intensity in humans. *Pain* 1999;80:257–263.

Le Bars D, Menetrey D, Conseiller C, Besson JM. Depressive effects of morphine upon lamina V cells activities in the dorsal horn of the spinal cat. *Brain Res* 1975;98:261–277.

Maixner W, Fillingim R, Booker D, Sigurdsson A. Sensitivity of patients with painful temporomandibular disorders to experimentally evoked pain. *Pain* 1995;63:341–351.

Mense S, Simons DG. *Muscle Pain: Understanding Its Nature, Diagnosis, and Treatment*. Philadelphia: Lippincott Williams & Wilkins; 2001.

Morch CD, Hu JW, Arendt-Nielsen L, Sessle B. Convergence of cutaneous, musculoskeletal, dural and visceral afferents onto nociceptive neurons in the first cervical dorsal horn. *Eur J Neurosci* 2007;26:142–154.

Mørk H, Ashina M, Bendtsen L, Olesen J, Jensen R. Experimental muscle pain and tenderness following infusion of endogenous substances in humans. *Eur J Pain* 2003;7:145–153.

Ness TJ, Gebhart GF Visceral pain: A review of experimental studies. *Pain* 1990;41:167–234.

Neugebauer V, Schaible HG. Evidence for a central component in the sensitization of spinal neurons with joint input during development of acute arthritis in cat's knee. *J Neurophysiol* 1990;64:299–311.

Olesen J. Clinical and pathophysiological observations in migraine and tension-type headache explained by integration of vascular, supraspinal and myofascial inputs. *Pain* 1991;46:125–132.

O'Neill S, Manniche C, Graven-Nielsen T, Arendt-Nielsen L. Generalized deep-tissue hyperalgesia in patients with chronic low-back pain. *Eur J Pain* 2007;11:415–420.

Pielsticker A, Haag G, Zaudig M, Lautenbacher S. Impairment of pain inhibition in chronic tension-type headache. *Pain* 2005;118:215–223.

Qerama E, Fuglsang-Frederiksen A, Kasch H, Bach FW, Jensen TS. Evoked pain in the motor endplate region of the brachial biceps muscle: an experimental study. *Muscle Nerve* 2004;29:393–400.

Sandrini G, Rossi P, Milanov I, Serrao M, Cecchini AP, Nappi G. Abnormal modulatory influence of diffuse noxious inhibitory controls in migraine and chronic tension-type headache patients. *Cephalalgia* 2006;26:782–789.

Schaible H-G, Schmidt RF. Mechanosensibility of joint receptors with fine afferent fibers. *Exp Brain Res Suppl* 1984;9:284–297.

Schmidt-Hansen PT, Svensson P, Bendtsen L, Graven-Nielsen T, Bach FW. Increased muscle pain sensitivity in patients with tension-type headache. *Pain* 2007;129:113–121.

Sessle BJ, Hu JW, Amano N, Zhong G. Convergence of cutaneous, tooth pulp, visceral, neck and muscle afferents onto nociceptive and non-nociceptive neurones in trigeminal subnucleus caudalis (medullary dorsal horn) and its implications for referred pain. *Pain* 1986;27:219–235.

Sessle BJ, Hu JW, Yu X-M. Brainstem mechanisms of referred pain and hyperalgesia in the orofacial and temporomandibular region. In: Vecchiet L, Albe-Fessard D, Lindblom U, Giamberardino MA, eds. *New Trends in Referred Pain and Hyperalgesia*. London: Elsevier Science Publishers; 1993:59–71.

Simons DG, Travell JG, Simons L. *Myofascial Pain and Dysfunction: The Trigger Point Manual*. Philadelphia: Lippincott Williams & Wilkins; 1999.

Sowman PF, Wang K, Svensson P, Arendt-Nielsen L. Diffuse noxious inhibitory control evoked by tonic craniofacial pain in humans. *Eur J Pain* 2011;15:139–145.

Svensson P, Graven-Nielsen T. Craniofacial muscle pain: review of mechanisms and clinical manifestations. *J Orofac Pain* 2001;15:117–145.

Svensson P, De Laat A, Graven-Nielsen T, Arendt-Nielsen L. Experimental jaw-muscle pain does not change heteronymous H-reflexes in the human temporalis muscle. *Exp Brain Res* 1998;121:311–318.

Svensson P, List T, Hector G. Analysis of stimulus-evoked pain in patients with myofascial temporomandibular pain disorders. *Pain* 2001;92:399–409.

Tommaso MD, Difruscolo O, Sardaro M, Libro G, Pecoraro C, Serpino C, Lamberti P, Livrea P. Effects of remote cutaneous pain on trigeminal laser-evoked potentials in migraine patients. *J Headache Pain* 2007;8:167–174.

Wang K, Svensson P, Sessle BJ, Cairns BE, Arendt-Nielsen L. Painful conditioning stimuli of the craniofacial region evokes diffuse noxious inhibitory controls in men and women. *J Orofac Pain* 2010;24:255–261.

Whitty CWM, Willison RG. Some aspects of referred pain. *Lancet* 1958;2:226–231.

Wolff HG. *Headache and Other Head Pain*. New York: Oxford University Press; 1963.

Yarnitsky D, Arendt-Nielsen L, Bouhassira D, Edwards RR, Fillingim RB, Granot M, Hansson P, Lautenbacher S, Marchand S, Wilder-Smith O. Recommendations on terminology and practice of psychophysical DNIC testing. *Eur J Pain* 2010;14:339.

A Comprehensive View of Migraine Pathophysiology

Andreas Gantenbein, MD, Peter Sándor, MD,
Franz Riederer, MD, and Jean Schoenen, MD, PhD

INTRODUCTION

Migraine is a recurrent neurologic dysfunction. Why this dysfunction occurs and where it occurs is not completely clear, but many pieces of the migraine "puzzle" have been identified during the last decade. Migraine occurs in many different phenotypical variants, and sometimes a different disease mimics the typical presentation of migraine.

What is the most important feature of migraine? Is it the severe unilateral throbbing headache? Is it the hypersensitivity to light, sound, odors, or movement? Is it the spreading scintillating scotoma? Is it the interictal lack of habituation to repeated stimuli? Is it the progressive appearance of radiological brain lesions? Or is it even the food craving and mood changes, the extensive yawning or the urinary urgency—all of which have been noted to precede the headache attack by several hours? Why do some migraine patients improve with preventive treatments, whereas others do not?

We know that migraine involves more than just severe throbbing pain and the usual accompanying symptoms. The episode of central nervous system dysfunction may start 24 hours or longer before the headache occurs (Blau, 1992; Giffin et al., 2003). The frequency of recurring attacks seems to be a result of a conflict of the individual's underlying genetic susceptibility and the environmental/internal triggering factors. At least in the episodic form of migraine, by far the most important factor could be the "migraine threshold," which seems to undergo rhythmic fluctuations, with a refractory period occurring after the attack and susceptibility then gradually increasing until the next attack, and being part of a long series of cycling changes of the brain's responsiveness to external stimuli associated with metabolic changes (Schoenen et al., 2003). This chapter provides comprehensive insights into a number of different historical and contemporary concepts about the mechanisms that lead to a migraine headache attack with all its symptoms and features.

THE DIFFERENT PATHOPHYSIOLOGICAL CONCEPTS

A Short Historical Note

First descriptions of conditions of what we would call migraine today date back to 3000–1000 BC. In the papyrus of Eber's writings, the unilateral headache was attributed to ghosts and demons, and the treatment of choice was wrapping young crocodiles around the head. Hippocrates described his headaches—what we would call migraine with aura—in 460 BC. He considered the stomach to be the origin of his distress, with vapors heading in a cranial direction and causing severe throbbing pain in the temples. Emesis was his treatment of first choice. Galen explained "hemicrania" (his naming accounts for the origin of the term "migraine") as an unbalance of the four humors (vital fluids), especially the yellow bile. This perspective persisted mostly unchanged into the Middle Ages (Isler, 2006).

The Vascular Theory

In 1664, Thomas Willis postulated a vascular cause for migraine for the first time—namely, the dilatation of cranial blood vessels as the origin of the pain (Isler, 1986). The same theory was supported by the Swiss pharmacist and pathologist Johann Jakob Wepfer (Isler, 1985), who also tried to explain the aura as being the result of overfilled cranial blood vessels. In 1849, Hall postulated another vascular theory, this time due to venous congestion ("phlebismus"). Later in the nineteenth century, P. W. Latham (1872) argued that cervical sympathetic overactivity might lead to cerebral ischemia, which would then generate the migraine aura, followed by a phase of sympathetic exhaustion resulting in cranial vasodilatation and the headache itself.

In the twentieth century, Harold G. Wolff (1963) conducted extensive investigations of migraine and came to the conclusion that its neurologic symptoms were associated with constriction of the cerebral arteries and the headache with dilatation of extracerebral arteries. It was only recently shown by Schoonman et al. (2008) with magnetic resonance (MR)–angiography imaging that there might be no vasodilatation during the migrainous headache phase. Nonetheless, extracerebral and intracerebral blood vessels may play some role in migraine pathophysiology. The large cranial vessels, the proximal cerebral vessels, venous sinuses, and meningeal blood vessels are the only intracranial pain-perceptive structures. Recent studies of vasodilating substances triggering migraine headaches (typically within 2–6 hours after exposure) give some support to vascular theory, as does the therapeutic effect of mechanical and pharmaceutical vasoconstrictors.

Vasodilators as Migraine Triggers

Based on the vascular theory, but also on incidental reports on drug side effects, it has become general knowledge that nitroglycerine (NTG), a nitric oxide (NO) donor, may cause headaches (Iversen et al., 1989). Further investigations along this line have shown that infusions of NTG reliably trigger a typical migraine attack and even premonitory symptoms (Afridi et al., 2004). Concordantly, NO synthase inhibitors may relieve migraine headaches. However, NTG also triggers cluster headache attacks, albeit with a shorter delay. Indeed, most persons taking NTG in any form may perceive an almost instant mild headache, though without migrainous features.

NTG is not the only vasodilating agent that can cause migraine and head pain. The same effect has been reported for other substances, such as CGRP, glutamate, dipyridamole, and sildenafil (Kruuse et al., 2003; Asghar et al., 2010), and the triggering mechanism of alcohol may equally be due to vasodilation (Panconesi, 2008; Bagdy et al., 2010). The exact mechanisms by which NO donors, such as NTG, induce migraine-like attacks are not fully understood. However, NO may easily penetrate the blood–brain barrier and other membranes, and may trigger migraine through peripheral or central modulation. Sildenafil, for instance, has been shown to trigger migraine-like attacks without immediate vasodilation, most probably through up-regulation of intracellular cGMP (Schytz et al., 2010).

Vasoconstrictors as Migraine Treatment

William H. Thompson induced the research into contemporary migraine treatment when, in 1884, he rediscovered the anti-migraine effect of ergots that Woakes had previously described for "neuralgia" in 1868 (see also Tfelt-Hansen & Koehler, 2008). In 1918, Stoll extracted ergotamine, an agent that is still in use for migraine treatment in some countries and seems to be administered as an inhaler (i.e., the "ergot inhaler"; Armer et al., 2007). In

1938, Wolff published a paper with Graham describing the use of ergotamine tartrate for the relief of migraine; this work was published before Wolff actually elaborated the vascular theory of migraine (Graham et al., 1938).

The mechanisms of action of ergotamine are complex. Its anti-migrainous effect seems to be due to constriction of the intracranial extracerebral blood vessels through the 5-HT$_{1B}$ receptor, and to the inhibition of trigeminal neurotransmission via 5-HT$_{1D}$ receptors. This agent also inhibits neurogenic inflammation in an animal model (Markowitz et al., 1988). However, ergotamine also has agonistic effects on the dopamine D$_2$ and norepinephrine receptors.

It was not until the 1980s that the dedicated research of Patrick A. Humphrey led to the discovery of the first specific 5-HT$_{1B/D}$ receptor agonist or triptan, sumatriptan. This substance has, compared to ergotamine, both a more cranioselective vasoconstrictive effect and a better oral bioavailability (Humphrey, 2007). Thus ergotamine lost its place as a standard drug for migraine attack treatment.

The Vasculature as a Risk Factor

In recent years, it has been recognized that migraine with aura is an independent risk factor for ischemic stroke, conferring an approximately twofold increase in stroke risk (Kurth et al., 2006). Migraine with aura also seems to increase the risk for angina pectoris, myocardial infarction (Teo et al., 2006), and intracranial bleeding (Kurth et al., 2010). Lee et al. (2008) have suggested that an endothelial dysfunction might be present in migraine, although this hypothesis was not confirmed in a recent study of forearm vessels (Vanmolkot & de Hoon, 2010). A decreased number and function of endothelial progenitor cells have been reported in patients with migraine. Consistent with the increased vascular risk, prevalence of white matter abnormalities and subclinical infarcts on brain MRI is increased in migraine (with aura) patients (Swartz & Kern, 2004; Scher et al., 2009). In the so-called CAMERA study (Kruit et al., 2005), the prevalence of subclinical infarcts was higher only in the posterior circulation territory, particularly in migraine with aura and in subjects with a high attack frequency.

In the context of the vascular risk of migraine with aura, it is interesting that this form of migraine is also associated with an increased prevalence of cardiac abnormalities, such as patent foramen ovale (PFO) and mitral valve prolapse (Del Sette et al., 1998; Anzola et al., 1999). Various theories have been proposed to explain how these cardiac abnormalities might potentially influence or trigger migraine: (1) triggering of CSD by paradoxical microemboli (Nozari et al., 2010); (2) a cerebral effect of vasoactive or other chemical substances that cannot be filtered in the lungs because of right–left shunt; and (3) a cerebral effect of hormones of cardiac origin owing to volume overload in the right atrium and change in its endocrine activity (e.g., increased ANP secretion).

An argument in favor of the microemboli theory is the observation that attacks of migraine with aura may occur during injection of agitated saline during a transcranial Doppler study to detect right–left shunts (Zaletel et al., 2008) and within several hours after endovascular closure of a PFO (Rigatelli et al., 2011). Several retrospective case series and open-label studies have suggested a beneficial effect of endovascular PFO closure (Morandi et al., 2003; Azarbal et al., 2005). In most of these studies, migraine was a comorbid condition and not the reason for PFO closure; instead, the procedure was most commonly performed in response to stroke. The only randomized sham-controlled trial to investigate the effect of PFO closure on migraine with aura yielded negative results (Dowson et al., 2008) and could be criticized from a methodological point of view. In a recent case-control study, the association between migraine (with and without aura) and PFO was challenged (Garg et al., 2010), however. Clinical trials are now under way trying to determine whether subgroups of patients with disabling migraine may benefit from PFO closure.

Abnormalities of Cortical Function

Deficient Habituation and Increased Cortical Responsiveness

Clinical, neurophysiological, and neuroimaging studies have disclosed abnormalities of cortical responsiveness to external stimuli in both types of migraine between attacks (Coppola et al., 2007a, 2007b). The first indication of this dysfunction was the photic driving response that seems to be prevalent in migraineurs (Golla & Winter, 1959), yet is not very specific for migraine. The most reproducible group abnormality in evoked potential studies is a deficit of habituation during stimulus repetition (Schoenen et al., 1995; Schoenen et al., 2003), of which the metabolic correlate was recently demonstrated in functional neuroimaging studies.

The underlying causes are not fully understood, but neuronal hyperexcitability may be an oversimplified and misleading explanation. On the one hand, some studies suggest that insufficient cortical inhibitory processes might be responsible for the lack of habituation (Aurora et al., 2005). On the other hand, converging evidence from clinical and electrophysiological data suggests that the pre-activation level of sensory cortices is reduced because of an inefficient thalamo-cortical drive (Coppola et al., 2007a). In reality, deficient inhibition and low pre-activation may coexist, as the latter can promote the former via reduction of lateral inhibition. The final consequence on the functional properties of the cerebral cortex is a heightened response to repeated stimuli (i.e., hyper-responsiveness), which results in exaggerated energy demands (Sandor et al., 2005) and possibly may lead to subtle cognitive dysfunction (Waldie et al., 2002; Camarda et al., 2007).

Some indirect evidence indicates that the thalamo-cortical dysrhythmia and ensuing decreased pre-activation level of sensory cortices might be due to hypoactivity of the so-called state-setting, chemically addressed subcortico-cortical projections (Mesulam, 1990). Among the latter, the serotonergic pathway seems to be the most relevant, but interactions between amines are well known (Hamel, 2007).

It is well established that cortical responsiveness fluctuates over time in relation to the migraine attack. It grows and leads to increased energy demands during the days immediately preceding the attack, when habituation of evoked potentials reaches its minimum and amplitude its maximum (Kropp & Gerber, 1998). By contrast, just before the attack, at a time point when premonitory symptoms may occur, and during the attack, habituation increases and normalizes; this effect is accompanied by an increased thalamo-cortical drive (Judit et al., 2000; Coppola et al., 2005). These electrophysiological changes could be due to further pre-ictal *decrease* of serotonergic neurotransmission and cortical pre-activation levels that change to *increased* serotonergic transmission and pre-activation levels during the attack. Interestingly, increased serotonin disposition (Evers et al., 1999), brain tryptophan uptake (Sakai et al., 2008), and activation in the area of the raphe serotonergic neurons (Weiller et al., 1995; Bahra et al., 2001) have all been reported during migraine attack.

Finally, as hypothesized previously (Schoenen, 1996), the cerebral metabolic homeostasis may be disrupted by the increased energy demands due to the ictal and even more so pre-ictal cortical hyper-responsiveness, because of a constitutional decrease of the mitochondrial energy reserve (Welch et al., 1989; Montagna et al., 1994). This phenomenon may ignite the major alarm-signaling system of the brain, the trigeminovascular system (discussed later), and/or favor the occurrence of cortical spreading depression (also discussed later). During the migraine attack itself, activation of the endogenous pain control systems will lead to increased central serotonergic transmission and normalization of cortical responsiveness, by which, as stated by Edward Liveing in 1873, after "the nerve storm . . . this condition is dispersed and the equilibrium for the time restored."

Cortical Spreading Depression: The Culprit Underlying the Migraine Aura?

In 1944, Leão published the first studies in animals of cortical spreading depression (CSD), a slowly progressing wave (3–5 mm/min) of neuron-glial depolarization, followed by a long-lasting suppression of neuronal activity and excitability. A few years earlier, K. C. Lashley (1941) had described in great detail the progression of his own migraine aura in the visual field. The similarity between the extension and speed of propagation of the scintillating scotoma and Leão's cortical spreading depression was first pointed out by Milner (1958). This concept was later revitalized by Olesen and colleagues, who performed single-photon emission tomography studies during carotid angiography-triggered attacks of migraine with aura and found posterior spreading oligemia at a pace similar to that of CSD (Lauritzen & Olesen, 1984). That blood flow and metabolic changes compatible with the CSD phenomenon occur during the migraine aura was subsequently confirmed with modern neuroimaging methods (Hadjikhani et al., 2001; Cao et al., 2002).

Attacks with aura can be triggered in susceptible individuals by trauma (Black, 2006), and in animal models, cortical spreading depression (CSD) can be triggered by trauma (Pietrobon & Striessnig, 2003). In both head trauma and severe stroke, repetitive episodes of CSD have been recorded; it is hypothesized that they might have protective functions (Fabricius et al., 2006; Dohmen et al., 2008). In fact, CSD can be elicited by a number of triggers, including high concentrations of K^+ or hypoxia, and it is considered a valid experimental model for the migraine aura (Bergerot et al., 2006). Recently, studies in animals showed that cerebral micro-emboli—which might, for instance, occur in case of a PFO—can trigger CSD (Nozari et al., 2010).

CSD in animals is able to activate the trigeminovascular nociceptive system thought to be responsible for the headache in migraineurs (Moskowitz, 1984; Moskowitz et al., 1993; Bolay et al., 2002). It is also common clinical knowledge that a substantial proportion of migraine patients present with both attacks with and without aura. Nevertheless, the precise relationship, if any, between CSD (i.e., the aura) and the migraine headache remains unclear. For instance, migraine auras without headache occur frequently, especially in elderly people; moreover, in migraine without aura (which affects 80 % of patients), there are no clinical signs suggestive of CSD. Based on the finding that chronic administration of various established preventive anti-migraine drugs suppresses CSD in the rat model of KCl-induced CSD (Ayata et al., 2006), it has been hypothesized that CSD suppression may be the common mechanism explaining the therapeutic action of anti-migraine drugs and, therefore, that CSD or CSD-like events play a causative role in all migraine types, including migraine without aura. This hypothesis cannot be accepted without reservation (Schoenen, 2006) because, as mentioned previously, there is no proof for the occurrence of CSD in migraine without aura. Moreover, several effective preventive anti-migraine drugs have only a weak or no suppressive effect on experimental CSD (Bogdanov et al., 2011), whereas others have a selective effect on CSD and the aura but no therapeutic action on migraine without aura (Steiner et al., 1997; D'Andrea et al., 1999; Lampl et al., 2005; Goadsby et al., 2009; Hauge et al., 2009; Bogdanov et al., 2011).

If CSD has no causative role in migraine without aura, then what causes this most prevalent type of migraine? This question is far from being resolved, and may have several answers. A common denominator seems to be activation of the peripheral and/or central parts of the major pain-signaling system of the brain, the trigeminovascular pain pathway, and dysfunction of its descending control mechanisms.

The Neurovascular Theory

Trigeminovascular Pain Pathways

The pivotal pathway for pain perception in the head is the trigeminovascular input from the meningeal vessels (**Figure 8.1**). Nociceptive input from first-order neurons belonging to the visceral part of the first division of the trigeminal nerve (ophthalmic nerve) is transferred to second-order nociceptors in the trigeminal nucleus caudalis (trigeminocervical complex), from whence it is transferred to the thalamus (quinto- or trigemino-thalamic pathway). Second-order nociceptors in the trigeminocervical complex receive convergent input from the somatic part of V_1 and from the C_2 dermatome, which explains referred pain to the fronto-temporo-orbital region and to the neck. The trigeminal nucleus caudalis has reciprocal connections with the pain control centers in the upper brainstem such as the periaqueductal gray matter (PAG) and with the hypothalamus (**Figure 8.2**). Via the nucleus

of the solitary tract, it has connections with the superior salivary nucleus, providing the parasympathetic innervation of meningeal blood vessels in addition to nasal mucosa and lacrymal gland, via the greater superficial petrosal nerve and the sphenopalatine ganglion (see Figure 8.1). This trigemino-autonomic reflex pathway is responsible for ipsilateral autonomic signs in trigeminal autonomic cephalalgias, such as cluster headache, SUNCT (short-lasting, unilateral, neuralgiform headache attacks with conjunctival injection and tearing), and paroxysmal hemicrania (Goadsby et al., 2002), but may also occur during a migraine attack.

One point of interest for migraine treatment is the fact that targets for all available effective acute anti-migraine drugs are present in the peripheral and central parts of the trigeminovascular system (see Figure 8.1). This is in particular the case for triptans and $5\text{-HT}_{1B/D}$ receptors, or gepants and CGRP receptors, or NOS inhibitors and NO, or NSAIDs and cyclo-oxygenases. Drugs acting on 5-HT_{1F} receptors that are mainly centrally located can also abort migraine attacks. The therapeutic potential of compounds acting on glutamate or TRVP1 receptors remains to be determined. To date, none of the NK1 antagonists studied so far has been found to be effective as a migraine therapy.

Neurogenic Inflammation and Neuropeptides

The concept of neurogenic inflammation/vasodilatation dates back to the late nineteenth century, when Goltz (1874) found vasodilation in tissue innervated by the stimulated sciatic nerve. It was introduced in migraine pathophysiology by Moskowitz and colleagues, who developed the rat model of dural plasma extravasation induced by electro-stimulation of the trigeminal ganglion (Markowitz et al., 1989). Several drugs that are able to inhibit plasma extravasation in the rat model were, however, ineffective for the treatment of migraine attacks, and meningeal inflammation was not convincingly demonstrated during migraine attacks in patients with modern neuroimaging methods.

Nevertheless, the possibility that the peripheral fibers of the trigeminovascular system are depolarized in migraine is suggested by the elevated CGRP level in the jugular vein blood observed during an attack (Goadsby et al., 1988). GCRP levels remain normal in chronic tension-type headache except in patients with a pulsating quality, suggesting a common pathophysiological denominator with migraine in these individuals (Ashina et al., 2000). In their study, Lassen et al. (2002) reported that migraine-like

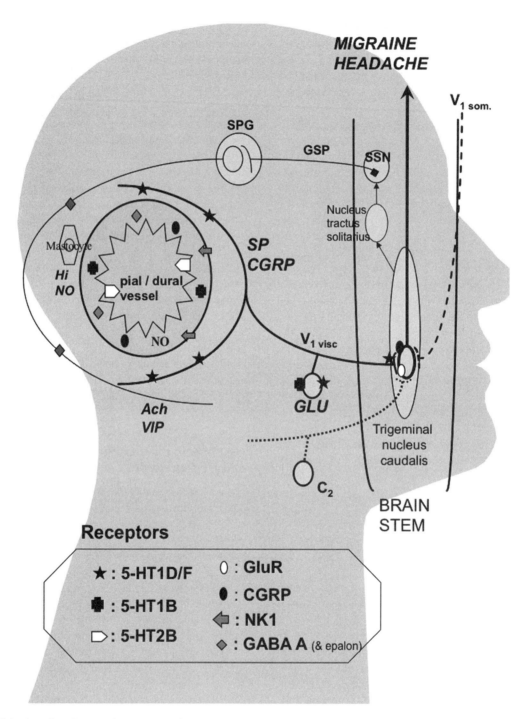

Figure 8.1 The Trigeminovascular System and Its Main Neurotransmitters and Receptors

attacks could be induced in 67 % of migraineurs by infusions of CGRP. Thus CGRP seems to play a key role in the process responsible for the migraine attack, via activation of mast cells, vasodilation, and activation of central receptors. It has been hypothesized that meningeal neurogenic inflammation may be responsible for the throbbing character of migraine headache, but this view has been challenged to some extent by a recent study showing poor correlation between arterial pulse and the subjective experience of throbbing pain (Ahn et al., 2010).

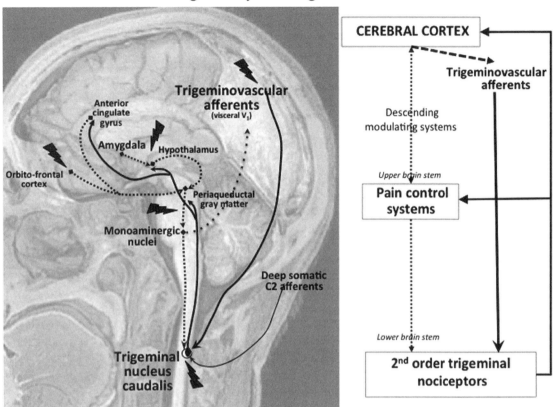

Figure 8.2 The Cortico-Trigemino-Ponto-Trigemino-Cortical Network Involved in Migraine Pathophysiology. Symbols indicate possible dysfunctions responsible for migraine attacks.

Central Sensitization

Allodynia, an experience of pain from non-noxious stimuli, which is explained by a central sensitization of second- or higher-order nociceptive neurons, is a commonly experienced symptom in migraine, suggesting that central sensitization plays a key role in migraine pathophysiology (see Chapter 6). In particular, the finding of allodynia in limbs during migraine attacks suggests involvement of third-order neurons in the thalamus. Originally, it was suggested that triptans would be ineffective in acute attacks if they were taken as late as when cutaneous allodynia is present (Strassmann et al., 1996; Burstein et al., 2004). Subsequent pharmacological studies, however, have shown that this issue can be overcome by using injectable sumatriptan. In such cases, the crucial factor predicting treatment outcome is not allodynia, but rather headache intensity at the time of treatment, to which it is proportionally related (Schoenen et al., 2008).

The Brainstem "Generator"

It has been proposed that the primary cause of migraine is a dysfunction in brainstem nuclei involved in the central control of nociception. This hypothesis is based on the observation that continuous migraine-like headaches can be triggered in non-migraineurs by electrode implantation into the PAG for treatment of chronic pain (Raskin et al., 1987). The brainstem "generator" hypothesis was subsequently supported by PET and functional magnetic resonance imaging (fMRI) studies showing increased blood flow in the midbrain during migraine attacks (Weiller et al., 1995; Cao et al., 2002). Concordantly, binding sites for migraine specific agents were localized in the brainstem (Goadsby et al., 1991). MRI studies have also provided evidence of iron accumulation in the mes-encephalic PAG in proportion to attack frequency (Welch et al., 2001). Although these brainstem areas are not specifically involved in migraine (May, 2009a, 2009b), a dysfunction of structures involved in central pain processing (i.e., the PAG, raphe nuclei, or locus coeruleus) might promote central trigeminovascular hyperexcitability and contribute to the pro-nociceptive state observed in migraine (Pietrobon et al., 2003). A dysfunction at the brainstem level could also explain the increased sensitivity to visual (photophobia), auditory (phonophobia), and olfactory (osmophobia) stimuli as well as to (head) movement.

Brain Plasticity in Migraine

Recent voxel-based morphometry (VBM) studies have shown various gray matter (GM) abnormalities in migraine patients. Rocca et al. (2006) reported GM increase in the PAG in patients with episodic migraine and subtle T2-hyperintense white matter lesions but decreased GM volume in frontal and temporal regions. Schmitz et al. (2008) found decreased frontal and parietal lobe GM density. Kim et al. (2008) reported significant GM reductions in several regions, such as the bilateral insula, motor/pre-motor, prefrontal, cingulate cortex, right posterior parietal cortex, and orbitofrontal cortex areas. Valfré et al. (2008) also reported significant GM reduction in temporal and frontal regions; these researchers paid special attention to patients with chronic migraine who showed a focal GM decrease in the bilateral anterior cingulate cortex, left amygdala, left parietal operculum, left middle and inferior frontal gyrus, right inferior frontal gyrus, and bilateral insula. Considering all the migraine patients, a significant correlation between GM reduction in anterior cingulate cortex and frequency of migraine attacks was found. Interestingly, Obermann et al. (2009) identified a midbrain GM increase in patients with chronic post-traumatic headache.

Contrasting with the GM density decreases found in most cortical areas, thickening of the somatosensory cortex (DaSilva et al., 2007a) and visual motion processing areas MT+ and V3a (Granziera et al., 2006) were shown with MRI in mixed groups of patients with and without aura. Using diffusion tensor (DT) tractography, selective diffusion changes with reduced fractional anisotropy were detected in optic radiations (Rocca et al., 2008) and the ventral trigemino-thalamic tract (DaSilva et al., 2007b) in patients having migraine with aura, in the ventro-lateral periaqueductal GM in patients having migraine without aura, and in the thalamo-cortical tract in patients with both migraine types (DaSilva et al., 2007b). Currently, the significance of these MRI findings is not clear. It is likely that most of the GM changes reported are not specific for migraine, but are more generally an indication of activation in the pain

neuro-matrix, as they can also be found in other chronic pain conditions (May, 2009a, 2009b). By the same token, the changes in visual areas and pathways could be due to repeated and excessive activation during migraine attacks. Moreover, it is unlikely that these abnormalities represent structural damage to brain tissue, although it remains to be determined if they might be reversed with successful treatment. Finally, the neural correlates of the MRI changes are as yet unclear. Gray matter alterations might reflect cell swelling, changes in neuronal or glial density, synaptic density, effects of blood flow, or a combination of these alterations (Draganski et al., 2004; Obermann et al., 2009). Gray matter increases in task specific regions have been observed after motor learning (Draganski et al., 2004) and painful stimuli (Teutsch et al., 2008) in healthy controls and are thought to reflect neuroplasticity in adults.

Genetics of Migraine

Several epidemiologic (and clinical) studies have shown that migraine has a strong genetic background. This evidence comes from family studies showing that first-degree relatives are at increased risk for similar recurrent headaches (Russell & Olesen, 1995), as well as from studies involving monozygotic twins (Ulrich et al., 1999). Contrary to the findings with familial hemiplegic migraine, however, the common forms of migraine seem to be polygenic disorders where single-nucleotide polymorphisms in several genes set a migraine threshold.

Numerous studies showing association of migraine with various markers for candidate genes have been published, though few have been successfully replicated. This was recently the case, especially in migraine with aura, for a marker on chromosome 8 that can modify the expression of neighboring genes coding for proteins involved in glutamate metabolism (Anttila et al., 2010). In addition, a dominant negative mutation in the TRESK potassium channel on chromosome 10 that modulates neuronal excitability was associated with familial migraine with aura (Lafrenière et al., 2010).

In the subtype of familial hemiplegic, migraine mutations in three different genes have been described: the *CACNA1A* gene on chromosome 19 coding for a subunit of a voltage-gated neuronal calcium channel (FHM-1) (Ophoff et al., 1996); the *ATP1A2* gene on chromosome 1 coding for the α subunit of the Na/K-ATPase-pump (FHM-2) (De Fusco et al., 2003); and the *SCN1A* gene on chromosome 2 coding for a voltage-gated sodium channel (FHM-3) (Swoboda et al., 2004). The functional result of these mutations is most probably increased neuronal excitability and susceptibility for cortical spreading depression (De Vries et al., 2009), but they do not seem to be linked to the remaining facets of migraine pathophysiology. In fact, to date no clear-cut abnormalities of the FHM genes have been found in the common types of migraine (Wessman et al., 2007).

Hormones and Migraine

The fact that migraine in childhood is almost evenly distributed but starts to diverge with puberty to a proportion of approximately 3:1 in women to men is a strong indicator that migraine susceptibility and initiation might be linked to hormonal changes (see Chapter 11). Furthermore, attacks of migraine without aura seem to be triggered by declining plasma levels of estrogens (e.g., in the premenstrual phase), whereas migraine with aura is more likely to begin with high levels of estrogens (e.g., during pregnancy or with use of estrogen-containing contraceptives or hormone replacement therapy). Evidence from a vast number of studies indicates that estrogens modulate a number of neurobiological processes relevant for migraine pathophysiology, such as neuronal excitability, synthesis and release of nitric oxide and neuropeptides, CGRP (Pardutz et al., 2002), and vasodilating mechanisms, pain processing (Multon et al., 2005), and the serotonergic, adrenergic, and GABA-ergic systems (Gupta et al., 2007; MacGregor, 2008).

COMORBIDITIES
Migraine and Affective Disorders

As discussed in Chapter 3, migraine and, to a lesser extent, non-migrainous headaches are clearly associated with mood and anxiety disorders (Merikangas et al., 1993; Saunders et al., 2008). This relationship seems somewhat stronger for migraine with aura. For one complication of migraine—medication-overuse headache—the association may even be stronger (Radat et al., 2005). Remarkably, affective disorders often coexist before headache chronification related to medication overuse. In contrast to affective disorders, migraine is generally accepted to be a somatic disease; thus its cause remains obscured, and shared pathways may well exist. For instance, frontal gray matter abnormalities have been observed in migraine and affective disorders. In particular, the most commonly reported trigger factors such as "stress," disturbed sleep pattern, and exhaustion/fatigue may well be associated with a similar autonomic or endocrine dysfunction. Critical changes in endogenous cortisol levels—due to

psychological alteration—may initiate migraine attacks as well (Ziegler et al., 1979). Furthermore, psychological stress may provoke mast cell degranulation, thereby influencing the probable neurogenic inflammation process. Finally, brainstem mechanisms—in particular, a dysfunction of the locus coeruleus—have been discussed as explanations for distractibility and anxiety (Sprenger & Goadsby, 2009).

Medication Overuse and Substance Abuse

For the development of medication-overuse headache (MOH), several mechanisms are discussed. From observations of MOH occurring in rheumatologic patients only when a history of migraine is present (Bahra et al., 2003), a strong association with the migraine has been suggested. Whether this association reflects a common genetic background (Cevoli et al., 2006) or the regulation of receptor and enzyme physiology remains unclear. Recent data indicate that most patients with MOH also meet the criteria for substance dependence in the *Diagnostic and Statistical Manual of Mental Disorders* (DSM-IV) (Fuh et al., 2005; Radat et al., 2008). Furthermore, physical withdrawal symptoms often occur in these individuals (Evers et al., 2010). In turn, neurobiological similarities between MOH and drug addiction have been proposed, and hypoactivity in the orbitofrontal cortex—a hallmark in patients with substance abuse—has been described in MOH patients (Fumal et al., 2006). In addition, sensitization of central nociceptive neurons and impairment of descending pain control pathways may play roles in headache chronification.

Migraine and Vascular Complications

Recent data from the Women's Health Study and a meta-analysis report an increased risk for cerebral stroke in female migraine patients with aura, albeit not in those without aura (Schürks et al., 2009; Kurth et al., 2010), although the absolute numbers are still very small. The same is true for the risk of cardiac ischemic events (Kurth et al., 2006). A different perspective comes from the Dutch cohort-study/CAMERA-study (Kruit et al., 2005) and the Reykjavik-cohort study (Scher et al., 2009): both showed an increased number of white matter lesions in the posterior circulation, though the clinical impact of these "silent infarcts" remains unclear. Although some studies suggest that migraine is a chronic disease, this hypothesis is negated by the natural course of the disorder; in the majority of cases, migraine improves in the third decade of life, and migraine patients have normal mortality.

MIGRAINE AND THE PLACEBO EFFECT

The placebo effect (discussed further in Chapter 23) in medical research seems to be psychologically related to expectation, conditioning, and therapeutic relation and empowerment (Hyland, 2003). Its neurobiological mechanisms are explained by both opioid and non-opioid (i.e., beta-adrenergic sympathetic, 5-HT-dependent) pathways. Especially in migraine, placebo responses are reported to be as high as almost 50% (Antonaci et al., 2007). While the placebo response in cluster headache has been considered to be small for a long time, this might not be true (Nilsson et al., 2003). The placebo effect also depends on the method of administration; it is far higher for injections and infusions than for oral or rectal application, for example. This finding is compatible with the results of recent large placebo-controlled trials related to the prophylaxis of migraine. In one of these studies, traditional acupuncture (Diener et al., 2006) was found not to be superior to either sham-acupuncture or standard treatment.

In the recent studies of botulinum toxin A (onabotulinumtoxinA; Botox) in chronic migraine (Diener et al., 2010), the headache episodes were not different in comparison to the placebo group, but the headache days per month improved by 9 and 6.7, respectively. Contrary to common belief, the placebo effect lasted for at least 6 months up to the end of the blinded phase.

CONCLUSIONS

Migraine appears to be a recurrent dysfunction of central information processing, which involves the main structures of pain processing: the trigeminovascular system, the brainstem, and the cortex. The susceptibility to suffer from migraine attacks seems to be partially inherited, and the initiation of the attack seems to be due to a combination of heterogeneous environmental and internal factors. The lifetime prevalence of migraine is estimated to be as high as 43% (Stewart et al., 2008) and the chance of suffering a single migraine attack in one's life might even be higher. Loder (2002) even went as far as explaining this high prevalence from an evolutionary point of view, equating it with reproductive or survival advantages.

Researchers continue their efforts to identify possible triggers and the impact of an individual's migraine and to search for migraine subtypes. This line of research might eventually lead to a better understanding of migraine pathophysiology. Comorbidities need to be taken into account to prescribe an optimal migraine treatment. Future advances in research on genetics potential treatments will certainly improve the management of migraine patients.

REFERENCES

Afridi SK, Kaube H, Goadsby PJ. Glyceryl trinitrate triggers premonitory symptoms in migraineurs. *Pain* 2004;110:675–680.

Ahn AH. On the temporal relationship between throbbing migraine pain and arterial pulse. *Headache* 2010;50:1507–1510.

Antonaci F, Chimento P, Diener HC, et al. Lessons from placebo effects in migraine treatment. *J Headache Pain* 2007;8:63–66.

Anttila V, Stefansson H, Kallela M, et al. Genome-wide association study of migraine implicates a common susceptibility variant on 8q22.1. *Nature Genetics* 2010;42:869–873.

Anzola GP, Magoni M, Guindani M, et al. Potential source of cerebral embolism in migraine with aura: a transcranial Doppler study. *Neurology* 1999;52:1622–1625.

Armer TA, Shrewsbury SB, Newman SP, et al. Aerosol delivery of ergotamine tartrate via a breath-synchronized plume-control inhaler in humans. *Curr Med Res Opin* 2007;23:3177–3187.

Asghar MS, Hansen A, Kapijimpanga T, et al. Dilation by CGRP of middle meningeal artery and reversal by sumatriptan in normal volunteers. *Neurology* 2010;26(75):1520–1526.

Ashina M, Bendtsen L, Jensen R, et al. Plasma levels of calcitonin gene-related peptide in chronic tension-type headache. *Neurology* 2000;55:1335–1340.

Aurora SK, Barrodale P, Chronicle EP, Mulleners WM. Cortical inhibition is reduced in chronic and episodic migraine and demonstrates a spectrum of illness. *Headache* 2005;45:546–552.

Ayata C, Jin H, Kudo C, et al. Suppression of cortical spreading depression in migraine prophylaxis. *Ann Neurol* 2006;59:652–661.

Azarbal B, Tobis J, Suh W, et al. Association of interatrial shunts and migraine headaches: impact of transcatheter closure. *J Am Coll Cardiol* 2005;45:489–492.

Bagdy G, Riba P, Kecskeméti V, et al. Headache-type adverse effects of NO donors: vasodilation and beyond. *Br J Pharmacol* 2010;160:20–35.

Bahra A, Matharu MS, Buchel C, et al. Brainstem activation specific to migraine headache. *Lancet* 2001;357:1016–1017.

Bahra A, Walsh M, Menon S, Goadsby PJ. Does chronic daily headache arise de novo in association with regular use of analgesics? *Headache* 2003;43:179–190.

Bergerot A, Holland PR, Akerman S, et al. Animal models of migraine: looking at the component parts of a complex disorder. *Eur J Neurosci* 2006;24:1517–1534.

Black DF. Sporadic and familial hemiplegic migraine: diagnosis and treatment. *Semin Neurol* 2006;26:208–216.

Blau JN. Migraine: theories of pathogenesis. *Lancet* 1992;339:1202–1207.

Bogdanov VB, Multon S, Chauvel V, et al. Migraine preventive drugs differentially affect cortical spreading depression in rat. *Neurobiol Disease* 2011;41:430–435.

Bolay H, Reuter U, Dunn AK, et al. Intrinsic brain activity triggers trigeminal meningeal afferents in a migraine model. *Nat Med* 2002;8:136–142.

Burstein R, Collins B, Jakubowski M. Defeating migraine pain with triptans: a race against the development of cutaneous allodynia. *Ann Neurol* 2004;55:19–26.

Camarda C, Monastero R, Pipia C, et al. Interictal executive dysfunction in migraineurs without aura: relationship with duration and intensity of attacks. *Cephalalgia* 2007;10:1094–1100.

Cao Y, Aurora SK, Nagesh V, et al. Functional MRI-BOLD of brainstem structures during visually triggered migraine. *Neurology* 2002;59:72–78.

Cevoli S, Mochi M, Scapoli C, et al. A genetic association study of dopamine metabolism-related genes and chronic headache with drug abuse. *Eur J Neurol* 2006;13:1009–1013.

Coppola G, Vandenheede M, Di Clemente L, et al. Somatosensory evoked high-frequency oscillations reflecting thalamo-cortical activity are decreased in migraine patients between attacks. *Brain* 2005;128:98–103.

Coppola G, Ambrosini A, Di Clemente L, et al. Interictal abnormalities of gamma band activity in visual evoked responses in migraine: an indication of thalamocortical dysrhythmia? *Cephalalgia* 2007a;27:1360–1367.

Coppola G, Pierelli F, Schoenen J. Is the cerebral cortex hyperexcitable or hyper-responsive in migraine? *Cephalalgia* 2007b;27:1427–1439.

D'Andrea G, Granella F, Cadaldini M, Manzoni GC. Effectiveness of lamotrigine in the prophylaxis of migraine with aura: an open pilot study. *Cephalalgia* 1999;19:64–66.

DaSilva AF, Granziera C, Snyder J, Hadjikhani N. Thickening in the somatosensory cortex of patients with migraine. *Neurology* 2007a;69:1990–1995.

DaSilva AF, Granziera C, Tuch DS, et al. Interictal alterations of the trigeminal somatosensory pathway and periaqueductal gray matter in migraine. *Neuroreport* 2007b;18:301–305.

De Fusco M, Marconi R, Silvestri L, et al. Haploinsufficiency of ATP1A2 encoding the Na$^+$/K$^+$ pump alpha$_2$ subunit associated with familial hemiplegic migraine type 2. *Nat Genet* 2003;33:192–196.

Del Sette M, Angeli S, Leandri M, et al. Migraine with aura and right-to-left shunt on transcranial Doppler: a case-control study. *Cerebrovasc Dis* 1998;8:327–330.

De Vries B, Frants RR, Ferrari MD, van den Maagdenberg AM. Molecular genetics of migraine. *Hum Genet* 2009; 126:115–132.

Diener HC, Kronfeld K, Boewing G, et al.; GERAC Migraine Study Group. Efficacy of acupuncture for the prophylaxis of migraine: a multicentre randomised controlled clinical trial. *Lancet Neurol* 2006;5:310–316.

Dohmen C, Sakowitz OW, Fabricius M, et al. Spreading depolarizations occur in human ischemic stroke with high incidence. *Ann Neurol* 2008;63:720–728.

Dowson A, Mullen MJ, Peatfield R, et al. Migraine Intervention with STARFlex Technology (MIST) trial: a prospective, multicenter, double-blind, sham-controlled trial to evaluate the effectiveness of patent foramen ovale closure with STARFlex septal repair implant to resolve refractory migraine headache. *Circulation* 2008;117:1397–1404.

Draganski B, Gaser C, Busch V, et al. Neuroplasticity: changes in grey matter induced by training. *Nature* 2004;427:311–312.

Evers S, Marziniak M. Clinical features, patho-physiology, and treatment of medication-overuse headache. *Lancet Neurol* 2010;9:391–401.

Evers S, Quibeldey F, Grotemeyer KH, et al. Dynamic changes of cognitive habituation and serotonin metabolism during the migraine interval. *Cephalalgia* 1999;19:485–491.

Fabricius M, Fuhr S, Bhatia R, et al. Cortical spreading depression and peri-infarct depolarization in acutely injured human cerebral cortex. *Brain* 2006;129:778–790.

Fuh JL, Wang SJ, Lu SR, Juang KD. Does medication overuse headache represent a behavior of dependence? *Pain* 2005;119:49–55.

Fumal A, Laureys S, Di Clemente L, et al. Orbitofrontal cortex involvement in chronic analgesic-overuse headache evolving from episodic migraine. *Brain* 2006;129:543–550.

Garg P, Servoss SJ, Wu JC, et al. Lack of association between migraine headache and patent foramen ovale: results of a case-control study. *Circulation* 2010;121:1406–1412.

Giffin NJ, Ruggiero L, Lipton RB, et al. Premonitory symptoms in migraine: an electronic diary study. *Neurology* 2003;60:935–940.

Goadsby PJ, Edvinsson L, Ekman R. Release of vasoactive peptides in the extracerebral circulation of humans and the cat during activation of the trigeminovascular system. *Ann Neurol* 1988;23:193–196.

Goadsby PJ, Zagami AS, Lambert GA. Neural processing of craniovascular pain: a synthesis of the central structures involved in migraine. *Headache* 1991;31:365–371.

Goadsby PJ, Lipton RB, Ferrari MD. Migraine: current understanding and treatment. *N Engl J Med* 2002;346:257–770.

Goadsby PJ, Ferrari MD, Csanyi A, et al. Randomized, double-blind, placebo-controlled, proof-of-concept study of the cortical spreading depression inhibiting agent tonabersat in migraine prophylaxis. *Cephalalgia* 2009;29:742–750.

Golla FL, Winter AL. Analysis of cerebral responses to flicker in patients complaining of episodic headache. *Electroencephalogr Clin Neurophysiol* 1959;11:539–549.

Goltz F. Über gefässerweiternde nerven. *Arch Gen Physiol* 1874;9:174–190.

Graham JR, Wolff HG. Mechanism of migraine headache and action of ergotamine tartrate. *Arch Neurol Psychiatr* 1938;39(7):37–63.

Granziera C, DaSilva AFM, Snyder J, et al. Anatomical alterations of the visual motion processing network in migraine with and without aura. *PLoS Med* 2006;3:e402.

Gupta S, Mehrotra S, Villalón CM, et al. Potential role of female sex hormones in the pathophysiology of migraine. *Pharmacol Therap* 2007;113:321–340.

Hadjikhani N, Sanchez Del Rio M, Wu O, et al. Mechanisms of migraine aura revealed by functional MRI in human visual cortex. *Proc Natl Acad Sci USA* 2001;98:4687–4692.

Hamel E. Serotonin and migraine: biology and clinical implications. *Cephalalgia* 2007;27:1295–1300.

Hauge AW, Asghar MS, Schytz HW, et al. Effects of tonabersat on migraine with aura: a randomised, double-blind, placebo-controlled crossover study. *Lancet Neurol* 2009;8:718–723.

Humphrey PP. The discovery of a new drug class for the acute treatment of migraine. *Headache* 2007;47:10–19.

Hyland ME. Using the placebo response in clinical practice. *Clin Med* 2003;3:347–350.

Isler H. History of the headache. In: Olesen J, Goadsby P, Ramadan N, Tfelt-Hansen P, Welch KMA, eds. *The Headaches*. 3rd ed. Philadelphia, PA: Lippincott Williams & Wilkins; 2006:1–7.

Isler H. Johann Jakob Wepfer (1620–1695): discoveries in headache. *Cephalalgia* 1985;5:423–425.

Isler H. Thomas Willis' chapters on headache of 1672. *Headache* 1986;25:95–98.

Iversen HK, Olesen J, Tfelt-Hansen P. Intravenous nitroglycerin as an experimental model of vascular headache: basic characteristics. *Pain* 1989;38:17–24.

Judit A, Sandor PS, Schoenen J. Habituation of visual and intensity dependence of auditory evoked cortical potentials tends to normalize just before and during the migraine attack. *Cephalalgia* 2000;20:714–719.

Kim JH, Suh SI, Seol HY, et al. Regional grey matter changes in patients with migraine: a voxel-based morphometry study. *Cephalalgia* 2008;28:598–604.

Kropp P, Gerber WD. Prediction of migraine attacks using a slow cortical potential, the contingent negative variation. *Neurosci Lett* 1998;257:73–76.

Kruit MC, Launer LJ, Ferrari MD, van Buchem MA. Infarcts in the posterior circulation territory in migraine: the population-based MRI CAMERA study. *Brain* 2005;128:2068–2077.

Kruuse C, Thomsen LL, Birk S, Olesen J. Migraine can be induced by sildenafil without changes in middle cerebral artery diameter. *Brain* 2003;126:241–247.

Kurth T, Gaziano JM, Cook NR, et al. Migraine and risk of cardiovascular disease in women. *JAMA* 2006;296:283–291.

Kurth T, Kase CS, Schürks M, et al. Migraine and risk of haemorrhagic stroke in women: prospective cohort study. *BMJ* 2010;341:c3659.

Lafrenière RG, Cader MZ, Poulin JF, et al. A dominant-negative mutation in the TRESK potassium channel is linked to familial migraine with aura. *Nat Med* 2010;16:1157–1160.

Lampl C, Katsarava Z, Diener HC, Limmroth V. Lamotrigine reduces migraine aura and migraine attacks in patients with migraine with aura. *J Neurol Neurosurg Psychiatry* 2005;76:1730–1732.

Lashley K. Patterns of cerebral integration indicated by scotomas of migraine. *Arch Neurol Psychiatry* 1941;46:331–339.

Lassen LH, Haderslev PA, Jacobsen VB, et al. CGRP may play a causative role in migraine. *Cephalalgia* 2002;22:54–61.

Latham PW. Nervous or sick headache. *Br Med J* 1872;i:305–306, 336–337.

Lauritzen M, Olesen J. Regional cerebral blood flow during migraine attacks by xenon-133 inhalation and emission tomography. *Brain* 1984;107:447–461.

Leão AAP. Spreading depression of activity in cerebral cortex. *J Neurophysiol* 1944;7:359–390.

Lee ST, Chu K, Jung KH, et al. Decreased number and function of endothelial progenitor cells in patients with migraine. *Neurology* 2008;70:1510–1517.

Liveing E. *On Megrim, Sick-Headache, and Some Allied Disorders: A Contribution to the Pathology of Nerve-Storms*. London: Churchill; 1873:512.

Loder E. What is the evolutionary advantage of migraine? *Cephalalgia* 2002;22:624–632.

MacGregor EA. Menstrual migraine. *Curr Opin Neurol* 2008;21:309–315.

Markowitz S, Saito K, Moskowitz MA. Neurogenically mediated plasma extravasation in dura mater: effect of ergot alkaloids. A possible mechanism of action in vascular headache. *Cephalalgia* 1988;8:83–91.

Markowitz S, Saito K, Buzzi MG, Moskowitz MA. The development of neurogenic plasma extra-vasation in the rat dura mater does not depend upon the degranulation of mast cells. *Brain Res* 1989;477:157–165.

May A. Morphing voxels: the hype around structural imaging of headache patients. *Brain* 2009a;132:1419–1425.

May A. New insights into headache: an update on functional and structural imaging findings. *Nat Rev Neurol* 2009b;5:199–209.

Merikangas KR, Merikangas JR, Angst J. Headache syndromes and psychiatric disorders: association and familial transmission. *J Psychiatr Res* 1993;27:197–210.

Mesulam MM. Large-scale neurocognitive networks and distributed processing for attention, language and memory. *Ann Neurol* 1990;28:597–613.

Milner PM. Note on a possible correspondence between the scotomas of migraine and spreading depression of Leao. *Electroencephalogr Clin Neurophysiol* 1958;10:705.

Montagna P, Cortelli P, Barbiroli B. Magnetic resonance spectroscopy studies in migraine. *Cephalalgia* 1994;14:184–193.

Morandi E, Anzola GP, Angeli S, et al. Transcatheter closure of patent foramen ovale: a new migraine treatment? *J Interv Cardiol* 2003;16:39–42.

Moskowitz MA. The neurobiology of vascular head pain. *Ann Neurol* 1984;16:157–168.

Moskowitz MA, Nozaki K, Kraig RP. Neocortical spreading depression provokes the expression of c-fos protein-like immunoreactivity within trigeminal nucleus caudalis via trigeminovascular mechanisms. *J Neurosci* 1993;13:1167–1177.

Multon S, Pardutz A, Mosen J, et al. Lack of estrogen increases pain in the trigeminal formalin model: a behavioural and immunocytochemical study of transgenic ArKO mice. *Pain* 2005;114:257–265.

Nilsson Remahl AI, Laudon Meyer E, Cordonnier C, Goadsby PJ. Placebo response in cluster headache trials: a review. *Cephalalgia* 2003;23:504–510.

Nozari A, Dilekoz E, Sukhotinsky I, et al. Microemboli may link spreading depression, migraine aura, and patent foramen ovale. *Ann Neurol* 2010;67:221–229.

Obermann M, Nebel K, Schumann C, et al. Gray matter changes related to chronic posttraumatic headache. *Neurology* 2009;73:978–983.

Ophoff RA, Terwindt GM, Vergouwe MN, et al. Familial hemiplegic migraine and episodic ataxia type-2 are caused by mutations in the Ca^{2+} channel gene CACNL1A4. *Cell* 1996;87:543–552.

Panconesi A. Alcohol and migraine: trigger factor, consumption, mechanisms. A review. *J Headache Pain* 2008;9:19–27.

Pardutz A, Multon S, Malgrange B, et al. Effect of systemic nitroglycerin on CGRP and 5-HT afferents to rat caudal spinal trigeminal nucleus and its modulation by estrogen. *Eur J Neurosci* 2002;15:1803–1809.

Pietrobon D, Striessnig J. Neurobiology of migraine. *Nat Rev Neurosci* 2003;4:386–398.

Radat F, Creac'h C, Swendsen JD, et al. Psychiatric comorbidity in the evolution from migraine to medication overuse headache. *Cephalalgia* 2005;25:519–522.

Radat F, Creac'h C, Guegan-Massardier E, et al. Behavioural dependence in patients with medication overuse headache: a cross-sectional study in consulting patients using the DSM-IV criteria. *Headache* 2008; 48:1026–1036.

Raskin NH, Hosobuchi Y, Lamb S. Headache may arise from perturbation of brain. *Headache* 1987;27:416–420.

Rigatelli G, Cardaioli P, Dell'Avvocata F, et al. May migraine post-patent foramen ovale closure sustain the microembolic genesis of cortical spread depression? *Cardio Revascul Med* 2011;12:217–219

Rocca MA, Ceccarelli A, Falini A, et al. Brain gray matter changes in migraine patients with T2-visible lesions: a 3-T MRI study. *Stroke* 2006;37:1765–1770.

Rocca MA, E Pagani, B Colombo, et al. Selective diffusion changes of the visual pathways in patients with migraine: a 3-T tractography study. *Cephalalgia* 2008;28:1061–1068.

Russell MB, Olesen J. Increased familial risk and evidence of genetic factor in migraine. *BMJ* 1995;311:541–544.

Sakai Y, Dobson C, Diksic M, et al. Sumatriptan normalizes the migraine attack-related increase in brain serotonin synthesis. *Neurology* 2008;70:431–439.

Sándor PS, Dydak U, Schoenen J, et al. MR-spectroscopic imaging during visual stimulation in subgroups of migraine with aura. *Cephalalgia* 2005;25:507–518.

Saunders K, Merikangas K, Low NC, et al. Impact of comorbidity on headache-related disability. *Neurology* 2008;70:538–547.

Scher AI, Gudmundsson LS, Sigurdsson S, et al. Migraine headache in middle age and late-life brain infarcts. *JAMA* 2009;301:2563–2570.

Schmitz N, Arkink EB, Mulder M, et al. Frontal lobe structure and executive function in migraine patients. *Neurosci Lett* 2008;440:92–96.

Schoenen J. Deficient habituation of evoked cortical potentials in migraine: a link between brain biology, behavior and trigeminovascular activation? *Biomed Pharmacother* 1996;50:71–78.

Schoenen J, Wang W, Albert A, Delwaide PJ. Potentiation instead of habituation characterizes visual evoked potentials in migraine patients between attacks *Eur J Neurol* 1995;2:115–122.

Schoenen J. Future preventive therapy: are there promising drug targets? *Headache Curr* 2006;3:108–111.

Schoenen J, Ambrosini A, Sandor PS, Maertens de Noordhout A. Evoked potentials and trans-cranial magnetic stimulation in migraine: published data and viewpoint on their patho-physiologic significance. *Clin Neurophysiol* 2003;114:955–972.

Schoenen J, De Klippel N, Giurgea S, et al. Almotriptan and its combination with aceclofenac for migraine attacks: a study of efficacy and the influence of auto-evaluated brush allodynia. *Cephalalgia* 2008;28:1095–1105.

Schoonman GG, van der Grond J, Kortmann C, et al. Migraine headache is not associated with cerebral or meningeal vasodilatation: a 3T magnetic resonance angiography study. *Brain* 2008;131:2192–2200.

Schürks M, Rist PM, Bigal ME, et al. Migraine and cardiovascular disease: systematic review and meta-analysis. *BMJ* 2009;339:b3914.

Schytz HW, Schoonman GG, Ashina M. What have we learnt from triggering migraine? *Curr Opin Neurol* 2010;23:259–265.

Sprenger T, Goadsby PJ. Migraine pathogenesis and state of pharmacological treatment options. *BMC Med* 2009;7:71.

Steiner TJ, Findley LJ, Yuen AW. Lamotrigine versus placebo in the prophylaxis of migraine with and without aura. *Cephalalgia* 1997;17:109–112.

Stewart WF, Wood C, Reed ML, et al.; AMPP Advisory Group. Cumulative lifetime migraine incidence in women and men. *Cephalalgia* 2008;28:1170–1178.

Strassman AM, Raymond SA, Burstein R. Sensitization of meningeal sensory neurons and the origin of headaches. *Nature* 1996;384:560–564.

Swartz RH, Kern RZ. Migraine is associated with magnetic resonance imaging white matter abnormalities: a meta-analysis. *Arch Neurol* 2004;61:1366–1368.

Swoboda KJ, Kanavakis E, Xaidara A, et al. Alternating hemiplegia of childhood or familial hemiplegic migraine? A novel ATP1A2 mutation. *Ann Neurol* 2004;55:884–887.

Teo KK, Ounpuu S, Hawken S, et al. Tobacco use and risk of myocardial infarction in 52 countries in the INTERHEART study: a case-control study. *Lancet* 2006;368:647–658.

Teutsch S, Herken W, Bingel U, et al. Changes in brain gray matter due to repetitive painful stimulation. *Neuroimage* 2008;42:845–849.

Tfelt-Hansen PC, Koehler PJ. History of the use of ergotamine and dihydroergotamine in migraine from 1906 and onward. *Cephalalgia* 2008;28:877–886.

Ulrich V, Gervil M, Kyvik KO, et al. Evidence of a genetic factor in migraine with aura: a population-based Danish twin study. *Ann Neurol* 1999;45:242–246.

Valfrè W, Rainero I, Bergui M, Pinessi L. Voxel-based morphometry reveals gray matter abnormalities in migraine. *Headache* 2008;48:109–117.

Vanmolkot FH, de Hoon JN. Endothelial function in migraine: a cross-sectional study. *BMC Neurol* 2010;10:119.

Waldie KE, Hausmann M, Milne BJ, Poulton R. Migraine and cognitive function: a life-course study. *Neurology* 2002;59:904–908.

Weiller C, May A, Limmroth V, et al. Brain stem activation in spontaneous human migraine attacks. *Nat Med* 1995;1:658–660.

Welch KM, Levine SR, D'Andrea G, et al. Preliminary observations on brain energy metabolism in migraine studied by in vivo phosphorus 31 NMR spectroscopy. *Neurology* 1989;39:538–541.

Welch KM, Nagesh V, Aurora SK, Gelman N. Periaqueductal gray matter dysfunction in migraine: cause or the burden of illness? *Headache* 2001;41:629–637.

Wessman M, Terwindt GM, Kaunisto MA, et al. Migraine: a complex genetic disorder. *Lancet Neurol* 2007;6:521–532.

Woakes E. On ergot of rye in the treatment of neuralgia. *Br Med J* 1868;2:350–361.

Wolff HG. *Headache and Other Head Pain.* 2nd ed. New York: Oxford University Press; 1963.

Zaletel M, Zvan B, Koželj M, et al. Migraine with aura induced by artificial microbubbles. *Cephalalgia* 2008;29:480–483.

Ziegler DK, Hassanein RS, Kodanaz A, Meek JC. Circadian rhythms of plasma cortisol in migraine. *J Neurol Neurosurg Psychiatry* 1979;42:741–748.

Pharmacotherapy for Migraine

Acute Anti-Migraine Drugs

Fabio Antonaci, MD, PhD, and Marta Allena, MD

EFFICACY AND ADVERSE-EFFECT PROFILES

Traditionally, the management of migraine is divided into acute and/or symptomatic strategies (to mitigate attack) and preventive strategies (to reduce frequency, duration, and intensity of the attacks). The goals of the acute treatment are to treat the attacks rapidly and to prevent their recurrence with minimal or no adverse events and costs so as to restore the patient's ability to function (Silberstein, 2000). To meet these objectives it is important to follow some general principles:

1. Stress early intervention when the pain is still mild, which can result in shortening the time to achieve a pain-free response.
2. Provide adequate doses and/or appropriate route of administration so that the therapy is fully effective in a migraine attack.
3. Co-administration of antiemetic or prokinetic drugs is recommended to treat vegetative symptoms, but is likely to facilitate the absorption of the primary drug and, therefore, ameliorate speed of action and efficacy.
4. Guard against chronification and medication-overuse headache through the frequent use of acute drugs. Many experts limit acute therapy to two headache days per week on a regular basis for simple analgesics or nonsteroidal anti-inflammatory drugs (NSAIDs) and to no more than one day per week of triptan, ergotamine, or combination analgesics.

In terms of acute symptomatic treatment, a variety of options are available to stop migraine attacks. Acute therapies are generally divided into two categories: (1) nonspecific treatments, such as paracetamol (acetaminophen), NSAIDs (including aspirin), opioids, and combinations of analgesics, which are the medications most commonly used for the treatment of mild or moderate attacks; and (2) specific anti-migraine treatments, including ergotamine derivates and triptans (almotriptan, naratriptan, sumatriptan, zolmitriptan), which are usually first-line drugs for the treatment of severe migraine attacks.

New strategies in acute treatment appear promising. Some of these, such as calcitonine gene-related peptide (CGRP) receptor antagonists, and serotonin 5-HT$_{1F}$ agonists, are now in the late stages of clinical trial evaluation.

Nonspecific Anti-Migraine Drugs

Simple analgesic drugs or NSAIDs are the first choice for mild or moderate migraine attacks. They may be the acute treatment of choice when triptans or ergots are contraindicated. Not all NSAIDs are useful as symptomatic treatment for migraine crisis, however. Those with proven efficacy and tolerability demonstrated in clinical placebo-controlled studies, when used at the recommended doses and in the absence of contraindications, are acetylsalicylic acid (ASA) up to 1,000 mg; ibuprofen 200–800 mg; diclofenac 50–100 mg; phenazon 1,000 mg; metamizol, a widely used product in some countries, 1,000 mg; and tolfenamic acid 200 mg orally (Evers et al., 2006) (**Table 9.1**).

A primary action of NSAIDs is the inhibition of the synthesis of prostaglandins (PGs) from arachidonic acid by blocking cyclo-oxygenase. Their effect in migraine has long been linked to this capacity to inhibit PGs' synthesis at the peripheral level. In the last decade, a central action of NSAIDs has been also suggested to play a role in these agents' anti-migraine effects (Tfelt-Hansen & McEwen, 2000). Together with the inhibition of PGs' synthesis in brain neurons, a direct action on serotonergic or opiatergic systems had been assumed for the central action.

NSAIDs are well-tolerated drugs; their side effects are usually minor and mostly related to the gastrointestinal tract, such as epigastric pain. In comparative trials with ergotamine, the differences mainly reflected tolerability; in particular, lower rates of nausea and vomiting were noted in patients treated with NSAIDs. Contraindications for use of NSAIDs include peptic ulcer and hemorrhagic diatesis.

Selective cyclo-oxygenase 2 (Cox-2) inhibitors have also proved effective in migraine treatment and offer similar efficacy to NSAIDs (Silberstein et al., 2004). It remains for researchers to demonstrate whether Cox-2 inhibitors have an advantage besides better gastric tolerance. Notably, patients with high risk of cardiovascular disease should not use cyclo-oxygenase inhibitors frequently.

Antiemetics or prokinetics (such as domperidone 10 mg orally and metoclopramide 10 mg orally) are indicated in addition to analgesics or NSAIDs when treating attacks with nausea and vomiting. However, these agents might enhance the effectiveness of the acute drug, facilitating its absorption, and have an independent antinociceptive effect.

In some countries, formulations containing NSAIDs (acetylsalicylic acid or paracetamol) with metoclopramide are available. Paracetamol 1,000 mg in combination with metoclopramide 10 mg has proved superior to placebo in studies.

Combining analgesics and/or NSAIDs with caffeine increases their efficacy (Di Monda et al., 2003; Diener et al., 2005; Goldstein et al., 2006). Unfortunately, the risk of medication-overuse headache development in susceptible patients with frequent migraine attacks becomes higher with these drugs' associations.

Specific Anti-Migraine Drugs

Specific and more effective anti-migraine treatments are required when analgesic measures fail to avert disability. These medications include ergotics and triptans. In this chapter, we also discuss new strategies in acute treatment relating to specific anti-migraine agents.

Ergotamine and Derivates

Ergotamine was the first drug introduced in migraine attack treatment (Maier, 1926), and it remains the most widely used specific symptomatic product in many countries, probably due to its low cost and its long duration of action. This drug is still very helpful in the treatment of long-lasting attacks with headache recurrence.

Ergotamine can no longer be considered the drug of choice, however, because the risk of overuse especially when combined with caffeine, associated with the many vascular problems generated by its potent generalized vasoconstrictor effect, is high if dosing has not been carefully monitored.

Dihydroergotamine (DHE), introduced in migraine therapy in 1945, is usually better tolerated than ergotamine, but has a poor oral bioavailability that impairs its efficacy. Intranasal DHE has a better bioavailability (approximately 40%), but the onset of action is relatively slow. Moreover, in two trials focused on its comparison with intranasal and subcutaneous sumatriptan, DHE's inferiority to the triptan has been clearly demonstrated (Touchon et al., 1996; Boureau et al., 2000). Parenteral DHE (injectable, intravenous, and subcutaneous solution) is more effective on severe migraine attacks but produces more side effects (Colman et al., 2005). Also, when compared with sumatriptan, this formulation's

Table 9.1 Recommended Doses for NSAIDs in Acute Migraine Treatment

Drug	Starting Dose (mg)	Maximum Daily Dose (mg)
Aspirin	1,000	2,000
Aspirin + metoclopramide	900 + 10	1,800 + 20
Tolfenamic acid	200	400
Ibuprofen	400–1,200	1,600
Naproxen sodium	825	1,375
Diclofenac	75	150
Ketoprofen	100	200

efficacy was inferior to the triptan for the first 2 hours and apparently comparable thereafter (Tfelt-Hansen & Saxena, 2000).

Ergotics share with triptans an agonist action on 5-HT receptors, for a factor that explains their anti-migraine effect. Because of their complex pharmacology and interaction with many other receptors (5-HT$_{1A}$, 5-HT$_5$, 5-HT$_2$, 5-HT$_7$, α-adrenoceptors, and dopamine D$_2$ receptors), beyond their long duration of action, they generate frequent and varied adverse effects (nausea and vomiting are the most common, but cramps, sleepiness, and transient muscular pain in the lower limbs have also been noted). The powerful and spreading vasoconstrictor action of ergotamine and DHE also underlies their contraindications, which include cardiac and peripheral vascular diseases, hypertension, liver and kidney diseases, sepsis, peptic ulcer, concomitant use of triacetyloleandomicyn, and pregnancy.

Triptans

During the last decade, the advent of a new class of selective and highly effective 5-HT$_{1B/1D}$ receptor agonists, the triptans, has shaped one strategy employed for the acute treatment of migraine. In particular, these potent vasoconstrictors have largely replaced the ergots. Triptans seem to act in migraine by three main mechanisms: intracranial extracerebral vasoconstriction, plus inhibition of neurotransmitters, release at the peripheral terminal as well as at the central terminal of trigeminal nociceptors mainly via 5-HT$_{1B/1D}$ receptors (trigeminovascular afferents and trigeminal nucleus caudalis) (Humphrey & Goadsby, 1994).

Sumatriptan was the pioneer triptan developed; it was soon followed by several newer 5-HT$_{1B/1D}$ agonists (zolmitriptan, naratriptan, rizatriptan, eletriptan, almotriptan, and frovatriptan), comprising the second-generation triptans, which were created to improve and correct some shortcomings and pharmacological properties. Although these agents are currently available in various formulations (tablets, nasal spray, subcutaneous injection, suppositories), most triptans are effective when delivered by the oral route of administration (**Table 9.2**).

Many randomized double-blind, placebo-controlled clinical trials, including the large meta-analysis of 53 eligible clinical trials conducted by Ferrari et al. (2001), have been performed to demonstrate the efficacy of triptans in migraine attack treatment and to define the optimal doses of these medications. Differences in head-to-head comparisons between oral triptans do exist for some outcome measures, but they are clinically relevant only for the individual patient. The decision about which triptan and which formulation to use depends on the patient's characteristics and preferences, the features of the individual's headache, convenience, and cost. Individual response to a triptan cannot be predicted.

The optimal benefit of triptans is achieved when they are taken at the very onset of headache, while pain is of only mild or moderate intensity (Antonaci et al., 2010). They are ineffective if taken during the aura phase. A key advantage of triptans over most other alternatives in migraine attacks is their more favorable side-effect profile. Side effects are similar for all triptans, and their variability depends on the route of delivery (the subcutaneous route is associated with greater side effects than the oral route) and drug preparation. The most common side effects, which are known as "triptan sensation," include paresthesias, flushing, tingling, neck pain, and mild transient chest pressure. They can sometimes be mitigated by switching to another triptan or to another

Table 9.2 Triptans: Routes of Administration and Recommended Doses

Drug	Available Formulations	Starting Dose (mg)	Maximum Daily Dose (mg)
Sumatriptan	Tablet	50–100	200
	Nasal spray	20	40
	Suppository	25	50
	Subcutaneous injection	6	12
Zolmitriptan	Tablet or wafer or nasal spray	2.5	5
Eletriptan	Tablet	40	80
Almotriptan	Tablet	12.5	25
Rizatriptan	Tablet or wafer	5 or 10	10 or 20
Naratriptan	Tablet	2.5	5
Frovatripan	Tablet	2.5	5

route of administration. Although rare, cardiovascular complications have occurred in some treated patients (Welch et al., 2000). Contraindications for the use of triptans include untreated arterial hypertension, coronary heart disease, Raynaud's disease, history of ischemic stroke, pregnancy, lactation, and severe liver or renal failure. The use of other vasoconstrictors, such as ergotamine and its derivate and also other triptans, is contraindicated within 24 hours after administration of a triptan.

Despite improved pharmacokinetics and dynamics, as many as 40% of all attacks and 25% of all patients do not respond to any of the triptans. Moreover, headache recurrence (return of pain after initial treatment success) occurs in 15% to 40% of the patients taking oral triptans.

The efficacy of triptans could be improved, after switching from one substance to another has failed, by the association with an NSAID. This combination produces more favorable benefits than either monotherapy or placebo. It also reduces headache recurrence, as demonstrated in recent placebo-controlled trials for sumatriptan/naproxen sodium (Brandes et al., 2007) and almotriptan/aceclofenac combinations (Schoenen et al., 2008).

For the headache recurrence, a second dose of the triptan is effective in most cases (Cady et al., 2006).

The Newest Acute Treatments

When specific anti-migraine therapies (i.e., triptans or ergots) fail (i.e., patients do not respond or experience headache recurrence), or when their use is limited (e.g., in cases of multiple vascular risk factors or important adverse effects), other therapeutically non-vasoconstrictor alternatives may be offered (**Table 9.3**).

On the basis of the complex pathogenic mechanisms involved in the migraine attack, substantial effort has been expended to search for other targets that might be addressed by acute therapies. Candidates for acute treatment of migraine currently include CGRP receptor agonists (Goadsby, 2005), nitric oxide synthase inhibitors (Lassen et al., 1997), vanilloid-receptor modulators (Rami et al., 2006), and 5-HT$_{1F}$ receptor agonists (Goldestein et al., 2001).

The most recent experimental and clinical studies have focused on the role of the neuropeptide α-calcitonine gene-related peptide (CGRP) and on its receptor agonists as new targets for acute treatment. Two CGPR receptor agonists (called "gepant") have shown clinical efficacy as acute migraine therapies. In a phase II trial, intravenous 2.5–5 mg olcegepant proved effective at aborting migraine attack (Olesen et al., 2004). Telcagepant, an orally available potent CGRP receptor antagonist, is currently in late-stage clinical testing for migraine-attacks treatment. Clinical studies have demonstrated that telcagepant relieves migraine pain, improves the associated symptoms, and is well tolerated; its efficacy is comparable to that of the triptans, and it seems to have a better safety and tolerability profile.

CUSTOMIZED ACUTE TREATMENT STRATEGIES

Before starting the management process, and once a diagnosis of migraine has been made accurately, it is important to focus on patient information and education. This approach is helpful for patients because it involves them in their own care and in the therapeutic decision-making process, which in turn facilitates management. Monitoring of headache attacks and their features using a daily diary and recording of triggers for each attack, if identifiable, are subsequent key steps to establish the choice of the acute therapy and to determine the need for preventive treatment. In fact, in the majority of patients, only acute (abortive or symptomatic) treatment for migraine attacks is required. Once the various trigger factors and the situations that could worsen migraine have been identified, patients need to be encouraged to avoid or limit them, as far as possible.

As mentioned earlier, adherence to some key principles will increase the chance of success in alleviating migraine attack. In particular, it is necessary to identify the best drug for each individual patient, choosing the drug that proves to be completely effective in relieving pain and associated symptoms in the shortest possible time, and choosing the most appropriate route of administration. To achieve this goal, the clinical characteristics of the attacks, the contraindications to the use of various preparations, the presence of any concomitant therapies, the pharmacological properties of the various preparations, and the possible pharmacological interactions with other drugs used by the patient, must all be taken into account.

Drugs must always be taken early, at the onset of migraine attack, at the appropriate dosage. Following this plan will prevent recurrent headache and reduce adverse effects, thereby enabling the patient to continue with his or her daily activities.

Two broad management approaches have been introduced in recent years for the acute treatment of migraine (Lipton et al., 2000): (1) a stepwise approach in which

Table 9.3 New Drugs for Acute Migraine Treatment

Acute Treatment	Developer	Mechanism of Action	Clinical Trial Phase
Telcagepant	Merck	CGRP receptor antagonist	III
BI-44370	Boehringer Ingelheim	CGRP receptor antagonist	II
Sumatriptan, iontophoretic transdermal patch	Nupathe	Triptan, 5-HT_1 receptor agonist	II
Sumatriptan, oral spray	NovaDel Pharma	Triptan, 5-HT_1 receptor agonist	II
Sumatriptan, intranasal	OptiNose	Triptan, 5-HT_1 receptor agonist	II
Sumatriptan, DPI	Vectura Group	Triptan, 5-HT_1 receptor agonist	I
Sumatriptan, oral film	IntelGenx	Triptan, 5-HT_1 receptor agonist	I
Sumatriptan, needleless injectable SDI	GLIDE	Triptan, $5\text{-HT}-$ receptor agonist	I
COL-144	CoLucid	5-HT_{1F} receptor agonist	II/III
Inhaled dihydroergotamine (MAP-0004; Levadex)	MAP Pharmaceuticals	Ergot derivate	III
Inhaled loxapine (AZ-104)	Alexza Pharmaceuticals	5-HT_2 receptor antagonist: dopamine D_2 receptor antagonist	II
Tazampanel (IV/NGX-426 (oral)	Raptor Pharmaceuticals	Glutamate AMPA/kainate receptor antagonist	II
IGlueR5 receptor antagonist	Eli Lilly	Iontropic glutamate receptor 5 antagonist	II
NXN-188	NeurAxon	Nitric oxide synthase inhibitor and 5-HT receptor agonist	II
Intranasal CO_2 (Capella)	Capnia		II

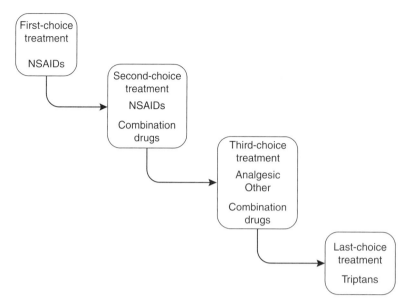

Figure 9.1 Symptomatic Therapy: "Stepped Care." Sequence of treatments with ongoing more specific drugs given in different visits or at the first visit to use in sequence at the first attack.

Modified from Lipton RB, Steward WF, Ryan RE Jr, et al. Stratified care vs step care strategies for migraine. The Disability in Strategies of Care (DISC) Study: a randomized trial. *JAMA* 2000;284:2599–2605.

initially acute attacks are treated with the safest, least expensive therapies, and migraine-specific medication is used only if the initial treatment fails (**Figure 9.1**); and (2) a stratified strategy that is based on severity of illness and matches the patient's needs to the characteristics of the migraine (i.e., severity, frequency, disability, symptoms, and time to peak; **Figure 9.2**). The latter approach recommends use of migraine-specific drugs for severe

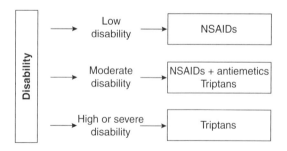

Figure 9.2 Symptomatic Therapy: "Stratified Care." The treatment is based on a disability assessment of the patient's headache.

Modified from Lipton RB, Steward WF, Ryan RE Jr, et al. Stratified care vs step care strategies for migraine. The Disability in Strategies of Care (DISC) Study: a randomized trial. *JAMA* 2000;284:2599–2605.

attacks (Silberstein, 2000). This approach, in fact, stratifies attacks and patients according to their therapeutic needs. Lipton et al. (2000), in their prospective study, showed that the stratified care approach provides the optimal clinical outcome, and a post hoc analysis suggested stratified care was associated with lower costs and lower migraine disability compared with other approaches (Sculpher et al., 2002).

CONCLUSIONS

Primary objectives of the acute migraine treatment are to abort the attacks and treat associated symptoms, with minimal and or no adverse events. Optimum management of acute migraine requires pharmacological treatment for rapid resolution, using the correct drug, formulation, and dose. Nonspecific anti-migraine drugs like nonsteroidal anti-inflammatory drugs and anti-emetics are usually helpful in mild to moderate attacks. Older nonspecific drugs, particularly butalbital and opioids, contribute to medication overuse and are to be avoided. Specific anti-migraine drugs, like triptans and ergots, are useful for moderate to severe attacks. In a step care approach, the patients start with the simplest options, such as simple analgesics followed by nonsteroidal agents, then proceed with ergot preparations and eventually triptans if they do not respond. In a stratified care approach, the patients and their attacks are stratified according to severity and therapeutic response. Those with severe disabling episodes are given specific anti-migraine medications like triptans, whereas patients with mild or low disability are treated with simple analgesics.

REFERENCES

Antonaci F, De Cillis I, Cuzzoni MG, Allena M. Almotriptan for the treatment of acute migraine: a review of early intervention trials. *Expert Rev Neurother* 2010;10:351–364.

Boureau F, Kappos L, Schoenen J, Esperanca P, Ashford E. A clinical comparison of sumatriptan nasal spray and dihydro-ergotamine nasal spray in the acute treatment of migraine. *Int J Clin Pract* 2000;54:281–286.

Brandes JL, Kudrow D, Stark SR, et al. Sumatriptan–naproxen for acute treatment of migraine: a randomized trial. *JAMA* 2007;297:1443–1454.

Cady R, Martin V, Mauskop A, et al. Efficacy of rizatriptan 10 mg administered early in a migraine attack. *Headache* 2006;46:914–924.

Colman I, Brown MD, Innes GD, et al. Parenteral dihydroergotamine for acute migraine headache: a systematic review of the literature. *Ann Emerg Med* 2005;45:393–401.

Diener HC, Pfaffenrath V, Pageler L, Peil H, Aicher B. The fixed combination of acetylsalicylic acid, paracetamol and caffeine is more effective than single substances and dual combination for the treatment of headache: a multicentre, randomized, double-blind, single-dose, placebo-controlled parallel group study. *Cephalalgia* 2005;25:776–787.

Di Monda V, Nicolodi M, Aloisio A, et al. Efficacy of a fixed combination of indomethacin, prochlorperazine, and caffeine versus sumatriptan in acute treatment of multiple migraine attacks: a multicenter, randomized, crossover trial. *Headache* 2003;43:835–844.

Evers S, Afra J, Frese A, et al. EFNS guidelines on the drug treatment of migraine: report on EFNS task force. *Eur J Neurol* 2006;13:560–572.

Ferrari MD, Roon KI, Lipton RB, Goadsby PJ. Oral triptans (serotonin 5-HT$_{1B/1D}$ agonists) in acute migraine treatment: a meta-analysis of 53 trials. *Lancet* 2001;358:1668–1675.

Goadsby PJ. Calcitonine gene-related peptide antagonists as treatment of migraine and other primary headaches. *Drugs* 2005;65:2557–2567.

Goldestein DJ, Roon KI, Offen WW, et al. Selective serotonin 1F (5HT-1F) receptor agonist LY334370 for acute migraine: a randomized controlled trial. *Lancet* 2001;358:1230–1234.

Goldstein J, Silberstein SD, Saper JR, Ryan RE Jr, Lipton RB. Acetaminophen, aspirin, and caffeine in combination versus ibuprofen for acute migraine: results from a multicenter, double-blind, randomized, parallel-group, single-dose, placebo-controlled study. *Headache* 2006;46:444–453.

Humphrey PPA, Goadsby PJ. The mode of action of sumatriptan is vascular? A debate. *Cephalalgia* 1994;14:401–410.

Lassen LH, Ashina M, Christiansen I, Ulrich V, Olesen J.

Nitric oxide synthesis inhibition in migraine. *Lancet* 1997;349:401–402.

Lipton RB, Steward WF, Ryan RE Jr, et al. Stratified care vs step care strategies for migraine. The Disability in Strategies of Care (DISC) Study: a randomized trial. *JAMA* 2000;284:2599–2605.

Maier HW. L'ergotamine inhibiteur du sympathique étudie en clinique, comme moyen d'exploration et comme agent therapeutique. *Rev Neurol* 1926;33:1104–1108.

Olesen J, Diener HC, Husstedt IW, et al. Calcitonin gene-related peptide receptors agonist BIBN 4096BS for the acute treatment of migraine. *N Eng J Med* 2004;350:1104–1110.

Rami HK, Thompson M, Stemp G, et al. Discovery of SB-705498: a potent, selective and orally bioavailable TRPV1 antagonist suitable for clinical development. *Bioorg Med Chem Lett* 2006;16:3287–3291.

Schoenen J, De Klippel N, Giurgea S, et al. On behalf of the Belgian Headache Society. Almotriptan and its combination with aceclofenac for migraine attacks: a study of efficacy and the influence of auto-evaluated brush allodynia. *Cephalalgia* 2008;28:1095–1105.

Sculpher M, Millson D, Meddis D, Poole L. Cost-effectiveness analysis of stratified versus stepped care strategies for acute treatment of migraine: the Disability in Strategies of Care (DISC) Study. *Pharmacoeconomics* 2002;20:91–100.

Silberstein SD. Practice parameter: evidence-based guidelines for migraine headache (an evidence-based review): report of the Quality Standards Subcommittee of the American Academy of Neurology. *Neurology* 2000;55:754–762.

Silberstein S, Tepper S, Brandes J, et al. Randomized, placebo- controlled trial of recoxib in the acute treatment of migraine. *Neurology* 2004;62:1552–1557.

Tfelt-Hansen P, McEwen J. Nonsteroidal anti-inflammatory drugs in the acute treatment of migraine. In: Olesen J, Tfelt-Hansen P, Welch KMA, eds. *The Headaches*. 2nd ed. Philadelphia: Lippincott Williams & Wilkins, 2000;391–397.

Tfelt-Hansen P, Saxena PR. Ergot alkaloids in the acute treatment of migraine. In: Olesen J, Tfelt-Hansen P, Welch KMA, eds. *The Headaches*. 2nd ed. Philadelphia: Lippincott Williams & Wilkins, 2000;399–409.

Touchon J, Bertin L, Pilgrim AJ, Ashfod E, Bes A. A comparison of subcutaneous sumatriptan and dihydroergotamine nasal spray in the acute treatment of migraine. *Neurology* 1996;47:361–365.

Welch KMA, Mathew NT, Stone P, et al. Tolerability of sumatriptan: clinical trials and post-marketing experience. *Cephalalgia* 2000;20:687–695.

Preventive Anti-Migraine Drugs

Stephen Silberstein, MD, Meryl Latsko,
MD, MPH, and Jean Schoenen, MD, PhD

INTRODUCTION

The pharmacological treatment of migraine headache may be acute (abortive) or preventive (prophylactic). Patients with frequent severe headaches often require both types of approaches. Preventive therapy is used to try to reduce the frequency, duration, or severity of attacks.

Additional benefits include enhancing the response to acute treatments, improving a patient's ability to function, and reducing disability (Lipton & Silberstein, 1994). Preventive treatment may also result in health-care cost reductions (Silberstein et al., 2003). Recent U.S. and European guidelines (Silberstein, 2004; Lipton et al., 2005) have established the circumstances that might warrant preventive treatment: (1) recurring migraine that significantly interferes with a patient's quality of life and daily routine despite acute treatment; (2) four or more attacks per month; (3) failure of, contraindication to, or troublesome side effects from acute medications; and (4) frequent, very long, or uncomfortable auras (Silberstein, 2004; Lipton et al., 2005).

A migraine preventive drug is considered successful if it reduces migraine attack frequency by at least 50% within 3 months. A migraine diary is highly recommended for treatment evaluation (Silberstein, 2004; Lipton et al., 2005) (**Table 10.1**).

Prevention is not being utilized to the extent it should be; only 13% of all migraineurs currently use preventive therapy to control their attacks (Lipton et al., 2005). According to the American Migraine Prevalence and Prevention (AMPP) Study, 38.8% of patients with migraine should be considered for (13.1%) or offered (25.7%) migraine preventive therapy (Silberstein et al., 2005a).

Table 10.1 U.S. Evidence-Based Guidelines for Migraine: Indications for Preventive Treatment

1. Recurring migraine that significantly interferes with the patient's daily routine despite acute treatment (e.g., two or more attacks a month that produce disability that lasts 3 or more days, or headache attacks that are infrequent but produce profound disability)

2. Failure of, contraindication to, or troublesome side effects from acute medications

3. Overuse of acute medications

4. Special circumstances, such as hemiplegic migraine or attacks with a risk of permanent neurologic injury

5. Very frequent headaches (more than two per week) or a pattern of increasing attacks over time, with the risk of developing medication-overuse headache

6. Patient preference—that is, the desire to have as few acute attacks as possible

The major medication groups for preventive migraine treatment include anticonvulsants, antidepressants, β-adrenergic blockers, calcium-channel antagonists, serotonin antagonists, botulinum neurotoxins, nonsteroidal anti-inflammatory drugs (NSAIDs), and others (including riboflavin, magnesium, and Petasites). If preventive medication is indicated, the agent should be chosen from one of the first-line categories based on the drug's relative efficacy in double-blind, placebo-controlled trials, its side-effect profile, and the patient's preference, as well as coexistent and comorbid conditions (Tfelt-Hansen, 2000). The next section describes general principles of preventive therapy, based on the authors' experience.

PRINCIPLES OF PREVENTIVE THERAPY

When preventive therapy is prescribed, it is important to start the chosen drug at a low dose and increase it slowly until therapeutic effects develop, the ceiling dose for the chosen drug is reached, or adverse events (AEs) become intolerable.

- Give each treatment an adequate trial. The full benefit of the drug may not be realized until 6 months have elapsed.

- Set realistic goals. Success is defined as a 50% reduction in attack frequency, a significant decrease in attack duration, or an improved response to acute medication.

- Set realistic expectations regarding AEs. The risk and extent of AEs vary greatly from patient to patient, and there is currently no way to predict the presence or severity of AEs for an individual patient. Most AEs are self-limited and dose-dependent, and patients should be encouraged to tolerate the early AEs that may develop when a new medication is started.

- Avoid acute headache medication overuse and drugs that are contraindicated because of coexistent or comorbid illnesses.

- Reevaluate therapy and, if possible, taper or discontinue the drug after a sustained period of remission (6 to 9 months).

- Make a woman of childbearing potential aware of any potential risks associated with the drug, and choose the medication that will have the least potential for adverse effect on a fetus (Silberstein, 1997).

- To maximize compliance, involve patients in their own care. Take patient preferences into account when deciding between drugs of relatively equivalent efficacy and tolerability.

- Consider comorbidity, which is the presence of two or more disorders whose association is more likely than chance. Conditions that are comorbid with migraine are shown in **Table 10.2** (Ryan & Sudilovsky, 1983; Ryan, 1984; Olerud et al., 1986; Sudilovsky et al., 1986).

Preventive treatment is often recommended for only 6 to 9 months, but few randomized, placebo-controlled trials have been performed to investigate migraine frequency after the preventive treatment has been

Table 10.2 Migraine Comorbid Diseases

Cardiovascular	Psychiatric	Neurologic	Gastrointestinal	Other
Hypertension/hypotension	Depression	Epilepsy	Irritable bowel syndrome	Asthma
Raynaud's syndrome	Mania	Positional vertigo (may be migrainous vertigo)		Allergies
In migraine with aura:	Panic disorder			Other chronic pain disorders
• Patent foramen ovale	Anxiety disorder	Restless legs syndrome		
• Mitral valve prolapse, stroke		Essential tremor (controversial)		
• Myocardial infarction (controversial)				

discontinued. Diener et al. (2007) assessed 818 migraine patients who were treated with topiramate for 6 months to see the effects of topiramate discontinuation. Patients received topiramate in a 26-week open-label phase. They were then randomly assigned to continue this dose or switch to placebo for a 26-week, double-blind phase. Of the 559 patients who completed the open-label phase, 514 entered the double-blind phase and were assigned to topiramate ($n = 255$) or placebo ($n = 259$). The mean increase in number of migraine days was greater in the placebo group (1.19 days in 4 weeks; 95% CI: 0.71 to 1.66; $P <0.001$) than in the topiramate group (0.10 day in 4 weeks; 95% CI: –0.36 to 0.56; $P = 0.5756$). Patients in the placebo group had a greater number of days on acute medication than did those in the topiramate group (mean difference between groups: –0.95; 95% CI:–1.49 to –0.41; $P = 0.0007$). A sustained benefit was reported after topiramate was discontinued, although the number of migraine days did increase. These findings suggest that patients should be treated for 6 months, with the option to continue to 12 months.

SPECIFIC MIGRAINE PREVENTIVE AGENTS

β-Adrenergic Blockers

β-blockers (**Table 10.3**), the most widely used class of drugs in prophylactic migraine treatment, are approximately 50% effective in producing a greater than 50% reduction in attack frequency. Evidence has consistently demonstrated the efficacy (Gray et al., 1999; Silberstein, 2000) of the nonselective β-blocker propranolol (Ryan & Sudilovsky, 1983; Ryan, 1984; Cortelli et al., 1985; Koella, 1985; Sudilovsky et al., 1986; Andersson & Vinge, 1990; Gray et al., 1999; Silberstein, 2000; Ramadan, 2004) and of the selective β1-blocker metoprolol (Ryan & Sudilovsky, 1983; Ryan, 1984; Tfelt-Hansen et al., 1984; Sudilovsky et al., 1987; Andersson & Vinge, 1990; Panerai et al., 1990). Atenolol (Kishore-Kumar et al., 1990), bisoprolol (Feinmann, 1985; Panerai et al., 1990), nadolol (Baldessarini, 1990; Richelson, 1990), and timolol (Abramowicz, 1990; Gray et al., 1999) are also likely to be effective. β-blockers with intrinsic sympathomimetic activity (e.g., acebutolol, alprenolol, oxprenolol, pindolol) are not effective for migraine prevention. Propranolol is effective for migraine prevention in a daily dose of 120 to 240 mg, but no correlation has been found between its dose and its clinical efficacy.

The action of β-blockers is probably central and could be mediated by three approaches: (1) inhibiting central β-receptors that interfere with the vigilance-enhancing

Table 10.3 Beta-Blockers and Antidepressants in the Preventive Treatment of Migraine

Agent	Daily Dose	Comment
Beta-Blockers		
Atenolol	50 mg to 200 mg	Use QD Fewer side effects than propranolol
Bisoprolol	5 mg to 10 mg	Use QD
Metoprolol	100 mg to 200 mg	Use the long-acting form QD
Nadolol	20 mg to 160 mg	Use QD Fewer side effects than propranolol
Propranolol	40 mg to 400 mg	Use the long-acting form QD or BID 1 to 2 mg/kg in children
Timolol	20 mg to 60 mg	Divide the dose Short half-life
Antidepressants		
Tertiary Amines		
Amitrip-tyline	10 mg to 400 mg	Start at 10 mg at bedtime
Doxepin	10 mg to 300 mg	Start at 10 mg at bedtime
Secondary Amines		
Nortrip-tyline	10 mg to 150 mg	Start at 10 to 25 mg at bedtime If insomnia, give early in the morning
Protriptyline	5 mg to 60 mg	Start at 10 to 25 mg at bedtime
Selective Serotonin and Norepinephrine Reuptake Inhibitors		
Venlafaxine	75 to 225 mg	Start 37.5 mg in the morning

adrenergic pathways; (2) interaction with 5-HT receptors (although not all effective β-blockers bind to these receptors); and (3) cross-modulation of the serotonin system (Koella, 1985). Propranolol inhibits nitrous oxide production by blocking inducible nitric oxide synthase. This agent also inhibits kainate-induced currents and is synergistic with N-methyl-ᴅ-aspartate blockers, which reduce neuronal activity and have membrane-stabilizing properties (Ramadan, 2004). β-Blockers tend to normalize habituation of cortical evoked potentials that is reduced in migraine patients between attacks (Sándor et al., 2000).

Contraindications to the use of β-blockers include asthma and chronic obstructive lung disease, congestive heart failure, atrioventricular conduction defects, Raynaud's disease, peripheral vascular disease, and brittle diabetes. All β-blockers can produce behavioral AEs, such as drowsiness, fatigue, lethargy, sleep disorders, nightmares, depression, memory disturbance, and hallucinations (Gray et al., 1999). Other potential AEs include gastrointestinal complaints, decreased exercise tolerance, orthostatic hypotension, bradycardia, and impotence. Although stroke has been reported to occur after patients with migraine with aura were started on β-blockers, there is neither an absolute nor a relative contraindication to their use in patients with migraine, either with or without aura.

Evidence for β-Blockers in the Prevention of Migraine

The strength of the evidence supporting the use of β-blockers as migraine prophylaxis is summarized here and in Appendix 10.1 (Silberstein et al., 2000; Evers et al., 2009; Silberstein et al., 2012):

- Strong evidence exists (Level A) establishing the effectiveness of metoprolol, propranolol, and timolol.
- Evidence exists (Level B) to suggest that the following agents are probably effective and should be considered: bisoprolol, atenolol, and nadolol.
- The following is possibly effective (Level C) and may be considered: nebivolol.
- There is inadequate evidence to support or refute the use of the following: pindolol.

Tolerability

Besides the known contraindications, the major limiting adverse effects of β-blockers are fatigue, depressive mood, and hypotension (and erectile dysfunction in males).

Antidepressants

Antidepressants (see Table 10.3) consist of a number of different drug classes with different mechanisms of action. Only one member of the class of tricyclic antidepressants (TCAs)—amitriptyline—has some proven efficacy in migraine (Silberstein, 2000). Although the mechanism by which antidepressants work to prevent migraine headache is uncertain, it does not result from treating masked depression. Antidepressants are useful in treating many chronic pain states, including headache, independent of the presence of depression, and the response occurs sooner than the expected antidepressant effect (Kishore-Kumar et al., 1990; Panerai et al., 1990). In animal pain models, antidepressants have been shown to potentiate the effects of co-administered opioids (Feinmann, 1985). The antidepressants that are clinically effective in headache prevention either inhibit noradrenaline and 5-HT reuptake or are antagonists at the 5-HT_2 receptors (Richelson, 1990).

The TCA dose range is wide and must be individualized. Most TCAs are sedating. Start with a low dose of the chosen TCA at bedtime, except when using protriptyline, which should be administered in the morning. If the TCA is too sedating, switch from a tertiary TCA (e.g., amitriptyline, doxepin) to a secondary TCA (e.g., nortriptyline, protriptyline, clomipramine). AEs are common with TCA use. Antimuscarinic AEs include dry mouth, a metallic taste, epigastric distress, constipation, dizziness, mental confusion, tachycardia, palpitations, blurred vision, and urinary retention. Other AEs include weight gain (rarely seen with protriptyline), orthostatic hypotension, reflex tachycardia, and palpitations. Antidepressant treatment may change depression to hypomania or frank mania (particularly in bipolar patients). Older patients may develop confusion or delirium (Baldessarini, 1990). The muscarinic and adrenergic effects of these agents may pose increased risks for patients with cardiac conduction abnormalities, especially in elderly individuals, and these patients should be carefully monitored or other agents considered.

Amitriptyline and doxepin are both known to be sedating. Patients with coexistent depression may require higher doses of these drugs to treat underlying depression. Start these drugs at a dose of 10 to 25 mg at bedtime. The usual effective dosage for migraine ranges from 25 to 200 mg. Nortriptyline, a major metabolite of amitriptyline, is a secondary amine that is less sedating than amitriptyline. It is started at a dose of 10 to 25 mg at bedtime, with the total dose ranging from 10 to 150 mg per day. Protriptyline is a secondary amine that is similar to nortriptyline. It is started at a dose of 5 mg in the morning; the total dose ranges from 5 to 60 mg per day, given as either a single or split dose.

Evidence for the use of selective serotonin reuptake inhibitors (SSRIs) or other antidepressants for migraine prevention is poor. Fluoxetine in doses between 10 and 40 mg proved effective in three placebo-controlled trials and not effective in one placebo-controlled trial (Mathew et al., 1995b; Silberstein et al., 1995; Silberstein et al., 2001). Other antidepressants not effective in placebo-controlled trials include clomipramine and sertraline; for other antidepressants, only data from open or not placebo-controlled trials are available. Because their tolerability profile is superior to that of TCAs, SSRIs may be helpful for patients with comorbid depression (Lipton et al., 2002). The most common AEs noted with these agents include sexual dysfunction, anxiety, nervousness, insomnia, drowsiness, fatigue, tremor, sweating, anorexia, nausea, vomiting, and dizziness or lightheadedness. The combination of an SSRI and a TCA can be beneficial in treating refractory depression (Bowden et al., 1994) and, in our experience, resistant cases of migraine. Such a combination may require the TCA dose to be adjusted, because TCA plasma levels may significantly increase.

Venlafaxine, a selective serotonin and norepinephrine reuptake inhibitor, has been shown to be effective in a double-blind, placebo-controlled trial (Ozyalcin et al., 2005) and a separate placebo- and amitriptyline-controlled trial (Bulut et al., 2004). The usual effective dose is 150 mg per day. Start with the extended-release 37.5-mg tablet for 1 week, then give 75 mg for 1 week, and then give the extended-release 150-mg tablet in the morning. AEs associated with venlafaxine include insomnia, nervousness, mydriasis, and seizures.

Evidence for Antidepressants in the Prevention of Migraine

The strength of the evidence supporting use of antidepressants as migraine prophylaxis is summarized here (Silberstein et al., 2000; Evers et al., 2009; Silberstein et al., 2012):

- There is no strong evidence (Level A) for any antidepressants.
- The following are probably effective (Level B) and should be considered: amitriptyline and venlafaxine.
- There is Level C evidence that fluoxetine may be considered, but available data are controversial.
- There is inadequate evidence to support or refute (Level U) the use of the following: fluvoxamine and protriptyline.

Tolerability

Dry mouth, sedation, and weight gain are the major limiting AEs for tricyclic antidepressants.

Calcium-Channel Antagonists

Two types of calcium channels exist: calcium entry channels, which allow extracellular calcium to enter the cell, and calcium release channels, which allow intracellular calcium (in storage sites in organelles) to enter the cytoplasm (Greenberg, 1997). Calcium entry channel subtypes include voltage-gated channels, which are opened by depolarization; ligand-gated channels, which are opened by chemical messengers, such as glutamate; and capacitative channels, which are activated by depletion of intracellular calcium stores. The mechanism of action of the calcium-channel antagonists (**Table 10.4**) in migraine prevention is uncertain, but possibilities include inhibition of 5-HT release, neurovascular inflammation, or the initiation and propagation of cortical spreading depression (Wauquier et al., 1985).

Flunarizine, a nonselective calcium-channel antagonist with antidopaminergic properties, was reported to be superior to placebo in six of seven randomized clinical trials investigating its use in migraine prevention (Riopelle & McCans, 1982; Markley et al., 1984; Tfelt-Hansen et al., 1984; Smith & Schwartz, 1984; Cortelli et al., 1985; Wauquier et al., 1985; Solomon, 1986; Greenberg, 1997;

Table 10.4 Selected Calcium-Channel Blockers and Anticonvulsants Used in the Preventive Treatment of Migraine

Agent	Daily Dose	Comment
Calcium-Channel Blockers		
Verapamil	120 mg to 640 mg	Start 80 mg BID or TID Sustained-release formulation can be given QD or BID
Flunarizine	5 mg to 10 mg	QD at bedtime Better tolerated in children and adolescents than in adults
Anticonvulsants		
Topiramate	100 mg	Start 15 to 25 mg at bedtime Increase 15 to 25 mg per week Attempt to reach 50 to 100 mg Increase further if necessary Associated with weight loss, not weight gain
Valproate/divalproex	500 mg to 1,500 mg/day	Use long-acting form QD Start 250 to 500 mg per day Monitor blood levels if compliance is an issue Maximum dose is 60 mg/kg per day

Reveiz-Herault et al., 2003; Bulut et al., 2004; Ozyalcin et al., 2005). Its usual dose is 5 to 10 mg given at night (women seem to need lower doses than men). The most prominent AEs associated with this agent include weight gain, somnolence, dry mouth, dizziness, hypotension, occasional extrapyramidal reactions, and exacerbation of depression. Because of its side-effect profile, flunarizine should be considered as a second-line drug for migraine prevention, after β-blockers. Flunarizine is widely used in Europe, but is not available in the United States, where verapamil is the recommended calcium-channel antagonist.

Verapamil was found to be more effective than placebo in two of three migraine prevention trials, but both positive trials were very small and dropout rates were high, rendering the findings of uncertain validity (Rompel & Bauermeister, 1970; Hanston & Horn, 1985; Mathew et al., 2001). Rigorous, randomized, controlled trial evidence to support the use of verapamil for migraine is lacking, as is the case for most older anti-migraine drugs. Nimodipine, nicardipine, diltiazem, and cyclandelate—other nonselective calcium-channel antagonists—have not shown superiority over placebo in well-designed clinical trials and cannot be recommended for migraine prophylaxis.

Evidence for Calcium-Channel Blockers in the Prevention of Migraine

The strength of the evidence supporting the use of calcium-channel blockers for migraine prophylaxis is summarized here (Silberstein et al., 2000; Evers et al., 2009; Silberstein et al., 2012):

- One agent has strong evidence (Level A): flunarazine. European guidelines are used for this agent because it is not marketed in the United States.
- The following is probably effective (Level B) and should be considered: verapamil.
- There is inadequate evidence (Level U) to support or refute the use of the following: nicardipine, nifedipine, cyclandelate, and nimodipine.

Tolerability

Fatigue, depression, and weight gain are the major limiting AEs with flunarizine. Flunarizine is better tolerated in children and adolescents than in adults; it can induce (or reveal) Parkinsonian symptoms in elderly patients. Fatigue, constipation, leg edema, and hypotension are the limiting factors for verapamil.

Anticonvulsants

Anticonvulsants (see Table 10.4) are being increasingly recommended for migraine prevention as more data from well-conducted placebo-controlled trials become available. With the exception of valproic acid, topiramate, and zonisamide, anticonvulsants may substantially interfere with the efficacy of oral contraceptives (Coulam & Annagers, 1979; Hanston & Horn, 1985).

Carbamazepine

The only placebo-controlled trial of carbamazepine that suggested a significant benefit suffered from methodologic issues in several important respects (Rompel & Bauermeister, 1970). Thus there is no credible evidence that carbamazepine, 600 to 1,200 mg per day, is an effective preventive migraine treatment, and it is rarely used in clinical practice for this purpose.

Gabapentin

Gabapentin (1,800 to 2,400 mg) showed efficacy in a placebo-controlled, double-blind trial only when a modified intent-to-treat analysis was used. Migraine attack frequency was reduced by 50% in approximately one-third of patients (Mathew et al., 2001). The most common AEs were dizziness or giddiness and drowsiness.

Valproic Acid

Valproic acid is a simple 8-carbon, 2-chain fatty acid; divalproex sodium (which has been approved by the U.S. Food and Drug Administration [FDA]) is a combination of valproic acid and sodium valproate. Both agents are effective in preventing migraine (Klapper, 1995, 1997), as is an extended-release form of divalproex sodium (Freitag et al., 2003). In 1992, Hering and Kuritzky evaluated sodium valproate's efficacy in migraine treatment in a double-blind, randomized, cross-over study. Sodium valproate was effective in preventing migraine or reducing the frequency, severity, and duration of attacks in 86.2% of 29 patients, whose attacks were reduced from 15.6 to 8.8 per month. In 1994, Jensen et al. (1994) studied 43 patients with migraine without aura in a triple-blind, placebo- and dose-controlled, cross-over study of slow-release sodium valproate. In the valproate group, 50% of the patients had a reduction in migraine frequency to 50% or less of their initial rate, compared with a reduction of 18% achieved with placebo.

Several subsequent randomized, placebo-controlled studies have confirmed these results, with significant responder rates ranging between 43 % and 48 % (Smith & Schwartz, 1984; Jensen et al., 1994) being achieved with dosages ranging from 500 to 1,500 mg per day. Extended-release divalproex sodium has also been shown to be effective for migraine prevention, and both compliance and side-effect profile may be more favorable with this formulation (Mathew et al., 1995a).

Nausea, vomiting, and gastrointestinal distress are the AEs that occur most commonly with valproic acid; their incidence decreases, however, particularly after 6 months. Tremor and alopecia can occur later. Valproate has little effect on cognitive functions and rarely causes sedation. Rare, severe AEs include hepatitis and pancreatitis; their frequency varies with the number of concomitant medications used, the patient's age, the presence of genetic and metabolic disorders, and the patient's general state of health. These idiosyncratic reactions are unpredictable (Pellock & Willmore, 1991). Valproate is also teratogenic (Silberstein, 1996). Hyperandrogenism, ovarian cysts, and obesity are of concern in young women with epilepsy who use valproate (Vainionpaa et al., 1999). Absolute contraindications are pregnancy and a history of pancreatitis or a hepatic disorder; relative contraindications include thrombocytopenia, pancytopenia, and bleeding disorders.

Valproic acid is available as 250-mg capsules and as syrup (250 mg/5 mL). Divalproex sodium is available as 125-, 250-, and 500-mg capsules and as a sprinkle formulation. Slow-release sodium valproate is available in Europe in 300- and 500-mg capsules. The recommended regimen is to start with 250 to 500 mg per day in divided doses and slowly increase the dose. Monitor serum levels if a question of toxicity or compliance arises. The maximum recommended dose is 60 mg/kg/day.

Topiramate

Topiramate was originally synthesized as part of a research project to discover structural analogues of fructose-1,6-diphosphate capable of inhibiting the enzyme fructose-1,6-bisphosphatase, thereby blocking gluconeogenesis. Researchers discovered, however, that this agent has no hypoglycemic activity. Topiramate and divalproex sodium are the only two anticonvulsants that have received FDA approval for migraine prevention. Topiramate is not associated with significant reductions in estrogen exposure at doses of less than 200 mg per day. At doses greater than 200 mg per day, there may be a dose-related reduction in exposure to the estrogen component of oral contraceptives.

Two large, pivotal, multicenter, randomized, double-blind, placebo-controlled clinical trials assessed the efficacy and safety of topiramate (50, 100, and 200 mg/day) in migraine prevention. In the first trial, the responder rate (patients with 50 % or greater reduction in monthly migraine frequency) was 52 % with topiramate 200 mg/day ($P < 0.001$), 54 % with topiramate 100 mg ($P < 0.001$), and 36 % with topiramate 50 mg/day ($P = 0.039$), compared with 23 % with placebo (Silberstein et al., 2004). The 200-mg dose was not significantly more effective than the 100-mg dose. The second pivotal trial (Brandes et al., 2004) had significantly more patients who exhibited at least a 50 % reduction in mean monthly migraines in the groups treated with 50 mg/day of topiramate (39 %; $P = 0.009$), 100 mg/day of topiramate (49 %; $P = 0.001$), and 200 mg/day of topiramate (47 %; $P = 0.001$).

A third randomized, double-blind, parallel-group, multicenter trial (Diener et al., 2004) compared two doses of topiramate (100 mg/day or 200 mg/day) to placebo or propranolol (160 mg/day). Topiramate 100 mg/day was superior to placebo as measured by average monthly migraine period rate, average monthly migraine days, rate of rescue medication use, and percentage of patients with a 50 % or greater decrease in average monthly migraine period rate (responder rate = 37 %). The topiramate 100 mg/day and propranolol groups were similar in change from baseline to the core double-blind phase in average monthly migraine period rate and other secondary efficacy variables.

Topiramate's most common AE is paresthesia; other AEs associated with this agent include fatigue, decreased appetite, nausea, diarrhea, weight decrease, taste perversion, hypoesthesia, and abdominal pain. In the migraine trials, body weight was reduced by an average of 2.3 % in the 50-mg group, 3.2 % in the 100-mg group, and 3.8 % in the 200-mg group. Patients on propranolol gained 2.3 % of their baseline body weight. The AEs most commonly reported in this study were somnolence, insomnia, mood problems, anxiety, difficulty with memory, language problems, and difficulty with concentration. Renal calculi can also occur with topiramate use; the reported incidence of this condition is approximately 1.5 %, representing a twofold to fourfold increase over the estimated occurrence in the general population (Sachedo et al., 1997).

A very rare AE reported with topiramate is acute myopia associated with secondary angle closure glaucoma. No cases of this condition were reported in the clinical studies (Thomson Healthcare, 2003). Oligohidrosis has been reported in association with an elevation in body temperature; most of these reports have involved children.

When topiramate is given, it is recommended to start at a dose of 15 to 25 mg given at bedtime, and then increase by a dose of 15 to 25 mg/week. Do not increase the dose if bothersome AEs develop; wait until they resolve (they usually do). If they do not resolve, decrease the drug to the last tolerable dose, then increase by a lower dose more slowly. Attempt to reach a dose of 50 to 100 mg/day given twice daily. It is our experience that patients who tolerate the lower doses with only partial improvement often have increased benefit with higher doses. The dose can be increased to 600 mg/day or higher.

Lamotrigine

Lamotrigine blocks voltage-sensitive sodium channels, leading to inhibition of neuronal glutamate release of glutamate. Chen et al. (2001) have reported the use of this drug in two patients with migraine with persistent aura-like visual phenomena for months to years. After 2 weeks of lamotrigine treatment, both had resolution of their visual symptoms.

Although open-label studies have suggested that lamotrigine may have a select role in the treatment of patients with frequent or prolonged aura, results from a placebo-controlled study in migraine without aura were negative. Steiner et al. (1997) compared the safety and efficacy of lamotrigine (200 mg/day) and placebo in migraine prophylaxis in a double-blind, randomized, parallel-groups trial. Improvements were greater on placebo, and these changes, which were not statistically significant, indicate that lamotrigine was ineffective for migraine prophylaxis. More AEs were observed among patients on lamotrigine than on placebo, most commonly rash. With slow dose escalation, their frequency was reduced and the rate of withdrawal due to AEs was similar in both treatment groups.

Several open-label studies have suggested that lamotrigine may have a select role in the treatment of migraine with aura, but no placebo-controlled studies have been conducted as yet in this patient population. Both lamotrigine and topiramate (Freitag, 2003) may have a special role in the treatment of migraine with aura. A more recent Class I cross-over trial comparing lamotrigine 50 mg/day to placebo or topiramate 50 mg/day in a mixed group of patients (30% of whom had migraine with aura) reported that lamotrigine was not more effective than placebo (Gupta et al., 2007). The primary outcome measure (responder rate of 50% or greater reduction in monthly migraine frequency) was 46% for lamotrigine versus 34% for placebo ($P = 0.093$; 95% CI: 0.02–0.26), and 63% for topiramate versus 46% for lamotrigine ($P = 0.019$; 95% CI: 0.03–0.31).

Lamotrigine, however, was more effective than placebo on the secondary outcome measure monthly headache frequency (−1.13; $P = 0.002$), but less effective than topiramate (−1.98; $P < 0.001$).

Evidence for Anticonvulsants in the Prevention of Migraine

The strength of the evidence supporting the use of anticonvulsants in migraine prophylaxis is summarized here (Silberstein et al., 2000; Evers et al., 2009; Silberstein et al., 2012):

- There is strong evidence (Level A) establishing the effectiveness of the following: divalproex sodium, sodium valproate, and topiramate.
- The following anticonvulsant is possibly effective (Level C): gabapentin.
- Lamotrigine is ineffective in migraine prevention overall (Level A Negative), but Level C evidence supports consideration of its use in migraine with aura. There is no proven efficacy of carbamazepine in migraine prevention (Level U).

Tolerability

Anticonvulsants have a high prevalence of side effects. For sodium valproate, both the number needed to treat (1.6) and the number needed to harm (2.4) are low (Schoenen et al., 1998). The major limiting AEs for valproate are GI problems (early), fatigue, weight gain, alopecia, and tremor (late). For topiramate, these effects are mood changes, cognitive disturbances, anorexia, dysgeusia, and paresthesias.

Other Drugs

Other drugs used to prevent migraine are summarized in **Table 10.5**.

Angiotensin-Converting Enzyme Inhibitors and Angiotensin II Receptor Antagonists

Schrader et al. (2001) conducted a double-blind, placebo-controlled, cross-over study of lisinopril, an angiotensin-converting enzyme inhibitor, in migraine prophylaxis. Days with migraine were reduced by at least 50% in 14 participants for active treatment versus placebo and in 17 patients for active treatment versus run-in period. Days with migraine were cut by at least 50% in 14 participants for active treatment versus placebo.

Tronvik et al. (2003) have performed a randomized, double-blind, placebo-controlled, cross-over study of candesartan (16 mg), an angiotensin II receptor blocker, in migraine prevention. In a period of 12 weeks, the mean number of days with headache was 18.5 with placebo versus 13.6 with candesartan ($P = 0.001$) in the intention-to-treat analysis ($n = 57$). The number of candesartan responders (reduction of 50% or more compared with placebo) was 18 of 57 (31.6%) for days with headache and 23 of 57 (40.4%) for days with migraine. AEs were similar in the two periods. In this study, the angiotensin II receptor blocker candesartan was effective, with a tolerability profile comparable to that of placebo.

Evidence for ACE Inhibitors and Angiotensin II Receptor Antagonists in the Prevention of Migraine
The strength of the evidence supporting the use of ACE inhibitors and angiotensin II receptor antagonists in migraine prophylaxis is summarized here (Silberstein et al., 2000; Evers et al., 2009; Silberstein et al., 2012):

- The following are probably effective (Level B) and may be considered: candesartan and telmisartan.
- Lisinopril is possibly effective (level C).

Tolerability   An advantage of the angiotensin II receptor antagonists (sartans) is their excellent tolerance. The major limiting AE of lisinopril is cough.

Botulinum Toxin Type A

Botulinum toxin type A is discussed in detail in Chapter 27.

Vitamins and Medicinal Herbs

A major problem with vitamins and herbal extracts is that the concentration and bioavailability of the active compound may greatly vary between the various commercialized preparations (see **Table 10.5**).

Feverfew (*Tanacetum parthenium*) is a medicinal herb whose effectiveness has not been totally established (Vogler et al., 1998). Different preparations of feverfew containing various concentrations of parthenolide, the active component, are available in some countries.

Riboflavin (400 mg) was effective in migraine prevention in one placebo-controlled, double-blind trial. More than half of the patients responded (Schoenen et al., 1998).

Petasites hybridus root (butterbur) is a perennial shrub (Lipton et al., 2001). A standardized extract of this plant (75 mg twice daily) was effective in preventing migraine in two double-blind, placebo-controlled studies (Grossmann & Schmidramsl, 2000; Lipton et al., 2002, 2004). The most common AE was belching.

Table 10.5 Miscellaneous Medications Used in the Preventive Treatment of Migraine

Agent	Daily Dose	Comment
Angiotensin-Converting Enzyme (ACE) Inhibitors and Angiotensin Receptor Antagonists		
Lisinopril	10 to 40 mg	Positive small controlled trial
Candesartan	16 mg	Positive small controlled trial
Others		
Feverfew	50 to 82 mg	Controversial evidence
Petasites	50 to 100 mg	75 and 100 mg better than placebo in independent trials
Riboflavin	400 mg QD	Positive small controlled trial. Intake during a meal for better absorption GI tolerance
Coenzyme Q	200 to 300 mg	Two positive small controlled trials. Dosage depends on bioavailability of preparation
Magnesium	400 to 600 mg	Controversial evidence

Coenzyme Q10 (Co-Q10) may be effective for the prevention of migraine. One small Class II study showed that a patented nanodispersion of well-characterized, very small nanoparticles containing Co-Q10 100 mg three times daily was significantly more effective than placebo in reducing attack frequency from baseline to 4 months following treatment (Sándor et al., 2005).

A phytoestrogen preparation of 60 mg soy isoflavones, 100 mg dong quai, and 50 mg black cohosh (each component standardized to its primary alkaloid) reduced menstrual migraine attack frequency versus placebo in a small Class II study (Burke et al., 2002).

Evidence for Vitamins and Medicinal Herbs in the Prevention of Migraine   The strength of the evidence supporting the use of vitamins and medicinal herbs in migraine prophylaxis is summarized here (Silberstein et al., 2000; Evers et al., 2009; Silberstein et al., 2012):

- Petasites (butterbur) is established as effective (Level A) and should be offered.
- Riboflavin (400 mg/day in adults) and feverfew are probably effective (Level B) and should be considered.

- Co-Q10 and magnesium are possibly effective (Level C) and may be considered.
- Omega-3 is possibly ineffective (Level C Negative) and may not be considered.

Tolerability   Feverfew occasionally produces AEs, the most frequent of which are mouth ulcerations and oral inflammation with loss of taste. Riboflavin may have rarely gastrointestinal AEs, and in exceptional cases may produce an allergic cutaneous rash. In Schoenen et al.'s (1998) riboflavin trial, the number needed to treat for effectiveness was 2.3 and the number needed to harm 33.3. The most prevalent AE with use of butterbur is burping. Butterbur is known to contain pyrrolizidines—alkaloid substances with hepatotoxic properties that may cause liver cancer and that must be completely removed during the manufacturing process (Danesch & Rittinghausen, 2003).

Aspirin and Other NSAIDs

The following NSAIDs are probably effective (Level B) for the prevention of migraine: aspirin, fenoprofen, ibuprofen, ketoprofen, naproxen, and naproxen sodium (Pradalier et al., 1988; Bensenor et al., 2001; Diener et al., 2001). Regular or daily use of selected NSAIDs for the treatment of frequent migraine attacks may exacerbate headache, however, due to development of a condition called medication-overuse headache (Silberstein et al., 2005b). Therefore, using aspirin, selected analgesics, and NSAIDs may exacerbate headache, which may confound the clinical interpretation of study results in migraine prevention.

Evidence for Aspirin and Other NSAIDS in the Prevention of Migraine   The strength of the evidence supporting the use of aspirin and other NSAIDs in migraine prophylaxis is summarized here (Silberstein et al., 2000; Evers et al., 2009; Silberstein et al., 2012):

- Aspirin is possibly effective (Level C) for migraine prevention (multiple Class II studies). Caution against overuse and exacerbation of headache is warranted.
- Aspirin may be useful in the prevention of frequent migraine with aura attacks (Massiou, 2000), but controlled trials are lacking.

Serotonin Receptor Antagonists

Methysergide, a compound blocking 5-HT$_2$ receptors but also active on other serotonin receptor subtypes, is among the first and rare drugs specifically designed for migraine prevention. Although it is undoubtedly effective in clinical practice, trials of sufficient methodological quality to provide evidence of its efficacy are lacking.

Methysergide, an ergot derivative, may cause fibrosis after its long-term use. This serious complication can, in principle, be prevented by taking a 1-month drug holiday after every 6-month treatment period. The major limiting AEs in the short term are abdominal and leg pains, nausea, fatigue, and appetite increase. Methysergide is contraindicated in patients with cardiovascular disorders.

Because of its unfavorable side-effect profile, methysergide should be restricted to migraine patients who have not been satisfied with other preventive drugs such as beta-blockers, anticonvulsants, and calcium-channel blockers. Doses should be increased progressively, starting with 1 mg during dinner and increasing the dose if necessary to 2 mg two or three times daily. Although it is available in Europe and other parts of the world, methysergide is no longer available in the United States.

SETTING TREATMENT PRIORITIES AND MANAGING COMORBIDITIES

The goals of preventive treatment of migraine are to reduce the frequency, duration, or severity of attacks, improve responsiveness to acute attack treatment, improve function, and reduce disability. The preventive medications with the best-documented efficacy are the beta-blockers, divalproex/sodium valproate, and topiramate. The choice of an agent is made based on a drug's proven efficacy, the physician's informed belief about medications not yet evaluated in controlled trials, the drug's AEs (**Table 10.6**), the patient's preferences and headache profile, and the presence or absence of coexisting disorders (Silberstein et al., 2001). Coexistent diseases have important implications for treatment. The presence of a second illness provides therapeutic opportunities but also imposes certain therapeutic limitations. In some instances, two or more conditions may be treated with a single drug. Use of a single medication to treat two illnesses has limitations, however. Notably, giving a single medication may not treat two different conditions optimally: Although one of the two conditions may be adequately treated, the second illness may require a higher or lower dose, such that the patient is at risk of the second illness not being adequately treated. Therapeutic independence may be needed should monotherapy fail. Avoiding drug interactions or increased AEs is a primary concern when using polypharmacy.

Given that most preventive therapies used for migraine were developed and initially approved for other indications,

Table 10.6 Migraine Prevention Drugs Grouped According to the Efficacy/Adverse Effect Ratio

High Efficacy: Moderate to High AEs	Low Efficacy: Low to Moderate AEs	Low Efficacy: Moderate to High AEs	Unproven Efficacy: Low to Moderate AEs	Proven Not Effective or Selective Efficacy
Propranolol, metoprolol, timolol, bisoprolol Valproate, topiramate Flunarizine Methysergide	Aspirin, flurbiprofen, ketoprofen, naproxen sodium, fenoprofen Atenolol, nadolol candesartan, lisinopril Vitamin B$_2$, coenzyme Q10, Petasites, feverfew Pizotifen	Amitriptyline Verapamil	Gabapentin Doxepin, nortriptyline, imipramine, protriptyline, venlafaxine, fluvoxamine, mirtazepine, paroxetine, protriptyline, sertraline, trazodone	Acebutolol, carbamazepine, clomipramine, clonazepam, indomethacin, nabumetone, nicardipine, nifedipine, pindolol Lamotrigine (ineffective for migraine without aura; possibly effective for migraine aura)

these medications not surprisingly have effects on other disorders, many of which may be comorbid with migraine (e.g., epilepsy, depression). Some of the substances can be used against several different comorbidities at the same time, such as beta-blockers, which have both antihypertensive and anxiolytic effects. Antiepileptic drugs can, in general, be used in comorbid pain conditions, such as neuropathic pain, and, of course, also in comorbid epilepsy; compared to comorbid pain disorders, however, comorbid epilepsy is relatively rare. ACE inhibitors and sartans have antihypertensive effects and can be used in patients suffering from a variety of heart conditions. Antidepressants, being effective against depression and anxiety, are often also useful in the treatment of neuropathic pain and insomnia. Furthermore, metabolic enhancers—such as riboflavin, coenzyme Q10, and possibly magnesium—can be used in the absence of comorbidities, and have the characteristic of being well tolerated. This profile makes them the treatment of choice for some clinicians, when combination therapies with the other mentioned classes of substances are planned.

In clinical practice, it often happens that a patient already has a treatment for a disorder comorbid with migraine. For optimal management, adequate communication between medical specialists is necessary to coordinate the respective pharmacotherapies.

As shown schematically in **Table 10.7**, three situations can occur regarding the reciprocal influence of migraine and comorbidity therapies: neutral, positive/beneficial, and negative/deleterious. In the ideal situation (Table 10.7, first line, first column, shaded light gray—"green light"), the anti-migraine preventive treatment has a strong beneficial effect on the comorbid disorder and monotherapy is

sufficient to manage both conditions. This situation might occur in depressed migraineurs in whom both migraine and depression are satisfactorily improved by a tricyclic antidepressant. However, appropriate management of depression often requires higher doses of TCAs, which may be associated with more AEs (Silberstein et al., 1995). A better approach might be to treat the depression with an SSRI or serotonin–norepinephrine reuptake inhibitor (SNRI) and treat the migraine with an anticonvulsant. Divalproex and topiramate are the drugs of choice for the patient with migraine and bipolar illness (Bowden et al., 1994; Silberstein, 1996), but again they will not be sufficient to treat the psychiatric disorder.

At the other end of the spectrum (Table 10.7, third line, third column, shaded dark gray—"red light"), the anti-migraine therapy can worsen the comorbid disorder, and vice versa. Such could be the case in a depressed migraineur who receives flunarizine, which can worsen depression, or an SSRI such as trazodone, which can worsen migraine. If this happens, both treatments need to be modified. If the preventive treatment of first choice for migraine has no therapeutic effect for the comorbid disorder (e.g., use of a beta-blocker in a migraineur who also has depression) or if monotherapy is not sufficient (e.g., a TCA is effective for the patient's migraine but not for his or her depression; Table 10.7, second line, second column, shaded middle gray—"orange light"), the patient obviously needs treatment with two distinct medications targeting each disorder.

Although monotherapy is preferred, it is often not the best choice and it may be necessary to combine preventive medications. Unfortunately, only some observational studies have assessed the benefit of combining two drugs for

Table 10.7 Management of the Treatments for Migraine and a Comorbid Disorder

Therapeutic recommendations considering possible reciprocal influences of migraine and comorbid disorder treatments			
Influence of the migraine treatment on the *comorbid* disorder	Influence of the *comorbid disorder* treatment on migraine		
	Beneficial	**Neutral**	**Deleterious**
Beneficial	*Monotherapy may suffice*	Migraine Ther ok (but add *Comorbid Ther* if necessary)	Migraine Ther ok but **Change** *Comorbid Ther*
Neutral	*Comorbid Ther ok* (but add MIG Ther if necessary)	**Migraine Ther** *combined to Comorbid Ther*	Change *Comorbid Ther*
Deleterious	*Comorbid Ther ok* but **Change** Migraine Ther	Change Migraine Ther	*Change* **Migraine** and *Comorbid Ther*

migraine prevention. In clinical practice, nonetheless, antidepressants are often used with beta-blockers or calcium-channel blockers, and topiramate or divalproex sodium may be used in combination with any of these medications.

CONCLUSIONS

Preventive therapy plays an important role in migraine management. With the addition of a preventive medication, patients may experience reduced attack frequency and improved response to acute treatment, which can result in reduced health-care resource utilization and improved quality of life. Despite research suggesting that a large percentage of migraine patients are candidates for prevention, only a fraction of these patients are receiving or have ever received preventive migraine medication.

Many preventive medications are available, and guidelines for their selection and use have been established. Nevertheless, these recommendations may differ to some extent depending on the criteria used for assessing the methodological quality of older trials, clinical experience, and local availability of drugs. Because comorbid medical and psychological illnesses are prevalent in patients with migraine, one must consider comorbidity when choosing preventive drugs. Drug therapy may be beneficial for both disorders, but it is also a potential confounder of optimal treatment of either condition.

No clinical trial data exist to predict among the various therapeutic options and biologic or clinical parameters. The impact of prevention on the natural history of migraine remains to be fully investigated.

REFERENCES

Abramowicz M. Fluoxetine (Prozac) revisited. *Drugs Ther Medical Letter* 1990;83–85.

Andersson K, Vinge E. Beta-adrenoceptor blockers and calcium antagonists in the prophylaxis and treatment of migraine. *Drugs* 1990;39:355–373.

Baldessarini RJ. Drugs and the treatment of psychiatric disorders. In: Gilman AG, Rall TW, Nies AS, Taylor P, eds. *The Pharmacological Basis of Therapeutics.* New York: Pergamon; 1990:383–435.

Bensenor IM, Cook NR, Lee IM, Chown MJ, Hennekens CH, Buring JE. Low-dose aspirin for migraine prophylaxis in women. *Cephalalgia* 2001;21:175–183.

Bowden CL, Brugger AM, Swann AC. Efficacy of divalproex vs lithium and placebo in the treatment of mania. *JAMA* 1994;271:918–924.

Brandes JL, Saper JR, Diamond M, Couch JR, Lewis DW, Schmitt J, Neto W, Schwabe S, Jacobs D, MIGR-002 Study Group. Topiramate for migraine prevention: a randomized controlled trial. *JAMA* 2004;291:965–973.

Bulut S, Berilgen MS, Baran A, Tekatas A, Atmaca M, Mungen B. Venlafaxine versus amitriptyline in the prophylactic treatment of migraine: randomized, double-blind, crossover study. *Clin Neurol Neurosurg* 2004;107:44–48.

Burke BE, Olson RD, Cusack BJ. Randomized, controlled trial of phytoestrogen in the prophylactic treatment of menstrual migraine. *Biomed Pharmacother* 2002;56:283–288.

Chen WT, Fuh JL, Lu SR, Wang SJ. Persistent migrainous visual phenomena might be responsive to lamotrigine. *Headache* 2001;41:823–825.

Cortelli P, Sacquegna T, Albani F, Baldrati A, D'Alessandro R, Baruzi A, Lugaresi E. Propranolol plasma levels and relief of migraine. *Arch Neurol* 1985;42:46–48.

Coulam CB, Annagers JR. New anticonvulsants reduce the efficacy of oral contraception. *Epilepsia* 1979;20:519–525.

Danesch U, Rittinghausen R. Safety of a patented special butterbur root extract for migraine prevention. *Headache* 2003;43(1):76–78.

Diener HC, Agosti R, Allais G, Bergmans P, Bussone G, Davies B, Ertas M, Lanteri-Minet M, Reuter U, Del Rio MS, Schoenen J, Schwalen S, van Oene J. Cessation versus continuation of 6-month migraine preventive therapy with topiramate (PROMPT): a randomised, double-blind, placebo-controlled trial. *Lancet Neurol* 2007;6:1054–1062.

Diener HC, Hartung E, Chrubasik J, Evers S, Schoenen J, Eikermann A, Latta G, Hauke W. A comparative study of oral acetylsalicylic acid and metoprolol for the prophylactic treatment of migraine: a randomized, controlled, double-blind, parallel group phase III study. *Cephalalgia* 2001;21:120–128.

Diener HC, Tfelt-Hansen P, Dahlof C, Lainez MJ, Sandrini G, Wang SJ, Neto W, Vijapurkar U, Doyle A, Jacobs D. Topiramate in migraine prophylaxis: results from a placebo-controlled trial with propranolol as an active control. *J Neurol* 2004;251:943–950.

Evers S, Áfra J, Frese A, Goadsby PJ, Linde M, May A, Sándor PS. EFNS guideline on the drug treatment of migraine: revised report of an EFNS task force. Eur J Neurol 2009;16:968–981.

Feinmann C. Pain relief by antidepressants: possible modes of action. *Pain* 1985;23:1–8.

Freitag FG. Topiramate prophylaxis in patients suffering from migraine with aura: results from a randomized, double-blind, placebo-controlled trial. *Adv Stud Med* 2003;3:S562–S564.

Freitag FG, Collins SD, Carlson HA, Goldstein J, Saper J, Silberstein SD, Mathew N, Winner PK, Deaton R, Sommerville K. A randomized trial of divalproex sodium extended-release tablets in migraine prophylaxis: for the Depakote ER Migraine Study Group. *Neurology* 2003;58:1652–1659.

Gray RN, Goslin RE, McCrory DC, Eberlein K, Tulsky J, Hasselblad V. *Drug Treatments for the Prevention of Migraine Headache.* Prepared for the Agency for Health Care Policy and Research, Contract No. 290-94-2025. Available from the National Technical Information Service Accession 1999; No. 127953.

Greenberg DA. Calcium channels in neurological disease. *Ann Neurol* 1997;42:275–282.

Grossmann M, Schmidramsl H. An extract of *Petasites hybridus* is effective in the prophylaxis of migraine. *Intl J Clin Pharmacol Therapeut* 2000;38:430–435.

Gupta P, Singh S, Goyal V, Shukla G, Behari M. Low-dose topiramate versus lamotrigine in migraine prophylaxis: the Lotolamp study. *Headache* 2007;47:402–412.

Hanston PP, Horn JR. Drug interaction. *Newsletter* 1985;5:7–10.

Hering R, Kuritzky A. Sodium valproate in the prophylactic treatment of migraine: a double-blind study versus placebo. *Cephalalgia* 1992;12:81–84.

Jensen R, Brinck T, Olesen J. Sodium valproate has prophylactic effect in migraine without aura: a triple-blind, placebo-controlled crossover study. *Neurology* 1994;44:241–244.

Kishore-Kumar R, Max MB, Schafer SC, Gaughan AM, Smoller B, Gracely RH, Dubner R. Desipramine relieves postherpetic neuralgia. *Clin Pharmacol Ther* 1990;47:305–312.

Klapper JA. An open label crossover comparison of divalproex sodium and propranolol HCl in the prevention of migraine headaches. *Headache Quarterly* 1995;5:50–53.

Klapper JA. Divalproex sodium in migraine prophylaxis: a dose-controlled study. *Cephalalgia* 1997;17:103–108.

Koella WP. CNS-related side-effects of β-blockers with special reference to mechanisms of action. *Eur J Clin Pharmacol* 1985;28:55–63.

Lipton RB, Silberstein SD. Why study the comorbidity of migraine? *Neurology* 1994;44:4–5.

Lipton RB, Hamelsky SW, Stewart WF. Epidemiology and impact of headache. In: Silberstein SD, Lipton RB, Dalessio DJ, eds. *Wolff's Headache and Other Head Pain.* New York: Oxford University Press; 2001:85–107.

Lipton RB, Gobel H, Wilks K, Mauskop A. Efficacy of Petasites (an extract from *Petasites rhizone*) 50 and 75mg for prophylaxis of migraine: results of a randomized, double-blind, placebo-controlled study. *Neurology* 2002;58:A472.

Lipton RB, Gobel H, Einhaupl KM, Wilks K, Mauskop A. *Petasites hybridus* root (butterbur) is an effective preventive treatment for migraine. *Neurology* 2004;63:2240–2244.

Lipton RB, Diamond M, Freitag F, Bigal M, Stewart WF, Reed ML. Migraine prevention patterns in a community sample: results from the American Migraine Prevalence and Prevention (AMPP) study [Abstract]. *Headache* 2005;45:792–793.

Markley HG, Cleronis JCD, Piepko RW. Verapamil prophylactic therapy of migraine. *Neurology* 1984;34:973–976.

Massiou H. [Prophylactic treatments of migraine]. *Rev Neurol (Paris)* 2000;156(suppl 4):4S79–4S86. [Article in French.]

Mathew NT, Saper JR, Silberstein SD, Rankin L, Markley HG, Solomon S, Rapoport AM, Silber CJ, Deaton RL. Migraine prophylaxis with divalproex. *Arch Neurol* 1995a;52:281–286.

Mathew NT, Saper JR, Silberstein SD, Tolander LR, Markley H, Solomon S, Rapoport A, Turkewitz LJ, Silber CJ, Deaton R. Prophylaxis of migraine headaches with divalproex sodium. *Arch Neurol* 1995b;52:281–286.

Mathew NT, Rapoport A, Saper J, Magnus L, Klapper J, Ramadan N, Stacey B, Tepper S. Efficacy of gabapentin in migraine prophylaxis. *Headache* 2001;41:119–128.

Olerud B, Gustavsson CL, Furberg B. Nadolol and propranolol in migraine management. *Headache* 1986;26:490–493.

Ozyalcin SN, Talu GK, Kiziltan E, Yucel B, Ertas M, Disci R. The efficacy and safety of venlafaxine in the prophylaxis of migraine. *Headache* 2005;45:144–152.

Panerai AE, Monza G, Movilia P, Bianchi M, Francussi BM, Tiengo M. A randomized, within-patient, cross-over, placebo-controlled trial on the efficacy and tolerability of the tricyclic antidepressants chlorimipramine and nortriptyline in central pain. *Acta Neurol Scand* 1990;82:34–38.

Pellock JM, Willmore LJ. A rational guide to routine blood monitoring in patients receiving antiepileptic drugs. *Neurology* 1991;41:961–964.

Pradalier A, Clapin A, Dry J. Treatment review: nonsteroid antiinflammatory drugs in the treatment and long-term prevention of migraine attacks. *Headache* 1988;28:550–557.

Ramadan NM. Prophylactic migraine therapy: mechanisms and evidence. *Curr Pain Headache Rep* 2004;8:91–95.

Reveiz-Herault L, Cardona AF, Ospina EG, Carrillo P. [Effectiveness of flunarizine in the prophylaxis of migraine: a meta-analytical review of the literature]. *Rev Neurol* 2003;36:907–912.

Richelson E. Antidepressants and brain neurochemistry. *Mayo Clin Proc* 1990;65:1227–1236.

Riopelle R, McCans JL. A pilot study of the calcium channel antagonist diltiazem in migraine syndrome prophylaxis. *Can J Neurol Sci* 1982;9:269.

Rompel H, Bauermeister PW. Aetiology of migraine and prevention with carbamazepine (Tegretol). *S Afr Med J* 1970;44:75–80.

Ryan RE. Comparative study of nadolol and propranolol in prophylactic treatment of migraine. *Am Heart J* 1984;108:1156–1159.

Ryan RE, Sudilovsky A. Nadolol: its use in the prophylactic treatment of migraine. *Headache* 1983;23:26–31.

Sachedo RC, Reife RA, Lim P, Pledger G. Topiramate monotherapy for partial onset seizures. *Epilepsia* 1997;38:294–300.

Sándor PS, Áfra J, Ambrosini A, Schoenen J. Prophylactic treatment of migraine with beta-blockers and riboflavin: differential effects on the intensity dependence of auditory evoked cortical potentials. *Headache* 2000;40:30–35.

Sándor PS, Di CL, Coppola G, Saenger U, Fumal A, Magis D, Seidel L, Agosti RM, Schoenen J. Efficacy of coenzyme Q10 in migraine prophylaxis: a randomized controlled trial. *Neurology* 2005;64:713–715.

Schoenen J, Jacquy J, Lenaerts M. Effectiveness of high-dose riboflavin in migraine prophylaxis: a randomized controlled trial. *Neurology* 1998;50:466–470.

Schrader H, Stovner LJ, Helde G, Sand T, Bovim G. Prophylactic treatment of migraine with angiotensin converting enzyme inhibitor (lisinopril): randomized, placebo-controlled, crossover study. *Br Med J* 2001;322:19–22.

Silberstein SD. Divalproex sodium in headache: literature review and clinical guidelines. *Headache* 1996;36:547–555.

Silberstein SD. Migraine and pregnancy. *Neurol Clin* 1997;15:209–231.

Silberstein SD. Practice parameter: evidence-based guidelines for migraine headache (an evidence-based review). Report of the Quality Standards Subcommittee of the American Academy of Neurology for the United States Headache Consortium. *Neurology* 2000;55:754–762.

Silberstein SD. Headaches in pregnancy. *Neurol Clin* 2004;22:727–756.

Silberstein SD, Lipton RB, Breslau N. Migraine: association with personality characteristics and psychopathology. *Cephalalgia* 1995;15:337–369.

Silberstein SD, Saper JR, Freitag F. Migraine: diagnosis and treatment. In: Silberstein SD, Lipton RB, Dalessio DJ, eds. *Wolff's Headache and Other Head Pain*. New York: Oxford University Press; 2001:121–237.

Silberstein SD, Winner PK, Chmiel JJ. Migraine preventive medication reduces resource utilization. *Headache* 2003;43:171–178.

Silberstein SD, Neto W, Schmitt J, Jacobs D. Topiramate in the prevention of migraine headache: a randomized, double-blind, placebo-controlled, multiple-dose study. For the MIGR-001 Study Group. *Arch Neurol* 2004;61:490–495.

Silberstein S, Diamond S, Loder E, Reed ML, Lipton RB. Prevalence of migraine sufferers who are candidates for preventive therapy: results from the American migraine study (AMPP) [Abstract]. *Headache* 2005a;45:770–771.

Silberstein SD, Olesen J, Bousser MG, Diener HC, Dodick D, First M, Goadsby PJ, Gobel H, Lainez MJ, Lance JW, Lipton RB, Nappi G, Sakai F, Schoenen J, Steiner TJ. The International Classification of Headache Disorders, 2nd edition (ICHD-II): revision of criteria for 8.2 medication-overuse headache. *Cephalalgia* 2005b;25:460–465.

Silberstein S, Freitag F, Dodick D, Ashman E, Pearlman S. Evidence-based guideline update: OTC treatments for migraine prevention in adults. Report of the Quality Standards Subcommittee of the American Academy of Neurology and the American Headache Society. *Neurology* 2012.

Smith R, Schwartz A. Diltiazem prophylaxis in refractory migraine. *N Engl J Med* 1984;310:1327–1328.

Solomon GD. Verapamil and propranolol in migraine prophylaxis: a double-blind crossover study. *Headache* 1986;26:325.

Steiner TJ, Findley LJ, Yuen AW. Lamotrigine versus placebo in the prophylaxis of migraine with and without aura. *Cephalalgia* 1997;17:109–112.

Sudilovsky A, Stern MA, Meyer JH. Nadolol: the benefits of adequate trial duration in the prophylaxis of migraine. *Headache* 1986;26:325.

Sudilovsky A, Elkind AH, Ryan RE, Saper JR, Stern MA, Meyer JH. Comparative efficacy of nadolol and propranolol in the management of migraine. *Headache* 1987;27:421–426.

Tfelt-Hansen P. Prioritizing acute pharmacotherapy of migraine. In: Olesen J, Tfelt-Hansen P, Welch KMA, eds. *The Headaches*. New York: Lippincott Williams & Wilkins; 2000:453–456.

Tfelt-Hansen P, Standnes B, Kangasniemi P, Hakkarainen H, Olesen J. Timolol vs propranolol vs placebo in common migraine prophylaxis: a double-blind multicenter trial. *Acta Neurol Scand* 1984;69:1–8.

Thomson Healthcare. *Physicians' Desk Reference.* Montvale, NJ: Thomson PDR; 2003.

Tronvik E, Stovner LJ, Helde G, Sand T, Bovim G. Prophylactic treatment of migraine with an angiotensin II receptor blocker: a randomized controlled trial. *JAMA* 2003;289:65–69.

Vainionpaa LK, Rattya J, Knip M, Tapanainen JS, Pakarinen AJ, Lanning P, Tekay A, Myllyla W, Isojarvi JI. Valproate-induced hyperandrogenism during pubertal maturation in girls with epilepsy. *Ann Neurol* 1999;45:444–450.

Vogler BK, Pittler MH, Ernst E. Feverfew as a preventive treatment for migraine: a systematic review. *Cephalalgia* 1998;18:704–708.

Wauquier A, Ashton D, Marranes R. The effects of flunarizine in experimental models related to the pathogenesis of migraine. *Cephalalgia* 1985;5:119–120.

Appendix 10.1

AAN Classification of Evidence for the Rating of a Therapeutic Study

Class I: A randomized, controlled clinical trial of the intervention of interest with masked or objective outcome assessment, in a representative population. Relevant baseline characteristics are presented and substantially equivalent among treatment groups or there is appropriate statistical adjustment for differences.

The following are also required:

a. Concealed allocation.
b. Primary outcome(s) clearly defined.
c. Exclusion/inclusion criteria clearly defined.
d. Adequate accounting for dropouts (with at least 80% of enrolled subjects completing the study) and cross-over with numbers sufficiently low to have minimal potential for bias.
e. For non-inferiority or equivalence trials claiming to prove efficacy for one or both drugs, the following are also required:*
  1. The authors explicitly state the clinically meaningful difference to be excluded by defining the threshold for equivalence or non-inferiority.
  2. The standard treatment used in the study is substantially similar to that used in previous studies establishing efficacy of the standard treatment (e.g., for a drug, the mode of administration, dose, and dosage adjustments are similar to those previously shown to be effective).

3. The inclusion/exclusion criteria for patient selection and the outcomes of patients on the standard treatment are comparable to those of previous studies establishing efficacy of the standard treatment.
4. The interpretation of the results of the study is based on a protocol analysis that takes into account dropouts or cross-overs.

Class II: A randomized, controlled clinical trial of the intervention of interest in a representative population with masked or objective outcome assessment that lacks one of the criteria a–e given previously, or a prospective, matched cohort study with masked or objective outcome assessment in a representative population that meets the criteria b–e. Relevant baseline characteristics are presented and substantially equivalent among treatment groups or there is appropriate statistical adjustment for differences.

Class III: All other controlled trials (including well-defined natural history controls or patients serving as own controls) in a representative population, where outcome is independently assessed, or independently derived by objective outcome measurement.†

Class IV: Studies not meeting Class I, II, or III criteria including consensus or expert opinion.

---

*Note that numbers 1–3 in Class Ie are required for Class II in equivalence trials. If any one of the three is missing, the class is automatically downgraded to Class III.
†Objective outcome measurement: an outcome measure that is unlikely to be affected by an observer's (patient, treating physician, investigator) expectation or bias (e.g., blood tests, administrative outcome data).

Appendix 10.2

Classification of Recommendations

Level A: Established as effective, ineffective, or harmful (or established as useful/predictive or not useful/predictive) for the given condition in the specified population. (Level A rating requires at least two consistent Class I studies.)*

Level B: Probably effective, ineffective, or harmful (or probably useful/predictive or not useful/predictive) for the given condition in the specified population. (Level B rating requires at least one Class I study or two consistent Class II studies.)

Level C: Possibly effective, ineffective, or harmful (or possibly useful/predictive or not useful/predictive) for the given condition in the specified population. (Level C rating requires at least one Class II study or two consistent Class III studies.)

Level U: Data inadequate or conflicting; given current knowledge, the treatment (test, predictor) is unproven.

*In exceptional cases, one convincing Class I study may suffice for an "A" recommendation if (1) all criteria are met and (2) the magnitude of effect is large (the relative rate of the improved outcome is greater than 5 and the lower limit of the confidence interval is greater than 2).

Management Specificities in Female Migraineurs

Hélène Massiou, MD, and Geneviève Plu-Bureau, MD, PhD

INTRODUCTION

Links between female hormones and migraine are strong. Both endogenous and exogenous hormones may play a role: the female preponderance in migraine appears after puberty; in many patients, migraine occurs at the time of menses, and menstrual migraine may benefit from specific therapeutic approaches, including hormonal treatments. Migraine, especially without aura, often improves during pregnancy. Hormonal contraception and postmenopausal hormone therapy may modify the course of the migrainous disease, and require specific attention in view of their potential to increase cerebral ischemic risk, especially in women suffering from migraine with aura. Hence, the management of a female migraineur requires a precise knowledge of her past and present hormonal status.

FEMALE HORMONES AND MIGRAINE

Whereas the prevalence of migraine is similar in boys and girls before puberty, it rises after this age to become approximately threefold higher in adult females (25%) than in males (8%) (Rasmussen et al., 1991). Our knowledge of the mechanisms explaining the influence of steroidal hormones on migraine has been enriched by experiments in transgenic mice expressing familial hemiplegic mutations migraine type 1 (FHM1) (Eickermann-Haerter et al., 2009b). Spreading depression susceptibility is strikingly higher in female FHM1 mutant strains than in males, but not in wild-type mice. This sex difference is abrogated by ovariectomy, implicating the effects of female steroidal hormones in the adult brain as the culprit, rather than sex chromosome–related developmental differences in synaptic organization and structure. Spreading depression frequencies and propagation speed are significantly reduced in senescent female mutant mice after cessation of estrous cycle. Chronic estrogen replacement by subcutaneous implantation of 17β-estradiol is associated with a small increase in spreading depression susceptibility in ovariectomized mutants. Neither gonadectomy nor advanced age nor estrogen replacement influences spreading depression susceptibility in wild-type mice, which suggests that steroidal hormones modulate spreading depression susceptibility predominantly in brains made susceptible by gene mutations.

Enhancement of spreading depression susceptibility by estrogen is only one mechanism by which steroidal hormones may influence migraine. A large body of evidence also suggests that estrogen, progesterone, and androgen modulate the neurotransmitter systems and pain processing networks thought to be involved in the pathogenesis of migraine (Martin & Behbehani, 2006; Eickermann-Haerter et al., 2009a).

MENSTRUAL MIGRAINE
Definition

Migraine is frequently associated with menstruation in female migraineurs, during a period between the 2 days before menstruation and the first 3 days of bleeding (Johannes et al., 1995; Stewart et al., 2000; MacGregor & Hackshaw, 2004). Migraine without aura but not migraine with aura shows a significant association with menstruation (Johannes et al., 1995; Russell et al., 1996). The second edition of the *International Classification of Headache Disorders* (ICHD-II; Headache Classification Committee of the International Headache Society, 2004) defines two different diagnoses:

- *Menstrually related migraine* meets the diagnostic criteria for migraine without aura, and attacks occur on day –2 to +3 of menstruation in at least two out of three menstrual cycles as well as at other times in the cycle.
- *Pure menstrual migraine* meets the diagnostic criteria for migraine without aura, and attacks occur on day –2 to +3 of menstruation in at least two out of three menstrual cycles and at no other time of the month.

Epidemiology and Clinical Characteristics

The prevalence rate for menstrually related migraine is approximately 50% (35% to 54%), and that for pure

menstrual migraine is 7% (3.5% to 21%) (review in Martin & Lipton, 2008). Menstrual attacks have been found to be more severe, of longer duration, and more resistant to therapy than other attacks in several studies, most of which were clinic based (Couturier et al., 2003; Granella et al., 2004; MacGregor & Hackshaw, 2004; Martin et al., 2005; MacGregor et al., 2010).

In one population-based survey, however, few significant differences were observed between menstrual and nonmenstrual attacks (Stewart et al., 2000). These discrepant findings may reflect differences between the populations included in these surveys: subjects selected in clinic-based studies, especially in tertiary referral centers, may suffer from more severe headache. Unlike migraineurs in population-based studies, they often receive preventive medications, which may reduce the severity of migraine at other times of the month but leave menstrual migraine unabated. In a study comparing migraine features and acute therapy response in women with menstrually related migraine who were not taking migraine prophylaxis, Pinkerman and Holroyd (2010) found that menstrual attacks were longer, more likely associated with disability, and less responsive to acute therapy, and demonstrated higher rates of recurrences than nonmenstrual attacks.

Biology

The evidence indicates that estrogen withdrawal may trigger attacks of migraine. Somerville (1972, 1975a, 1975b) noted that a period of estrogen priming with several days of exposure to high estrogen levels is necessary for migraine to result from estrogen withdrawal, such as occurs in the late luteal phase of the menstrual cycle. This finding was confirmed by Lichten et al. (1996) and by MacGregor et al. (2006a) (**Figure 11.1**).

Pharmacological Management
Acute Medications

The initial strategy to treat menstrual attacks consists of the use of acute medications only—the same agents as are used for nonmenstrual attacks. These nonspecific drugs include analgesics, nonsteroidal anti-inflammatory drugs (NSAIDs), and specific acute treatments of migraine (triptans and ergot derivatives). Some of them have been studied in specific trials for menstrually related migraine. In a systematic review and meta-analysis of double-blind, randomized, controlled trials for the symptomatic relief or prevention of menstrually related

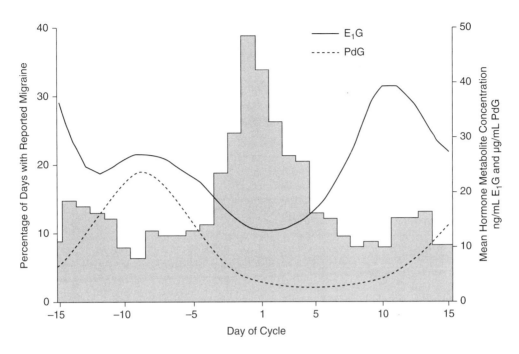

Figure 11.1 Incidence of Migraine, Urinary Estrone-3-Glucuronide (E1G) Levels, and Pregnanediol-3-Glucuronide (PdG) Levels on Each Day of the Menstrual Cycle in 120 Cycles from 38 Women

Adapted from MacGregor EA, Frith A, Ellis J, et al. Incidence of migraine relative to menstrual cycle phases of rising and falling estrogen. *Neurology* 2006a;67:2154–2158.

migraine, Pringsheim et al. (2008) proposed evidence-based recommendations based on the quality criteria of the U.S. Preventive Services Task Force. Specifically, for acute treatment of menstrual migraine, sumatriptan 50 and 100 mg, mefenamic acid, and rizatriptan 10 mg were rated as grade B options, and zolmitriptan was rated as grade C. More recently, two trials showed the efficacy of sumatriptan–naproxen combination therapy for menstrual migraine and dysmenorrhea (Mannix et al., 2009).

Short-Term Prevention

When acute treatments are not sufficient to bring significant relief of menstrual attacks, or when they are not well tolerated or are contraindicated by comorbidities, short-term prevention is required. Agendas then become important tools to ensure that migraine attacks are related to menses, and to determine at what time they occur during the perimenstrual period. Short-term prevention therapies are to be started 2 days before the expected onset of headache and continued for 6 or 7 days. Some NSAIDs (naproxen, mefenamic acid, flurbiprofen, ketoprofen, meclofenamate) have been

suggested as effective in this indication in small trials (review Silberstein & Hutchinson, 2008). In their systematic review, Pringsheim et al. (2008) made grade B recommendations for the perimenstrual use of frovatriptan 2.5 mg twice daily and naratriptan 1 mg twice daily. Zolmitriptan 2.5 mg, given three times daily and twice daily, was also found to be more effective than placebo in the prevention of menstrual migraine attacks (Tuchman et al., 2008). Nevertheless, some concern about drug overuse persists, especially in women who also suffer from nonmenstrual attacks, and additional information about the risks and benefits of triptan prophylaxis for menstrual migraine is required.

Considering that estrogen withdrawal triggers attacks of migraine, it appeared logical to try estrogen supplements as a short-term preventive treatment for menstrual migraine. Transdermal estradiol gel 1.5 mg given perimenstrually was found to be more effective in the prevention of menstrual attacks than placebo in three small studies (De Lignières et al., 1986; Dennerstein et al., 1988; MacGregor et al., 2006b) and rated as a grade B option in the review conducted by Pringsheim et al. (2008). In MacGregor et al.'s (2006b) study, however, 15 of the 22 women who benefited from the estradiol gel experienced an increased number of migraine days during the 5 days after estradiol discontinuation compared to the 5 days after placebo.

Before prescribing estradiol, physicians must confirm that the patient has no contraindications to this therapy, especially those related to the risk of breast cancer. Transdermal patches delivering 50 μg of estradiol over a period of 24 hours (TTS 50) have been studied in one controlled trial (Smits et al., 1994) but were not found to be superior to placebo for the prevention of menstrual migraine, perhaps because serum levels were too low. TTS 100 was found superior to TTS 25 in one open trial (Pradalier et al., 1994). Currently, the evidence is insufficiently strong to recommend the use of estradiol patches in the prevention of menstrual migraine. In women who take an oral contraceptive containing estrogen and progestin for 21 days out of a 28-day cycle and experience migraine during the pill-free or placebo-pill week, a continuous regimen of the combined contraceptive may lead to an improvement of their menstrual attacks (Edelman et al., 2006; Sulak et al., 2007).

MIGRAINE AND HORMONAL CONTRACEPTION

Prescribing hormonal contraceptives to migrainous women raises two main issues:

- What is the influence of this contraception on the course of migraine?
- What is the risk of stroke in migraineurs who take hormonal contraceptives, and should this contraception be contraindicated in some cases?

Influence of Hormonal Contraception on the Course of Migraine

The influence of hormonal contraception on the course of migraine appears largely variable in the literature. In a systematic review of trials published between 1966 and 2004, Loder et al. (2005) included trials with a control group and prospective cohort trials, so as to assess the headache risk that was attributable to combined estrogen–progestin oral contraceptives, and to determine the natural history and treatment response of these headaches. They concluded that because of differences in study populations, oral contraceptive formulations, trial endpoints, and trial duration, it was not possible to pool data.

Headache related to use of combined oral contraceptives (COCs) generally is precipitated by estrogen

withdrawal during the pill-free week. However, switching to COCs that contain a very low dose of estrogen (e.g., 20 or 25 μg of ethinyl-estradiol), which minimizes the magnitude of estrogen withdrawal, does not improve headache, perhaps because COCs with very low estrogen doses do not suppress ovarian function completely. Strategies that reduce estrogen withdrawal, via continuous or extended-duration COCs or through estrogen supplementation during the pill-free week, may provide benefit.

In the Head-HUNT study (Aegidius et al., 2006), 13,944 premenopausal women responded to questions regarding the use of contraceptives. A significant association was found to exist between migraine and COC use (OR: 1.4; 95% CI: 1.2–1.7), but no relationship was noted between headache and the amount of estrogen. No significant association between headache and progestin-only contraceptives (POCs) was found. In migraineurs who complain from a worsening of their headaches when taking COCs, it might then be of interest to switch to POCs, although specific studies are required to demonstrate the benefit of this strategy.

Stopping oral contraceptives when migraine starts with their use may have a variable effect: the relief may occur immediately, or after a delay of 6 to 12 months. In some patients migraine may continue on a long-term basis. In the Head-HUNT study (Aegidius et al., 2006), the researchers observed an increased prevalence of migraine among previous users of oral contraceptives.

Migraine, Hormonal Contraception, and Risk of Stroke

Stroke is rare in young women. The baseline incidence of stroke in women younger than 35 years is estimated to be 6 to 20 per 100,000 woman-years, and the incidence increases with age (Petitti et al., 1997).

Hormonal Contraception and Risk of Stroke

Concerns about a link between COC use and stroke were first raised in the early 1960s. Many case-control studies and some cohort studies have been undertaken to address this question. Because of methodological shortcomings and changes in the doses of estrogen and the type of progestogen, results have been somewhat conflicting. Early epidemiologic studies on COCs containing high doses of estrogen (at least 50 μg of ethinyl-estradiol) found that these drugs increased the risk of cardiovascular disease (review in Bousser & Kittner, 2000). In the last 40 years, however, the formulations of oral contraceptives have dramatically changed. The newer pills contain 35 to 15 µg of ethinyl-estradiol combined with new progestins, including second-generation (levonorgestrel) or third-generation progestins (desogestrel, gestodene, and norgestimate).

Past users of COCs have a risk of stroke that approximates that of never-users. With respect to the dose of estrogen, analysis reveals that the risk of stroke is higher among women taking COCs containing 50 µg or more than among those using COCs containing less than 50 µg of ethinyl-estradiol. Nevertheless, recent meta-analyses (Gillum et al., 2000; Chan et al., 2004; Baillargeon et al., 2005) have found that the risk of ischemic stroke remains significant among current users of low-dose COCs (i.e., RR: 2.12; 95% CI: 1.56–2.86 in Baillargeon et al., 2005).

Regarding the type of progestins, studies indicate a significant association of stroke with both types of progestins (second- or third-generation COCs). The strongest association was found in women 35 years or older, in smokers, and in women with hypertension (Chan et al., 2004). The results of a recent cohort Swedish study (Yang et al., 2009) provide a different take on this issue, however: among 45,699 women, 193 ischemic strokes and 72 hemorrhagic strokes occurred during follow-up (average length, 12.9 years) and neither ischemic nor hemorrhagic stroke risk was related to oral contraceptive (OC) use, duration, or type of OC use. These findings are consistent with the meta-analysis published by Chan et al. (2004), where the pooled odds ratio from four cohort studies demonstrated no increased stroke risk with OC use, whereas the pooled odds ratio from the case-control studies showed a significant association.

Regarding the new routes of administration, the association between vaginal contraceptive use and ischemic stroke has not yet been evaluated. Two studies have compared the rates of ischemic stroke between users of 35 µg of ethinyl-estradiol combined with norgestimate administered either by patch or by oral pill (Jick & Jick, 2007; Dore et al., 2010). Neither study indicated that the risk level differed for these two routes of administration. However, only 18 and 17 strokes occurred in the studies, respectively, and imprecise data limited the researchers' ability to make inferences about the products' effects on the risk of stroke.

Based on six epidemiologic studies, the risk of stroke in relation to the use of POCs was evaluated in a recent meta-analysis (Chaktoura et al., 2009). The combined odds ratio showed no increase in the risk of stroke among POC users (OR: 0.96; 95% CI: 0.70–1.31). This result

was similar for each route of administration considered (either implant or injectable or oral POC). However, these results were based on limited data, and further investigations are needed in women with risk factors for stroke.

Migraine and Risk of Stroke

A link between migraine and stroke has been established in several case-control and cohort studies. The most recent meta-analysis, which included nine studies investigating the association between migraine and stroke, found a relative risk of ischemic stroke of 1.73 (95% CI: 1.31–2.29) for any type of migraine (Schürks et al., 2009). The risk was significantly increased for migraine with aura (RR: 2.16; 95% CI 1.53–3.03), but not for migraine without aura (RR: 1.23; 95% CI: 0.9–1.69). Further analysis for any migraine type suggested an increased risk among women (RR: 2.08; 95% CI: 1.13–3.84), compared with men (RR: 1.37; 95% CI: 0.88–2.11), and for people younger than age 45 (RR: 2.62; 95% CI: 1.41–4.97)—an effect that was more pronounced among women (RR: 3.65; 95% CI: 2.21–6.04). The risk of ischemic stroke seemed to be further increased among smokers (RR: 9.03; 95% CI: 4.22–19.33) and women currently using OCs (RR: 7.02; 95% CI: 1.51–32.68). In women suffering from migraine with aura, currently using OCs, and smoking, the relative risk was 10 (95% CI: 1.4–73.7).

Recommendations

The following recommendations have been issued regarding the use of hormonal contraception in women with migraine (Bousser et al., 2000):

1. There is no contraindication to the use of COCs in women with migraine in the absence of migraine aura or other risk factors. Women should be counseled and regularly assessed for the development of additional risk factors.
2. There is a potentially increased risk of ischemic stroke in women with migraine who are using COCs and have additional risk factors, which cannot easily be controlled, including migraine with aura. Health-care providers must individually assess and evaluate these risks. COC use may be contraindicated.
3. Women suffering from migraine, especially with aura, should be strongly advised to stop smoking.
4. In women with migraine with aura, methods of birth control other than COCs must be considered, including POCs.

5. Some situations require cessation of combined hormonal contraception:
   • New persisting headache
   • New onset of migraine aura
   • Increased headache frequency or intensity
   • Development of unusual aura symptoms, particularly prolonged aura

MIGRAINE AND MENOPAUSE

Course of Migraine During Menopause

Data about menopause and migraine are conflicting. The prevalence of migraine decreases with age in both sexes, and the feminine preponderance, although less important, persists after menopause. The female–male incidence ratio of migraine is still 2.5:1 after 70 years of age.

The classical statement that claims there is a worsening of migraine during perimenopause and an improvement after menopause needs to be reconsidered in view of recent studies. In a study by Neri et al. (1993), two-thirds of the women reported an improvement of their migraine after spontaneous menopause, whereas a worsening occurred in two-thirds of the women after surgical menopause. This improvement of migraine after menopause was not confirmed in a cross-sectional study performed in Sweden on 728 women aged 40 to 74 years (Mattson, 2003). A crude odds ratio of 0.47 (95% CI: 0.24–0.86) indicated a decrease in risk for migraine without aura in postmenopausal women; however, after adjusting for differences in age and the use of hormonal therapy (HT), this association was not statistically significant. A longitudinal follow-up of women starting at the perimenopausal period is warranted to demonstrate the pattern of change in migraine prevalence throughout the menopause transition.

Migraine and Menopausal Hormonal Therapy

Hormonal therapy (HT) varies widely from one country to another. Various types of estrogens are used: conjugated equine estrogen, estradiol, and synthetic ethinyl-estradiol. Estrogens are available orally and parenterally in the form of injections, percutaneous gels, transdermal patches, and vaginal creams. Adjunct hormones include progestogens and sometimes androgens. Unopposed estrogens and combined regimens are administered either continuously or sequentially for 25 days per month.

The association between HT and migraine was examined in the large population-based Women's Health Study (Misakian et al., 2003). In this study, current HT use in postmenopausal women was associated with higher rates of migraine headache than non-use (OR: 1.42; 95% CI: 1.24–1.62). Odds ratios were similar for users of estrogen alone and users of both estrogen and progestin. In the Head-HUNT study (Aegidius et al., 2007), migraine among postmenopausal women was also significantly associated with current use of HT (OR: 1.6; 95% CI: 1.4–1.9), whether the HT was delivered systemically or by the local route. Whether HT caused headache or was used partly because of headache could not be determined in this cross-sectional study.

Two longitudinal studies also assessed the influence of HT on migraine. In the first investigation, after a 1-month run-in period, women received two different HT regimens: transdermal estradiol 50 μg every 7 days for 28 days plus medroxyprogesterone acetate (MPA) 10 mg/day from days 15 to 28, or oral conjugated estrogens 0.625 mg/day for 28 days plus MPA 10 mg/day for the last 14 days (Nappi et al., 2001). The route of HT significantly affected the course of migraine: both frequency of attacks and days with headache significantly increased during the span when HT was delivered in the subgroup receiving an oral formulation, but not in the subgroup who received HT via the transdermal route. In the other trial (Facchinetti et al., 2002), after a 1-month run-in period, women were assigned to one of three regimens of HT: estradiol hemihydrate 1 mg/day plus norethisterone 0.5 mg/day for 28 days, in a continuous combined scheme; oral conjugated estrogens 0.625 mg/day for 28 days plus medroxyprogesterone acetate 10 mg/day in the last 14 days, in a sequential continuous scheme; and estradiol valerate 2 mg/day for 21 days plus cyproterone acetate 1 mg/day from day 12 to 21 in a sequential cyclical scheme. Overall, a progressive increase in attack frequency, days with headache, and analgesic consumption (from 3.4 ± 1.3 to 5.6 ± 2.2, $P < 0.001$) was observed after 6 months. The increase in number of days with headache and number of analgesics used was smaller in the group receiving the continuous combined regimen than in the other two groups.

In view of these results, it appears that continuous HT, with the transdermal route being used for delivery of estrogen, should be proposed in cases of worsening of migraine with another regimen. Continuous administration is especially indicated in case of estrogen withdrawal migraine.

Hormone Therapy and Risk of Stroke in Postmenopausal Women with Migraine

During the 20 last years, trials focusing on the risk of ischemic stroke with HT have produced conflicting results. A meta-analysis (Bath & Gray, 2005) found that HT is associated with an increased risk of ischemic stroke (OR: 1.29; 95% CI: 1.06–1.56). Odds ratios were similar for users of estrogen alone and users of both estrogen and progestin. The currently available data do not show any differences between the different types of oral estrogens in this regard. The recent data provided by the Women's Health Initiative—a large, randomized trial evaluating conjugated equine estrogen alone or in combination with MPA—confirmed these results, showing an increased risk for combined estrogen and progestogen use (RR: 1.34; 95% CI: 1.05–1.71), and for estrogen alone use (RR: 1.37; 95% CI: 1.10–1.77) (Wassertheil-Smoller et al., 2003; Anderson et al., 2004; Hendrix et al., 2006). The risk of stroke associated with HT use increases from the first year and remains elevated afterward.

In a recent study, Renoux et al. (2010) performed a nested case-control study based on data from a cohort of women in the U.K. General Practice Research Database. Current use of oral and transdermal HT was compared to no use in 15,710 cases and 59,958 controls. The adjusted rate ratio for stroke for current use of transdermal estrogens, with or without progestin, was not increased (RR: 0.95; 95% CI: 0.75–1.20), but a significant increase was associated with use of oral estrogen, with or without progestin (RR: 1.28; 95% CI: 1.15–1.42). There was an indication of a dose-response relationship: a significant increase in risk was observed with transdermal estrogen doses greater than 50 µg. This study was the first major analysis to compare transdermal and oral HT. Its results support the growing perception that transdermal HT at standard doses is free of the cardiovascular risks associated with oral therapy. Whether the risk of stroke differs according to the type of progestogen remains unknown.

Migraine in women older than age 45 years does appear to be a weaker risk factor for ischemic stroke than migraine in younger women, however, and there is no evidence to show that this risk increases with use of HT. Consequently, the usual indications and contraindications for HT should be applied in migrainous postmenopausal women. To be on the safe side, if new onset of migraine aura or worsening of auras occur in patients taking HT, it is recommended to reduce or discontinue estrogens.

MIGRAINE, PREGNANCY, AND THE POSTPARTUM PERIOD
Effects of Migraine on Pregnancy Outcome

Several associations have been proposed between migraine and complications in pregnancy, including low birth weight, birth defects, and preeclampsia. Most studies in this area have suffered from methodological limitations, however, including retrospective designs and lack of standardized criteria for the diagnosis of migraine. A recent prospective study found an increased risk in migraineurs for development of hypertensive disorders (OR: 2.85; 95% CI: 1.40–5.81) (Facchinetti et al., 2009). In another large population-based, case-control study, an association was observed between active peripartum migraine and vascular diagnoses during pregnancy, including stroke, myocardial infarction, venous thromboembolism, and preeclampsia (Bushnell et al., 2009). Nevertheless, these studies failed to establish a causal relationship between migraine and the vascular events.

Influence of Pregnancy on the Course of Migraine

An improvement in migraine during pregnancy has been observed in several studies, occurring in 55% to 90% of cases; in 10% to 20% of women, attacks completely disappear (Maggioni et al., 1997; Granella et al., 2000; Sances et al., 2003). The rate of reduction of attacks increases with the progression of pregnancy, reaching a high of 89% of women with fewer or no attacks by the third trimester in a recent large prospective study (Melhado et al., 2007). This beneficial effect of pregnancy is observed more frequently in women who suffered from menstrual attacks before their pregnancy. Nevertheless, migraine patterns may remain unchanged during pregnancy, or worsen or even occur for the first time during this period, especially migraine with aura (Cupini et al., 1995; Granella et al., 2000). Stable plasma levels of estrogen during pregnancy might at least partially explain the improvement of migraine without aura during this period, whereas high levels of estrogen may induce auras. Other suggestions to explain the pregnancy–migraine link focus on changes of the metabolism of serotonin and endogenous opioids during pregnancy.

Postpartum Migraines

Approximately 30% to 40% of women suffer from headache during the first postpartum week. These headaches occur most often between day 3 and day 6 postpartum. Some of them are migraine attacks, which are more likely to occur in women with a prior history of migraine. Migraine can also begin de novo in the postpartum period. These attacks might be triggered by the estrogen withdrawal observed during the postpartum period. Postpartum headaches may potentially have multiple etiologies, including eclampsia, cerebral venous thrombosis, reversible angiopathy (which may be triggered by bromocriptine), and post–dural puncture headache complicating an epidural anesthesia (Sharshar et al., 1995; Marcus et al., 1999; Singhal, 2004).

Treatment of Migraine During Pregnancy

Although migraine often improves during pregnancy, the need for treating migraine during this period is not a rare situation. Among 60,435 pregnant women assessed in a large population-based cohort study (Nevzalova-Henriksen et al., 2009), 3,480 (5.8%) reported having migraine during the first 5 months of pregnancy. Of these women, 2,525 (72.6%) reported using migraine pharmacotherapy, mostly non-narcotic analgesics (54.1%) and triptans (25.4%); 0.9% used a prophylactic agent.

This study highlighted the fact that many women take drug treatments for migraine during pregnancy, which makes it essential to know the teratogenic risks of antimigraine drugs and their effects on pregnancy. These risks can be evaluated by referring to several databases that include recommendations for treatment strategies, including the U.S. Food and Drug Administration (FDA) system, the Teratogen Information System (TERIS), the European Network Teratology Information Service (ENTIS), and the Centre de Référence sur les Agents Tératogènes (CRAT) in France. There is limited agreement between these databases and recommendations, however, and no single method of assessing drug risk in pregnancy provides complete or perfect information.

Acute Treatments

Paracetamol (acetaminophen) is the first-line choice for acute treatment of migraine during pregnancy (FDA rating: B, TERIS: no risk), although the grade of evidence for its efficacy is low. If this agent provides no benefit, opioids may be the treatment of choice during pregnancy, whereas this is not the case outside pregnancy (Goadsby et al., 2008). Antiemetics can be used during pregnancy, and are often necessary given that pregnancy-associated nausea may exacerbate the nausea and vomiting associated with migraine attacks. Aspirin may be used occasionally until the end of the fifth month of pregnancy (24 weeks of amenorrhea) and is contraindicated at doses of 500 mg/day or higher after this point. NSAIDs are contraindicated after 24 weeks of amenorrhea because of the risk of closure of the fetal ductus arteriosus and kidney lesions; it is preferable to avoid these medications during the 5 first months of pregnancy (FDA, TERIS, CRAT).

From January 1996 to October 2008, information from the sumatriptan and naratriptan pregnancy registry showed no statistically significant difference between the rate of birth defects in pregnancies where first-trimester exposure to sumatriptan occurred and the background rate of birth defects in the general population (Cunnington et al., 2009). Data on naratriptan are too sparse to draw definite conclusions regarding this agent, however. The rizatriptan registry produced no signal of teratogenicity, but again data on this usage remain scarce. In a recent large cohort study, no significant association between triptan therapy during the first trimester and major congenital malformations or adverse pregnancy outcomes was found; the authors, however, stated that such a link cannot be excluded because a difference in the risk between triptan use and individual or rare congenital malformations may exist (Nevzalova-Henriksen et al., 2010). A slight increase in the risk of atonic uterus (OR: 1.4; 95% CI: 1.1–1.8) and blood loss of more than 500 mL during labor (OR: 1.3; 95% CI: 1.1–1.5) was associated with triptan use during the second and/or third trimesters. In the authors' view, the current classification of triptans within Category C in the FDA Pregnancy Classification remains appropriate (for drugs in Category C, "safety in human pregnancy has not been determined and potential benefits should justify potential risks if used in pregnancy"). However, the consistency of information from multiple sources of data is reassuring for the woman whose fetus has been inadvertently exposed to triptans during the first trimester of pregnancy.

Ergotamine—a nonselective serotonin agonist—is contraindicated in pregnancy based on evidence suggesting it increases prenatal mortality, may be linked to fetal hypoxia and growth retardation, and produces pronounced effects on blood flow to the placenta as well as an increase in uterine muscle tone (Czeizel, 1989).

The recommendations of the FDA and the CRAT for the use of acute migraine treatments during pregnancy are summarized in **Table 11.1**.

Preventive Treatments

Prophylactic drugs for migraine should ideally be stopped in women who are planning to conceive. As migraine usually improves during pregnancy, prophylaxis is rarely necessary, although it may be required in patients whose attacks cannot be adequately managed with acute therapy alone. Relaxation strategies and other nonpharmacologic methods of treatment should be proposed as a first choice for prevention; if possible, drug treatments

Table 11.1 Safety Profiles in Pregnancy for Drugs Commonly Used to Treat Acute Migraine Attacks According to FDA and CRAT Recommendations

	FDA	CRAT
Paracetamol (acetaminophen)	B	Possible
Aspirin	C[a]	Occasionally until the end of the fifth month of pregnancy; contraindicated afterward if dose is more than 500 mg/day
NSAIDs		Avoid until the end of the fifth month of pregancy; contraindicated afterward
Ibuprofen	B[a]	
Naproxen	B[a]	
Codeine	C[b]	Possible
Caffeine	B	Possible
Metoclopramide	B	Possible
Domperidone		Possible
Triptans	C	Sumatriptan possible
Ergotamine	X	Contraindicated
Dihydroergotamine	X	Contraindicated

United States Food and Drug Administration Categories of Medication Risk in Pregnancy
Category A: Controlled human studies show no risk.
Category B: No evidence of risk in humans, but there are no controlled human studies.
Category C: Risk to humans has not been ruled out.
Category D: Positive evidence of risk to humans from human or animal studies.
Category X: Contraindicated in pregnancy.

a. D if third trimester.
b. D if prolonged or at term.

should be delayed until the second trimester or later, because the risk of adverse effects is less once the fetus's major organ systems have formed.

Propranolol and metoprolol are preferred agents for migraine prevention during pregnancy (MacGregor, 2007; Goadsby et al., 2008; CRAT), but should be used at the lowest possible dose and stopped a few days before delivery to avoid fetal bradycardia and reduction of uterine contractions. Tricyclic antidepressants can also be used for this indication; although rated as grade C by the FDA, they appear safe when used at doses between 10 and 50 mg—the range recommended for migraine prophylaxis (Koren et al., 1998; CRAT; TERIS). These agents should be stopped at least 2 weeks before delivery to avoid the risk of tachycardia, muscular spasms, and convulsions in the newborn. Methysergide and dihydroergotamine are contraindicated as well as sodium valproate, which is a known teratogen; flunarizine, oxetorone, pizotifen, indoramin, topiramate, and gabapentin have not been established as safe and should not be used during pregnancy. Angiotensin-converting enzyme inhibitors and angiotensin receptor blockers are contraindicated during pregnancy. Finally, women must be informed that over-the-counter herbal medicines for migraines and nausea may contain substances that are contraindicated during pregnancy (Buckner et al., 2005; Marcus & Snodgras, 2005).

Lactation

The major concern regarding lactation in migraineurs using medication is the possible effect of drugs on the infant, through transmission in breast milk. The amount of a maternal medication dose that appears in breast milk varies depending on the lipid solubility of the drug and other pharmacokinetic factors. The recommendations of the American Academy of Pediatrics (AAP) Committee on Drugs (http://www.aap.org) and of the CRAT regarding the compatibility of acute treatments of migraine with breastfeeding appear in **Table 11.2**. NSAIDs and sumatriptan will be the preferred drugs in such women. If prophylaxis is required, propranolol, rather than metoprolol, can be used (CRAT). Other prophylactic drugs should be avoided.

Table 11.2 Safety Profiles During Breastfeeding for Drugs Commonly Used to Treat Acute Migraine Attacks According to AAP Ratings and CRAT Recommendations

	AAP	CRAT
Paracetamol (acetaminophen)	Compatible	Possible
Aspirin	Caution	Possible occasionally
Metoclopramide	Caution	Possible
Domperidone		Possible
Caffeine	Compatible	Possible
Ibruprofen	Compatible	Possible
Naproxen	Compatible	
Ketoprofen		Possible
Codeine	Compatible	Caution, low doses, fewer than 2 to 3 days
Sumatriptan	Probably compatible	Possible
Ergotamine	Contraindicated	
Dihydroergotamine	Contraindicated	

CONCLUSIONS

Knowing about the influence of female hormones on migraine plays a major role in our understanding of migraine pathophysiology and the management of female migraineurs. Recent experiments in transgenic mice expressing familial hemiplegic migraine have demonstrated the enhancing effect of estrogen on spreading depression. Menstrual attacks are, in some women, resistant to usual acute treatments; because the pain attacks are related to estrogen withdrawal, hormonal treatments may then be proposed. Although migraine usually improves during pregnancy, the need for treating migraine during this period is not a rare situation and requires the identification of authorized drugs. The risk of stroke in females suffering from migraine with aura is increased by the use of combined contraceptives containing ethinyl-estradiol, therefore necessitating other methods of birth control in these patients, including progestogen-only hormonal contraception.

REFERENCES

Aegidius K, Zwart JA, Hagen K, et al. Oral contraceptives and increased headache prevalence: the Head-HUNT Study. *Neurology* 2006;66:349–353.

Aegidius KL, Zwart JA, Hagen K, et al. Hormone replacement therapy and headache prevalence in postmenopausal women: the Head-HUNT study. *Eur J Neurol* 2007;14:73–78.

Anderson GL, Limacher M, Assaf AR, et al. Women's Health Initiative Steering Committee. Effects of conjugated equine estrogen in postmenopausal women with hysterectomy: the Women's Health Initiative randomized controlled trial. *JAMA* 2004;291:1701–1712.

Baillargeon JP, McClish DK, Essah PA, Nestler JE. Association between the current use of low-dose oral contraceptives and cardiovascular arterial disease: a meta-analysis. *J Clin Endocrinol Metab* 2005;90:3863–3870.

Bath PM, Gray LJ. Association between hormone replacement therapy and subsequent stroke: a meta-analysis. *BMJ* 2005;330:342.

Bousser MG, Conard J, Kittner S, et al. Recommendations on the risk of ischaemic stroke associated with use of combined oral contraceptives and hormone replacement therapy in women with migraine. *Cephalalgia* 2000;20:155–166.

Bousser MG, Kittner SJ. Oral contraceptives and stroke. *Cephalalgia* 2000;20:183–189.

Buckner KD, Chavez ML, Raney EC, Soteher J. Health food stores' recommendations for nausea and migraines during pregnancy. *Ann Pharmacother* 2005;39:274–279.

Bushnell CD, Jamison M, James AH. Migraines during pregnancy linked to stroke and vascular diseases: US population based case-control study. *BMJ* 2009;338:664.

Chakhtoura Z, Canonico M, Gompel A, et al. Progestogen-only contraceptives and the risk of stroke: a meta-analysis. *Stroke* 2009;40:1059–1062.

Chan WS, Ray J, Wai EJ, et al. Risk of stroke in women exposed to low-dose oral contraceptives. *Arch Intern Med* 2004;164:741–747.

Couturier E, Bomhof M, Knuistingh Neven A, van Duijn N. Menstrual migraine in a representative Dutch population sample: prevalence, disability and treatment. *Cephalalgia* 2003;23:302–308.

Cunnington M, Ephross S, Churchill P. The safety of sumatriptan and naratriptan in pregnancy: what have we learned? *Headache* 2009;49:1414–1422.

Cupini L, Matteis M, Troisi E, et al. Sex-hormone–related events in migrainous females: a clinical comparative study between migraine with aura and migraine without aura. *Cephalalgia* 1995;15:140–144.

Czeizel AE. Teratogenicity of ergotamine. *J Med Genet* 1989;26:69–70.

De Lignières B, Vincens M, Mauvais-Jarvis P, et al. Prevention of menstrual migraine by percutaneous estradiol. *BMJ* 1986;293:1540.

Dennerstein L, Morse C, Burrows G, et al. Menstrual migraine: a double-blind trial of percutaneous estradiol. *Gynecol Endocrinol* 1988;2:113–120.

Dore DD, Norman H, Loughlin J, Seeger JD. Extended case-control study results on thromboembolic outcomes among transdermal contraceptives users. *Contraception* 2010;81:408–413.

Edelman A, Gallo MF, Nichols MD, et al. Continuous versus cyclic use of combined oral contraceptives for contraception: systematic Cochrane review of randomized controlled trials. *Hum Reprod* 2006;21:573–578.

Eikermann-Haerter K, Baum MJ, Ferrari MD, et al. Androgenic suppression of spreading depression in familial hemiplegic migraine type 1 mutant mice. *Ann Neurol* 2009a;66:564–568.

Eikermann-Haerter K, Dileköz E, Kudo C, et al. Genetic and hormonal factors modulate spreading depression and transient hemiparesis in mouse models of familial hemiplegic migraine type 1. *J Clin Invest* 2009b;119:99–109.

Facchinetti F, Nappi RE, Tirelli A, et al. Hormone supplementation differently affects migraine in postmenopausal women. *Headache* 2002;42:924–929.

Facchinetti F, Allais G, Nappi RE, et al. Migraine is a risk factor for hypertensive disorders in pregnancy: a prospective cohort study. *Cephalalgia* 2009;29:286–292.

Gillum LA, Mamidipudi SK, Johnston SC. Ischemic stroke risk with oral contraceptives: a meta-analysis. *JAMA* 2000;284:72–78.

Goadsby PJ, Golberg J, Silberstein SD. Migraine and pregnancy. *BMJ* 2008;336:1502–1504.

Granella F, Sances G, Pucci E, et al. Migraine with aura and reproductive life events: a case control study. *Cephalalgia* 2000;20:701–707.

Granella F, Sances G, Allais G, et al. Characteristics of menstrual and non-menstrual attacks in women with menstrually related migraine referred to headache centres. *Cephalalgia* 2004;24:707–716.

Headache Classification Subcommittee of the International Headache Society (IHS). The International Classification of Headache Disorders (2nd ed.). *Cephalalgia* 2004;24(suppl 1): 1–160.

Hendrix SL, Wassertheil-Smoller S, Johnson KC, et al. Effects of conjugated equine estrogen on stroke in the Women's Health Initiative. *Circulation* 2006;113:2425–2434.

Jick SS, Jick H. The contraceptive patch in relation to ischemic stroke and acute myocardial infarction. *Pharmacotherapy* 2007;27:218–220.

Johannes C, Linet M, Stewart W, et al. Relationship of headache to the phase of the menstrual cycle among young women: a daily diary study. *Neurology* 1995;45:1076–1082.

Koren G, Pastuzak A, Ito S. Drugs in pregnancy. *N Engl J Med* 1998;338:1128–1137.

Lichten EM, Lichten JB, Whitty A, Pieper D. The confirmation of a biochemical marker for women's hormonal migraine: the depo-oestradiol challenge test. *Headache* 1996;36:367–371.

Loder EW, Buse DC, Golub JR. Headache as a side effect of combination estrogen–progestin oral contraceptives: a systematic review. *Am J Obstet Gynecol* 2005;193:636–649.

MacGregor EA. Migraine in pregnancy and lactation: a clinical review. *J Fam Plan Reprod Health Care* 2007;33:83–93.

MacGregor EA, Hackshaw A. Prevalence of migraine on each day of the natural menstrual cycle. *Neurology* 2004;63:351–353.

MacGregor EA, Frith A, Ellis J, et al. Incidence of migraine relative to menstrual cycle phases of rising and falling estrogen. *Neurology* 2006a;67:2154–2158.

MacGregor EA, Frith A, Ellis J, et al. Prevention of menstrual attacks of migraine: a double-blind placebo-controlled crossover study. *Neurology* 2006b;67:2159–2163.

MacGregor EA, Victor TW, Hu X, et al. Characteristics of menstrual vs non menstrual migraine: a post hoc, within-woman analysis of the usual-care phase of a nonrandomized menstrual migraine clinical trial. *Headache* 2010;50:528–538.

Maggioni F, Alessi C, Maggino T, Zanchin G. Headache during pregnancy. *Cephalalgia* 1997;17:765–769.

Mannix LK, Martin VT, Cady RK, et al. Combination treatment for menstrual migraine and dysmenorrhea using sumatriptan–naproxen: two randomized controlled trials. *Obstet Gynecol* 2009;114:106–113.

Marcus DM, Snodgras WR. Do not harm: avoidance of herbal medicines during pregnancy. *Obstet Gynecol* 2005;105:1119–1122.

Marcus DA, Scharff L, Turk D. Longitudinal prospective study of headache during pregnancy and postpartum. *Headache* 1999;39:625–632.

Martin VT, Behbehani M. Ovarian hormones and migraine headache: understanding mechanisms and pathogenesis. Part I. *Headache* 2006;46:3–23.

Martin VT, Lipton RB. Epidemiology and biology of menstrual migraine. *Headache* 2008;48(suppl 3):S124–S130.

Martin VT, Wernke S, Mandell K, et al. Defining the relationship between ovarian hormones and migraine headache. *Headache* 2005;45:1190–1201.

Mattson P. Hormonal factors in migraine: a population-based study of women aged 40 to 74 years. *Headache* 2003;43:27–35.

Melhado EM, Maciel JA Jr, Gerreiro CA. Headache during gestation: evaluation of 1101 women. *Can J Neurol Sci* 2007;34:187–192.

Misakian AL, Langer RD, Bensenor IM, et al. Postmenopausal hormone therapy and migraine headache. *J Women Health* 2003;12:1027–1036.

Nappi RE, Cagnacci A, Granella F, et al. Course of primary headaches during hormone replacement therapy. *Maturitas* 2001;38:157–163.

Neri I, Granella F, Nappi R, et al. Characteristics of headache at menopause: a clinico-epidemiologic study. *Maturitas* 1993;17:31–37.

Nevzalova-Henriksen K, Spigset O, Nordeng H. Maternal characteristics and migraine pharmacotherapy during pregnancy: cross-sectional analysis of data from a large cohort study. *Cephalalgia* 2009;29:1267–1276.

Nevzalova-Henriksen K, Spigset O, Nordeng H. Triptan exposure during pregnancy and the risk of major congenital malformations and adverse pregnancy outcomes: results from the Norwegian mother and child cohort study. *Headache* 2010;50:563–575.

Petitti DB, Sidney S, Quesenberry CP Jr, Bernstein A. Incidence of stroke and myocardial infarction in women of reproductive age. *Stroke* 1997;28:280–283.

Pinkerman B, Holroyd K. Menstrual and non-menstrual migraines differ in women with menstrually-related migraine. *Cephalalgia* 2010;30:1187–1194.

Pradalier A, Vincent D, Beaulieu P, et al. Correlation between estradiol plasma level and therapeutic effect on menstrual migraine. In: Rose F, ed. *New Advances in Headache Research*. London: Smith-Gordon; 1994:129–132.

Pringsheim T, Davenport WJ, Dodick D. Acute treatment and prevention of menstrually related migraine headache: evidence-based review. *Neurology* 2008;70:1555–1563.

Rasmussen B, Jensen R, Schroll M, Olesen J. Epidemiology of headache in a general population: a prevalence study. *J Clin Epidemiol* 1991;44:1147–1157.

Renoux C, Dell'Aniello S, Garnbe E, Suissa S. Transdermal and oral hormone replacement therapy and the risk of stroke: a nested case-control study. *BMJ* 2010;340:C2519.

Russell MB, Rasmussen BK, Fenger K, Olesen J. Migraine without aura and migraine with aura are distinct clinical entities: a study of four hundred and eighty-four male and female migraineurs from the general population. *Cephalalgia* 1996;16:239–245.

Sances G, Granella F, Nappi R, et al. Course of migraine during pregnancy and postpartum: a prospective study. *Cephalalgia* 2003;23:197–205.

Schürks M, Rist PM, Bigal ME, et al. Migraine and cardiovascular disease: systematic review and meta-analysis. *BMJ* 2009;339:3914.

Sharshar T, Lamy C, Mas JL. Incidence and causes of strokes associated with pregnancy and puerperium: a study in public hospitals of Ile de France. Stroke in Pregnancy Study Group. *Stroke* 1995;26:930–936.

Silberstein SD, Hutchinson SL. Diagnosis and treatment of the menstrual migraine patient. *Headache* 2008;48(suppl 3):S115–S123.

Singhal AB. Postpartum angiopathy with reversible posterior leukoencephalopathy. *Arch Neurol* 2004;61:411–416.

Smits MG, van der Meer YG, Pfeil JP, et al. Perimenstrual migraine: effect of Estraderm TTS and the value of contingent negative variation and exteroceptive temporalis muscle suppression test. *Headache* 1994;34:103–106.

Somerville BW. The role of estradiol withdrawal in the etiology of menstrual migraine. *Neurology* 1972;22:355–365.

Somerville BW. Estrogen-withdrawal migraine. I. Duration of exposure required and attempted prophylaxis by premenstrual estrogen administration. *Neurology* 1975a;25:239–244.

Somerville BW. Estrogen-withdrawal migraine II. Attempted prophylaxis by continuous estradiol administration. *Neurology* 1975b;25:245–250.

Stewart W, Lipton R, Chee E, et al. Menstrual cycle and headache in a population sample of migraineurs. *Neurology* 2000;55:1517–1523.

Sulak P, Willis S, Kuehl T, et al. Headaches and oral contraceptives: impact of eliminating the standard 7-day placebo interval. *Headache* 2007;47:27–37.

Tuchman MM, Hee A, Emeribe U, Silberstein S. Oral zolmitriptan in the short-term prevention of menstrual migraine: a randomized, placebo-controlled study. *CNS Drugs* 2008;22:877–886.

Wassertheil-Smoller S, Hendrix SL, Limacher M, et al. Effects of estrogen plus progestin on stroke in postmenopausal women. *JAMA* 2003;289:2673–2684.

Yang L, Kuper HK, Sandin S, et al. Reproductive history, oral contraceptives use, and the risk of ischemic and hemorrhagic stroke in a cohort study of middle-aged Swedish women. *Stroke* 2009;40:1050–1058.

Pharmacoeconomic Aspects of Drug Treatment for Migraine

Fabio Antonaci, MD, PhD, Cristina Tassorelli, MD, PhD, and Marta Allena, MD

INTRODUCTION

Migraine is a highly prevalent and disabling pain disorder that affects millions of individuals worldwide and significantly impairs patients' ability to function. The World Health Organization includes migraine among the 10 most disabling conditions for the two genders, and among the five most disabling conditions for women (Leonardi et al., 2005). Indeed, migraine is most prevalent in the productive years of a person's life, generating substantial lost work time.

Nevertheless, headache patients remain poorly diagnosed and treated in most countries. Recently, the European Headache Federation, in conjunction with Lifting the Burden (the global campaign to reduce the burden of headache worldwide), has published guidelines for the management of common headache disorders in primary care (Stovner et al., 2007). These measures include accurate diagnosis, appropriate treatment and follow-up, and referral for specialist care when needed.

Appropriate management and treatment of migraine can substantially reduce the costs associated with this disorder. While effective treatments that could alleviate these burdens are within reach, however, many of the available treatments are not accessible, not optimized, not effective, or simply not tolerated. The new guidelines are intended to provide strategies and practical considerations for physicians in the management of migraine and prompt a better education for more efficient therapies and for greater support from national health systems.

Usually, costs associated with migraine are divided into indirect costs (loss or reduction of productivity) and direct costs related to the use of medical care resources. There is general agreement that indirect costs are predominant over the direct ones, making up approximately 93% of the total economic burden of migraine (Lipton et al., 1994; Hu et al., 1999).

COSTS RELATED TO ACUTE TREATMENTS

Direct costs concern mainly expenses for drugs, consultations, and instrumental examinations. In 2006, Hawkins et al. published data on direct costs for migraine, reporting that the estimated national direct costs totaled $11 billion, of which $4.5 million was spent on prescription acute treatment and preventive drugs. This figure, of course, does not include the cost of nonprescription acute treatment drugs (i.e., over-the-counter drugs), which might significantly contribute to the direct costs of migraine.

The analytical evaluation of the cost of migraine therapies became an issue of interest only recently, and the first analyses of the migraine pharmacoeconomic burden coincided with the introduction in the market of triptans for the acute treatment of headache. On the one hand, sumatriptan—the prototype of the 5-HT$_{1B/1D}$ agonist class—was quite an expensive treatment as compared to the other available drugs (ergotamine and nonsteroidal anti-inflammatory drugs [NSAIDs]). On the other hand, sumatriptan met the acute treatment goal of providing rapid relief, therefore proving highly effective in reducing time of disability and consequently the indirect costs of the disease.

In 2005, Goldberg reported that expenditures on triptans accounted for the majority of the total annual costs associated with the treatment of migraine. This relationship may reflect the tendency, as noted in recent studies, to emphasize early intervention in acute migraine treatment, when the pain is still mild, because acute drugs (and triptans in particular), when administered early in the migrainous process, can bring about a shortened time to pain-free response. In turn, the prescription and the use of triptans increased and contributed to the amplifications of direct costs for migraine.

Pharmacoeconomic analyses have compared the costs related to the use of different triptans. In their analysis of utilization and reimbursement data from state Medicaid programs in the United States, Mullins et al. (2007) showed that eletriptan 20 mg and eletriptan 40 mg represent the two triptans associated with the lowest cost to treat 100 migraine attacks (ranges of $1,549–$1,658 and $1,578–$1,661, respectively). Using a composite measure of effectiveness, the "successfully treated" migraine (defined as requiring only one triptan dose to treat one migraine attack during a 24-hour period), Perfetto et al. (2005) showed that eletriptan 40 mg was associated with both the lowest total triptan cost for treating 100 migraine attacks ($1,560) and the lowest cost per successfully treated patient ($56.39).

At variance, when using a composite efficacy/tolerability endpoint based on the number of patients who achieved sustained pain-free relief and sustained pain-free relief without adverse events, Kelman and Von Seggern (2006) calculated that almotriptan 12.5 mg was the most cost-effective triptan. Another analysis conducted on the U.S. population calculated the cost per attack when sustained pain-free relief without adverse events was achieved with almotriptan 12.5 mg and sumatriptan 50 and 100 mg (Williams & Reeder, 2004). Again, this analysis showed that almotriptan was the most cost-effective agent ($82, $133, and $138 per sustained pain-free patient without adverse events, respectively). Further analysis exploring the impact of other health-care costs, doses required, and variability in cost and using different outcome results than those used in the original analysis confirmed that almotriptan was the most cost-effective agent. An Italian study Almotriptan (Gori et al., 2006) showed that almotriptan 12.5 mg was the most cost-effective acute drug for migraine, closely followed by rizatriptan 10 mg.

In a recent study conducted in Spain (Slof et al., 2009), the authors combined the cost of the drugs with the resulting disability and reduction of productivity and also evaluated health-related quality of life. Using this composite evaluation system, the authors showed that almotriptan was more cost-effective than the combination of ergotamine plus caffeine. Indeed, this agent was the dominant option in terms of clinical efficacy, being more economical from a societal perspective.

COSTS OF PROPHYLACTIC TREATMENTS

Very few data are available on the evaluation of cost-effectiveness of preventive treatment for migraine. Prophylactic medication for migraine is usually underused. In the American Migraine and Prevention study conducted by Diamond et al. (2007), 38.8% of migraine patients needed preventive treatment, yet only 12.4% reported that they were taking a migraine preventive treatment for the disease. Nevertheless, 17.2% of patients were using therapies for other concomitant conditions that could be used to prevent migraine (i.e., beta-blockers for hypertension).

According to Silberstein (2005), in patients with high frequency of migraine or comorbid diseases, prophylactic therapy is effective in reducing overall resource utilization, including use and overuse of other migraine medications and subsequent clinical visits and hospitalizations. Adelman et al. (2002) found that the costs of topiramate, an anti-migraine preventive treatment, could be offset by gains achieved by reducing headache frequency, disability, and lost productivity, along with an improvement in the quality of life. More recently, the pattern of headache-related resource utilization and costs before and after initiation of preventive migraine treatment with topiramate was evaluated in a sample of a large managed-care population in a retrospective, longitudinal, cohort study analysis of medical and pharmacy claims using the HealthCore Integrated Research Network Database (Wertz et al., 2009). During and following topiramate intake, outpatient visits decreased by 30%, diagnostic procedures decreased by 74%, emergency room visits decreased by 27%, and abortive prescriptions decreased by 25%. Total headache-related inpatient costs and outpatient costs decreased by 43% and 46%, respectively.

Yu et al. (2010) compared the cost-effectiveness of adding preventive treatment (five agents used for migraine, including amitriptyline, topiramate, timolol, sodium valproate, and propranolol) to the acute therapy versus abortive therapy alone for headache in a primary care setting. The expected total annual cost for the use of preventive treatments in migraine was determined to be lower than the cost for acute therapy only, and amitriptyline results the most cost-effective option (Yu et al., 2010).

Very recently, prophylactic treatment of patients with chronic migraine who overused an acute drug containing botulinum toxin induced a decrease in costs for acute prescription headache medications, including significant reductions in triptan costs (mean reduction of US $100.88 ± $116.57, Canadian $106.32 ± $122.87/month) (Christie et al., 2010). Furthermore, the observed reduction in the percentage of patients with severe disability (as measured with the Migraine Disability Assessment Score [MIDAS]) led researchers to envisage that this approach might also result in a reduction in lost productivity (which was not calculated in the study).

CONCLUSIONS

Migraine is a serious disabling disorder that imposes a substantial burden upon society. The exact size of this burden remains to be defined, especially in terms of pharmacoeconomic costs and benefits. The goals of migraine treatment include relieving pain and restoring ability to function. Migraine treatment programs may reduce the total economic costs of illness by decreasing the indirect costs associated with such headaches: effective migraine therapy reduces absenteeism and improves the productivity of individuals at work. Education of patients and physicians involved in the management of migraine is mandatory for improving the burden of the disease.

REFERENCES

Adelman JU, Adelman LC, Von SR. Cost-effectiveness of antiepileptic drugs in migraine prophylaxis. *Headache* 2002;42:978–983.

Christie SN, Giammarco R, Gawel M, et al. Botulinum toxin type A and acute drug costs in migraine with triptan overuse. *Can J Neurol Sci* 2010;42:978–983.

Diamond S, Bigal ME, Silberstein S, et al. Patterns of diagnosis and acute and preventive treatment for migraine in the United States: results from the American Migraine and Prevention Study. *Headache* 2007;47:355–363.

Goldberg LD. The costs of migraine and its treatment. *Am J Manage Care* 2005;11:S62–S67.

Gori S, Morelli N, Acuto G, et al. A pharmaco-economic evaluation of oral triptans in the treatment of migraine in Italy. *Minerva Med* 2006;97:467–477.

Hawkins K, Rupnow M, Wang S. Direct costs of burden of migraine among member of US employers. *Value Health* 2006;9:A85

Hu XH, Markson LE, Lipton RB, et al. Burden of migraine in the United States: disability and economic costs. *Arch Intern Med* 1999;159:813–818.

Kelman L, Von Seggern RL. Using patient-centered endpoints to determine the cost-effectiveness of triptans for acute migraine therapy. *Am J Ther* 2006;13:411–417.

Leonardi M, Steiner TJ, Scher AT, Lipton RB. The global burden of migraine: measuring disability in headache disorders with WHO's classification of functioning, disability and health (ICF). *J Headache Pain* 2005;6:429–440.

Lipton RB, Stewart WF, Von Korff M. The burden of migraine: a review of cost to society. *Pharmacoeconomics* 1994;6:215–221.

Mullins CD, Subedi PR, Healey PJ, Sanchez RJ. Economic analysis of triptan therapy for acute migraine: a Medicaid perspective. *Pharmacotherapy* 2007;27:1092–1101.

Perfetto EM, Weis KA, Mullins CD, et al. An economic evaluation of triptan products for migraine. *Value Health* 2005;8:647–655.

Silberstein S. Preventive treatment of headaches. *Curr Opin Neurol* 2005;18:289–292.

Slof J, Láinez J, Comas A, Heras J. Almotriptan vs. ergotamine plus caffeine for acute migraine treatment: a cost–efficacy analysis. *Neurologia* 2009;24:147–153.

Stovner LJ, Hagen K, Jensen R, et al. The global burden of headache: a documentation of headache prevalence and disability worldwide. *Cephalalgia* 2007;27:193–210.

Wertz DA, Quimbo RM, Yaldo AZ, Rupnow MF. Resource utilization impact of topiramate for migraine prevention in the managed-care setting. *Curr Med Res Opin* 2009; 25: 499–503.

Williams P, Reeder CE. A comparison of the cost-effectiveness of almotriptan and sumatriptan in the treatment of acute migraine using a composite efficacy/tolerability end point. *J Manage Care Pharm* 2004;10:259–265.

Yu J, Smith K, Brixner D. Cost effectiveness of pharmacotherapy for the prevention of migraine: a Markov model application. *CNS Drugs* 2010;24:695–712.

Pediatric and Juvenile Migraine

Donald W. Lewis, MD, FAAP, FAAN

INTRODUCTION

Migraine is an inherited, chronic, debilitating neurologic disorder that affects the lives of millions of individuals. The origins of this disability can be traced into childhood or adolescence in many of the most severely affected adult migraine sufferers (Bigal & Lipton, 2008). Accurate diagnosis and aggressive treatment *during childhood and adolescence* can prevent decades of suffering and diminished quality of life that are directly attributable to migraine.

This chapter focuses on the clinical manifestations and management options for the broad spectrum of migraine through childhood and adolescence, beginning with the earliest manifestations in early childhood and the evolution toward adult forms during adolescence. A case-based format is used, and emphasis is placed on those clinical entities peculiar to young children. Much of the pharmacological commentary will involve "off-label" use of medications.

A newborn child may be genetically predisposed to migraine (Antilla et al., 2010). The clinical expression of that gene or genes may begin to manifest during early childhood, or it may be delayed until adolescence. When it is expressed in young children or infants, making the diagnosis of migraine can be a particular challenge. Not only do the clinical manifestations vary widely during the various phases of childhood, but the gene may also be expressed incompletely or in unusual forms.

Because the child's nervous system is developing and maturing, the expression may begin with one of the periodic syndromes that are precursors to migraine, before evolving to one of the more characteristic clinical patterns. The diagnostic landscape may be further clouded by mimickers of migraine—that is, other episodic disorders—that also emerge during childhood. For example, mitochondrial or metabolic disturbances, epilepsy syndromes, vascular anomalies, and congenital malformations may present with episodic symptoms, including headache. In addition, the medical history can be limited by the child's ability to articulate the symptoms, complicated by parental interpretation, distortion, and editorial. Further, children are often brought for medical evaluation at the *onset* of transient neurologic, autonomic, gastrointestinal (GI), or visual symptoms, before the characteristic recurrent pattern is established. Curiously, headache may *not* be the primary symptom in such patients. The key aspect to recognizing the spectrum of migraine in children is to appreciate that the migraine is an episodic disorder, separated by symptom-free intervals.

MIGRAINE IN INFANTS, TODDLERS, AND YOUNG CHILDREN

> A mother presents with her 9-month-old child, describing episodes of "head cocking." Several times per month, the child will tilt her head off to one direction, fixed in one position for minutes to hours, tilting her head toward her shoulder and chin up and outward. The position does not appear painful, it may tilt to either direction, and there is no distortion of alertness. The child will occasionally vomit, and once or twice the mother has noted that the baby's eyes will jiggle.

Benign Paroxysmal Torticollis

Perhaps the earliest manifestation of migraine, benign paroxysmal torticollis (BPT) is an uncommon paroxysmal dyskinesia characterized by attacks of head tilt alone or head tilt accompanied by vomiting, nystagmus, and ataxia that may last hours to days. Attacks first manifest during infancy between 2 and 8 months of age, but typically resolve before age 2 years. Other torsional or dystonic features may also be observed during these episodes, including truncal or pelvic posturing (Cohen et al., 1993).

BPT was omitted from the 2004 ICHD classification, but compelling molecular genetic data may result in its inclusion in future editions. Giffin et al. (2002) reported two patients from kindred with familial hemiplegic migraine (FHM) linked to calcium-channel gene (*CACNA1A*) mutation. This report suggests that BPT may be a migraine with aura equivalent. This report broadens our understanding of the varying phenotypic expression of calcium-channelopathies at different stages of development.

BPT is likely an early-onset variant of basilar-type migraine. Nevertheless, the differential diagnosis must include gastroesophageal reflux (i.e., Sandifer syndrome), idiopathic torsional dystonia, and complex partial seizure. In addition, particular attention must be paid to anatomic disturbances in the posterior fossa or craniocervical junction, where congenital or acquired lesions may produce torticollis. Once the diagnosis is established and the benign nature of the condition confirmed, there may be no requirement for treatment beyond reassurance.

Periodic Syndromes of Childhood That Represent Precursors of Migraine

This aptly named group of disorders occurs in toddlers and young children. These conditions are episodic in nature (ergo "periodic") and represent early manifestations of migraine with an evolution toward more typical migraine, at least in some children (ergo "precursors of migraine"). Currently, the ICHD includes three conditions in the category of "periodic syndromes": benign paroxysmal vertigo, cyclic (or cyclical) vomiting syndrome, and abdominal migraine (Cuvellier & Lépine, 2010).

> An 18-month-old child presents with episodes of intense unsteadiness. He is sitting, standing, or walking and then suddenly becomes wildly imbalanced, grabs onto any nearby furniture for support, or drops to the floor. He will occasionally vomit, but there is no loss of consciousness. The child may have as many as 10 episodes in a day, and the length of an attack will typically be measured in minutes; in all cases, it lasts less than an hour. He was not taking or ingesting any drugs. If he has a day with a cluster of spells, his mother comments that the cluster will end following a nap. His father has episodes of headache with vertigo.

Benign Paroxysmal Vertigo

Benign paroxysmal vertigo (BPV) occurs in young children and is characterized by abrupt episodes of unsteadiness or ataxia (**Table 13.1**) (Dunn & Snyder, 1976). The child may appear startled or frightened by the sudden loss of balance. Witnesses may report nystagmus or pallor. Older children may describe a sense of dizziness, imbalance, and nausea. The spells may occur in clusters that typically resolve with sleep.

Table 13.1 Diagnostic Criteria for Benign Paroxysmal Vertigo

Description

This probably heterogeneous disorder is characterized by recurrent, brief, episodic attacks of vertigo occurring without warning and resolving spontaneously in otherwise healthy children.

Diagnostic Criteria

A. At least five attacks fulfilling criterion B
B. Multiple episodes of severe vertigo,* occurring without warning and resolving spontaneously after minutes to hours
C. Normal neurologic examination; audiometric and vestibular functions between attacks
D. Normal electroencephalogram

*BPV attacks are often associated with nystagmus or vomiting, and unilateral throbbing headache may occur in some attacks.

It was long thought that BPV was a precursor for basilar-type migraine and that some proportion of affected children would evolve to develop BTM. Lindskog et al. (1999) reported the results of a 13- to 20-year follow-up on 19 children who experienced onset of BPV symptoms between the ages of 5 months and 8 years; these researchers stated that none were found to have had basilar-type migraine and only 21% evolved to develop more typical migraine.

The diagnosis of BPV is based on a characteristic clinical history, although caution must be exercised to exclude seizure disorders (e.g., benign occipital epilepsy), otological or vestibular pathology, posterior fossa malformations or neoplasms, cervical spine abnormalities, and metabolic disorders (i.e., urea-cycle defects).

A 7-year-old girl presents with an abrupt onset of dramatic vomiting that began when she awakened at 5 A.M. She was pale, photophobic, diaphoretic, and dehydrated, and complained of a vague frontal headache. Emergent head CT was normal. Electrolytes reflected a moderate dehydration with acidosis but no elevation of ammonia levels and a negative toxicological screen. This child was rehydrated and given an antiemetic. She fell asleep and awoke approximately 2 hours later back to her baseline, eager to eat. The astute resident noticed on the electronic medical record that the child had visited the emergency department on eight previous occasions, always at the beginning of the month, with the same history; a diagnosis of "viral gastroenteritis" had been made. Following the most recent prior episode,

social services had investigated the family with a suspicion of "Munchhausen's by proxy" and the case was still open.

Cyclic Vomiting Syndrome

A recurring pattern of episodic vomiting may be seen with a variety of gastrointestinal, neurologic, and metabolic disorders. A subset of these children with stereotyped episodes of vomiting has a migraine precursor known as cyclic or cyclical vomiting syndrome (CVS). The key clinical feature of CVS is recurrent episodes of severe vomiting, interspersed with intervals of wellness (**Table 13.2**).

CVS episodes occur on a regular, often predictable basis every 2 to 4 weeks, lasting 1 to 2 days. The attacks usually begin in the early morning hours or on awakening. The age of onset is approximately 5 years, and boys and girls are affected equally. Generally, a several-year time lag separates the onset of attacks and the recognition of the diagnosis, as the average age of diagnosis is approximately 8 years. Although the majority of children will outgrow their symptoms by age 10, some patients continue to have persistent symptoms through adolescence, and even as young adults (Li et al., 2008).

A complete diagnostic investigation is necessary to exclude other causes of the cyclic vomiting pattern, including upper GI studies, metabolic testing, electroencephalography (EEG), and brain magnetic resonance imaging (MRI).

A comprehensive treatment plan includes acute interventions and prophylactic measures. For acute treatment of attacks, aggressive hydration, sedation, and an

Table 13.2 Diagnostic Criteria for Cyclic Vomiting Syndrome

Description

Recurrent episodic attacks, usually stereotypical in the individual patient, of vomiting and intense nausea. Attacks are associated with pallor and lethargy. There is complete resolution of symptoms between attacks.

Diagnostic Criteria

A. At least five attacks fulfilling criteria B and C
B. Episodic attacks, stereotypical in the individual patient, of intense nausea and vomiting lasting 1 to 5 days
C. Vomiting during attacks occurs at least five times per hour for at least 1 hour
D. Symptom free between attacks
E. Not attributed to another disorder*

*In particular, the patient's history and physical examination do not show signs of gastrointestinal disease.

antiemetic agent represent the first-line choices. Oral or intravenous (IV) hydration with a glucose-containing solution is essential. Antiemetic choices may include ondansetron (0.3–0.4 mg/kg IV or 4–8 mg oral disintegrating or tablet), promethazine (0.25–0.5 mg/kg/dose), metoclopramide (1–2 mg/kg up to 10 mg twice daily), or prochlorperazine (2.5–5 mg twice daily).

During an attack, sedation with a benzodiazepine (lorazepam 0.05–0.1 mg/kg, up to 5 mg) or diphenhydramine (0.25–1 mg/kg) is often necessary. While this indication is off label, nasal (5 mg) or subcutaneous sumatriptan (approximately 0.07 mg/kg) preparations may be considered.

Initiation of a migraine prophylactic agent for CVS should be strongly considered, given that CVS is an extraordinarily disabling condition for both the child and the family. Daily options include cyproheptadine (2–4 mg/day), amitriptyline (5–25 mg/day), anticonvulsants such as valproate (10–14 mg/kg/day) or topiramate (1–10 mg/kg/day), beta-blockers (e.g., propranolol), or calcium-channel blockers (e.g., verapamil).

> A 10-year-old girl presents with recurrent episodes of vague, periumbilical abdominal pain. She has undergone repeated GI and renal work-ups without a diagnosis. The episodes typically last several hours and are not usually associated with vomiting or diarrhea. During the episodes, the child is pale, diaphoretic, and photophobic, and she occasionally complains of a frontal headache. Her mother has suffered from migraine since her teenage years.

Abdominal Migraine

Abdominal migraine is characterized by episodic, vague, midline, or periumbilical abdominal pain (**Table 13.3**). Abdominal migraine generally occurs in school-aged children, who report recurrent attacks of midline, or upper abdominal, pain that is dull in nature and generally lasts for hours (Lewis et al., 2005).

As with CVS, the key to diagnosing this entity is to recognize the recurrent pattern of the symptoms and to exclude other gastrointestinal or renal diseases by appropriate investigations. Approximately 5% to 15% of children with idiopathic, recurrent abdominal pain will fulfill criteria for abdominal migraine.

An up-to-date reference list for CVS and abdominal migraine is available online at www.cvsaonline.org.

> A 6-year-old girl is referred to child psychiatry for "hallucinations." She has experienced several

Table 13.3 Diagnostic Criteria for Abdominal Migraine

Description

An idiopathic recurrent disorder seen mainly in children and characterized by episodic midline abdominal pain, manifesting in attacks lasting 1 to 72 hours, with normality between episodes. The pain is of moderate to severe intensity and is associated with vasomotor symptoms, nausea, and vomiting.

Diagnostic Criteria

A. At least five attacks fulfilling criteria B–D
B. Attacks of abdominal pain lasting 1 to 72 hours
C. Abdominal pain has all of the following characteristics:
   1. Midline location, periumbilical or poorly localized
   2. Dull or "just sore" quality
   3. Moderate or severe intensity
D. During abdominal pain—at least two of the following:
   1. Anorexia
   2. Nausea
   3. Vomiting
   4. Pallor
E. Not attributed to another disorder. History and physical examination do not show signs of gastrointestinal or renal disease, or such disease has been ruled out by appropriate investigations.

episodes during which she "sees funny things" and her pediatrician is concerned she might be psychotic. The visual illusions include facial distortions in which the eyes or ears are large or detached, or the doors appear small or low. The child once described her dog as flying; on another occasion, she was seen dropping bread crumbs onto the carpet which she thought was "a pond and I was feeding the fish."

Following these bizarre episodes, the child was pale and withdrawn, and complained of a frontal headache.

"Alice in Wonderland" Syndrome

While not included among the ICHD classification system, the "Alice in Wonderland" syndrome is a long-recognized clinical entity in children and is now viewed as residing within the spectrum of migraine with aura. The aura most likely arises from spreading cortical depression and oligemia in the parieto-occipital region. The resulting visual aura may include bizarre visual illusions and spatial distortions preceding an otherwise nondescript headache. Patients will describe distorted visual perceptions such as micropsia, macropsia, metamorphopsia, teleopsia, and macro/microsomatognopsia.

MIGRAINE IN OLDER CHILDREN

As children age and mature, more characteristic and recognizable patterns of headache emerge and familiar forms of migraine become more easily identifiable and quantifiable. Bille's landmark epidemiologic survey, conducted in the 1950s and involving 6,000 schoolchildren, reported the prevalence of frequent or recurring patterns of headache, of which migraine represents a significant subset. Such headaches occurred in 2.5% of 7-year-olds, with the rate increasing to 15% of 15-year-olds based on the strict migraine criteria of the time (Bille, 1962).

Subsequent epidemiologic studies have found that the prevalence of migraine headache steadily increases through childhood, peaking in adolescence. Depending on the diagnostic criteria utilized, the prevalence increases from 3% in preschool-aged children, to 4% to 11% in elementary school-aged children, and then to 8% to 23% during the high school years. Before puberty, boys have more headaches than girls; after puberty, migraine headaches occur more frequently in girls (Dalsgaard-Nielsen, 1970; Deubner, 1977; Sillanpaa, 1983).

The incidence of migraine peaks earlier in boys than in girls (Stewart et al., 1991). The mean age of onset of migraine is 7 years for boys and 11 years for girls; the gender ratio also shifts during the adolescent years (**Table 13.4**). The incidence of migraine with aura peaks earlier than the incidence of migraine without aura (Valquist, 1955; Small & Waters, 1974; Sillanpaa, 1976; Mortimer et al., 1992; Stewart et al., 1992; Lipton et al., 1994; Laurell et al., 2004).

The *International Classification of Headache Disorders* (ICHD-2; Olesen, 2004) for migraine is shown in **Table 13.5** and is available online at www.i-h-s.org.

Migraine Without Aura

An 8-year-old boy presents for evaluation of recurring headache that he describes as feeling as if "my heart is pounding in my head." He places his hand across his forehead when asked where the pain is located. His mother reports that he stops

Table 13.4 The Prevalence of Migraine Headache Through Childhood

By Age	3–7 Years	7–11 Years	15 Years
Prevalence	1.2–3.2%	4–11%	8–23%
Gender ratio	Boys > girls	Boys = girls	Boys < girls

Table 13.5 Migraine Classification

Migraine without aura
Migraine with aura
   Typical aura with migraine headache
   Typical aura with non-migraine headache
   Typical aura without headache
   Familial hemiplegic migraine
   Sporadic hemiplegic migraine
   Basilar-type migraine
Childhood periodic syndromes that are commonly precursors of migraine
   Cyclical vomiting
   Abdominal migraine
   Benign paroxysmal vertigo of childhood
Retinal migraine
Complications of migraine
   Chronic migraine
   Status migraine
   Persistent aura without infarction
   Migrainous infarction
   Migraine-triggered seizure
Probable migraine

playing, turns very pale, goes into a cool, dark, quiet room, and occasionally vomits. The child says his tummy hurts but describes no change in vision. After a nap or a period of rest, the pain will be gone in about an hour. The patient has these episodes two or three times per week. His mother and sister have recurring "sinus headaches" with photophobia and nausea.

Migraine without aura is the most frequent form of migraine in children and adolescents (60% to 85%). The key feature of migraine without aura in children consists of episodes of intense, disabling headache separated by symptom-free intervals. The criteria for diagnosis require at least five distinct attacks, lasting 1 to 72 hours, and permit attacks to be shorter in duration in children than in adults (4 to 72 hours) (Dooley & Pearlman, 2010). The location of the pain may be unilateral or, in children younger than 15 years of age, bilateral (bifrontal, bitemporal). The quality of pain is typically pulsing or throbbing, a symptom that may require specific questioning to elicit in young children. By definition, the pain is moderate to intense, and is aggravated by routine physical activity such as walking, running, or climbing stairs. The autonomic features—nausea, vomiting, photophobia, and phonophobia—may be as disabling as the pain. The latter two features may be *inferred* by the patient's behavior if the child withdraws to a quiet, dark place during the attack.

The ICHD diagnostic criteria for this disorder (**Table 13.6**) include three modifications to increase sensitivity of diagnosis in young children: short duration (1 to 72 hours), bilateral/bifrontal location in children younger than 15 years of age, and the inference of photophobia and phonophobia by behavioral response (i.e., withdrawing to a dark quiet room), rather than verbal report. The IHS criteria also include the statement that the headache should "not be attributed to another disorder," implying that the prudent physician will carefully consider other possible causes for the recurrent headaches.

Migraine with Aura

A 9-year-old girl presents with recurring episodes of "fuzzy" vision and headache. The episodes have occurred approximately four times. The child describes seeing dots or rainbows in the middle of her vision so that she cannot read or watch TV until the episode passes, which happens in approximately 20 minutes. Within 30 minutes, she will turn pale, feel nauseated, go into a quiet room, and ask for a cool washcloth to put on her forehead. The girl is anorectic during the episodes and wants to be left alone. The episodes last approximately 4 hours and typically begin at 3 to 4 P.M. (after school). Her mother has menstrual migraine and her maternal grandmother has "retinal" migraine.

Approximately 15% to 30% of children and adolescents with migraine will report visual disturbances, distortions, or obscurations before, or as, the headache begins. The visual symptoms begin gradually and last for several minutes (*typical aura*), as noted in **Table 13.7**. The most frequent forms are binocular visual impairment with scotoma (77%), distortion or hallucinations (16%), and monocular visual impairment or scotoma (7%) (Hachinski et al., 1973). Formed illusions (e.g., spots, balloons, colors, rainbows) or other bizarre visual distortions (e.g. "Alice in Wonderland" syndrome) may be described, albeit infrequently.

A group of disorders are now included within the spectrum of migraine with aura on the basis that the focal symptoms such as visual disruptions, hemiparesis, and aphasia are viewed as manifestations of the regional neuronal depolarization and oligemia caused by CSD (see Table 13.5). In particular, several clinical entities with focal neurologic symptoms, such as hemiplegic and basilar type, are included within this category of migraine with aura.

Sudden images and complicated visual perceptions should prompt consideration of benign occipital epilepsy, specifically Panayiotopoulos syndrome (Parisi et al., 2007). In addition, transient visual obscurations may also be described with idiopathic intracranial hypertension, so not all visual symptoms with headache are due to migraine with aura.

Table 13.6 Diagnostic Criteria for Pediatric Migraine Without Aura

A. At least five attacks fulfilling criteria B through D
B. Headache attacks lasting 1 to 72 hours
C. Headache has at least two of the following characteristics:
    1. Unilateral location, but may be bilateral; fronto-temporal (not occipital)
    2. Pulsing quality
    3. Moderate or severe pain intensity
    4. Aggravation by or causing avoidance of routine physical activity (e.g., walking or climbing stairs)
D. During the headache, at least one of the following:
    1. Nausea and/or vomiting
    2. Photophobia and phonophobia, which may be inferred from the patient's behavior
E. Not attributed to another disorder

Table 13.7 Diagnostic Criteria for Pediatric Migraine with Aura

A. At least two attacks fulfilling criteria B through D
B. Aura consisting of at least one of the following, but no motor weakness:
    1. Fully reversible visual symptoms including positive features (i.e., flickering lights, spots, or lines) and/or negative features (i.e., loss of vision)
    2. Fully reversible sensory symptoms including positive features (i.e., pins and needles) and/or negative features (i.e., numbness)
    3. Fully reversible dysphasic speech disturbance
C. At least two of the following:
    1. Homonymous visual symptoms and/or unilateral sensory symptoms
    2. At least one aura symptom develops gradually over 5 minutes or longer and/or different aura symptoms occur in succession over 5 minutes or longer
    3. Each symptom lasts between 5 and 60 minutes
D. Headache fulfilling the criteria for migraine without aura begins during the aura or follows the aura within 60 minutes
E. Not attributed to another disorder

Basilar-Type Migraine

A 5-year-old presents with dizziness. The child reports spells in which he feels "funny in my head" and his "head spins." The family describes brief, 10- to 15-minute periods of unsteadiness and clumsiness, after which the boy vomits and complains of a "sore" in the back of his head. He feels "weak" all over, particularly in his legs, and refuses to walk during these spells. There is no loss or distortion of consciousness. The head pain lasts about an hour. The child is irritable and pale and prefers to lie down and be very still during the episodes.

Basilar-type migraine (BM) accounts for 3% to 19% of all childhood migraine and has a mean age of onset of 7 years. Attacks are characterized by episodes of dizziness, vertigo, visual disturbances, and ataxia or diplopia as the aura, followed by the headache phase. The pain of BM may be occipital in location, unlike the usual frontal or bitemporal pain of typical migraine. The diagnostic criteria require two or more symptoms and emphasize the bulbar and bilateral sensorimotor features of the migraine (**Table 13.8**). Familiar forms of BM linked to

Table 13.8 Diagnostic Criteria for Basilar-Type Migraine

A. Fulfills criteria for migraine with aura
B. Accompanied by two or more of the following types of symptoms:
    1. Dysarthria
    2. Vertigo
    3. Tinnitus
    4. Hypacusia
    5. Diplopia
    6. Visual phenomena in both the temporal and nasal fields of both eyes
    7. Ataxia
    8. Decreased level of consciousness
    9. Decreased hearing
    10. Double vision
    11. Simultaneous bilateral paresthesias
C. At least one of the following:
    1. At least one aura symptom develops gradually over 5 minutes or longer and/or different aura symptoms occur in succession over 5 minutes or longer.
    2. Each aura symptom lasts more than 5 minutes but less than 60 minutes.
D. Headache fulfilling the criteria for migraine without aura begins during the aura or follows the aura within 60 minutes.

the same genes as familial hemiplegic migraine types 1 and 2 have been reported (Kirchmann et al., 2006).

Familial Hemiplegic Migraine

A 16-year-old presents to the emergency department (ED) following an episode of speech disturbance and right-sided weakness. The event began at school at approximately 9 A.M. The girl noticed first that her right hand became numb, and then it became difficult to hold her pen or to text on her phone. Her teacher asked the girl what was wrong, and she was unable to make the words to respond. The words that "came out were slurred." She began to hyperventilate and tried to stand but her whole right side was weak. Emergency medical services (EMS) was summoned, and the patient was delivered to a nearby ED, where noncontrast computed tomography (CT) studies were normal. The ED team was convinced that the event was a stroke and wanted to start tissue plasminogen activator (TPA) infusion, but hesitated when the girl's mother arrived and said this episode was very similar to the attacks she and her father had experienced as teenagers.

Familial hemiplegic migraine falls into the category of migraine with aura. This type of migraine is heralded by an aura that has "stroke-like" qualities producing some degree of hemiparesis (**Table 13.9**). The transient episodes of focal neurologic deficits precede the headache phase by 30 to 60 minutes, but occasionally extend well beyond the headache itself (hours to days). The location of headache is often, but not invariably, contralateral to the focal deficits. Many children and adolescents will report transient somatosensory symptoms heralding an attack, with focal paresthesias noted around the mouth and hand (e.g., chiro-oral) without weakness; this does not fulfill the criteria for hemiplegic migraine, however. Genetic testing is commercially available to determine whether a person has FHM type 1.

No form of migraine has yielded more information about the underlying molecular genetics of migraine than FHM. FHM type 1 is an uncommon autosomal dominant form of migraine with aura caused by a missense mutation in the calcium-channel gene (*CACNA1A*) linked to chromosome 19p13. FHM types 2 and 3 are clinically quite similar but have distinctly different molecular mechanisms. FHM type 2 is due to a point mutation of the alpha$_2$ subunit of the sodium–potassium pump (*ATP1A2*) gene on chromosome 1q21–23, whereas

Table 13.9 Diagnostic Criteria for Familial Hemiplegic Migraine

A. Fulfills the criteria for migraine with aura
B. Aura consists of fully reversible motor weakness and at least one of the following:
   1. Fully reversible visual symptoms including positive features (e.g., flickering lights, spots, or lines) and/or negative features (e.g., loss of vision)
   2. Fully reversible sensory symptoms including positive features (e.g., pins and needles)
   3. Fully reversible dysphasic speech disturbance
C. At least two of the following:
   1. At least one aura symptom develops gradually over more than 5 minutes
   2. The aura symptom lasts more than 5 minutes and less than 24 hours
   3. Headache that fulfills the criteria for migraine without aura begins during the aura or follows the onset of aura within 60 minutes
D. At least one first-degree or second-degree relative has had an attack
E. At least one of the following:
   1. History and physical and neurologic examinations not suggesting any organic disorder
   2. History or physical or neurologic examinations suggesting such disorder, but ruled out by appropriate investigations

type 3 is due to a sodium-channel gene mutation (*SCN1A*) (DeFusco et al., 2003; Dichgans et al., 2005).

Diagnosis of sporadic hemiplegic migraine is made in patients who present with an abrupt onset of focal neurologic signs or repetitive episodes of focal neurologic symptoms *without* family history.

Other Forms of Migraine Seen in Children and Adolescents

Confusional Migraine

A 14-year-old high school football player is brought to the ED following a scrimmage, after he experienced disorientation, confusion, agitation, and slurred speech. The boy was tackled following a punt return, got up, and returned slowly to the bench; within approximately 15 minutes, he became dazed, irritable, and combative. EMS was called. Although the patient resisted leaving the field of play, he was convinced by teammates to get into the ambulance. In the ED, noncontrast CT was normal, as was a urine toxicology screen. By the time his parents arrived, the patient had a global

pounding headache with nausea, but mentation and agitation were returning to baseline. His father reported two prior episodes of "concussion."

Headache and altered mental status following head injury constitute a neurologic emergency, and the ED performance of a noncontrast CT cited in the preceding case was appropriate. Likewise, laboratory studies including serum electrolytes and toxicology assessment are indicated for a teenage patient with altered sensorium. While clearly a diagnosis of exclusion, confusional migraine is a strong consideration in this clinical picture and within the spectrum of trauma-triggered migraine. Confusional migraine often occurs following a seemingly innocuous head injury that occurs in the context of sports (e.g., soccer, football, skating).

The key features of confusional migraine are altered mental status and perceptual distortions (Shaabat, 1996). Affected patients—usually boys—abruptly become agitated, restless, disoriented, and occasionally combative. The confusion phase may last minutes to hours. Later, once consciousness returns to baseline, the patients describe an inability to communicate, frustration, confusion, and loss of orientation to time, and they may *not* recall a headache phase at all.

Confusional migraine is not included in the ICHD classification system and most likely represents an overlap between hemiplegic migraine and basilar-type migraine. Patients who present with unilateral weakness or language disorders should be classified as having hemiplegic migraine, whereas patients with vertiginous or ataxic patterns should be classified as having basilar-type migraine.

Ophthalmoplegic Migraine

A 10-year-old girl presents with a "droopy" eyelid on the left side of her face, which has persisted for the past 2 days. She describes double vision when she looks to the right and has a boring pain in the left retro-orbital region. There was no antecedent trauma or illness. A neuro-ophthalmological examination demonstrates partial third nerve palsy on the left side. CT of the head and sinuses is normal. Six months earlier, the girl experienced a similar episode affecting the left eye, for which she received a 10-day course of prednisone and which resolved completely.

The key clinical feature of this case is painful ophthalmoparesis, and the differential diagnosis must include intraorbital infectious or inflammatory processes, brain tumor, demyelinative disorders, and post-infectious oculomotor disorders. The case presented here is consistent with ophthalmoplegic migraine (OM). OM has actually been removed from the migraine spectrum and is now included in the category of "cranial neuralgias"—a change prompted by elegant neuro-imaging evidence that demonstrated an underlying demyelinating–remyelinating mechanism (**Table 13.10**). Because OM is no longer viewed as migraine, eventually the term "ophthalmoplegic migraine" will likely evolve to become "ophthalmoplegic neuralgia" or "neuralgiform disorder."

The pain of OM may be a nondescript ocular or retro-ocular discomfort. Ptosis, limited adduction, and vertical displacement (e.g., effects on cranial nerve III) are the most common objective findings. The oculomotor symptoms and signs may appear well into the headache phase, rather than heralding the headache, contrary to the sequence observed with the more typical migraine. The signs may persist for days or even weeks after the headache has resolved.

The migraine precursors and these unusual forms of migraine with aura are unique to pediatrics and represent a challenging group of disorders characterized by the abrupt onset of focal neurologic signs and symptoms (e.g., hemiparesis, altered consciousness, nystagmus, or ophthalmoparesis) followed by headache. Frequently,

these ominous neurologic signs initially point the clinician in the direction of epileptic, cerebrovascular, traumatic, or metabolic disorders; only after thorough neuro-diagnostic testing does the migraine diagnosis become apparent. Some of these entities occur in infants and young children, in whom history is limited. Only after careful history, physical, and appropriate neuro-diagnostic studies can these diagnoses be comfortably entertained.

MANAGEMENT OF CHILDHOOD AND ADOLESCENT MIGRAINE

Once the diagnosis of migraine is established, a balanced, flexible, and individually tailored treatment plan can be put in place. It is important to educate the patient and the family about the diagnosis and to provide reassurance about the absence of other life-threatening disorders. The first step in developing the treatment plan is to appreciate the degree of disability imposed by the patient's headache. Understanding of the headache's impact on the quality of life will aid the clinician in identifying the most appropriate therapeutic course of action (Powers et al., 2003, 2004).

Goals of Treatment

Six fundamental goals of long-term migraine treatment have been established:

1. Reduction of headache frequency, severity, duration, and disability
2. Reduction of reliance on poorly tolerated, ineffective, or unwanted acute pharmacotherapies
3. Improvement in the quality of life
4. Avoidance of acute headache medication escalation
5. Education and enablement of patients to manage their disease to enhance personal control of their migraine
6. Reduction of headache-related distress and psychological symptoms (Silberstein, 2000)

To achieve these goals, the treatment regimen typically includes both biobehavioral strategies and pharmacological measures. Biobehavioral treatments may consist of biofeedback, stress management, sleep hygiene, exercise, and dietary modifications (**Table 13.11**). The value of these interventions cannot be overstated. Virtually all migraine sufferers will benefit from review of these measures, but certainly those patients who experience more frequent attacks, even daily migraine, will have

Table 13.10 Diagnostic Criteria for Ophthalmoplegic Migraine

Description
Recurrent attacks of headache with migrainous characteristics associated with paresis of one or more ocular cranial nerves (commonly the oculomotor nerve) in the absence of any demonstrable intracranial lesion other than MRI changes within the affected nerve.

Diagnostic Criteria
A. At least two attacks fulfilling criterion B
B. Migraine-like headache accompanied or followed within 4 days of its onset by paresis of one or more of the third, fourth, or sixth cranial nerves
C. Parasellar, orbital fissure and posterior fossa lesions ruled out by appropriate investigations

ICHD notes: Ophthalmoplegic "migraine" is a variant of migraine in which the headache often lasts for a week or more and there is a latent period of up to 4 days from the onset of headache to the onset of ophthalmoplegia. Furthermore, in some cases, MRI shows gadolinium uptake in the cisternal part of the affected cranial nerve, which suggests that the condition may be a recurrent demyelinating neuropathy.

Table 13.11 Biobehavioral Therapies for Pediatric Migraine

Identification of migraine triggers (foods, aromas, emotional, stresses)
Biobehavioral
    Biofeedback
        Electromyographic biofeedback
        Electroencephalography
        Thermal hand warming
        Galvanic skin resistance feedback
    Relaxation therapy
        Progressive muscle relaxation
        Autogenic training
        Meditation
        Passive relaxation
        Self-hypnosis
    Cognitive therapy/stress management
        Cognitive control
        Guided imagery
Dietary measures
    "Avoidance diets"
    Caffeine moderation
    Herbs
        Butterbur root
        Feverfew (*Tanacetum parthenium*)
        Ginkgo
        Valerian root
    Minerals
        Magnesium
    Vitamins
        Riboflavin (vitamin B$_2$)
Acupuncture
Aroma therapy

a greater degree of disability and, therefore, a greater need to reinforce them. Biofeedback and stress management, both of which are underutilized therapies, have been subjected to controlled trials and have been recently reviewed (Eidlitz-Markus et al., 2010; Hershey et al., 2010).

Biobehavioral Strategies

The basic recommendations given to pediatric migraine sufferers include getting regular sleep and exercise, having only moderate caffeine intake, and ensuring adequate hydration. The role of diet in migraine prevention and mitigation is controversial (Millichap & Yee, 2003). Between 7% and 44% of patients report that a particular food or drink can precipitate a migraine attack (Van den Bergh et al., 1987; Stang et al., 1992). In children, the primary dietary triggers are cheese, chocolate, and citrus fruits. Wholesale dietary elimination schedules are not recommended, however. Such elimination diets are generally excessive and set the stage for a battleground at home when parents attempt to enforce a restrictive diet upon an unwilling, resistant adolescent. The ensuing family friction may ultimately heighten tensions at home, thereby worsening the headache pattern. A more reasonable approach is to provide the patient and the family with a list of foods that, in some patients, may be linked to migraine. We then encourage the patient to keep a headache diary to see whether a temporal relationship exists between ingestion of one or more of those foods and the development of headache. If a link is discovered, common sense dictates avoidance of the offending food substance.

Table 13.11 identifies some of the complementary and alternative treatment measures for pediatric and adult migraine. Although few of these therapies have been subjected to controlled trials in children, they have become commonly used and are widely recommended on patient-education websites. Both magnesium (400–800 mg/day) and riboflavin (vitamin B$_2$) (400 mg/day) have demonstrated efficacy in controlled prophylaxis trials and are currently recommended for the prevention of migraine in adults (Schurks et al., 2008). Data regarding the efficacy of other herbal remedies are limited in children. Butterbur root, for example, was compared to placebo and music therapy. Only music therapy showed superiority compared to placebo during the trial period, but during extended follow-up, both music therapy and butterbur showed value (Oelker, 2008).

An intriguing study was conducted by Hershey et al. (2007), who sought to explore the value of coenzyme Q10 (Co-Q10) in the management of migraine. When the authors measured the levels of Co-Q10 in 1,550 children with documented migraine, they found that 33% had values less than reference range. These patients were supplemented with 1–3 mg/kg/day of Co-Q10. Upon follow-up, their headache frequency had improved from 19 headaches (±10) to 12 (±11)/month (P <0.001). The authors proposed that Co-Q10 deficiency may be a common phenomenon in children with frequent migraine (Hershey et al., 2007). This issue clearly warrants further study.

Overuse of over-the-counter (OTC) analgesics (more than five times per week) can be a contributing factor to frequent, even daily, headache patterns. When recognized, patients who are overusing analgesics must be educated to discontinue the practice. Retrospective studies have suggested that this recommendation alone can decrease headache frequency (Reimschisel, 2003; Rothner & Guo, 2004).

Pharmacological Measures

The pharmacological management of pediatric migraine has been subjected to thorough review but controlled data are, unfortunately, limited. Consequently, recommendations for this population are all "off label" (Victor & Ryan, 2003; Lewis et al., 2004a, 2005a, 2005b; Hamalainen, 2006; Gunner et al., 2008).

Acute Therapies for Pediatric Migraine

Acute treatments represent the mainstay of migraine management. Patients should be offered several acute treatment options to explore after the initial office visit, so that they may determine what works most effectively for them. Regardless of the acute treatment selected, several basic guidelines should be followed regarding the use of acute treatments, which must be included as part of the patient's educational process. The essential message is *give enough and give it early*!

1. Take the medicine as soon as possible when the headache begins, even when the migraine is still mild, but within 20 to 30 minutes.
2. Take the appropriate dose based on the patient's weight (e.g., ibuprofen 10 mg/kg).
3. Ensure that the medicine is available at the location where the patient usually has headaches (e.g., school) and complete the school medicine forms to allow prompt administration at school.
4. Avoid analgesic overuse (more than three to five doses of analgesic per week).

For the acute treatment of migraine, the most rigorously studied agents are ibuprofen, acetaminophen, and selected triptans (rizatriptan and almotriptan tablets, sumatriptan and zolmitriptan nasal sprays), which have shown safety and efficacy in controlled trials (**Table 13.12**). While triptans have revolutionized acute migraine treatment for adults, only almotriptan (12.5 mg) has been approved by the FDA for use in adolescents, even though multiple studies have demonstrated this agent's safety in children (Major et al., 2003; Silver et al., 2008).

Acute Treatments for Young Children   For children younger than 12 years of age, ibuprofen (7.5–10 mg/kg) and acetaminophen (15 mg/kg) have demonstrated efficacy and safety for the acute treatment of migraine (Hamalainen et al., 1997a; Lewis et al., 2002).

Acute Treatments for Adolescents (Triptans)   For adolescents (12 to 17 years of age), in addition to ibuprofen and acetaminophen, sumatriptan (5 and 20 mg) and

Table 13.12 Acute Treatment for Pediatric Migraine

Drug	Dose	Available Form
Acetaminophen*	10–15 mg/kg/ dose	Tablets 80, 160, 325 mg Syrup 160 mg/tsp
Ibuprofen*	10 mg/kg/dose	Tablets 100 mg chewable; 200, 400, 600, 800 mg Syrup 100 mg/tsp
Naproxen sodium	2.5–5 mg/kg	Tablets 220 (OTC), 250, 375, 500 mg
5-HT Agonists		
Almotriptan*†		Tablets 12.5 mg
Sumatriptan*†		Tablets 25, 50,100 mg Subcutaneous injection 6 mg Nasal spray 5, 20 mg*
Zolmitriptan‡		2.5, 5 mg Disintegrating tablets 2.5, 5 mg
Rizatriptan		Tablets 5, 10 mg Disintegrating tablets 5, 10 mg

*Supportive efficacy and safety data in adolescents.
†Approved for use in adolescents 12 to 17 years of age with migraine pain and attacks of more than 4 hours' duration.
‡Not approved for pediatric use.

zolmitriptan (5 mg) in the nasal spray forms, and rizatriptan (5 and 10 mg) and almotriptan (6.25, 12.5, and 25 mg) in the tablet forms have demonstrated both safety and efficacy in controlled trials (see Table 13.12) (Hamalainen et al., 1997b; Winner et al., 2000; Ueberall, 2001; Ahonen et al., 2004, 2006; Charles, 2006; Evers et al., 2006; Lewis et al., 2007; Linder et al., 2008; Papetti et al., 2010).

In June 2009, almotriptan was approved by the FDA for the acute treatment of migraine pain in adolescents whose migraines typically last longer than 4 hours. This approval was based on data from a study of 866 adolescents who were randomized in a double-blind, placebo-controlled, parallel-group, multicenter clinical trial, to receive 6.25-, 12.5-, or 25-mg doses versus matched placebo. The results demonstrated headache relief (defined as a 2-point reduction in pain on a 4-point scale) at a 2-hour endpoint in 72%, 73%, and 67% of almotriptan recipients, respectively, versus 55% for the placebo group; statistical significance was reached with the 6.25-mg and the 12.5-mg doses ($P < 0.001$). Interestingly, the study designers used the bold composite primary endpoint of "migraine relief," meaning relief of pain *and* associated symptoms; the data failed to reach statistical significance in this regard, primarily because of almotriptan's lack of efficacy for nausea. Nonetheless, the gold standard for migraine trials has been headache relief at 2 hours, a secondary endpoint in this study, for which the findings did achieve statistical significance. Based on these results, almotriptan is now approved in the United States for the acute treatment of adolescent migraine.

Combination agents such as sumatriptan 85 mg plus naproxen 550 mg have demonstrated efficacy in adults. In an open-label safety study in adolescents (aged 12-17 years) with an average of 2–8 migraines per month (n = 622) who treated at least 1 migraine with sumatriptan/naproxen sodium, 42% of the patients were pain free within 2 hours of treatment with sumatriptan/naproxen sodium. In addition, subjects reported improvements from baseline in 2 of 3 quality of life domains over time and were generally satisfied with the efficacy and tolerability at the end of the study (McDonald et al., 2011).

Preventive Therapies for Pediatric Migraine

A variety of medications are used to prevent attacks of migraine **(Table 13.13)**. It is prudent for the primary care physicians to become comfortable with a few of these agents. Daily preventive therapy should be limited to those patients whose headaches occur with sufficient frequency and/or severity as to warrant a daily treatment program. Most clinical studies require a minimum of three headaches per month to justify use of a daily agent. A clear sense of functional disability must be established before committing to a course of daily medication.

When selecting a daily medicine to use, it is useful to identify the presence of "comorbid conditions," which may suggest that one agent will demonstrate a relative benefit over another option. For example, if there is comorbid sleep disorder, amitriptyline or melatonin may be helpful. If there is a problem with the child being underweight, cyproheptadine or valproate might be

Table 13.13 Preventive Treatment for Pediatric Migraine

Drug	Dose	Available Form	Toxicity
Antihistamines			
Cyproheptadine	0.25–1.5 mg/kg	Syrup 2 mg/tsp Tablets 4 mg	Sedation, weight gain
Anticonvulsants			
Topiramate*	1–10 mg/kg/day	Sprinkles 15, 25 mg Tablets 25, 100 mg	Anorexia, paresthesias, weight loss, glaucoma, kidney stones
Valproic acid	20–40 mg/kg/day	Syrup 250 mg/tsp Sprinkles 125 mg Tablets 250, 500 mg Extended release 500 mg	Weight gain, hair loss, bruising, hepatotoxicity, ovarian cysts
Levetiracetam	125–250 mg bid	Tablets 250, 500, 750, 1,000 mg	Sedation, dizziness, irritability
Antidepressants			
Amitriptyline	5–25 mg qhs	Tablets 10, 25, 50 mg	Sedation
Nortriptyline	10–75 mg qhs	Tablets 10, 25, 50, 75 mg	Weight gain
Nonsteroidal Anti-Inflammatory Agents			
Naproxen sodium	250–500 bid	Tablets 220, 250, 375, 500 mg	Gastritis, nephritis
Calcium-Channel Blockers			
Flunarizine*	5–10 mg qhs	Capsules 5 mg	Drowsiness, weight gain
Verapamil	4–10 mg/kg/day tid	Tablets 40, 80, 120 mg SR tablets 120, 180, 240 mg	Nausea, hypotension, atrioventricular block, weight gain
Beta-Blockers			
Propranolol†	2–4 mg/kg/day	10, 20, 40, 60, 80 mg LA caplets 60, 80, 120, 160 mg	Hypotension, sleep disorder, decreased stamina, depression

*Supportive efficacy and safety data in adolescents.

†Avoid in patients with asthma, diabetes, and depression.

considered. In contrast, if the adolescent is overweight or obese, topiramate may be a good choice.

Once preventive treatment is initiated, both family and patient must be encouraged to permit enough time to elapse so that the beneficial effects can be appreciated. Generally, an 8- to 12-week course is required before the chosen agent can be called either a success or a failure. This point must be emphasized when the prescriptions are provided, because many impatient families will expect immediate effects after the first days of treatment. It is not uncommon to see families who state that multiple drugs that "failed" in the child, only to discover that the therapeutic trials lasted only a few days each.

The duration of treatment is controversial. Migraine in children and adolescents exhibits both seasonality and a cycling nature in many patients. For this reason, daily agents should be used for a finite period of time. The general recommendation is to provide treatment through the school year, then gradually eliminate daily agents during summer vacation. Another option in younger children is to use a shorter course (e.g., 6 to 8 weeks), followed by a slow wean off the medicine.

For preventive and/or prophylactic treatment in children and adolescents with frequent, disabling migraine, efficacy and safety data in children are available for only two agents—flunarizine, which is not available in the United States, and topiramate. These two agents with evidence-based data will be discussed next. Encouraging data are also emerging regarding several other agents, including the antiepileptic agents sodium valproate and levetiracetam, as well as the antihistamine cyproheptadine and the antidepressant amitriptyline (see Table 13.13) (Serdaroglu et al., 2002; Damen et al., 2006; Eiland et al., 2007).

Flunarizine Flunarizine is a calcium-channel blocker that has been studied in well-controlled trials for its ability to prevent pediatric migraine. Two double-blind, placebo-controlled trials using 5-mg bedtime doses of flunarizine ($n = 105$) produced a significant reduction in headache frequency, and one of the trials also demonstrated decreased headache duration (Sorge & Marano, 1985; Sorge et al., 1988). In this first trial, the frequency of migraine headaches was reduced from a baseline of 8.66 episodes over 3 months to 2.95 attacks during treatment. Approximately 76% of the patients taking flunarizine experienced greater than 50% improvement, whereas only 19% taking placebo had greater than 50% improvement. Another open-label trial of 13 patients showed decreased headache frequency (Guidetti et al., 1987). Other than sedation (9.5%) and weight gain (22.2%), side effects were minimal.

Based on these strong data, the 2004 AAN Practice Parameter for the treatment of pediatric migraine found that "flunarizine is *probably effective* for preventive therapy and can be considered for this purpose but it is not available in the United States."

Topiramate Topiramate is gaining wide acceptance for pediatric migraine, and a mounting body of evidence, based on well-designed controlled trials, supports its use for this indication. A 26-week trial of 50-, 100-, and 200-mg doses of topiramate found this agent produced a reduction in monthly migraine frequency of 46%, 63%, and 65%, respectively, versus a reduction of 16% with placebo (Winner et al., 2006). A second trial, in which 44 children were evenly randomized to receive either 100 mg divided twice a day or placebo, found a reduction in mean monthly migraine attacks from 16 per month to 4 per month in the treatment group versus 13 per month to 8 per month in the placebo group ($P = 0.025$) (Lakshmi et al., 2007). In this study, researchers identified a significant reduction in overall disability and in school absenteeism as well.

A third, recent report comparing doses of 50 mg/day, 100 mg/day, and matched placebo found statistically significant improvement from the prospective baseline period in migraine frequency in the 100-mg group (75% decrease in monthly migraine), but not in the 50-mg group (46% decrease) or the placebo group (45%) ($P = 0.016$). The greatest benefit was appreciated in the 100-mg group (50 mg oral dose, given twice daily), in which it was observed that more than 80% of patients experienced a greater than 50% reduction in headache burden after approximately 8 weeks of treatment (Lewis et al., 2009).

Typically, for teenagers, a dose of 15 to 25 mg of topiramate is initiated as a single bedtime dose and then gradually titrated toward 50 mg twice a day incrementally on a weekly or every-other-week basis. Clinical experience has demonstrated that many patients will respond with doses as low as 25 mg at bedtime, so it is valuable to "titrate to effect." Cognitive effects must be monitored quite carefully, and more evidence is needed to assess the educational impact of topiramate for prevention of adolescent migraine. It is counterproductive to reduce headache burden at the expense of academic performance.

Other Preventive Options Uncontrolled data and a wealth of clinical experience suggest that some other agents may have value in preventing pediatric migraine, including cyproheptadine, amitriptyline, beta-blockers, and divalproex sodium. In addition, uncontrolled data from small series suggest a possible role for the antiepilepsy agents levetiracetam and zonisamide.

For young children (younger than 10 years) who are not overweight, cyproheptadine at a starting dose of 2 to 4 mg as a single bedtime dose is a simple and safe strategy. Although the dosing schedule may be gradually changed to twice or even three times a day, most children become overly sedated at doses higher than 4 to 8 mg per day.

Amitriptyline is one of the most widely used agents for the prophylactic treatment of pediatric migraine. While amitriptyline has never been assessed in blinded, controlled trials, two open-label studies in children have found that this agent offers both safety and beneficial effects. The first study (n = 192) treated patients with doses up to 1/mg/kg/day; the researchers found that 84% of the patients experienced reductions in both frequency and severity of their headaches (Hershey et al., 2000). The second study (n = 73) found a "positive response rate" of 89% (Lewis et al., 2004b).

Typical starting dose of amitriptyline is 5 to 10 mg at bedtime, but may be gradually increased toward 1 mg/kg/day. The issue of whether a pretreatment ECG is needed remains a source of controversy.

Once the "drugs of choice" for pediatric migraine, beta-blockers now have a quite limited role in children and adolescents. Propranolol has been studied in three randomized, double-blind studies, but the results failed to consistently demonstrate its effectiveness in this indication (Ludvigsson, 1974; Forsythe, 1984; Olness et al., 1987). Propranolol may be used in a single daily dose ("LA") form or dosed on a two or three times per day schedule. The starting dose of 1–2 mg/kg/day is slowly escalated to 3 mg/kg/day as tolerated. Dosing adjustments can be made every 2 to 3 weeks. The selective beta-blockers atenolol, metoprolol, and nadolol are alternatives to propranolol, but there are no data to suggest any relative advantage of one versus the others.

Beta-blockers as a group are contraindicated in the presence of reactive airway disease, diabetes mellitus, orthostatic hypotension, and cardiac disorders associated with bradyarrhythmias. Curiously, a subset of patients with both neurocardiogenic syncope and comorbid migraine respond favorably to propranolol treatment.

Special caution must be taken when contemplating use of beta-blockers in either athletes or patients with affective disorders, particularly depression. Athletes may experience a lack of stamina and decreased performance when taking these medications. Those children with comorbid affective disorders can experience

deterioration of mood, and even suicidal depression, with propranolol.

Studies of divalproex sodium have yielded strong efficacy data in adults, and this agent is approved for use as a migraine preventive agent. No controlled trials for this indication exist in children or adults, however. Four open-label trials have shown beneficial effects from divalproex sodium in migraine. In one study of 42 children (7 to 16 years; mean: 11.3 years old), a 50% headache reduction was seen in 78.5% of patients, a 75% reduction was seen in 14.2% of patients, and 9.5% of patients became headache free. These open-label trial results indicate that this medication has the potential to be an effective and well-tolerated treatment for the prophylaxis of migraine in children (Caruso et al., 2000; Pakalnis et al., 2001; Serdaroglu et al., 2002).

Likewise, use of levetiracetam is supported by open-label data from 19 patients (mean: 11.9 years old) whose mean migraine frequency decreased from 6.3 migraines per month to 1.7 attacks per month at doses ranging from 125 to 250 mg twice a day. Ten patients (52.6%) had complete resolution of headache. The authors concluded that levetiracetam appeared to be a promising candidate for well-controlled clinical trials in pediatric patients with migraine (Miller, 2004). In a second open-label trial involving 20 patients, 18 patients had a 50% or greater reduction in monthly migraine frequency and had lowered disability scales at levetiracetam doses of approximately 20 mg/kg/day (Pakalnis et al., 2007).

In one small open-label study, children (10 to 17 years) with mixed, refractory headache conditions (50% migraine) were treated with an average dose of 6 mg/kg/day of zonisamide (Pakalnis & Kring, 2006). Two-thirds had a greater than 50% reduction in headache frequency from baseline.

PROGNOSIS

The long-term prognosis of adolescents with migraine has not been well studied. Five- to 7-year follow-up studies have revealed that 20% to 25% of adolescents originally diagnosed with migraine have remission of symptoms, 50% to 60% have persistence of their migraine with aura, and 25% convert to tension-type headache (TTH). Twenty percent who are originally diagnosed with TTH convert to migraine (Camarda et al., 2002; Kienbacher et al., 2006). When Monastero et al. (2006) evaluated 55 adolescents with migraine who were available for 10-year follow-up, they found that 42% had persistent migraine, 38% had experienced remission, and 20% had transformed to TTH. Interestingly, only migraine without aura persisted through the 10-year follow-up period, whereas other migrainous disorders and nonclassifiable headaches did not (Monastero et al., 2006).

The longest follow-up available came from Brna et al. (2005), who provided 20-year information on 60 patients out of an original cohort of 95 from 1983. Of the 60 individuals, 27% were headache free, 33% had TTH, 17% had migraine, and 23% had both TTH and migraine. Of those with persistent headache, 80% described their headaches as moderate to severe, although an overall improvement was described in 66%. TTH was more likely to remit. Headache severity at diagnosis was the most predictive of headache outcome at 20 years (Brna et al., 2005).

Collectively, these data indicate that female gender, worse migraine severity at diagnosis, and longer duration from time of onset of headache until time of initial medical examination are suggestive of an unfavorable prognosis. Given our current understanding of the long-term neuropathological and psychosocial consequences of persistent, frequent migraine, longitudinal epidemiologic studies of the evolution of adolescent migraine are imperative.

CONCLUSIONS

Migraine is a common disorder in children and adolescents. A wide spectrum of clinical forms are recognized, but the most frequently encountered variant is migraine without aura, which is characterized by attacks of frontal or bitemporal pounding, nauseating headache lasting 1 to 72 hours. A fascinating and challenging subset of disorders known as migraine with aura and the "periodic syndromes" can be associated with frightening focal neurologic disturbances and may require careful consideration for the possibility of neoplastic, vascular, metabolic, or toxic disorders.

Migraine treatment philosophy now embraces a balanced approach including both biobehavioral interventions and pharmacological measures. Treatment decisions must be based on the disability produced by the headaches—that is, the headache burden. A growing body of controlled pediatric data is beginning to emerge regarding the acute and preventive agents, thereby lessening clinicians' dependence upon extrapolated adult data for this indication.

For acute treatment of pediatric migraine, controlled data demonstrate the efficacy of acetaminophen, ibuprofen, tablet forms of almotriptan and rizatriptan, and nasal spray forms of sumatriptan and zolmitriptan. Only almotriptan is approved in the United States for the treatment of acute migraine pain in children ages 12 to 17 years. For preventive therapies, a wide variety of agents are used, but only flunarizine and topiramate have controlled data demonstrating their efficacy and safety.

In the near future, we anticipate further advances in understanding the molecular genetics of migraine, advances that will eventually translate into improved care of the pediatric patient with migraine headache. Further, the therapeutic energy expended on our pediatric patients will translate into decreased disability as our patients progress into adulthood, lessening the lifespan burden of migraine.

CASE REPORTS

Case 1

A 6-year-old boy presents with two to three intense frontal pounding headaches per week, during which he withdraws to a quiet, dark room and occasionally vomits. He is otherwise healthy except for mild reactive airway disease, and there has been no deterioration in school performance or behavior. His mother has menstrual migraine. The child's examination is normal except for his weight, which is below the fifth percentile.

> Diagnosis: migraine without aura
> Neuro-imaging: not warranted
> Institute biobehavioral regimen (see Table 13.11)
> Acute treatment:
> - Ibuprofen 10 mg/kg at onset of headache
> - Naproxen sodium 220 mg orally at onset of headache
> - If NSAIDs are ineffective, oral disintegrating or nasal spray triptan*
>
> Preventive treatment:
> - Cyproheptadine 2–4 mg orally at bedtime; option: up to 6–8 mg/day divided bid-tid
> - Amitriptyline 5 mg at bedtime; option: gradually increasing up to 1 mg/kg/day weekly
> Caution: propranolol (asthma), topiramate (weight < 5%)

Case 2

A 16-year-old girl presents with two episodes of intense temporal, pounding headaches per week, during which she complains that bright lights and loud music make her headache worse. She describes a flickering light in her lateral visual field that begins approximately 20 minutes before the pain emerges. On occasion, she

---

*Triptans are not approved for children younger than 12 years.

experiences numbness and tingling in her hand and around her mouth before the headache begins. She is otherwise healthy. There has been no deterioration in school performance or behavior changes. Her aunt has related migraine and father had migraine as a child. The patient's examination is normal except that her weight is above the 90th percentile.

> Diagnosis: migraine with aura
> Neuro-imaging: not warranted
> Institute biobehavioral regimen (see Table 13.11)
> Acute treatment options:
> - Ibuprofen 400–800 mg at onset of headache
> - Naproxen sodium 500 mg at onset of headache
> - If NSAIDs are ineffective, oral or intranasal triptan*
>
> Preventive treatment:
> - Topiramate 25 mg at bedtime, gradually titrating upward by 25-mg increments toward 50 mg bid every 1–2 weeks
> - Amitriptyline 10 mg at bedtime; option: gradually increasing up to 1 mg/kg/day weekly (usually not more than 50 mg/day)

Case 3

A 12-year-old boy presents following three stereotyped episodes of intense frontal pounding headaches, during which he complains of feeling weak and clumsy on his right side and has slurred speech. During these events, he goes into a dark room and occasionally vomits. He is otherwise healthy. There has been no deterioration in school performance or behavior. His mother and maternal grandmother have had similar attacks with weakness, slurred speech, and intense headache. The patient's examination is normal.

> Diagnosis: familial hemiplegic migraine
> Neuro-imaging: warranted (MRI, MRA, or CTA)
> Other testing: specific genetic testing for FHM
> If genetic testing is unrevealing, consider cardiac and coagulation evaluation
> Institute a biobehavioral regimen (see Table 13.11)
> Acute treatment:
> - Ibuprofen 10 mg/kg at onset of headache
> - Naproxen sodium 220–375 mg at onset of headache

> Preventive treatment:
> - With three attacks, daily prophylaxis is probably not warranted
> - Consider ASA (low dose) daily
> Caution: Triptans have not been studied adequately in the FHM population.

Case 4

A 16-year-old girl presents with 6 months of near-daily headache. At least four or five times per week, she experiences 6- to 8-hour-long episodes of intense frontal pounding headaches, during which she feels nauseated. She is otherwise healthy. There is no related trauma or illness. She has been unable to attend school for the past 3 months because of the headache, but maintains an A average on a homebound program. The patient complains of difficulty falling asleep. She began oral contraceptives about 6 months ago and is taking ibuprofen two to three times per day. Her mother and sister have frequent migraine. The patient's examination is normal except that her weight is at the 90th percentile.

> Diagnosis: chronic migraine (chronic daily headache) with analgesic overuse
> Neuro-imaging: not warranted
> Institute a biobehavioral regimen (see Table 13.11):
> - Strategy/contract to return to school
> - Psychological intervention
> - Biofeedback
> - Stress management
> - Discuss cessation of oral contraceptives and alternative birth control measures
>
> Acute treatment: learn to recognize the onset of intense headache from background daily pattern and use an oral triptan
> Preventive treatment:
> - Naproxen sodium 375–500 mg orally bid for 2–4 weeks (Lewis et al., 1994)
> - Topiramate 25 mg at bedtime, gradually titrating upward by 25-mg increments toward 50 mg bid every 1–2 weeks
> - Amitriptyline 5 mg at bedtime; option: gradually increasing up to 1 mg/kg/day weekly
> - Melatonin 3–6 mg orally at bedtime
> - Consider magnesium 400 mg/day and riboflavin 400 mg/day

---

*The only triptan approved in the United States for patients aged 12–17 is almotriptan.

REFERENCES

Ahonen K, Hamalainen ML, Rantala H, et al. Nasal suma-triptan is effective in the treatment of migraine attacks in children. *Neurology* 2004;62:883–887.

Ahonen K, Hämäläinen ML, Eerola M, et al. A randomized trial of rizatriptan in migraine attacks in children. *Neurology* 2006;67:1135–1140.

Antilla V, Stefansson H, Kallela M, et al. International Headache Genetics Consortium Genome-wide association study of migraine implicates a common susceptibility variant on 8q22.1. *Nat Genet* 2010; 42: 869–873.

Bigal ME, Lipton RB. The prognosis of migraine. *Curr Opin Neurol* 2008;21:301–308.

Bille B. Migraine in school children. *Acta Paediatr* 1962; 51(suppl 136):1–151.

Brandes JL, Kudrow D, Stark SR, et al. Sumatriptan–naproxen for acute treatment of migraine: a randomized trial. *JAMA* 2007;297:1443–1454.

Brna P, Dooley J, Gordon K, et al. The prognosis of childhood headache: a 20 year follow up study. *Arch Pediatr Adolesc Med* 2005;158:1157–1160.

Camarda R, Monastero R, Santangela G, et al. Migraine headaches in adolescents: a five year follow up study. *Headache* 2002;42:1000–1005.

Caruso JM, Brown WD, Exil G, et al. The efficacy of divalproex sodium in the prophylactic treatment of children with migraine. *Headache* 2000;40:672–676.

Charles J. Almotriptan in the acute treatment of migraine in patients 12–17 years old: an open label pilot study of efficacy and safety. *J Headache Pain* 2006;7:95–97.

Cohen HA, Nussinovitch M, Ashkenasi A, et al. Benign paroxysmal torticollis in infancy. *Pediatr Neurol* 1993; 9:488–490.

Cuvellier JC, Lépine A. Childhood periodic syndromes. *Pediatr Neurol* 2010;42:1–11.

Dalsgaard-Nielsen T. Some aspects of the epidemiology of migraine in Denmark. *Headache* 1970;10:14–23.

Damen L, Bruijn J, Verhagen AP, et al. Prophylactic treatment of migraine in children: a systematic review of pharmacological trials. *Cephalalgia* 2006;26:497–505.

DeFusco M, Marconi R, Silvestri L, et al. Haploinsufficiency of ATP1A2 encoding Na$^+$/K$^+$ pump alpha-2 subunit associated familial hemiplegic migraine, type 2. *Nat Genetics* 2003;33:192–196.

Deubner DC. An epidemiologic study of migraine and headache in 10–20 year olds. *Headache* 1977;17:173–180.

Dichgans M, Freilinger T, Eckstein G, et al. Mutation in the neuronal voltage-gated sodium channel SCN1A in familial hemiplegic migraine. *Lancet* 2005;366:371–377.

Dooley JM, Pearlman EM. The clinical spectrum of migraine in children. *Pediatr Ann* 2010;39:408–415.

Dunn DW, Snyder CH. Benign paroxysmal vertigo of childhood. *Am J Dis Child* 1976;130:1099–1100.

Eidlitz-Markus T, Haimi-Cohen Y, Steier D, Zeharia A. Effectiveness of nonpharmacologic treatment for migraine in young children. *Headache* 2010;50:219–223.

Eiland LS, Jenkins LS, Durham SH. Pediatric migraine: pharmacological agents for prophylaxis. *Ann Pharmacotherapy* 2007;41:1181–1190.

Evers S, Rahmann A, Kraemer C, et al. Treatment of childhood migraine attacks with oral zolmitriptan and ibuprofen. *Neurology* 2006;67:497–499.

Forsythe WI, Gillies D, Sills MA. Propranolol (Inderal) in the treatment of childhood migraine. *Dev Med Child Neurol* 1984;26:737–741.

Giffin NJ, Benton S, Goadsby PJ. Benign paroxysmal torticollis of infancy: four new cases and linkage to CACNA1A mutation. *Dev Med Child Neurol* 2002;44:490–493.

Guidetti V, Moscato D, Ottaviano S, et al. Flunarizine and migraine in childhood. An evaluation of endocrine function. *Cephalalgia* 1987;7:263–266.

Gunner KB, Smith HD, Ferguson LE. Practice guideline for the diagnosis and management of migraine headaches in children and adolescents: part two. *J Pediatr Health Care* 2008;22:52–59.

Hachinski VC, Porchawka J, Steele JC. Visual symptoms in the migraine syndrome. *Neurology* 1973;23:570–579.

Hamalainen ML. Migraine in children and adolescents: a guide to drug treatment. *CNS Drugs* 2006; 20: 813–820.

Hamalainen M, Hoppu K, Santavuori P. Sumatriptan for migraine attacks in children: a randomized placebo controlled study. *Neurology* 1997a;48:1100–1103.

Hamalainen ML, Hoppu K, Valkeila E, et al. Ibuprofen or acetaminophen for the acute treatment of migraine in children: a double-blind, randomized, placebo-controlled, crossover study. *Neurology* 1997b;48:102–107.

Hershey AD, Powers SW, Bentti AL, Degrauw TJ. Effectiveness of amitriptyline in the prophylactic management of childhood headaches. *Headache* 2000;40:539–549.

Hershey AD, Powers SW, Vockell AL, et al. Coenzyme Q10 deficiency and response to supplementation in pediatric and adolescent migraine. *Headache* 2007;47:73–80.

Hershey AD, Kabbouche MA, Powers SW. Treatment of pediatric and adolescent migraine. *Pediatr Ann* 2010;39:416–423.

Kienbacher C, Wober C, Zesch HE, et al. Clinical features, classification and prognosis of migraine and tension-type headache in children and adolescents: a long term follow up study. *Cephalalgia* 2006;26:820–830.

Kirchmann M, Thomsen LL, Olesen J. Basilar-type migraine: clinical, epidemiologic, and genetic features. *Neurology* 2006;66:880–886.

Lakshmi CV, Singhi P, Malhi P, et al. Topiramate in the prophylaxis of pediatric migraine: a double-blind placebo-controlled trial. *J Child Neurol* 2007;22:829–835.

Laurell K, Larsson B, Eeg-Olofsson O. Prevalence of headache in Swedish schoolchildren, with a focus on tension-type headache. *Cephalalgia* 2004;24:380–388.

Lewis D, Middlebrook M, Deline C. Naproxen sodium for chemoprophylaxis of adolescent migraine. *Ann Neurol* 1994;36:542.

Lewis DW, Kellstein D, Burke B, et al. Children's ibuprofen suspension for the acute treatment of pediatric migraine headache. *Headache* 2002;42:780–786.

Lewis D, Ashwal S, Hershey A, et al. Practice parameter: pharmacological treatment of migraine headache in children and adolescents. *Neurology* 2004a;63:2215–2224.

Lewis DW, Diamond S, Scott D, Jones V. Prophylactic treatment of pediatric migraine. *Headache* 2004b;44:230–232.

Lewis DW, Gozzo YF, Avner MT. The "other" primary headaches in children and adolescents. *Pediatr Neurol* 2005a;33:303–313.

Lewis DW, Yonker M, Winner P, et al. The treatment of pediatric migraine. *Pediatr Ann* 2005b;34:448–460.

Lewis DW, Winner P, Hershey AD, Wasiewski WW. Efficacy of zolmitriptan nasal spray in adolescent migraine. *Pediatrics* 2007;120:390–396.

Lewis D, Winner P, Saper J, et al. Randomized, double-blind, placebo-controlled study subjects 12 to 17 years of age to evaluate the efficacy and safety of topiramate for migraine prevention in pediatric. *Pediatrics* 2009;123:924–934.

Li BU, Lefevre F, Chelimsky GG, et al. North American Society for Pediatric Gastroenterology, Hepatology, and Nutrition consensus statement on the diagnosis and management of cyclic vomiting syndrome. American Society for Pediatric Gastroenterology, Hepatology, and Nutrition. *J Pediatr Gastroenterol Nutr* 2008;47:379–393.

Linder SL, Mathew NT, Cady RK, et al. Efficacy and tolerability of almotriptan in adolescents: a randomized, double-blind, placebo-controlled trial. *Headache* 2008;48:1326–1336.

Lindskog U, Odkvist L, Noaksson L, et al. Benign paroxysmal vertigo in childhood: a long-term follow-up. *Headache* 1999;39:33–37.

Lipton RB, Silberstein SD, Stewart WF. An update on the epidemiology of migraine. *Headache* 1994;34:319–328.

Ludvigsson J. Propranolol used in prophylaxis of migraine in children. *Acta Neurologica* 1974;50:109–115.

McDonald SA, Hershey AD, Pearlman E, et al. Long-term evaluation of sumatriptan and naproxen sodium for the acute treatment of migraine in adolescents. *Headache* 2011;51:1374–1378.

Major P, Grubisa H, Thie N. Triptans for the treatment of acute pediatric migraine: a systematic literature review. *Pediatr Neurol* 2003;29:425–429.

Miller GS. Efficacy and safety of levetiracetam in pediatric migraine. *Headache* 2004;44:238–243.

Millichap J, Yee M. The diet factor in pediatric and adolescent migraine. *Pediatr Neurol* 2003;28:9–15.

Monastero R, Camarda C, Pipia C, et al. Prognosis of migraine headaches in adolescents: a 10 year follow-up study. *Neurology* 2006;67:1353–1356.

Mortimer MJ, Kay J, Jaron A. Epidemiology of headache and childhood migraine in an urban general practice using Ad Hoc, Vahlquist and IHS criteria. *Dev Med Child Neurol* 1992;34:1095–1101.

Oelker A. Butterbur root extract and music therapy in the prevention of childhood migraine: an explorative study. *Euro J Pain* 2008;12:301–313.

Olesen J. The international classification of headache disorders (ICHD-2). *Cephalalgia* 2004;24:1–151.

Olness K, MacDonald JT, Uden DL. Comparison of self-hypnosis and propranolol in the treatment of juvenile classic migraine. *Pediatrics* 1987;79:593–597.

Pakalnis A, Kring D. Zonisamide prophylaxis in refractory pediatric headache. *Headache* 2006;46:804–807.

Pakalnis A, Greenberg G, Drake ME, Paolichi J. Pediatric migraine prophylaxis with divalproex. *J Child Neurol* 2001;16:731–734.

Pakalnis A, Kring D, Meier L. Levetiracetam prophylaxis in pediatric migraine: an open label study. *Headache* 2007;47:427–430.

Papetti L, Spalice A, Nicita F, et al. Migraine treatment in developmental age: guidelines update. *J Headache Pain* 2010;11:267–276.

Parisi P, Villa MP, Pelliccia A, et al. Panayiotopoulos syndrome: diagnosis and management. *Neurol Sci* 2007;28:72–79.

Powers S, Patton S, Hommel K, et al. Quality of life in childhood migraine: clinical aspects and comparison to other chronic illness. *Pediatrics* 2003;112:e1–e5.

Powers S, Patton S, Hommell, K, et al. Quality of life in paediatric migraine: characterization of age-related effects using PedsQL 4.0. *Cephalalgia* 2004;24:120–127.

Reimschisel T. Breaking the cycle of medication overuse headache. *Contemp Pediatr* 2003;20:101.

Rothner A, Guo Y. An analysis of headache types, over-the-counter (OTC) medication overuse and school absences in a pediatric/adolescent headache clinic. *Headache* 2004;44:490.

Schurks M, Diener HC, Goadsby P. Update on the prophylaxis of migraine. *Curr Treat Options Neurol* 2008;10:20–29.

Serdaroglu G, Erhan E, Tekgul H, et al. Sodium valproate prophylaxis in childhood migraine. *Headache* 2002;42:819–822.

Shaabat A. Confusional migraine in childhood. *Pediatr Neurol* 1996;15:23–25.

Silberstein SD. Practice parameter: evidence-based guidelines for migraine headache (an evidence-based review). *Neurology* 2000;55:754–762.

Sillanpaa M. Prevalence of migraine and other headache in Finnish children starting school. *Headache* 1976;15:288–290.

Sillanpaa M. Changes in the prevalence of migraine and other headache during the first seven school years. *Headache* 1983;23:15–19.

Silver S, Gano D, Gerretsen P. Acute treatment of paediatric migraine: a meta-analysis of efficacy. *J Paediatr Child Health* 2008;44:3–9.

Small P, Waters WE. Headache and migraine in a comprehensive school. In: Waters WE, ed. *The Epidemiology of Migraine*. Bracknell-Berkshire, UK: Boehringer Ingelheim; 1974:56–67.

Sorge F, Marano E. Flunarizine v. placebo in childhood migraine: a double-blind study. *Cephalalgia* 1985;5(suppl 2):145–148.

Sorge F, DeSimone R, Marano E, et al. Flunarizine in prophylaxis of childhood migraine: a double-blind, placebo-controlled crossover study. *Cephalalgia* 1988;8:1–6.

Stang P, Yanagihar P, Swanson J, et al. Incidence of migraine headache: a population based study in Olmsted County, Minn. *Neurology* 1992;42:1657–1662.

Stewart WF, Linet MS, Celentano DD, et al. Age and sex-specific incidence rates of migraine with and without visual aura. *Am J Epidemiol* 1991;34:1111–1120.

Stewart WF, Lipton RB, Celentano DD, et al. Prevalence of migraine headache in the United States. *JAMA* 1992;267:64–69.

Ueberall M. Sumatriptan in paediatric and adolescent migraine. *Cephalalgia* 2001;21:210–224.

Valquist B. Migraine in children. *Int Arch Allergy* 1955;7:348–355.

Van den Bergh V, Amery W, Waelkens J. Trigger factors in migraine: a study conducted by the Belgian Migraine Society. *Headache* 1987;27:191–196.

Victor S, Ryan S. Drugs for preventing migraine headaches in children. *Cochrane Database System Reviews* 2003;4:CD 002761.

Winner P, Rothner AD, Saper J, et al. A randomized, double-blind, placebo-controlled study of sumatriptan nasal spray in the treatment of acute migraine in adolescents. *Pediatrics* 2000;106:989–997.

Winner P, Gendolla A, Stayer C, et al. Topiramate for migraine prevention in adolescents: a pooled analysis of efficacy and safety. *Headache* 2006;46:1503–1510.

MANUAL THERAPIES FOR MIGRAINE

Neck and Thoracic Spine in Migraine

Clinical Exploration and Interventions

Peter Huijbregts, PT, MSc, MHSc, DPT, OCS,
FAAOMPT, FCAMT, Paul Glynn, PT, DPT, OCS, FAAOMPT,
John R. Krauss, PT, PhD, OCS, FAAOMPT, Bryan S. Dennison,
PT, DPT, MPT, OCS, CSCS, FAAOMPT, and Edgar Savidge, PT, DPT, OCS

INTRODUCTION

Parts I and II of this book discussed the medical–pharmacological management of patients with migraine pain. However, patients also seek nonpharmacological interventions for this pain. In many cases, these interventions are classified as complementary and alternative medicine (CAM). The boundary between allopathic medicine and CAM often is ill defined, arbitrary, and shifting. This blurring of boundaries is perhaps best illustrated by the manual therapy interventions discussed in this chapter. In day-to-day clinical practice, such interventions are provided not only by physical therapists and medical physicians, but also by chiropractors, osteopaths, naturopaths, massage therapists, and traditional Chinese medicine clinicians.

Epidemiologic data on the number of people seeking manual therapy for migraine headache from allopathic and CAM providers are lacking. Nevertheless, we do know that every year 62% of U.S. adults use some form of CAM. Of those individuals, 3.1% seek CAM interventions for severe headaches or migraines (Barnes et al., 2004). Twelve percent of patients visiting a U.S. chiropractor do so for headache and facial pain (National Board of Chiropractic Examiners [NBCE], 2010). Again not differentiating between migraine and other headaches, in a U.S. survey some 22% of outpatient physical therapy patients reported that they experienced headaches, although this condition was not necessarily the primary reason for which they sought physical therapy management (Boissonnault et al., 1999).

It is a mistake to assume that patients seek non-pharmacological treatments, including manual therapy interventions, for migraine because they reject drugs. As Linde (2006) noted, many patients choose these interventions with the intent of activating endogenous mechanisms for symptom control and to increase participation in their own recovery. They do so in addition to seeking medical–pharmacological management, rather than as a replacement for it. In the survey on U.S. adults using CAM, 54.9% indicated that they believed that a combination of CAM and allopathic intervention would work best (Barnes et al., 2004).

The American Physical Therapy Association (APTA) has defined manual therapy techniques as "skilled hand movements intended to improve tissue extensibility, increase range of motion, induce relaxation, mobilize or manipulate soft tissue and joints, modulate pain, and reduce soft-tissue swelling, inflammation or restriction." Techniques matched with these proposed indications for manual therapy include massage, manual lymphatic drainage, manual traction, mobilization/manipulation,

and passive range of motion (APTA, 2001). Within physical therapy in the United States, manual therapy techniques are often described as constituting a continuum of skilled passive movements to joints and related soft tissues. These techniques are applied at varying speeds and amplitudes, including via a small-amplitude/high-velocity therapeutic movement, commonly termed thrust or manipulation, as well as in the form of nonthrust, sustained or oscillatory, low-velocity movements referred to as mobilizations (APTA, 2001). Additional specified manual therapy interventions include soft-tissue and neural mobilization, joint stabilization, and self-mobilization exercises (Sluka & Milosavljevic, 2009).

This chapter discusses evidence- and clinical-informed physical therapy clinical diagnosis of patients with migraine and management by joint manipulation and mobilization techniques. Other manual therapy interventions will be discussed in subsequent chapters in Part III of this book.

Pathophysiological Rationale

Under the evidence-informed paradigm emphasized in this book, clinical decisions are not driven solely by research evidence, but rather are informed by this evidence. In other words, the clinician takes the evidence from research into account when making a clinical decision with regard to patient management, but evidence does not dictate this decision (Bohart, 2005; Pencheon, 2005). With this paradigm, extrapolation from basic science knowledge or a pathophysiological rationale provides a valid source for clinical decision making. In this context, we suggest four plausible explanations for the reported effects of manual therapy interventions of the cervical and thoracic spine in patients with migraine headache:

- Alterations of the input into the trigeminocervical complex
- Effects on central sensitization
- Regional interdependence
- Psychological or placebo effect

The role of the trigeminocervical complex in patients with migraine was discussed in Chapter 5. With afferent input from the C1–C3 spinal segments into the pars caudalis of the spinal nucleus of the trigeminal nerve (Bogduk, 1994; Linde, 2006), nociceptive input resulting from upper cervical motion segment dysfunction should be considered as one possible trigger in the multifactorial etiology of migraine headaches. Indirectly (and discussed in more detail as part of the consideration of regional interdependence), dysfunction in the mid- and lower cervical spine and even the thoracic spine may lead or contribute to upper cervical dysfunction. Manual therapy to dysfunctional cervical and thoracic motion segments may decrease nociceptive afferent input by way of both mechanical and neurophysiological mechanisms.

Disruption of (peri) articular adhesions, release of entrapped synovial folds or plicae, reduction of displaced nuclear fragments, and unbuckling of motion segments have all been suggested as mechanical effects of thrust techniques (Evans, 2002). The peak force magnitudes used during spinal thrust techniques are attained within 100 to 200 milliseconds (Herzog, 2005). Increased strain rates with thrust techniques, as compared to lower-velocity techniques, may lead to increased stiffness in collagenous tissues, possibly resulting in failure or disruption of adhesions with decreased joint excursion. Alternatively, mobility restrictions due to collagenous shortening, fibrosis, or hyperplasia may respond better to the viscoelastic deformation produced by sustained or oscillatory nonthrust mobilization techniques (Evans, 2002). Stimulation of cutaneous, musculo-tendinous, and capsule-ligamentous receptors and the associated thick-fiber afferent neurons may explain neurophysiologically mediated manual therapy-induced analgesia by way of activation of the gate control mechanism (Melzack & Wall, 1965). A persistent post-cavitation distention of the joint capsule causing depolarization of the thick-fiber afferent type III articular mechanoreceptors may lead to inhibition of peri-articular muscles (Paris & Loubert, 1999). Manipulation research has shown that decreased motor neuron excitability in healthy subjects is even more pronounced in subjects with chronic pain (Sluka & Milosavljevic, 2009). This reduction in excitability may be attributed to segmental mechanisms, as it occurs contrary to the increased motor neuron excitability attributed to higher-level neurologic systems.

Central sensitization in the etiology of migraine headache was discussed in Chapter 6. Manual therapy interventions to the cervical and thoracic spine may, in some patients, result in a decrease in this central sensitization through mechanisms other than the locally mediated mechanical and neurophysiological effects on nociceptive afferent input discussed previously. Because of the synaptic connections between low-threshold joint and muscle mechanoreceptors, the dorsal periaquaductal gray (PAG) area of the midbrain may play a role in producing manipulation-induced analgesia by way of descending inhibitory mechanisms.

The PAG is also likely involved in a disinhibitory mechanism contributing to the central sensitization relevant to migraine (Goadsby, 2005). This area of the brain plays an important integrative role with regard to the response to stress, pain, and other stimuli via coordination of the nociceptive, autonomic, and motor systems. Its hypothesized role in manipulation-induced analgesia has been supported by manipulation studies showing sympatho-excitation and central post-manipulation motor facilitation—the latter also evidenced by muscle activation remote from the area of manipulation occurring some 50 to 200 milliseconds after manipulation (Dishman et al., 2002; Wright, 2005). The ventrolateral PAG exerts its descending inhibitory influence through an opioid mechanism, although research has been equivocal when it has come to detecting elevated plasma β-endorphin levels after spinal thrust manipulation. Similarly, intravenously administered opioid antagonists do not reverse the hypoalgesic effect of at least nonthrust manual therapy interventions (Paungmali et al., 2004). Nevertheless, given that endorphins are too large to penetrate the blood–brain barrier, one might question the relevance of plasma samples to extrapolate a central role for endorphins in manipulation-induced analgesia.

Recently the endocannabinoid system has been suggested as relevant to both the analgesic and mood-enhancing effects of manual therapy interventions (McPartland et al., 2005). Animal research has also implicated central mechanisms involving serotonin and norepinephrine in the analgesia produced by nonthrust joint mobilization, but has not identified any role for gamma-aminobutyric acid (GABA) or—again—endorphins (Skyba et al., 2003).

The concept of regional interdependence means that we cannot regard motion segment dysfunction in isolation. Rather, areas remote to the primary complaint should be investigated for their potential contributing influence. The current best evidence indicates the importance of such a regional approach to examining and treating individuals with musculoskeletal dysfunction (Wainner et al., 2007). Due to the correlation identified between migraine headaches and neck pain (Tfelt-Hansen et al., 1981; Blau et al., 1994), the evidence-informed clinician should examine the many areas thought to influence the cervical spine. Recent research has identified the thoracic spine as one such area (Flynn et al., 2001; Fernández-de-las-Peñas et al., 2004; Cleland et al., 2005, 2007a, 2007b; Gonzalez-Iglesias et al., 2009). In a sample of 161 female laundry workers, Norlander et al. (1997) identified C7–T1 hypomobility as a predictor of neck and shoulder pain with a relative risk of 3.1 (CI 95%: 1.1–6.9). In a follow-up cross-sectional study, hypomobility of both C7–T1 and

T1–T2 was noted as significant contributors to neck and shoulder pain (Norlander et al., 1998). Fernández-de-las-Peñas et al. (2004) found that 13% of individuals with mechanical neck pain demonstrated thoracic spine dysfunction defined as hypomobility or an active range of motion flexion restriction. Cleland et al. (2007a) identified a decreased thoracic kyphosis in the upper thoracic spine (T3–T6) as a predictor variable of individuals with mechanical neck pain who were likely to benefit from upper and mid-thoracic manipulation.

Through careful and comprehensive history taking and physical examination, manual identification of the patient complaint, along with manual contact involving patient consent and cooperation during subsequent treatment, is likely to produce beneficial psychological or placebo effects. The reader is referred to the reports published by Price et al. (2008) and Roche (2007) for a more detailed discussion of the neurobiological aspects of the placebo response and its potential use in securing improved outcomes in clinical practice. Chapter 23 of this textbook summarizes placebo effects related to migraine.

Clinical research evidence supporting the use of joint mobilization and manipulation in patients with migraine (often in combination with additional manual therapy interventions, other modalities, education, and specific exercise instruction) varies from retrospective case reports to systematic reviews of randomized controlled trials (RCT). In a case report, Cattley and Tuchin (1999) noted improvement at 8-week follow-up in terms of headache frequency, intensity, and duration and in medication use in a 41-year-old male patient with migraine without aura treated five times over 5 weeks with C0–C1, C2–C3, and T3–T4 manipulation, massage of the upper trapezius and levator scapulae muscles, and home stretching exercises. Davis (2003) reported on a 22-year-old female patient with recurrent migraine headaches for 2 years; after 17 visits over 12 weeks consisting of cervical and thoracic thrust manipulation, moist heat, and strengthening and neuromuscular reeducation exercises, the patient reported no pain or headache-related disability. Elster (2004) described a 23-year old-male with a 6-year history of migraine who was treated with upper cervical manipulation. At 4 months after treatment was begun, the patient reported a reduction in headache frequency from three attacks per week to two migraines per month. At 7 months, the patient was completely symptom free and remained so at the 18-month follow-up.

Peters-Harris (2005) reported decreased headache frequency and intensity in a 49-year-old female patient with a 17-year history of migraine with aura after 20 treatments over 12 weeks consisting of C2–C3 and C5–C6 rotational manipulation, moist heat, and high-voltage electrical muscle stimulation; cervico-thoracic massage; strengthening, range of motion, endurance, and neuromuscular reeducation exercises; and education.

Tuchin (2008) reported on a 72-year-old female patient with a history of experiencing migraine headaches once or twice a week for 60 years who was treated with C0–C1 and T2–T7 manipulation, massage, and stretching of hypertonic muscles initially twice a week for 4 weeks, then once a week for 8 weeks, followed by treatment every 2 to 4 weeks. After 1 month of treatment, the patient reported no more headaches. After 12 weeks, she reported 100% reduction in medication use. During 7 years of ongoing treatment, the patient reported not a single headache.

A prospective cohort study of 32 patients with migraine headache consisted of a 2-month baseline period, 2 months of thrust interventions as deemed indicated by the clinician to the whole spine, and 2 months of post-treatment follow-up. The study showed significant (all $P < 0.05$) improvements in headache frequency (46% reduction), intensity (12%), duration (20%), and disability (14%) as compared to baseline after 2 months of intervention. At 6 months, 24 patients noted significant improvements as compared to baseline for headache frequency (60% reduction, $P < 0.005$), intensity (14% reduction, $P < 0.01$), and duration (20% reduction, $P < 0.05$), and medication use (36% reduction, $P < 0.01$) (Tuchin, 1999).

In an RCT, 85 subjects were randomized to receive cervical manipulation by a medical physician or physical therapist, cervical manipulation by a chiropractor, or cervical mobilization by a medical physician or physical therapist twice weekly over 8 weeks. The RCT yielded no significant between-group differences in migraine symptoms, but did produce within-group pre-test to post-test differences for all groups with regard to frequency, duration, or headache-related disability during migraine attacks. Only the chiropractic patients reported a significant reduction in pain intensity associated with migraine attacks (Parker et al., 1978).

In an extension of the previously described RCT, Parker et al. (1980) randomized 88 patients to either cervical manipulation or mobilization twice weekly for 8 weeks. At 8 weeks post treatment, a nonsignificant trend favored manipulation over mobilization in decreasing pain. At 20-months follow-up, a trend toward decreased headache frequency was observed in the chiropractic group.

In another RCT, Nelson et al. (1998) randomized 218 patients after a 4-week baseline period to 8 weeks of cervical and thoracic manipulation no more than twice a week, oral amitriptyline (titrated upward weekly during the first month and continued at 100 mg daily over the second month), or both. Subjects then were followed up for 4 weeks post treatment. All subjects were allowed to take over-the-counter (OTC) analgesics as needed, and no advice on behavior modification was provided. With a 49% reduction found in the amitriptyline group, 40% reduction in the spinal manipulation group, and 41% reduction in the combined-therapy group, there were no significant ($P = 0.66$) between-group differences in the headache index (a weekly sum of average 24-hour 0–10 headache intensity scores) in the last 4 weeks of treatment. There was also no significant between-group difference ($P = 0.35$) with regard to OTC medication use during the treatment period. A month after both therapies were stopped, a nonsignificant trend ($P = 0.05$) toward a lower headache index was found in the group whose members had received manipulation as compared to the group who had received amitriptyline, with a 24% reduction in the headache index in the amitriptyline group, a 42% reduction in the manipulation group, and a 25% reduction in the combined-therapy group. There was also a significant decrease in OTC medication use favoring the manipulation group ($P < 0.01$). Ten percent of the medication group withdrew from this study due to side effects, but only minor adverse effects, including transient muscle soreness and neck stiffness, were reported in the manipulation group.

An RCT in 127 patients with migraine after an initial baseline period of 2 months compared 2 months of thrust interventions as deemed indicated by the clinician to the whole spine to interferential current, with patients being followed during a 2-month post-treatment period. The study showed significant between-group differences favoring manipulation for headache frequency ($P < 0.005$), duration ($P < 0.01$), disability ($P < 0.05$), and medication use ($P < 0.001$) during the 2-month post-intervention follow-up (Tuchin et al., 2000).

Based on the Parker et al. (1978, 1980) and Nelson et al. (1998) RCTs, the systematic review by Bronfort et al. (2001) noted moderate evidence for short-term efficacy of spinal manipulation similar to amitriptyline in patients with migraine. Based on the Parker et al. (1978), Nelson et al. (1998), and Tuchin et al. (2000) RCTs, Astin and Ernst (2002) in their systematic review noted, to the contrary, that research did not support manipulation as an effective treatment for headache (including migraine) and suggested future research might address the possibility of placebo effects and also longer-term outcomes. In a Cochrane systematic review, Bronfort et al. (2004) reviewed the Parker et al. (1980), Nelson et al. (1998),

and Tuchin et al. (2000) RCTs. This review concluded that the evidence supports the contention that spinal manipulation might be an effective treatment option with a short-term effect similar to that of a commonly used, effective drug (amitriptyline) for the prophylactic treatment of migraine headache, but determined that further study on (cost) effectiveness was required; it also noted that, due to study heterogeneity, higher-quality studies could easily alter the present findings and recommendations.

When assessing the level of evidence, we must acknowledge that cervical manipulation and mobilization have been associated with a small risk of serious adverse events, most notably vertebral and internal carotid arterial dissection. Hurwitz et al. (1996) pointed out an underreporting bias and suggested that the estimated risk should be adjusted to account for the only 10% reporting rate in the literature at 5 to 10 events per 10 million patient encounters for all complications, 6 in 10 million for serious complications, and 3 in 10 million for death. Haneline et al. (2003) found 13 cases of internal carotid artery dissection temporally associated with cervical manipulation in a 1966–2000 Medline review and estimated the chance of developing dissection in this artery post manipulation to be 1 in 601,145,000. Most adverse events, however, are minor and transient. Epidemiologic data on serious adverse events with thoracic manual interventions are lacking, but in some reports rib fractures and pathological vertebral fractures with cord compression have been noted (Oppenheim et al., 2005; Huijbregts, 2011).

In summary, with risks of cervical and thoracic manual therapy interventions being relatively low and evidence of effectiveness being found in at least one higher-quality RCT (Nelson et al., 1998) and three lower-quality RCTs, we would suggest that cervical and thoracic joint manipulation and mobilization in the prophylactic treatment of patients with migraine warrant an evidence score of 1B+ and, therefore, a positive recommendation (Van Kleef et al., 2009).

CERVICAL SPINE PHYSICAL EXAMINATION

The patient with migraine presents a diagnostic challenge for the physical therapist. Local cranial structures (muscle, nerve, vascular structures) can be at fault when a patient experiences migraine symptoms. Distal to the cranium, the neck should be considered in the physical therapy differential diagnosis for the patient with headache.

The prudent physical therapy clinician will entertain multiple hypotheses during the patient interview, which will be teased out during the physical exam. While such an etiology is rare, the physical therapist evaluating a patient with headache should at least consider the possibility of pathological sources for the patient's presenting symptoms (i.e., central nervous system tumors, aneurysms, abscesses, hemorrhages) (Detsky et al., 2006). In keeping with a recently suggested framework for interviewing and examining patients in the physical therapy setting, it is recommended that the primary goal of the first patient encounter be to determine whether the patient is an appropriate candidate for physical therapy services (Childs et al., 2004).

A thorough questioning and comprehensive review of each patient's medical history will help inform hypothesis generation as it pertains to the patient's presenting migraine symptoms. Recently, a cluster of five historical items was found to create a large and conclusive shift in the probability of diagnosing a migraine:

1. Is it a pulsating headache?
2. Does it last between 4 and 72 hours?
3. Is it unilateral?
4. Is there nausea?
5. Is the headache disabling? (Detsky et al., 2006)

Identifying the presence of any of these findings can help shift the clinician's confidence that the patient presents with a migraine, allowing the clinician to proceed with the physical therapy investigation of the patient's local and remote areas that may be contributing to the current symptoms (i.e., the cervical spine or thoracic spine). Conversely, an evaluating physical therapist has cause to be concerned with the presence of (1) abnormal findings on neurologic examination, (2) cluster-type headache, (3) headache with aura, (4) headache that could not be clearly defined by a clinician, and (5) headache with vomiting and headache aggravated by exertion or Valsalva-like maneuvers (Detsky et al., 2006). The most significant finding in this group of variables is the presence of abnormal neurologic findings. Alternatively, these findings may pique the clinician's suspicion that something more sinister is present, necessitating the need to refer the patient to the appropriate medical provider for additional work-up.

Once the diagnosis of a migraine has been made, the clinician may proceed with evaluation of the cervical spine. Physical examination items may include postural assessment (i.e., forward head posture) (Fernández-de-las-Peñas et al., 2007a), range of motion testing, segmental springing, intersegmental motion assessment (Tuchin & Bonello, 1996; Tuchin et al., 2000), and palpation of the sub-occipital, upper cervical, and postural musculature (Tuchin et al., 2000; Fernández-de-las-Peñas et al., 2007a). Regarding range of motion, Zwart (1997) did not find any

difference in neck mobility between individuals with headache (migraine without aura, tension-type headache, and cervicogenic headache) and healthy controls. These findings were corroborated by Bevilaqua-Grossi et al. (2008) and Fernández-de-las-Peñas et al. (2006). In these two studies, individuals with migraine did not exhibit range of motion impairments compared to controls. In contrast to this finding, Fernández-de-las-Peñas et al. (2006) identified specific trigger points (upper trapezius, sternocleidomastoid, temporalis, and sub-occipital muscles) in the neck and head region that were more prevalent in individuals with migraine as compared to healthy subjects.

Posture

Although not a differentiating factor between tension-type, cervicogenic, and migraine headaches, forward head posture is a common finding in individuals with migraine (Marcus et al., 1999). The ability to reliably detect subtle postural deviations remains controversial; however, a gross screen of postural symmetry and deviation from normal anatomic alignment can provide insight into areas of cervical spine dysfunction, hypomobility, and neck pain. Postural observation is performed while the patient is in either a sitting or standing position and should be viewed posteriorly as well as laterally. Kendall et al. (1993) describe a forward head posture as a displacement of the external auditory meatus anterior to the acromion. Such a position may be associated with extension of the occiput on C1 and the upper cervical spine. Subsequently, dysfunction may occur in the upper cervical region, altering trigeminocervical input that arises from the C1–C3 afferents. Deviations in the frontal and transverse plane have also been correlated with middle and lower cervical hypomobility and pain, which may further contribute to central sensitization.

Active Range of Motion

While restricted neck range of motion does not appear to have a direct effect on the production of migraines, it has been associated with neck pain. Neck pain has been identified as a predictor of disability in individuals with migraine. As a consequence, it has been recommended to include cervical active range of motion (AROM) as part of a comprehensive examination. As with altered posture, painful AROM may identify those patients who would benefit from manual therapy due to cervical dysfunction, regional interdependence, and central sensitization. AROM testing should include flexion/extension, lateral flexion, and rotation, with careful attention being paid to pain provocation and restriction. The use of an inclinometer can reliably objectify restriction and onset of pain (Youdas et al., 1991; Hole et al., 2000) and should be used for test/retest purposes before and after the application of manual techniques.

Segmental Mobility Testing

In the presence of positive findings with restricted cervical AROM, testing of passive motions is typically used to further clarify the quality and quantity of motion in the regions and segments in question. Motion is rated as hypomobile, normal, or hypermobile, and the clinician should note the provocation of pain. Positive findings in this region may correlate with altered afferent input and abnormal trigeminocervical response contributing to migraine symptoms. Segmental mobility assessment may be assessed with passive physiological intervertebral movements (PPIVM) and passive accessory intervertebral motions (PAIVM). The following section describes PPIVMs and PAIVMs for the occipito-atlas and C2–C7.

Passive Motion Testing of the Occipito-Atlas

PPIVM OA Flexion and Extension The patient is placed in a supine position. The therapist faces the top of the patient's head, with the therapist's right and left hands positioned behind the patient's occiput and his or her thumbs pressing in the direction of the anterior aspect of the transverse processes of C1 bilaterally. Flexion PPIVM is generated by the combination of cranial motion with the posterior occiput by both hands, ventral motion of the top of the head with the abdomen, and posterior motion with the thumbs (**Figure 14.1**).

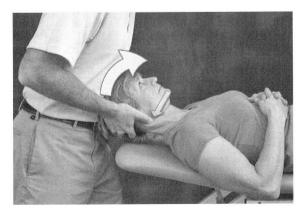

Figure 14.1 Passive Physiological Intervertebral Movements of the Occipito-Atlas in Flexion

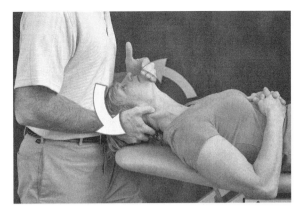

Figure 14.2 Passive Physiological Intervertebral Movements of the Occipito-Atlas in Extension

Extension PPIVM is generated by the combination of caudal motion with the posterior occiput by both hands, dorsal motion of the top of the head with the abdomen, and posterior motion with the thumbs (**Figure 14.2**).

During this testing, all points of contact on the patient are used to judge the quantity and quality of motion. The thumbs are used to judge the end-feel by pressing dorsally at the end of the motion.

PAIVM OA Dorsal Glide, Ventral Glide, and Medial to Lateral Glide All PAIVM tests for the OA joint are the same as the manipulation and mobilization techniques described in Figures 14.11 through 14.13 later in this chapter in terms of patient positions, body mechanics, and stabilization. When assessing the quantity, quality, and end-feel for the various tests, the examiner uses the same line of force as described for those techniques; however, the motion is applied at varying speeds (slow/gradual to rapid) and with an emphasis on sensing change in resistance (relative to speed) throughout the motion and the quality of resistance for the end-feel.

Passive Motion Testing C2–C7

PPIVM C2–C7 Flexion and Extension The patient is placed in a supine position. The therapist faces the top of the patient's head, with his or her left or right hand behind the occiput. The index finger of the therapist's other hand palpates the interspinal space of the tested segment. The therapist's chest/abdomen gently contacts the top of patient's head. Flexion PPIVM is generated by the ventral cranial motion of the left hand combined with a ventral

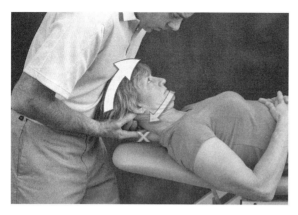

Figure 14.3 Passive Physiological Intervertebral Movements of C2–C7 in Flexion

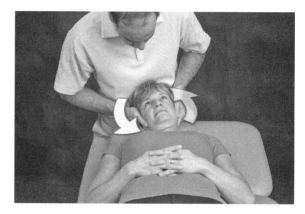

Figure 14.5 Passive Physiological Intervertebral Movements of C2–C7 in Side-Bending

motion with the abdomen (**Figure 14.3**). During flexion, the palpating finger presses into the interspinal space with enough pressure to palpate spinal process separation.

Extension PPIVM is generated by a dorsal caudal motion of the left hand combined with a dorsal, slightly caudal motion with the abdomen (**Figure 14.4**). During extension, the palpating finger presses into the interspinal space to create a slight fulcrum for extension and to palpate spinal process approximation.

During this testing, all points of contact on the patient are used to judge the quantity and quality of motion.

PPIVM C2–C7 Side-Bending   The patient is placed in a supine position. The therapist faces the top of the patient's head, with his or her right and left hands positioned with the radial border of the index fingers and radial side of the second metacarpal (MCP) contacting the articular processes, laminae, and lateral aspect of the spinous process of the cranial vertebra (e.g., C2) in the tested

segment (e.g., C2–C3). The therapist's chest/abdomen gently contacts the top of patient's head. Side-bending PPIVM to the right is generated by the combination of a ventral cranial motion of the left hand and dorsal caudal motion with the right hand, accompanied by movement of the top of the head to the right with the abdomen (**Figure 14.5**). End-feel is generated by adding additional dorsal caudal and ventral cranial pressures with the right and left testing hands, respectively.

PAIVM C2–C7 Translatoric Joint Play: Side-Lying
The patient is placed in a side-lying position. The therapist stands facing the patient, with the cranial arm and hand placed under the patient's head and neck (table side). The ulnar border of the cranial hand is cupped and contacts the cranial vertebra in the spinal segment. The therapist's left arm reaches over the top of the patient's upper thorax, with the forearm aligned roughly in line with the spinal column (**Figure 14.6**). The

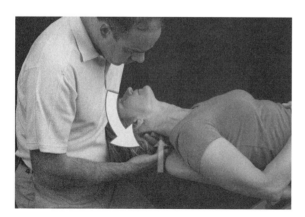

Figure 14.4 Passive Physiological Intervertebral Movements of C2–C7 in Extension

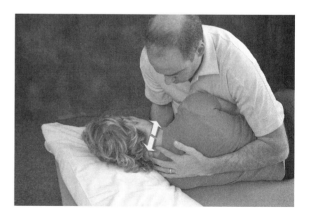

Figure 14.6 Passive Accessory Intervertebral Movements of C2–C7 Translatoric Joint Play in Side-Lying Position

therapist palpates the tested segments in the interspinal space with his or her left hand's index or middle finger. Translatoric joint play testing is performed by pressing dorsally and then pulling ventrally on the cranial vertebra in the tested segment. The segment is tested first in the resting position, but may also be tested in ventral and dorsal flexion.

The side-lying version of joint play testing offers the examiner an opportunity to assess the full anterior to posterior motion of the segment; in contrast, the prone test assesses anterior translation only. This test is usually performed at varying speeds (slow/gradual to rapid), with an emphasis on sensing changes in resistance (relative to speed) throughout the motion in addition to the quality of the end-feel.

C2–C7 Facet Separation   The patient is placed in a supine position, with the cervical spine positioned in left side-bending and right rotation (testing separation of the right facets). The therapist faces the top of the patient's head, with his or her left hand, forearm and the left side of the chest supporting the cervical position. The radial border of the therapist's right second MCP and index finger contacts the posterior lateral lamina and superior articular process of the caudal vertebra in the tested segment (**Figure 14.7**). The test is performed by pressing in a ventral, medial, and caudal manner with the right hand, while maintaining the cervical spine position with the left hand and left side of the chest.

Muscle Length Testing

Restricted cervical musculature may contribute to altered afferent input to the trigeminocervical nucleus, in turn stimulating the trigeminovascular system (Shevel &

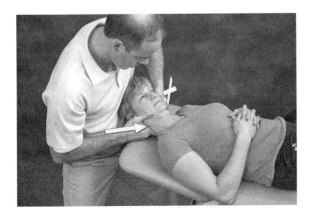

Figure 14.7 Passive Accessory Intervertebral Movements of C2–C7 Facet Separation

Spierings, 2004; Sorrell, 2006). For this reason, muscle length testing of the cranio-cervico-thoracic musculature should occur during examination. While the patient is in the supine position, the examining therapist should assess the length of the scalenes (anterior, middle), sternocleidomastoids (SCM), and upper trapezius muscles.

As described by Childs et al. (2004), the length of the scalenes is assessed by stabilizing the first rib and clavicle with one hand, while translating the head and neck into slight extension with the opposite hand and shoulder. The cervical spine is then side-bent away from the side to be tested. The upper trapezius and SCM length is assessed by depressing the lateral aspect of the scapula as the clinician flexes and side-bends the subject's head away while rotating toward the side to be tested. Further emphasis on the SCM can be placed by asking the patient to perform a chin tuck. The levator scapulae, splenius cervicis, and the posterior scalenes are tested while the patient is in side-lying position. The head and neck are placed in flexion, side-bending, and rotation away by lowering the head of the plinth. This position is stabilized with one hand, while the opposite hand depresses, posteriorly tilts, and upwardly rotates the scapula until a stretch is felt. Cleland et al. (2006) found that this technique achieves moderate to excellent interrater reliability ($k = 0.50–0.90$) of muscle length assessment in individuals with mechanical neck pain.

As noted earlier in this chapter, the use of manipulation and mobilization of the cervical spine may improve migraine headaches through four means: (1) alterations in the input into the trigeminocervical nucleus, (2) effects on central sensitization, (3) regional interdependence, and (4) psychological or placebo effect. The selection of manipulation or mobilization for a given patient or spinal segment depends on the presence and degree of pain, the number of spinal segments involved, and the nature of the end-feel determined during PPIVM and PAIVM. In cases in which the end-feel is firm/capsular and may be reached with little force or effort (a condition typically associated with little to no pain in the treatment segment), manipulation is indicated. In cases in which greater pain or discomfort is reported in the treatment segment or during the positioning for the technique, or in which the end-feel is more elastic/less firm or requires significant effort to reach, then mobilization is indicated.

THORACIC SPINE PHYSICAL EXAMINATION

While neck pain has been correlated with migraine headache (Tfelt-Hansen et al., 1981; Blau & MacGregor, 1994), impairments of the thoracic spine have not been directly correlated with migraine symptoms. Despite the current lack of research validating this proposed link, regional interdependence suggests that the evidence-based practitioner should examine areas thought to influence the cervical spine and neck pain. Due to the potential biomechanical and soft-tissue influences of the thoracic spine on the cervical region, it is suggested that this area be assessed as part of a comprehensive examination.

Posture

Although the biomechanical link between the thoracic spine and neck pain has been established, the ability of the examining therapist to reliably determine any impairment through visual inspection remains controversial (Fedorak et al., 2003). Despite this debate, the authors believe that a postural screen is beneficial, as it may detect segmental regions (upper, middle, lower) of hypomobility through comparison with the overall thoracic curvature. The postural screen should occur with the patient in a standing position, facing away from the examining therapist. The thoracic spine is inspected for excessive (increased convexity) or diminished (decreased convexity-flattening) kyphosis in the upper and middle thoracic spine. Particular attention should be paid to the cervicothoracic junction (C7–T2) owing to its biomechanical link with the cervical spine, as well as the middle thoracic spine (T3–T8). Hypomobility detected in the middle thoracic spine has been identified as predicting mechanical neck pain in individuals who may benefit from manipulative therapy aimed at the thoracic spine (Cleland et al., 2007a; Fernández-de-las-Peñas et al., 2007b). Postural assessment in this manner has been studied by Cleland et al. (2006) and has been found reliable, with k values ranging from moderate to substantial (0.58–0.9).

Frontal plane postural deviations, although not well studied, may also contribute to regional hypomobility. In a quick screen approach to identify these deviations, the examining therapist runs his or her index and middle fingers down the intervertebral gutter just off the spinous processes. This technique can also be used to identify areas of thoracic paraspinal tenderness. Local areas of thoracic paraspinal tenderness may be an indication of increased motor activity via EMG analysis (Fryer et al., 2006). Areas identified as possessing increased motor activity may be well served by manual therapy to inhibit the local musculature.

Active Range of Motion

Active range of motion of the thoracic spine can be performed with the patient in either a standing or sitting

position to decrease the contributions of the lower body. Flexion, extension, and side-bending can be measured with an inclinometer. The device is placed in the sagittal plane for flexion/extension and in the frontal plane for side-bending. The inclinometer is first placed over the T1 segment and the motion is recorded. This process is then repeated at the T12 segment, with this value being subtracted from the first to arrive at the total thoracic motion. Lee et al. (2003) found good reliability with the single-inclinometer approach to measuring thoracic spine motion.

In addition to recording range of active motion, the examining therapist should record the effect of the motion on the subject's symptoms. Due to the gravitational requirement of the inclinometer, thoracic rotation range of motion is typically not formally measured in the clinic. Instead, a visual estimate is made as the patient rotates from side to side in the sitting position.

Segmental Mobility Testing

Next, the upper and middle thoracic spine is assessed for segmental mobility and pain provocation. Segments T1–T8 are assessed while the patient is in a prone position by placing the examining therapist's hypothenar eminence over the target segment and applying a posterior to anterior pressure (**Figure 14.8**). The assessment should be repeated both at the spinous processes and at the costotransverse/costovertebral (CT/CV) junctions bilaterally. Hypomobility in the CT/CV area is particularly important due to the proximity of the thoracic sympathetic chain to the anterior head of the ribs. Current theory suggests that migraines may result from chronic stimulation of the sympathetic nervous system resulting in subsequent sympathetic hypofunction (Kuritzky, 1987; Peroutka, 2004). For this reason, it is important to identify and address restriction in this area. Mobility restrictions may be graded as normal, hypomobile, or hypermobile, and pain provocation should be identified as either "painful" or "nonpainful." When Cleland et al. (2006) utilized this approach for individuals with mechanical neck pain, they found slight to moderate interrater reliability, with weighted k values for mobility ranging from 0.13 to 0.82. Pain provocation was also studied and demonstrated less reliability, with a wider range of k values, from –0.10 to 0.90 (Cleland et al., 2006).

The assessment of thoracic spine mobility for potential contributions to neck pain and migraines should also include the rib cage. The thoracic sympathetic chain sits anterior to the rib heads, thus necessitating the identification of restrictions in this area. Segmental mobility should be assessed via the application of posterior

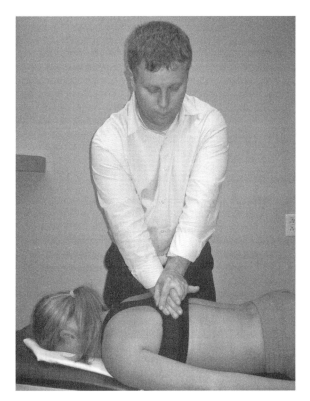

Figure 14.8 Segmental Mobility Testing of the Thoracic Spine

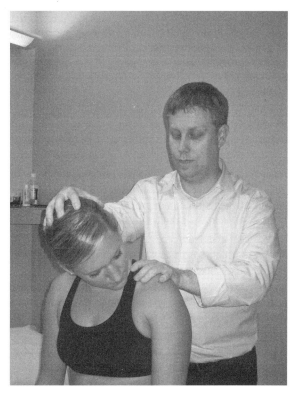

Figure 14.9 The Cervical Rotation Lateral Flexion Test for Assessing the First Rib

to anterior graded pressure to the rib angle while the patient is in a prone position. Particular attention should be paid to the first rib, as it has been implicated in multiple upper-quarter dysfunctions (Bookhout, 1996). The cervical rotation lateral flexion test has been proposed by Lindgren et al. (1989) as a means of assessing first-rib elevation and hypomobility (**Figure 14.9**). It is performed with the patient in the sitting position. The cervical spine is passively rotated away from the side that is being tested. It is then flexed forward toward the chest, with a positive test indicated by a bony block to the motion. The theory behind this test suggests that contralateral rotation and cervical flexion will maximize anterior translation of the lower cervical transverse processes, which will in turn be blocked by an elevated and hypomobile first rib. When Lindgren et al. (1992) have studied the interrater reliability of this test in a group of individuals with brachialgia, they found it yielded excellent results, with a *k* value of 1.0.

To date, the importance and potential contribution of the thoracic spine to migraine headaches has yet to be elucidated. Many possible mechanisms have been proposed, including the biomechanical and soft-tissue influence of the thoracic spine on the cervical spine as well as its potential influence on sympathetic hypofunction via the thoracic sympathetic chain. Whether this influence is direct or indirect, evidence-based practitioners who utilize a regional interdependence model in the treatment of migraine headaches should incorporate examination and subsequent treatment of the thoracic spine to maximize outcomes for their patients.

CERVICAL SPINE INTERVENTIONS

The cervical techniques presented in this chapter are divided into three categories—disc traction, facet/joint separation, and facet/joint gliding—based on the direction of the applied mobilization or manipulation. Translatoric traction techniques are used to improve motion and to unload/decompress the disc joint and intervertebral foramen contents (nerves, arteries, veins, and lymphatic vessels). Disc traction manipulations are performed at a right angle to the disc joint using a cranially directed force. During disc traction, bilaterally applied manipulative forces are used in an attempt to generate equal movement or traction of all parts of the intervertebral joint.

Translatoric articular/facet separation techniques are used to unload/decompress the articular surfaces of occipito-atlanto joints and the facet joints in the lower cervical spine. Techniques grouped in this category generate separation of the articular surfaces (OA and C2–C7 facets) that differs from disc traction, in that separation of all points of the articular surface is not equal. This discrepancy arises in part from the use of unilaterally generated impulses in addition to the orientation of the facet surfaces. In the upper cervical spine, because the articular surfaces of the joints are positioned in the transverse plane, the manipulation is directed cranially and slightly medially to maintain bone contact. In the lower cervical spine, the facet joints are oriented approximately 45° from the horizontal plane. To generate the greatest amount of facet separation in the lower cervical spine, the treatment segment is positioned in opposite side-bending and rotation, and the manipulation is directed in a ventral, medial, and caudal direction.

Translatoric facet gliding techniques are directed parallel to the articular surfaces in the upper and lower cervical spines. In the upper cervical spine, the manipulative force is principally directed in a ventral and dorsal direction. In the lower cervical spine (C2–C7), it is directed ventral, medial and cranial, or dorsal, medial, and caudal. The decision regarding the direction of movement used for gliding techniques is determined by the direction of restricted motion. More specifically, dorsal gliding at the OA joint is used when ventral flexion of the joint is restricted, whereas ventral gliding at the OA joint is used when dorsal flexion is restricted. In the lower cervical spine, ventral cranial gliding is used when ventral flexion is limited, or in the case of a right unilateral restriction when ventral flexion, left side-bending, and left rotation are restricted. Dorsal caudal gliding is used when dorsal flexion is restricted, or in the case of a right unilateral restriction when dorsal flexion, right side-bending, and right rotation are restricted. When using these techniques, it is important to avoid application of compressive forces during gliding, through the use of a small amount of traction prior to gliding.

Techniques presented in this chapter are grouped according to spinal level and described using the American Academy of Orthopedic Manual Physical Therapy's (AAOMPT) recommended standardized terminology (Mintken et al., 2008). The decision to apply a given technique as a manipulation or mobilization is partially determined by the specifics of the technique (hand contact, patient/therapist position, and joint position) and the characteristics of the end-feel perceived by the therapist when taking up the slack in the treatment segment. When slack may be taken up with little effort and the end-feel is firm, then the joint may be considered "manipulatable." In contrast, when taking up the slack requires effort and is painful, and the end-feel is too soft, then the joint is not readily manipulatable and should be mobilized first.

Mobilization and Manipulation of the Occipito-Atlas

Occipito-Atlanto Separation in Supine

The patient is positioned supine, with the OA positioned with slight left side-bending, right rotation, and dorsal flexion of the occiput on the atlas. The therapist is positioned to the left of the patient's head, neck, and shoulder. The therapist's right hand and forearm are positioned behind the patient's head and against the right side of the patient's face. The therapist's left hand contacts the inferior edge of the patient's left mastoid process. The slack between occiput and atlas is taken up in a cranial direction by the therapist's right hand and chest. The manipulation is delivered by the left hand in a cranial direction (**Figure 14.10**). No attempt is made to stabilize the patient's anatomy caudally, so movement will occur below the point of contact.

This articulation typically generates a cavitation as a response when the technique is performed with the correct speed and prepositioning. Loosening the OA joint may result in immediate reduction in cervicogenic-related headache. The degree of prepositioning used in the OA joint is very small and relates to the use of the application of a single manipulative force from the left hand. The OA joint may be manipulated without any prepositioning if the therapist uses a bilateral thrust from both hands.

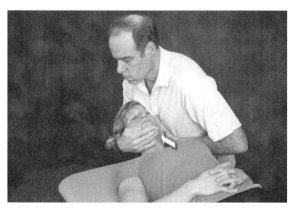

Figure 14.10 Occipito-Atlanto Separation in Supine Position

Occipito-Atlanto Unilateral Dorsal Glide in Supine

The patient is positioned supine, with slight left side-bending, right rotation, and ventral flexion of the occiput on the atlas. The therapist stands facing the head of the patient. The therapist's left hand is placed posteriorly under the patient's occiput. The therapist's left shoulder is positioned anteriorly on the patient's forehead superior to the patient's left eye. The therapist's right hand contacts and stabilizes the right transverse process and posterior arch of atlas with the MCP and radial border of the index finger. The slack in the right OA joint is taken up by applying a dorsal and medial pressure with the therapist's left shoulder in the direction of the stabilizing hand (**Figure 14.11**). The mobilization force is applied in a dorsal and medial direction by the therapist's left shoulder. This technique is considered moderate to very specific due to segmental prepositioning and the firm stabilization provided to the atlas by the therapist's hand positioned between the posterior arch of atlas and the treatment table.

When performed in this position, this technique is most suited as a mobilization. It may also be performed as a hold–relax muscle stretch/relaxation technique for the upper cervical muscles. In addition, this technique is a good choice for management of cervicogenic headache and restoration of upper cervical motion.

Occipito-Atlanto Unilateral Ventral Glide in Supine

The patient is positioned supine, with the OA joints in slight right side-bending, left rotation, and dorsal flexion, and the occiput positioned at the edge of the table.

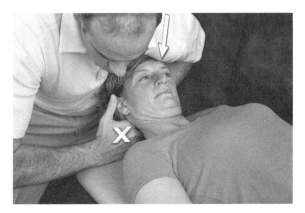

Figure 14.11 Occipito-Atlanto Unilateral Dorsal Glide in Supine Position

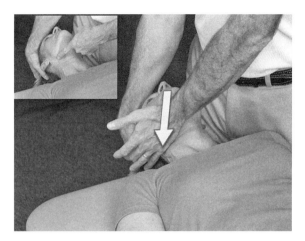

Figure 14.12 Occipito-Atlanto Unilateral Ventral Glide in Supine Position

The therapist stands facing the head of the patient. The therapist's right hand is placed against the right side of the patient's head and, along with the therapist's right thigh, supports the patient's head and neck position. The therapist's left hand presses in the direction of the anterior surface of the transverse process of atlas. Slack in the right OA joint is taken up by applying a dorsal and slightly medial pressure with the therapist's left hand (**Figure 14.12**). The mobilization force is applied in a dorsal direction. This technique is considered moderate to very specific due to segmental prepositioning and the firm stabilization provided to the occiput through the three-point contact of the right hand, right thigh, and treatment table.

When performed in this position, this technique is most suited as a mobilization. In addition, it may be adapted as a soft-tissue technique, with the massage applied by the ulnar side of the therapist's hypothenar eminence of the left hand.

Occipito-Atlanto Medial to Lateral Glide in Supine

The patient is positioned supine, with the head and neck in an actual resting position. The therapist stands facing the top of the patient's head. The therapist's left hand is placed against the left side of the patient's head and face and, along with the left side of the therapist's abdomen, supports the patient's head and neck position. The radial border of the therapist's right hand is placed against the right posterior-lateral transverse process and posterior arch of atlas. Slack in the OA joint is taken up by applying a medial pressure with the therapist's right hand.

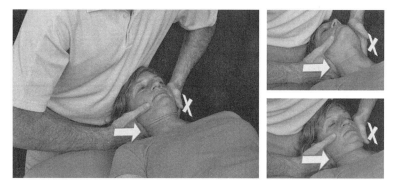

Figure 14.13 Occipito-Atlanto Medial to Lateral Glide in Supine Position

The mobilization force is applied in a medial direction (**Figure 14.13**). This technique is considered moderate to very specific due to segmental prepositioning and the firm stabilization provided to the occiput through the three-point contact of the left hand, abdomen, and treatment table.

When performed in this position, this technique is most suited as a mobilization. In addition, it may be applied at the point of greatest medial to lateral restriction in either dorsal or ventral flexion of the OA joints. While the side-bending available at the OA joints is relatively small, it is an important component of upper cervical coupled motion. Restoring coupled motion may contribute to reducing upper cervical stresses during active motion and subsequently reduce upper cervical contributions to cervicogenic headaches.

Mobilization and Manipulation of C2–C6

C2–C7 Disc Traction in Supine: General

The patient is placed supine in a position of greatest comfort, where signs and symptoms are most minimal. The therapist stands facing the top of the patient's head. The radial border of the therapist's left and right hands contact the posterior surface of the transverse processes, lamina, inferior articular processes, and spinous process of the cranial vertebra in the treatment segment. The therapist's thumbs press in the direction of the anterior aspect of the transverse processes of the cranial vertebra in the treatment segment. The slack in the treatment segment is taken up in a cranial direction with both hands, and the manipulation or mobilization is delivered using the same direction of motion (**Figure 14.14**). The specificity of this technique is generally low, with the degree to which traction occurs in the spinal segments caudal to the point of contact depending on factors such

as the amount of force used and the amount of motion available at each spinal segment.

Disc traction mobilization and manipulation are recommended in cases of multidirectional segmental movement restriction with or without cervical nerve irritation secondary to disc degeneration. Oscillatory mobilization techniques are recommended in patients in whom radicular discomfort is severe and variable. In cases of acute disc injury, traction may cause symptom irritation regardless of the amount of force applied. In this situation, it is recommended that the disc injury be protected (e.g., with use of a cervical collar and education regarding spinal loading and positioning) so that acute inflammation may resolve.

C2–C7 Disc Traction in Supine: Specific to Region

The patient is placed supine in a position of greatest comfort, where signs and symptoms are most minimal. The therapist stands facing the top of the patient's

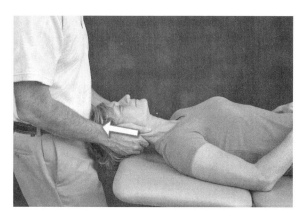

Figure 14.14 C2–C7 Disc Traction in Supine Position: General

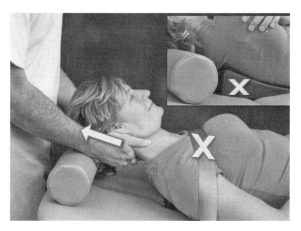

Figure 14.15 C2–C7 Disc Traction in Supine Position: Specific to Region

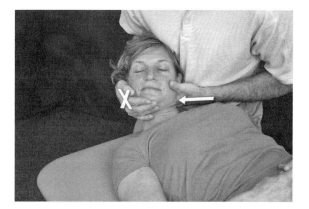

Figure 14.16 C2–C6 Facet Separation in Supine Position: Contralateral Gap

head. The therapist's left and right hands contact the posterior surface of the transverse processes, lamina, inferior articular processes, and spinous process of the cranial vertebra in the treatment segment. The therapist's thumbs press in the direction of the anterior aspect of the transverse processes of the cranial vertebra in the treatment segment. A wedge is placed under the upper thoracic spinal segments, and a belt is used to stabilize the patient's upper thoracic against the wedge and table (**Figure 14.15**). A roll or pillow is placed under the patient's head as needed to maintain the position of greatest comfort. The slack in the treatment segment is taken up in a cranial direction with both hands, and the manipulation or mobilization is delivered using the same direction of motion.

This technique is more specific to a region (i.e., the cervical spine) than the prior version, but is not specific to a segment. The degree to which traction occurs in the spinal segments caudal to the point of contact depends on factors such as the amount of force used and the amount of motion available at each spinal segment.

Patients generally perceive a greater amount of cervical traction when the belt and wedge are used to stabilize the thoracic spine. The extent to which the belt and wedge are able to make this technique more specific to the cervical region depends on the individual patient's sternal and rib cage shape and thoracic curve.

C2–C6 Facet Separation in Supine Contralateral Gap

With the patient supine, the patient's cervical spine down through the treatment segment is positioned in left side-bending and right rotation. The therapist stands

to the left of the patient's head, neck, and shoulder. The therapist's right forearm is placed against the right side of the patient's face, supporting the head position against the right side of the therapist's torso. The radial border of the therapist's left second MCP contacts the left inferior and superior articular processes of the treatment segment (**Figure 14.16**). The slack in the treatment segment is taken up through prepositioning in left side-bending and right rotation. The manipulation is delivered by the radial border of the therapist's left hand in a medial, slightly cranial, and slightly dorsal direction.

This technique is moderately specific in terms of the motion generated at the treatment segment. Specificity is enhanced by taking up soft-tissue slack in the treatment segment through prepositioning in side-bending and rotation. Impulses that are too long or movement of the support hand and therapist's body may generate unwanted movement in the spinal segments cranial and caudal to the treatment segment.

Due to the spinal prepositioning and the left hand contact used, this technique is best applied as a manipulation. In certain cases, patients may report tenderness under the manipulating hand when the therapist takes up the slack. This discomfort is often reduced by radial deviation of the wrist of the manipulating hand, thereby using a more posterior contact on the vertebrae.

Mobilization and Manipulation of C7

C7 Facet Separation Seated

The patient is positioned sitting in a chair with back support. The patient's C7 spinal segment is positioned in left side-bending and right rotation. The patient is seated with the upper thoracic spine positioned at the top of

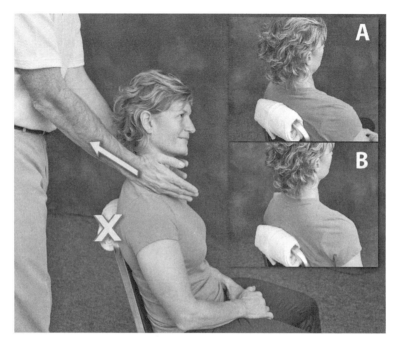

Figure 14.17 C7 Facet Separation in Seated Position

the chair back. The therapist stands behind the patient. The ulnar border of the therapist's right hand presses in the direction of the anterior surface of the patient's right transverse process of C7. The therapist's left hand supports the patient's head and neck position. The slack in the treatment segment is taken up through prepositioning, and a dorsal, slightly medial, and slightly cranial force is applied by the right hand on the right side of C7 (**Figure 14.17**). The manipulation or mobilization is delivered by the ulnar border of the therapist's right hand in a dorsal, lateral, and cranial direction.

The segmental specificity of this technique depends greatly on which thoracic vertebra is positioned to be stabilized against the top of the chair back. If a higher-level thoracic vertebra is positioned against the chair back (inset A in Figure 14.17), then the technique is more segmentally specific to the segments located between the chair contact and the manipulating hand. If a lower-level thoracic vertebra is stabilized against the chair back (inset B), then the technique treats a greater number of spinal segments.

In cases of multisegmental upper thoracic restrictions in addition to C7 restrictions, it is more efficient and effective to use this treatment in a less specific manner (e.g., with the patient positioned as shown in inset B). In cases of single C7 restrictions or thoracic restrictions, the more segmentally specific approach is recommended.

C7 Facet Ventral-Cranial Glide Seated

The patient is seated with the C7 in slight left side-bending, left rotation, and slight flexion. The therapist is positioned in front of the patient with his or her left knee positioned anteriorly, contacting the patient's right shoulder and chest (**Figure 14.18**). The ulnar border of the therapist's left hand contacts the posterior surface of the transverse process of C7 on the right. The radial border of the therapist's right hand contacts the left posterior laminae and facets of C7 and T1. The slack in the treatment segment is taken up during prepositioning.

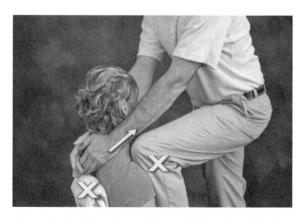

Figure 14.18 C7 Facet Ventral-Cranial Glide in Seated Position

The manipulation is applied by the therapist's left hand in a ventral, medial, and cranial direction.

This technique is moderate to very specific. Little movement should occur above or below the treatment segment.

This technique is most effective when applied as a mobilization. Patients whose cervical condition is less painful and more characterized by stiffness should respond well to this technique. It provides a strong stretch to the peri-articular structures at the C7–T1 articulation.

C7 Facet Dorsal-Caudal Glide Seated

The patient is positioned sitting in a chair with back support. The patient's C7 spinal segment is positioned in right side-bending, right rotation, and dorsal flexion. The patient is seated with the upper thoracic spine positioned at the top of the chair back. The therapist is positioned behind the patient, with the ulnar border of the therapist's right hand contacting the anterior lateral and posterior surface of the transverse process of C7 on the right (**Figure 14.19**). The radial border of the therapist's left hand contacts the left posterior laminae and facets of C7 and T1. The slack in the treatment segment is taken up during prepositioning. The manipulation is applied by the therapist's right hand in a dorsal, medial, and caudal direction.

The segmental specificity of this technique depends greatly on which thoracic vertebra is positioned to be stabilized against the top of the chair back. If a higher-level thoracic vertebra is positioned against the chair back (Figure 14.17A), the technique is more segmentally specific to the segments located between the chair contact and the manipulating hand. If a lower-level thoracic vertebra is stabilized against the chair back

(Figure 14.17B), then the technique treats a greater number of spinal segments.

This technique is an excellent choice for restoring dorsal caudal gliding for patients with a more stiffness-dominant C7 or multiple upper thoracic restrictions. It is particularly valuable in improving cervical rotation and dorsal flexion. This technique provides a strong stretch to the peri-articular structures at the C7–T1 articulation.

THORACIC SPINE INTERVENTIONS

The link between the thoracic spine and migraine may derive from this anatomic feature's ability to influence the cervical spine. Cervical spine impairments have been identified as potential contributors to migraine (Tfelt-Hansen et al., 1981; Blau & MacGregor, 1994). Therefore the astute, evidence-based practitioner should consider treatment of the thoracic spine as a potential means of achieving relief from this form of headache.

The body of literature supporting treatment of the thoracic spine in individuals with neck pain continues to grow. Currently studies have indicated the ability of manual physical therapy directed at this area to improve cervical range of motion, reduce pain, and improve function (Cleland et al., 2005, 2007a, 2007b, 2010; Fernández-de-las-Peñas et al., 2007b; Krauss et al., 2008; Gonzalez-Iglesias et al., 2009). In a randomized controlled trial, Cleland et al. (2005) demonstrated that thoracic thrust manipulation aimed at the hypomobile segments of the upper and middle thoracic spine produced statistically and clinically meaningful reductions in cervical pain as compared to the results in patients receiving placebo manipulations. Flynn et al. (2006) performed a prospective study in which subjects received thrust manipulation to the hypomobile segments of the upper and middle thoracic spine. Results included a significant reduction in pain as well as significant improvements in cervical range of motion for flexion, total rotation, and total side flexion.

Krauss et al. (2008) advanced clinical decision making in this area by demonstrating significant improvements in cervical rotation range of motion after upper thoracic thrust manipulations alone. Gonzalez-Iglesias et al. (2009) performed a trial in which electrothermal modalities were combined with middle thoracic thrust manipulations; this dual therapy produced significant improvements in pain and all cervical motions as compared to electrothermal modalities alone.

In a randomized controlled trial of thrust versus non-thrust manipulation, Cleland et al. (2007b) identified a significant between-group difference in neck pain

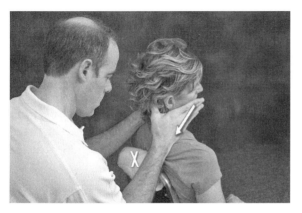

Figure 14.19 C7 Facet Dorsal-Caudal Glide in Seated Position

reduction as well as Neck Disability Index (NDI) improvement in those patients receiving thrust manipulation at a 48-hour follow-up. Additional analysis also demonstrated significantly higher perceived improvement in the thrust manipulation group as measured by the Global Ratings of Change Scale (GROC).

Currently, the characteristics that render individuals with neck pain more likely to respond favorably to thoracic thrust manipulation have not been identified (Cleland et al., 2010). Despite these shortcomings in understanding, research has indicated that this subgroup of patients seems to be large, suggesting that thoracic spine manipulation should be considered for most individuals in whom it is not specifically contraindicated. Current contraindications may best be considered as the exclusion criteria applied in many studies, which include individuals with a history of cancer, osteoporosis, infection, prolonged steroid use, rheumatoid arthritis, nerve root involvement, and recent fracture (Cleland et al., 2005, 2007a, 2007b, 2010; Krauss et al., 2008).

The addition of cervico-thoracic exercise to a manual physical therapy program has proved beneficial in individuals with cervicogenic as well as tension-type headache (Jull, 1997; Hammill et al., 1996; Jull et al., 2002; McDonnell et al., 2005; Issa & Huijbregts, 2006; Van Duijn et al., 2007). Furthermore, the combination of thoracic manipulation and cervico-thoracic exercise in individuals with mechanical neck pain has produced lower disability scores as measured by the NDI at 1 week ($P = 0.001$), 4 weeks ($P < 0.001$), and 6 months ($P < 0.001$) after treatment, as compared to individuals who received manipulation alone (Cleland et al., 2010). A combined treatment approach including both thrust manipulation and exercise is, therefore, recommended in the treatment of individuals with migraine. The following thoracic techniques are those that have been used most frequently in the current research.

Upper Thoracic Thrust Manipulation

Supine Upper Thoracic Thrust Manipulation

In the supine position, the patient clasps his or her hands together and places them at the base of the neck. The patient is rolled toward the therapist so that the therapist's hand, in a pistol-grip position, may be placed over the central upper thoracic region. The central position is identified by placing the spinous processes of the thoracic vertebrae between the flexed fingers and the thenar-hypothenar eminences. The therapist's

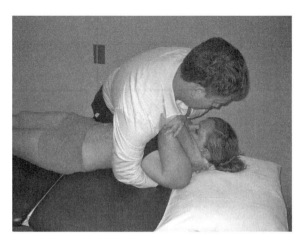

Figure 14.20 Supine Upper Thoracic Thrust Manipulation

manipulating hand stabilizes the inferior vertebrae of the targeted motion segments. The patient is then rolled back onto the flexed hand, downward pressure is applied through the patient's elbows until a firm endpoint is felt, and a thrust manipulation is applied within the restrictive barrier (**Figure 14.20**).

Middle Thoracic Thrust Manipulation

Seated Thoracic Distraction Thrust Manipulation

The patient is seated with his or her hands clasped behind the base of the neck. The therapist stands behind the patient and places his or her chest at the level of the thoracic spine that is targeted for manipulation. The therapist reaches around and holds the patient's elbows with clasped hands to avoid splaying during the thrust (**Figure 14.21**). Next, gentle anterior to posterior pressure is applied to take up the soft-tissue slack. Fine adjustments such as slight flexion may be added to further identify the firm endpoint. The therapist then applies a thrust manipulation by pulling the patient's elbows toward the therapist in a posterior and slight cranial direction.

Supine Middle Thoracic Thrust Manipulation (Figure 14.22)

The patient is placed in a supine position, with arms crossed over the chest. The therapist places his or her pistol-grip hand over the lower vertebrae of the motion segment. The patient is then rolled onto the hand, and

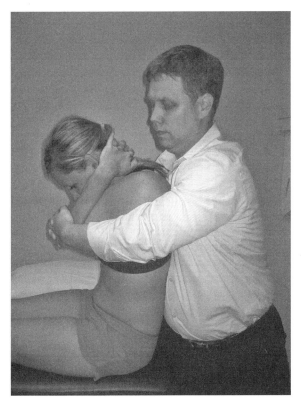

Figure 14.21 Seated Thoracic Distraction Thrust Manipulation

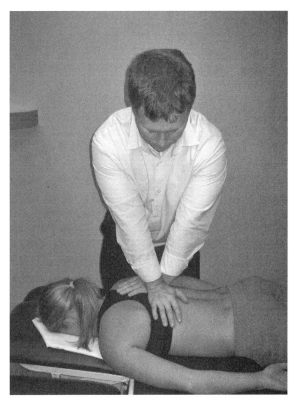

Figure 14.23 Prone Thoracic Thrust Manipulation

the patient's trunk is flexed upward until a firm endpoint is noted (**Figure 14.22**). The therapist applies anterior to posterior pressure through the patient's arms and onto the underlying hand. A downward thrust is applied into the restrictive barrier.

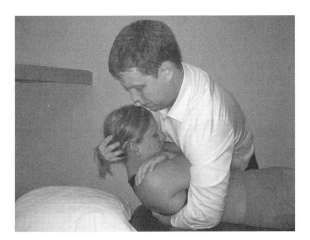

Figure 14.22 Supine Middle Thoracic Thrust Manipulation

Prone Thoracic Thrust Manipulation (Figure 14.23)

The patient is placed in a prone position, with arms by the sides of the body. The therapist stands off to the side, perpendicular to the patient. The therapist's proximal hand/pisiform bone is placed over the transverse process of the segment to be moved. His or her opposite hand/pisiform bone is placed on the opposite transverse process of the same vertebrae (**Figure 14.23**). Downward pressure is then applied through the extended elbows so that the soft-tissue slack is taken up. Final soft-tissue slack may be accounted for with slight rotation through both hands. Once the firm endpoint is noted, a thrust is applied from posterior to anterior.

CONCLUSIONS

The exact mechanism linking cervico-thoracic manual therapy intervention to the reduction of migraine has yet to be identified. Despite this uncertainty, one high-quality randomized controlled trial (Nelson et al., 1998) and at least three lower-quality trials have demonstrated a reduction in migraine symptoms with cervico-thoracic manual therapy, as compared to commonly prescribed medications. Considering the minimal side effects associated with cervico-thoracic manipulation and mobilization and the potential for headache intensity reduction as well as a reduction in medication use, the evidence-based practitioner should examine and subsequently manually intervene on identified impairments within the cervico-thoracic region. These recommendations are based on an evidence score of 1B+ (Van Kleef et al., 2009).

REFERENCES

American Physical Therapy Association (APTA). Guide to physical therapist practice. 2nd ed. *Phys Ther* 2001;81:9–744.

Astin JA, Ernst E. The effectiveness of spinal manipulation for the treatment of headache disorders: a systematic review of randomized clinical trials. *Cephalalgia* 2002;22:617–623.

Barnes PM, Powell-Griner E, McFann K, et al. Complementary and alternative medicine use among adults: United States, 2002. *Advance Data from Health Statistics* 2004(343):1–19.

Bevilaqua-Grossi D, Pegoretti KS, Goncalves MC, et al. Cervical mobility in women with migraine. *Headache* 2009;49:726–731.

Blau JN, MacGregor EA. Migraine and the neck. *Headache* 1994;34:88–90.

Bogduk N. Cervical causes of headache and dizziness. In: Boyling JD, Palastanga N, eds. *Grieve's Modern Manual Therapy.* 2nd ed. Edinburgh, UK: Churchill Livingstone; 1994:317–331.

Bohart A. Evidence-based psychotherapy means evidence-informed, not evidence-driven. *J Contemp Psychother* 2005;35:39–53.

Boissonnault WG. Prevalence of comorbid conditions, surgeries, and medication use in a physical therapy outpatient population: a multi-centered study. *J Orthop Sports Phys Ther* 1999;29:506–519.

Bookhout MR. Evaluation of the thoracic spine and ribcage. In Flynn TW, ed. *The Thoracic Spine and Ribcage.* Boston, MA: Butterworth-Heineman; 1996:147–167.

Bronfort G, Assendelft WJJ, Evans R, et al. Efficacy of spinal manipulation for chronic headache: a systematic review. *J Manipulative Physiol Ther* 2001;24:457–466.

Bronfort G, Nilsson N, Haas M, et al. Non-invasive physical treatments for chronic/recurrent headache. *Cochrane Database System Rev* 2004;3:CD001878.

Cattley P, Tuchin PJ. Chiropractic management of migraine without aura. *Aust Chiro Ost* 1999;8:85–90.

Childs JD, Fritz JM, Piva SR, et al. Proposal of a classification system for patients with neck pain. *J Orthop Sports Phys Ther* 2004;34:686–700.

Cleland JA, Childs JD, McRae M, et al. Immediate effects of thoracic manipulation in patients with neck pain: a randomized trial. *Man Ther* 2005;10:127–135.

Cleland JA, Childs JD, Fritz JM, et al. Interrater reliability of the history and physical examination in patients with mechanical neck pain. *Arch Phys Med Rehabil* 2006;87:1388–1395.

Cleland JA, Childs JD, Fritz JM, et al. Development of a clinical prediction rule for guiding treatment of a subgroup of patients with neck pain: use of thoracic spine manipulation, exercise and patient education. *Phys Ther* 2007a;87:9–23.

Cleland JA, Glynn PE, Whitman JM, et al. The short-term effects of thrust versus non-thrust mobilization/manipulation directed at the thoracic spine in patients with neck pain: a randomized clinical trial. *Phys Ther* 2007b;87:431–440.

Cleland JA, Mintken PE, Carpenter K, et al. Examination of a clinical prediction rule to identify patients with neck pain likely to benefit from thrust manipulation: a multi-site randomized clinical trial. *Phys Ther* 2010;90:1239–1250.

Davis RC. Chronic migraine and chiropractic rehabilitation: a case report. *J Chiro Med* 2003;2:55–59.

Detsky ME, McDonald DR, Baerlocher MO, et al. Does this patient with headache have a migraine or need neuroimaging? *JAMA* 2006;296:1274–1283.

Dishman JD, Ball KA, Burke J. Central motor excitability changes after spinal manipulation: a transcranial magnetic stimulation study. *J Manipulative Physiol Ther* 2002;25:1–9.

Elster EL. Treatment of bipolar, seizure, and sleep disorders and migraine headaches utilizing a chiropractic technique. *J Manipulative Physiol Ther* 2004;27:e5.

Evans DW. Mechanisms and effects of spinal high-velocity, low-amplitude thrust manipulation: previous theories. *J Manipulative Physiol Ther* 2002;25:251–262.

Fedorak CA, Ashworth N, Marshall J, et al. Reliability of visual assessment of cervical and lumbar lordosis: how good are we? *Spine* 2003;28:1857–1859.

Fernández-de-las-Peñas C, Fernandez-Carnero J, Plaza Fernandez A, et al. Dorsal manipulation in whiplash injury treatment: a randomized controlled trial. *J Whiplash Rel Disord* 2004;3:55–72.

Fernández-de-las-Peñas C, Cuadrado ML, Pareja JA. Myofascial trigger points, neck mobility and forward head posture in unilateral migraine. *Cephalalgia* 2006;26:1061–1070.

Fernández-de-las-Peñas C, Cuadrado ML, Pareja JA. Myofascial trigger points, neck mobility, and forward head posture in episodic tension-type headache. *Headache* 2007a;47:662–672.

Fernández-de-las-Peñas C, Palomeque-del-Cerro L, Rodriquez C, et al. Changes in neck pain and active range of motion after a single thoracic spine manipulation in patients with mechanical neck pain: a case series. *J Manipulative Physiol Ther* 2007b;330:312–320.

Flynn T, Wainner R, Whitman J. Immediate effects of thoracic spine manipulation on cervical spine range of motion and pain. *J Manual Manipulative Ther* 2001;9:165–166.

Fryer G, Morris T, Gibbons P, et al. The electromyographic activity of thoracic paraspinal muscles identified as abnormal with palpation. *J Manipulative Physiol Ther* 2006;29:437–447.

Goadsby PJ. Migraine, allodynia, sensitisation and all of that. *Eur Neurol* 2005;53:S10–S16.

Gonzalez-Iglesias J, Fernández-de-las-Peñas C, Cleland JA, et al. Thoracic spine manipulation for the management of patients with neck pain: a randomized clinical trial. *J Orthop Sports Phys Ther* 2009;39:20–27.

Hammill JM, Cook TM, Rosecrance JC. Effectiveness of a physical therapy regimen in the treatment of tension-type headache. *Headache* 1996;36:149–153.

Haneline MT, Croft AC, Frishberg BM. Association of internal carotid artery dissection and chiropractic manipulation. *Neurologist* 2003;9:35–44.

Herzog W. Physiological effects of manual therapy: Two commentaries. "High-speed–low-amplitude" spinal manipulative treatments. *Orthop Div Rev* 2005;10:29–31.

Hole DE, Cook JM, Bolton JE. Reliability and concurrent validity of two instruments for measuring cervical range of motion: effects of age and gender. *Man Ther* 2000;4:36–42.

Huijbregts PA. Manual therapy. In: Lennard TAL, ed. *Pain Procedures in Clinical Practice*. 3rd ed. Philadelphia, PA: Elsevier, 2001;578.

Hurwitz EL, Aker PD, Adams AH, et al. Manipulation and mobilization of the cervical spine: a systematic review of the literature. *Spine* 1996;21:1746–1759.

Issa TS, Huijbregts PA. Physical therapy diagnosis and management of a patient with chronic daily headache: a case report. *J Manual Manipulative Ther* 2006;14:E88–E123.

Jull G. Management of cervical headache. *Man Ther* 1997;2:144–149.

Jull G, Trott P, Potter H, et al. A randomized controlled trial of exercise and manipulative therapy for cervicogenic headache. *Spine* 2002;27:1835–1843.

Kendall FP, McCreary EK, Provance PG. *Muscles: Testing and Function*. 4th ed. Baltimore, MD: Williams & Wilkins; 1993.

Krauss J, Creighton D, Ely ED, et al. The immediate effects of upper thoracic translatoric spinal manipulation on cervical pain and range of motion: a randomized clinical trial. *J Manipulative Physiol Ther* 2008;16:93–99.

Kuritzky A. Autonomic nervous system imbalance in migraineurs. *Cephalalgia* 1987;7:539–541.

Lee CN, Robbins DP, Roberts HJ, et al. Reliability and validity of single inclinometer measurements for thoracic spine range of motion. *Physiother Can* 2003;55:73–78.

Linde M. Migraine: a review and future directions for treatment. *Acta Neurol Scand* 2006;114:71–83.

Lindgren KA, Leino E, Hakola M, et al. Cervical spine rotation and lateral flexion combined motion in the examination of the thoracic outlet. *Arch Phys Med Rehabil Med* 1989;71:343–344.

Lindgren KA, Leino E, Manninen H. Cervical rotation lateral flexion test in brachialgia. *Arch Phys Med Rehabil Med* 1992;73:735–737.

Marcus DA, Scharff L, Mercer S, et al. Musculoskeletal abnormalities in chronic headaches: a controlled comparison of headache diagnostic groups. *Headache* 1999;39:21–27.

McDonnell MK, Sahrmann SA, Van Dillen L. A specific exercise program and modification of postural alignment treatment of cervicogenic headache: a case report. *J Orthop Sports Phys Ther* 2005;35:3–15.

McPartland JM, Giuffrida A, King J, et al. Cannabimimetic effects of osteopathic manipulative treatment. *J Am Osteopath Assoc* 2005;105:283–291.

Melzack R, Wall PD. Pain mechanisms: a new theory. *Science* 1965;150:971–979.

Mintken PE, DeRosa C, Little T, Smith B. AAOMPT clinical guidelines: a model for standardizing manipulation terminology in physical therapy practice. *J Orthop Sports Phys Ther* 2008; 38:A1–6.

National Board of Chiropractic Examiners (NBCE). *Practice Analysis of Chiropractic 2010*. Greeley, CO: NBCE; 2010.

Nelson CF, Bronfort G, Evans R, et al. The efficacy of spinal manipulation, amitriptyline and the combination of both therapies for the prophylaxis of migraine headache. *J Manipulative Physiol Ther* 1998;21:511–519.

Norlander S, Nordgren B. Clinical symptoms related to musculoskeletal neck shoulder pain and mobility in the cervicothoracic spine. *Scand J Rehab Med* 1998;30:243–251.

Norlander S, Gustavsson BA, Lindell J, et al. Reduced mobility in the cervico-thoracic motion segment: a risk factor for musculoskeletal neck shoulder pain: a two year prospective follow-up study. *Scand J Rehab Med* 1997;29:167–174.

Oppenheim JS, Spitzer DE, Segal DH. Neurovascular complications following spinal manipulation. *Spine J* 2005;5:660–667.

Paris SV, Loubert PV. *Foundations of Clinical Orthopaedics*. 3rd ed. St. Augustine, FL: University Press; 1999.

Parker GB, Tupling H, Pryor DS. A controlled trial of cervical manipulation of migraine. *Aust NZ J Med* 1978;8:589–593.

Parker GB, Pryor DS, Tupling H. Why does migraine improve during a clinical trial? Further results from a trial of cervical manipulation for migraine. *Aust NZ J Med* 1980;10:192–198.

Paungmali A, O'Leary S, Souvlis T, et al. Naloxone fails to antagonize initial hypoalgesic effect of a manual therapy treatment for lateral epicondylalgia. *J Manipulative Physiol Ther* 2004;27:180–185.

Pencheon D. What's next for evidence-based medicine? *Evidence-Based Health Care & Public Health* 2005;9:319–321.

Peroutka SJ. Migraine: a chronic sympathetic nervous system disorder. *Headache* 2004;44:53–64.

Peters-Harris S. Chiropractic management of a patient with migraine headache. *J Chiropr Med* 2005;4:25–31.

Price DDF, Finniss DG, Benedetti F. A comprehensive review of the placebo effect: recent advances and current thought. *Annu Rev Psychol* 2008;59:565–590.

Roche PA. Pain and placebo analgesia: two sides of the same coin. *Phys Ther Rev* 2007;12:189–198.

Shevel E, Spierings EH. Cervical muscles in the pathogenesis of migraine headache. *J Headache Pain* 2004;5:12–14.

Skyba DA, Radhakrishnan R, Rohlwing JJ, et al. Joint manipulation reduces hyperalgesia by activation of monoamine receptors but not opioid or GABA receptors in the spinal cord. *Pain* 2003;136:159–168.

Sluka KA, Milosavljevic S. Manual therapy. In: Sluka KA, ed. *Mechanisms and Management of Pain for the Physical Therapist*. Seattle, WA: IASP Press; 2009:205–214.

Sorrell MR. The physical examination of migraine. *Curr Pain Headache Rep* 2006;10:350–354.

Tfelt-Hansen P, Lous I, Olesen J. Prevalence and significance of muscle tenderness during common migraine attacks. *Headache* 1981;21:49–54.

Tuchin PJ. A twelve-month clinical trial of chiropractic spinal manipulative therapy for migraine. *Aust Chiro Ost* 1999;8:61–65.

Tuchin PJ. A case of chronic migraine remission after chiropractic care. *J Chiro Med* 2008;7:66–70.

Tuchin PJ, Bonello R. Classic migraine or not classic migraine: that is the question. *Australas Chiropr Osteopathy* 1996;5:66–74.

Tuchin PJ, Pollard H, Bonello R. A randomized controlled trial of chiropractic spinal manipulative therapy for migraine. *J Manipulative Physiol Ther* 2000;23:91–95.

Van Duijn J, Van Duijn AJ, Nitsch W. Orthopaedic manual physical therapy including thrust manipulation and exercise in the management of a patient with cervicogenic headache: a case report. *J Manual Manipulative Ther* 2007;15:10–24.

Van Kleef M, Mekhail N, Van Zundert J. Evidence-based guidelines for interventional pain medicine according to clinical diagnoses. *Pain Pract* 2009;9:247–251.

Wainner RS, Whitman JM, Cleland JA, et al. Regional interdependence: a musculoskeletal examination model whose time has come. *J Orthop Sports Phys Ther* 2007;37:658–660.

Wright A. Physiological effects of manual therapy: two commentaries. "High-speed–low-amplitude" spinal manipulative treatments. *Orthop Div Rev* 2005;1:33–35.

Youdas JW, Carey JR, Garrett TR. Reliability of measurements of cervical spine range of motion: comparison of three methods. *Phys Ther* 1991;71:98–104.

Zwart JA. Neck mobility in different headache disorders. *Headache* 1997;37:6–11.

Manual Approaches for Myofascial Trigger Points

Robert D. Gerwin, MD, and César Fernández-de-las-Peñas, PT, DO, PhD

OVERVIEW: MYOFASCIAL TRIGGER POINTS

Myofascial trigger points (TrPs) constitute one of the most pervasive causes of chronic and recurrent pain, and one of the most common musculoskeletal pain conditions. As a primary problem, TrPs occur in the absence of other medical issues; they can be precipitated by underlying medical conditions such as certain metabolic, nutritional, and mechanical disorders (e.g., hypermobility states such as Ehlers-Danlos syndrome). As a comorbid condition, they are associated with and complicate other medical conditions such as osteoarthritis of the shoulder or hip, cervical or lumbar spondylosis, ureterolithiasis, and injuries such as whiplash. It could be said, however, that such conditions as arthritis, whiplash, and ureterolithiasis are precipitating conditions. The point is that pain induced by TrPs constitutes a separate and independent cause of chronic pain that both compounds the pain of other conditions and may long persist after the initiating condition, such as whiplash, has disappeared.

The Nature of Trigger Points and the Development of Sensitization and Referred Pain

TrPs are focal, localized regions within muscle that are extremely tender, and that can cause pain to be felt at distant sites or regions—that is, they can cause referred pain (Simons et al., 1999). The TrP is located on discrete bands of contracted muscle called taut bands. The discrete region of maximum tenderness is usually located at the point of maximum hardness on the taut band. Hardness and tenderness tend to diminish gradually with distance along the taut band away from the trigger zone. The trigger zone, however, is the most effective site for TrP treatment, whether that therapy takes the form of needling or manual interventions. Therefore, it is not only worthwhile, but also necessary, to learn to palpate muscle well enough to identify the trigger zone. In brief, the fastest and easiest way to identify TrPs is by manual palpation, which is always done by moving the fingers across the muscle, perpendicular to the direction of the muscle fibers in that particular muscle, searching for a discrete, hardened band of muscle fibers (**Figure 15.1**).

Taut Bands

Taut bands are palpable as tense strings within the belly of the muscle. Sometimes the regions of intense pain are found in nodular swellings of the taut band, although that is not necessarily the case in all taut bands. These contracted bands do not represent muscle spasms; indeed, the entire muscle is not tight or in spasm. Instead, the taut muscle bands represent groups of contracted muscle fibers. The taut bands are the site of pain; TrP tenderness occurs only in the taut band.

The current thinking is that the development of the taut band and subsequent pain is related to local muscle overload or overuse, to which the muscle cannot respond adequately (Simons et al., 1999; Gerwin et al., 2004; Mense & Gerwin, 2010). The failure of the muscle to respond to an acute or recurrent overload results from a local energy crisis. Muscle activation in response to a demand is always dispersed throughout the muscle among fibers that are the first to be contracted and the last to relax. These fibers are most vulnerable to muscle overload. Local muscle injury occurs with supra-maximal effort, or local biochemical changes occur without muscle breakdown, at those foci within the muscle that are most heavily worked. Delayed-onset muscle soreness (DOMS) can result, and may be associated with the development of myofascial TrPs.

Acetylcholine (ACh) leakage from the motor nerve terminal at the neuromuscular junction (NMJ) is thought to cause localized contraction of the muscle fiber under the motor endplate, albeit not enough to produce a fully propagated membrane depolarization resulting in an action potential and contraction of the entire muscle fiber. Leakage of ACh and consequent increase in intracellular ionized calcium concentration in the underlying muscle fiber is accelerated by sympathetic nervous system activation, but can be blocked by the alpha-adrenergic inhibitor phentolamine (Gerwin et al., 2004). Recent studies have found that TrP taut bands can be visualized using magnetic resonance elastography and sonographic elastography (Q. Chen et al., 2007, 2008; Sikdar et al., 2009).

Pain

Pain results from the release of neurotransmitters—substances such as protons (H$^+$), kinins such as bradykinin, and interleukins—that activate peripheral nociceptive receptors and potentiate dorsal horn neuron sensitization. Acid-sensing ion channels (ASIC), in responding to the presence of hydrogen ions (protons), can activate the nociceptive afferent system in the absence of inflammation (Sluka et al., 2009). Recent evidence suggests that glial cells may also play a role in inflammatory pain (Gosselin et al., 2010; O'Callaghan & Miller, 2010). Once the peripheral nociceptive receptors are activated, nociceptive impulses are transmitted through the second-order neurons in the dorsal horn, through the spinal cord, and to the primary and secondary sensory areas in the brain, including the amygdala, the anterior cingulated gyrus, and the primary sensory cortex. Niddam et al. (2007)

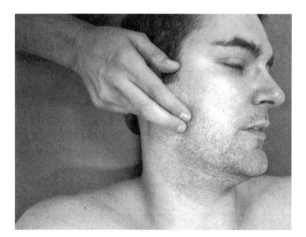

Figure 15.1 Perpendicular Palpation of a Trigger Point Taut Band on the Masseter Muscle

reported that pain from TrPs is at least partially processed at supraspinal levels. Modulation of nociceptive intensity takes place at all levels, either enhancing or inhibiting nociceptive transmission.

Referred pain, although not unique to myofascial TrPs, is nevertheless highly characteristic of myofascial pain. Occurring at the dorsal horn level, it results from the activation of otherwise quiescent axonal connections between affective nerve fibers and dorsal horn neurons that are activated by mechanisms of central sensitization (Mense & Gerwin, 2010). In fact, Kuan et al. (2007) found that TrPs were more effective in inducing neuroplastic changes in the dorsal horn neurons as compared to non-TrP regions.

The effect of multiple localized sites of muscle contraction throughout the muscle can compress regional capillaries, resulting in ischemia and hypoxia. The hypoxic and ischemic regions become acidic, and activate nociceptive ASICs, thereby initiating pain without muscle damage (Sluka et al., 2009). Local release of neurotransmitters—specifically, calcitonin gene-related peptide (CGRP), substance P, cytokines such as bradykinin, and an assortment of interleukins—results in activation of peripheral nociceptive receptors. When the nociceptive input to the spinal cord is intense or occurs repeatedly, peripheral and central sensitization occurs; subsequently, segmental spread of nociception at the spinal cord level results in referred pain (Hoheisel et al., 1993). Microdialysis studies indicate that the concentrations of bradykinin, CGRP, substance P, tumor necrosis factor alpha, interleukin-1β, serotonin, and norepinephrine are significantly higher in active TrPs as compared to latent TrP or control non-TrP points (Shah et al., 2005, 2008).

Trigger Points in Headache

Myofascial TrPs are also a problem in recurrent headache, including tension-type headache (Fernández-de-las-Peñas et al., 2007), cervicogenic headache (Roth et al., 2007), headaches associated with temporomandibular joint muscle dysfunction (Fernández-de-las-Peñas et al., 2010a), and migraine (Calandre et al., 2006; Fernández-de-las-Peñas et al., 2006a). In general, TrPs contribute to chronic daily headache more than episodic headache syndromes, whether or not they fall into any of the three previously mentioned categories. They can also be associated with acute headaches that arise from acute onset or worsening of TrP activity.

Myofascial TrPs may not be suspected in patients who complain of severe, but episodic headaches, because the patient and clinician may focus on the more severe headache that produces prominent migraine-associated symptoms of nausea, photophobia, and phonophobia. The same can be true for episodic tension-type headache and cervicogenic headache. However, careful questioning can uncover an underlying chronic daily or nearly daily headache in many of these patients. The headache intensity may be only a level 2 on a Likert scale where 0 represents no headache pain and 10 represents the most severe headache pain imaginable. Eliciting such a history of chronic, low-level, daily headache with episodic severe headache opens up a new thread of investigation into the nature of the headache and provides an additional approach to treatment.

This chapter discusses the role of myofascial TrPs in the generation of these headaches and outlines an approach to treatment that emphasizes manual techniques for management. Invasive treatment, emphasizing dry needling, is discussed in Chapter 21.

MYOFASCIAL TRIGGER POINTS IN MIGRAINE HEADACHE

Migraine headache is the result of activation of the trigeminovascular cascade that results in a sterile, neurogenic edema that initiates headache (see Chapter 5). Many potential triggers for activation of the trigeminovascular system exist, including vascular, psychological, chemical, and muscular etiologies. Muscle TrP nociceptive input from peri-cranial, cervical, and shoulder muscles is postulated to be such a trigger. Activation of the C2 dorsal root (the origin of the greater occipital nerve) secondarily activates the trigeminal nucleus caudalis. C1 and C2 are, therefore, considered part of the trigeminocervical complex (Bartsch & Goadsby, 2002).

The trigeminovascular system is activated by the nociceptive input to the trigeminal nucleus caudalis, which descends far down the cervical spinal cord—as far as the C5 level. This origin has been said to be the cause of neck pain in migraine, but the case is made here for the reverse concept—namely, that TrPs in the cervical musculature activate the trigeminocervical complex via the nucleus caudalis, thereby initiating migraine. Pressure pain thresholds appear to be significantly lower on the symptomatic side in individuals with strictly unilateral migraine in the sternocleidomastoid, sub-occipital, and temporalis muscles as compared to healthy controls (Fernández-de-las-Peñas et al., 2008). Active TrPs (i.e., TrPs that spontaneously cause pain) are more common in the upper trapezius, sternocleidomastoid, sub-occipital, and temporalis muscles in patients with unilateral migraine than in healthy control subjects (Fernández-de-las-Peñas et al.,

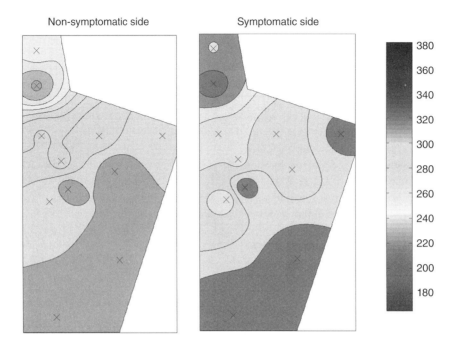

Figure 15.2 **Average Pain Threshold Maps for Patients with Unilateral Migraine.** X represents measurement sites.

Reprinted with permission from Fernández-de-las-Peñas C, et al. Generalized neck–shoulder hyperalgesia in chronic tension-type headache and unilateral migraine assessed by pressure pain sensitivity topographical maps of the trapezius muscle. *Cephalalgia* 2010;30:77–86.

2006a). The ipsilateral upper trapezius muscle has lower pain thresholds in persons with unilateral migraine than in healthy control subjects (Fernández-de-las-Peñas et al., 2010b) (**Figure 15.2**). Additionally, TrPs in the trochlear region, including the super oblique extra-ocular muscle, refer pain to the forehead and retro-orbital region in patients with unilateral migraine (Fernández-de-las-Peñas et al., 2006b) (**Figure 15.3**).

A study of 92 migraineurs showed that 93% had TrPs mostly in the temporalis and sub-occipital muscles,

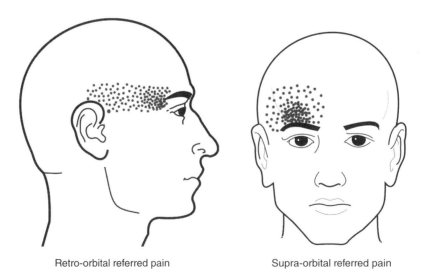

Retro-orbital referred pain   Supra-orbital referred pain

Figure 15.3 **Referred Pain Evoked from Myofascial Trigger Points in the Superior Oblique Muscle in Patients with Ipsilateral Unilateral Migraine**

Source: Adapted from Fernández-de-las-Peñas C, et al. Myofascial disorders in the trochlear region in unilateral migraine. *Clin J Pain* 2006;22:548–553.

compared to 29% in healthy controls (Calandre et al., 2006). The number of TrPs was related to the frequency of migraine headaches and the duration of the disease (Calandre et al., 2006). The association of TrPs with migraine does not constitute a causal relationship, but in 30.6% of the subjects with migraine, palpation of the TrPs provoked a migraine headache. That indicates that the peripheral nociceptive input into the trigeminal nucleus can act as a migraine trigger.

Further evidence to support this concept comes from the resolution of migraine headache by treating myofascial triggers in the neck and shoulders with lidocaine or saline injections (Tfelt-Hanson et al., 1981). Additionally, one author of this chapter terminated acute migraine headache within 15 minutes by lidocaine injection of pericranial, cervical, and shoulder myofascial TrPs in 15 of 15 consecutive patients, without recurrence of headache through the next day in all patients (Gerwin, unpublished data), suggesting that the TrP activates the trigeminocervical complex, rather than migraine activating cervical and shoulder TrPs. Moreover, inactivation of active myofascial TrPs that referred pain to the sites of headache complaint in migraine patients not only reduced the electrical pain threshold in the headache area of pain referral, but also reduced the number of headache attacks over the 60 days of the treatment period (Giamberardino et al., 2007). The results of this study strongly support the concept that cervical muscle TrPs initiate the trigeminovascular cascade that results in migraine headache.

TREATMENT OF MYOFASCIAL TRIGGER POINTS

Trigger Point Inactivation

Myofascial pain is treated by inactivation of the TrP. Inactivation of the TrP requires that the spontaneous generation of pain be diminished or eliminated, and that the TrP taut band be softened or eliminated. Local and referred pain diminish or are eliminated when the TrP is inactivated. TrPs can be inactivated manually, by needling with or without injection of a medication (the latter technique is commonly called "dry" needling), and by application of a low-level laser, although studies of laser treatment effectiveness have yielded mixed results (Gur et al., 2004; Ilbuldu et al., 2004; Dundar et al., 2007; K. H. Chen et al., 2008).

Local Twitch Response

A characteristic feature of TrP inactivation by dry needling (see Chapter 21) is the local twitch response (LTR) elicited

by the mechanical stimulation of the needle. Studies by Shah and colleagues (2005, 2008) have shown that this technique promotes a drop in the concentrations of local neurotransmitters such as CGRP and substance P, as well as cytokines and interleukins, in the extracellular fluid of the local milieu, starting immediately at the time of the local twitch, and lasting approximately 10 minutes, the concentrations approach, but never reach, the control levels. It is not known how these substances are removed, but the two likely candidates are increased cellular reuptake and washout by blood flow related to newly reopened capillaries.

The expanded integrated hypothesis of the TrP postulates that capillaries are compressed by the contraction of muscle caused by the taut band, which in turn creates local ischemia and hypoxia. Inactivation of the TrP is postulated to reduce muscle contraction and allow capillary blood flow to resume. This effect has not been demonstrated, however. Nevertheless, the washout of neurotransmitters and cytokines associated with nociception is consistent with the observed decrease in pain that immediately follows the LTR initiated by needling the TrP. The data presented by Shah et al. (2005), however, do not explain the immediate reduction in pain that occurs before the concentrations of these substances decline significantly. Moreover, the changes in concentrations of neurotransmitters, cytokines, and interleukins have never been examined following the manual induction of the local twitch, and certainly have never been examined after TrP manual inactivation.

Thus the rapid softening of the taut band with manual therapy has not been studied and remains a matter of conjecture. The cause of the rapid decrease in local pain with manual therapy also remains unexplained, although some sources speculate that it results from local stretching of the muscle fiber. Loss of referred pain is related to the decrease in nociceptive input to the dorsal horn of the spinal cord, and interruption of the segmental spread of pain through convergence and central sensitization. Nevertheless, the reversal in referred pain is amazingly rapid; indeed, it suggests that long-standing central sensitization can be reversed in less than 1 minute. This effect may be related to the effects over endocannabinoids that soft-tissue therapies can exert (McPartland, 2008).

MANUAL TREATMENT PRINCIPLES

Principles of Manual Therapy

The aim of manual inactivation of TrPs is the elimination of TrP pain, both local and referred. Following the reduction or elimination of pain, muscle function must be restored. Manual therapy is directed toward achieving these goals. Some of the techniques used in restoration of function, such as stretching the muscle to restore normal muscle length, can be uncomfortable when a TrP is actively causing pain. Hence, it is wise to use techniques such as TrP compression or needling that decrease pain before attempting to restore function. The techniques described in this chapter are specifically intended to inactivate TrPs, and may be used in any order, although there is logic to their sequential use as listed in this section. The logical order of the treatment sequence is based on relieving pain initially before introducing other techniques that might otherwise increase pain. Other, nonspecific therapies such as electrical stimulation and therapeutic ultrasound are also commonly used, albeit with variable outcomes (Fernández-de-las-Peñas, 2008).

Latent Trigger Points

It is intuitive to think that TrPs that actively cause pain should be treated and inactivated. However, it is not intuitive to think that only TrPs that are taut bands or that are painful only when mechanically stimulated (latent TrPs) should be treated. In reality, TrPs are dynamic and change back and forth between quiescent and spontaneously painful, depending on the degree of muscle activity or rest. Latent TrPs that do not spontaneously cause pain may still cause physiological and biomechanical problems (Lucas et al., 2004; Ge et al., 2008; Zhang et al., 2009; Fernández-Carnero et al., 2010; Xu et al., 2010; Wang et al., 2010) and, therefore, should be treated. If left untreated, they are likely to result in a recrudescence of TrP-induced pain.

Techniques of Manual Therapy

Inactivation of the TrP can be accomplished by a combination of several different techniques. The most commonly used are trigger point compression and stretch, the latter often with a vapocoolant spray. The technique of TrP compression is sometimes referred to as ischemic compression, although studies have not been conducted to prove that muscle ischemia results from this technique. In fact, gentle compression alone is sufficient to inactivate a TrP. Local stretching is applied to the muscle with some compression force, over a distance of 2 to 5 centimeters.

Muscle play is advocated by some sources as a means to reduce adhesions between muscle planes. Whether or not it actually achieves this goal, it certainly provides an additional form of local stretching to the muscle being treated. Myofascial release is intended to stretch the fascial covering of muscle. Therapeutic stretching is the controlled lengthening of the muscle to restore normal muscle length and facilitate restoration of muscle function. The patient's self-stretching is a home exercise designed to maintain normal muscle fiber length and decrease the likelihood of muscle shortening and recurrence of TrP.

These techniques may be used in any order. Nevertheless, because muscle stretching and myofascial release may be painful when TrPs are present, we prefer to inactivate the TrP by compression before using the other techniques.

Trigger Point Compression

TrP compression is the technique of direct compression of the TrP by the finger or with a handheld blunt-pointed or a knobby instrument. Simons (2002) proposed that compressing the sarcomeres by direct pressure in a vertical and perpendicular manner combined with active contraction of the involved muscle may equalize the length of the muscle sarcomeres in the involved TrP and consequently decrease the pain. Different studies have found that compression techniques are effective in reducing pain sensitivity of both latent (Fryer & Hogson, 2005) and active TrPs (Fernández-de-las-Peñas et al., 2006c; Gemmell et al., 2008). Vernon and Schneider (2009) reported moderately strong evidence supporting the use of compression interventions for immediate pain relief of muscle TrPs but only limited evidence for long-term pain relief.

Different compression techniques can be used depending on the amount of pressure applied and the presence or absence of pain (Hou et al., 2002; Fryer & Hodgson, 2005). The compression can be extremely gentle, yet still be effective (Lewit, 1999). In contrast, excessive force applied to the trigger zone may result in increased pain rather than dissolution of the TrP.

The point of compression is determined by examining the length of the TrP taut band to identify the region of greatest hardness. The taut band is identified by palpation of the muscle perpendicular to the fiber direction. The region of greatest hardness is usually also the region of greatest tenderness in an active TrP or in a latent TrP that is tender to palpation. In a nontender taut band, the region of greatest hardness is selected, regardless of the absence of tenderness. This region of greatest hardness is the site to treat by compression.

The treatment site is tender in active and latent TrPs, such that initial compression of this point elicits pain.

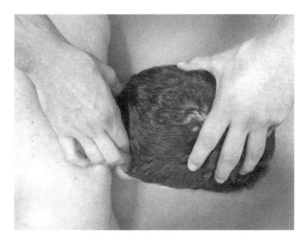

Figure 15.4 Flat Compression Technique over the Sub-Occipital Muscles

This pain should begin to subside in 15 to 20 seconds, and is usually gone, along with the referred pain, in 30 to 45 seconds. The muscle band can be felt to relax after 60 to 90 seconds of compression. Moving the muscle being treated through small, active, short-range movements that produce a contraction and relaxation of the muscle seems to facilitate the release of the TrP, although this technique has not been formally tested. We prefer to utilize TrP compression as the initial technique because it reduces pain and makes the other techniques more comfortable.

Figure 15.4 shows a flat compression technique over the sub-occipital muscles. **Figure 15.5** illustrates a pincer compression technique of the sternocleidomastoid muscle.

In patients with extremely higher hypersensitivity, the strain/counter-strain technique can be also applied (Jones, 1981; D'Ambrogio & Roth, 1997). In this technique, the therapist applies pressure until the pain threshold is reached. At that moment, the patient is passively placed in a position that reduces the tension under the palpating fingers and causes a subjective reduction of pain by 90% to 100%. This position is maintained for 90 seconds. Readers are referred to Chapter 17 for more data on this manual approach for the management of soft-tissues disorders.

Finally, a combination of manual approaches, referred as the integrated neuromuscular inhibition technique (Chaitow, 1994), has been applied over TrPs in the upper trapezius muscle with satisfactory results (Nagrale et al., 2010). The methodology of application of integrated neuromuscular inhibition technique is covered in Chapter 17.

Local Trigger Point Stretch

Local stretching is applied by the application of the index and long fingers to the taut band. The long finger pad is placed over the nail of the index finger to give additional force to the stretch. Force is applied along the long axis of the muscle fiber. The direction of the force is usually away from the nearest tendon attachment so as not to buckle the fibers, unless stretching is being applied in the mid-belly of the muscle, in which case the direction of stretching does not matter. The length of muscle fiber to which local stretching is applied is short, only 4 to 5 centimeters.

Local stretching is often the first manual technique applied after TrP compression. Pain that diminishes with local compression may transiently reoccur as local stretching is applied. This technique is particularly effective with pincer palpation (**Figure 15.6**).

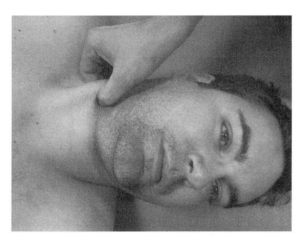

Figure 15.5 Pincer Compression Technique of the Sterno-cleidomastoid Muscle

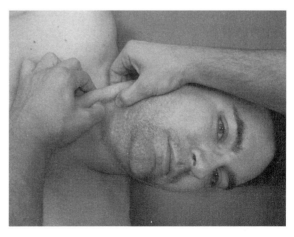

Figure 15.6 Local Stretch of the Sternocleidomastoid Muscle

Muscle Play

Muscle play is the term that has been applied to a technique originally designed to break up adhesions between adjacent muscle layers. Whether this method actually achieves this effect or not is debatable. However, the technique of working the fingers between muscles while putting the limb controlled by the muscle through a large arc of movement produces an effective local stretching of muscle.

An example is the attempted separation of the pectoralis major from the pectoralis minor muscle. To accomplish this, all four fingers are placed under the pectoralis major muscle at the anterior axillary fold, with the finger pad applied to the rib cage, on top of the pectoralis minor muscle (**Figure 15.7**). The fingers are vigorously moved in a sweeping motion under the pectoralis major muscle while the arm is moved in a wide arc of abduction–adduction. The result, at the very least, is an effective local stretch of the pectoralis major muscle.

Myofascial Release (Strokes)

The myofascial release technique is essentially a stretch of the fascial covering of the muscle. Firm force is applied with the heel of the hand or the knuckles, usually starting at the trigger zone, and extending toward the referred pain zone, but incorporating other directions of movement as the anatomy permits (**Figure 15.8**). Topical application of oil facilitates this stretch. Patients usually find this release soothing after TrP compression and local stretch.

Therapeutic Stretching

In therapeutic stretching, the clinician puts the affected part(s) through a larger stretch of the muscle(s), in

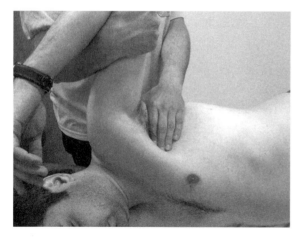

Figure 15.7 Muscle Play Between Pectoralis Major and Minor Muscles

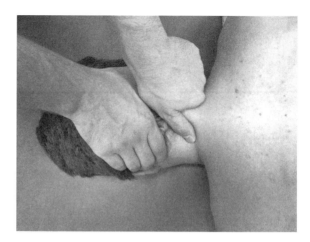

Figure 15.8 Myofascial Release over the Paraspinal Posterior Neck Muscles

contrast to the local stretch of just the muscle fiber described earlier in this section (**Figure 15.9**). Some evidence suggests that therapeutic stretching is effective for reducing pain sensitivity in active TrPs (Jaeger & Reeves, 1986; Hong et al., 1993; Hou et al., 2002). Restoration of

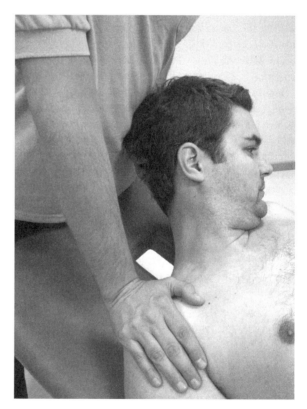

Figure 15.9 Therapeutic Stretching of the Levator Scapulae Muscle. The stretch is made more effective by abducting the ipsilateral arm in order to rotate the medial border of the scapula downward, which further lengthens the muscle.

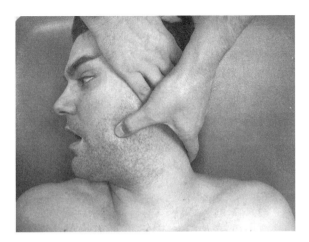

Figure 15.10 Dynamic Intervention over the Left Masseter Muscle

function through reestablishment of the normal range of motion, and subsequent muscle reeducation should be done after the trigger point is inactivated and the muscle is lengthened, but must be performed carefully to avoid joint injury in hypermobile subjects.

Dynamic Interventions

With dynamic interventions, the clinician applies either compression or myofascial release of the TrP, combined with contraction or stretching of the affected muscle. For instance, during TrP compression, the patient is asked to actively contract the muscle (Gröbli & Dommerholt, 1997; **Figure 15.10**). Another dynamic technique includes a myofascial release applied by the clinician to stretch the TrP taut band, with the patient being asked to move the segment (Gröbli & Dejung, 2003;

Figure 15.11). Although clinically effective, no scientific data are available for these techniques.

Self-Stretching

The patient's home exercise program should incorporate a reasonable stretching program designed to minimize the tendency of the muscle to shorten again with the reformation of muscle TrPs. Patients must be carefully instructed in how to perform each stretch so as to incorporate the various functions of the muscle (e.g., extension, flexion, abduction, adduction, rotation). The stretching is demonstrated to the patient, to ensure that it is done properly and that there is no overstretching. Hypermobile patients must be cautioned against excessive stretching that can injure joints.

Precautions

Manual therapy requires the application of pressure and stretching to various parts of the body. Care must be taken not to injure the tissue. Thus the pressure needed to inactivate TrPs is light, avoiding pressure that is too great and potentially damaging. Persons taking drugs that inhibit platelet function or taking warfarin are at increased risk for bruising, necessitating gentle force when compressing their TrPs. Areas that are infected, including cellulitis, and areas with hemorrhage, recent burns, fractures, or acute herpes zoster infections are avoided. Major arteries must be identified and avoided. Nerves must be identified and avoided to prevent nerve compression and injury. Joints should be mobilized to restore movement, but excessive stretching is to be avoided, particularly in persons who are hypermobile.

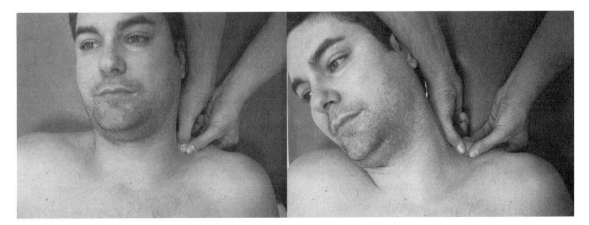

Figure 15.11 Dynamic Intervention over the Left Upper Trapezius Muscle

Functional Muscle Units

Muscles related to each other by function (i.e., agonist or antagonist muscles) should be examined and treated together. Muscles in a functional muscle unit work together to stabilize or to move a part of the body. An active or latent TrP may alter the pattern of muscle activation, thereby resulting in altered, compensatory muscle activity (Lucas et al., 2004; Hodges et al., 2009). A persistent TrP in an agonist or antagonist muscle may result in overload of the target muscle, inducing the return of TrPs in the target muscle that was treated.

MANUAL TREATMENT OF SPECIFIC MUSCLES

Principles Applicable to All Muscles

The patient is positioned comfortably and warmly, generally lying down, with the part to be treated well supported and accessible to the clinician's hands. The muscle to be treated is evaluated by palpation perpendicular to the direction of the muscle fibers. Given that muscle fiber direction often changes within a given muscle, the clinician must be knowledgeable about specific muscle anatomy. **Table 15.1** details the anatomy, function, and functional muscle unit, but does not address muscle fiber direction within any given muscle.

Next, the taut or hardened muscle band is identified. The hardest part of the band is located; it is usually the region of greatest tenderness. The examining finger maintains gentle pressure on the hardest part of the band. Referred pain, if present, will usually occur within 5 to 10 seconds. (**Table 15.2** summarizes the referred pain patterns of head and neck muscles relevant to migraine headache.) At that point, pressure is applied to the taut band. Referred pain and local pain usually begin to subside within 30 seconds. Softening of the taut band usually takes 60 to 90 seconds. Muscle play is performed, and local stretching applied. Myofascial release

Table 15.1 The Anatomy, Function, and Functional Unit Muscles of Head and Neck Muscles That Are Relevant to Migraine Headache

Muscle	Anatomy	Function	Functional Unit
Temporalis	Superior: temporal fossa Inferior: coronoid process of mandible	Elevate mandible to close mouth; laterally deviate and retrude jaw	Agonists: masseter, pterygoid Antagonists: digastric, omohyoid and myohyoid muscles, lateral pterygoid
Masseter (superficial and deep)	Superior: zygomatic arch and maxilla Inferior: mandible	Elevate mandible, close jaw	Agonist: temporalis; lateral pterygoid Antagonist: same as temporalis
Zygomatic		Raise corner of mouth in a smile	Obicularis orus
Corrugator and procerus		Frown and raise nose	Frontalis
Superior oblique muscle	Distal: globe of the eye	Move eye into medial downward gaze	Agonist: inferior oblique, inferior rectus Antagonist: Inferior oblique and superior and lateral rectus
Sternocleidomastoid	Superior: mastoid process Inferior: sternal head— sternum; clavicular head—clavicle	Flex neck against resistance, rotate head contralaterally, side-bend head ipsilaterally, elevate chin	Agonist: ipsilateral trapezius, scalene (side-bending) Contralateral oblique capitis inferior, splenius cervicis Antagonists: the above muscles on the opposite side and contralateral SCM
Levator scapula (neck)	Superior: transverse process of upper four cervical spines; Inferior: upper medial scapular border	Can rotate a contralaterally turned head back toward midline	Agonist: ipsilateral OCI and splenius cervicis, contralateral SCM and upper trapezius Antagonists: the same muscles cited as for agonists, but on the opposite side

Muscle	Anatomy	Function	Functional Unit
Splenius capitis	Superior: mastoid process, occiput Inferior: C3–C4 to T3–T4 vertebrae	Unilateral: rotate head to ipsilateral side Bilateral: neck extension	Agonist: rotation—contralateral upper trapezius and SCM; extension—SCM, longissimus capitis Antagonist: contralateral splenii, OCI, semispinalis cervicis
Splenius cervicis	Superior: transverse processes of C1–C3 Inferior: spinous processes of T2–T4	Unilateral: rotate head to ipsilateral side Bilateral: extend neck	Agonist: rotation—ipsilateral splenius capitis and OCI; extension—opposite splenii and upper trapezius
Sub-occipital muscles: the oblique capitis inferior	Superior/lateral: transverse process of C1 Inferior: spinous process of C2	Rotate head to ipsilateral side	Agonist: ipsilateral splenii, contralateral upper trapezius and SCM Antagonist: same as agonist muscles but on opposite side
Semispinalis	Capitis: superior—occiput to C4–C6; inferior—articular process C4–T6, transverse process of T1–T7 Cervicis: superior—spinous processes of C2; inferior—transverse process T1–T7	Capitis: head extension on neck Cervicis: neck extension and contralateral neck rotation	Agonist: extension—SCM; rotation—ipsilateral SCM and upper trapezius, contralateral splenii and semispinalis cervicis Antagonist: same as agonist muscles but on opposite side
Trapezius (upper)	Lateral: lateral clavicle Medial: medial nuchal line and cervical spine posterior spinous processes	Unilateral: rotates head to contralateral side Ipsilateral: side-bend Bilateral: extension	Agonist: rotation—ipsilateral SCM and contralateral splenii, OCI; extension—semispinalis and splenii; side-bend—scalene Antagonist: same as agonist muscles but on opposite side, and contralateral upper trapezius
Levator scapulae (shoulder)	See levator scapula (neck)	Rotate the medial border of the upper scapular cephalad Elevate the shoulder (with the upper trapezius)	Agonist: serratus anterior, upper trapezius Antagonist: lower serratus anterior, upper trapezius (in upward medial scapular rotation)

Abbreviations: SCM, sternocleidomastoid; OCI, oblique capitis inferior.

Table 15.2 Referred Pain Patterns of Head and Neck Muscles Relevant to Migraine Headache

Muscle	Referred Pain Pattern (Ipsilateral Unless Stated Otherwise)
Temporalis	Anterior fibers: anterior temple, eyebrow, and upper incisor and canine teeth Middle fibers: frontal temple, bicuspids and molars Posterior fibers: above and behind the ear
Masseter	Superficial: mandible, maxilla, molar teeth; above eye Deep: ear and tragus/cheek
Zygomatic	Alongside nose to eye, above eye
Corrugator and procerus	Local over eye and nose
Superior oblique muscle	Retro-orbital and forehead
Sternocleidomastoid	Sternal head: forehead over eye, deep within the orbit, vertex, occiput, cheek, chin, sternum Clavicular head: forehead (can be bilateral), deep in ear, retro-auricular
Upper trapezius	Neck, jaw, and temple
Levator scapulae	Occiput and retro-auricular, angle of neck and shoulder
Splenius capitis	Vertex
Splenius cervicis	Upper: band-like around head and straight through to eye Lower: to angle of neck and shoulder
Sub-occipital muscles	Occiput to eye (retro-orbital), forehead; deep, poorly localized intracranial pain

and therapeutic stretching can be performed next. The patient is instructed in home treatment, including a self-stretching and exercise program. Moist heat or cold can be applied at the end of treatment, as the patient desires. At this point, the manual treatment is considered complete.

The details for anatomy, fiber direction, use of muscle play and myofascial release, treatment precautions, and therapeutic stretching are unique to each muscle. Only the treatment template is universal.

Head Muscles

Temporalis Muscle

1. The patient is placed in either supine or side-lying position, with the pertinent temporalis muscle accessible to the clinician's hand. Taut bands are palpated perpendicular to the muscle fiber direction. The most firm and tender site in the band is selected (trigger zone). Referred pain, if present, is elicited.
2. Gentle pressure is applied to the taut bands until the TrP is released.
3. Local stretching is applied, followed by myofascial release (**Figure 15.12**).
4. There is no muscle play.
5. Therapeutic stretching is performed by grasping the patient's lower lip between the therapist's thumb and index finger, and gently lowering the mandible to an open position. The index finger can be hooked over the lower incisors, and the thumb under the mandible, to protract the open mandible. Note that pressure on the lower

incisors induces a tendency to bite and close the jaw, an effect opposite the desired stretch.

Masseter Muscle

1. The patient is placed in either supine or side-lying position, with the pertinent muscle accessible to the clinician's hand. Taut bands are identified by cross-fiber palpation, in both the superficial and deep masseter (**Figure 15.13**).
2. Direct compression is applied with the index or long finger pad.
3. Local stretching and myofascial release are performed, the latter with the direction of movement to the cheek and to the neck.
4. There is no muscle play.
5. Therapeutic stretching is the same as for the temporalis muscle, with the addition of a second stretch moving the jaw contralaterally.

Zygomatic Muscle

1. The patient is supine. The clinician uses flat palpation across muscle fibers, against the zygoma. The slips of the muscle are fine and may be difficult to identify. Alternatively, the index finger can be used to sweep the inside of the cheek and feel the firm bands of the muscle.
2. The taut bands are compressed with either flat palpation or pincer palpation.
3. Local stretching is applied by flat palpation directed away from the zygoma.
4. Myofascial release is applied downward from the zygoma

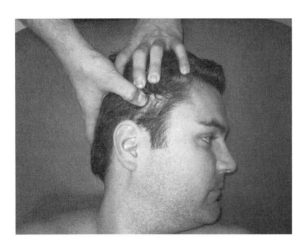

Figure 15.12 Myofascial Release of the Right Temporalis Muscle

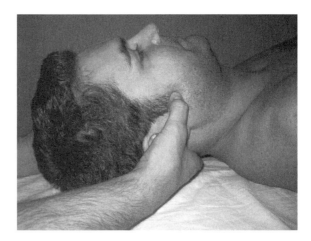

Figure 15.13 Compression of the Right Deep Masseter Muscle Trigger Point

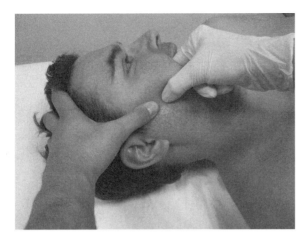

Figure 15.14 Therapeutic Stretching of the Right Zygomatic Muscle

5. Therapeutic stretching is performed by sweeping the index finger along the inside of the cheek, distending and stretching the cheek **(Figure 15.14)**.
6. Self-stretching is the same as therapeutic stretching.

Corrugator and Procerus Muscles

1. The patient is supine.
2. Compression is applied to the corrugator muscle or procerus muscle until referred and local pain subside.
3. Local stretching is directed in a medial to lateral direction for the corrugator muscles, and upward toward the forehead for the procerus muscle **(Figure 15.15)**.

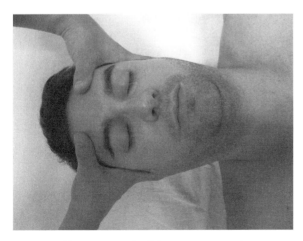

Figure 15.15 Local Stretch of the Corrugator and Procerus Muscles

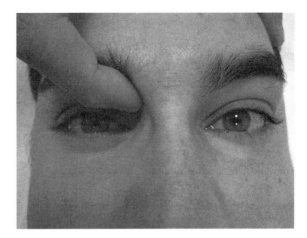

Figure 15.16 Compression of Right Superior Oblique Muscle Trigger Point

4. Myofascial release is directed similarly as local stretch.
5. There is no muscle play and no home exercise program.

Extra-Ocular Superior Oblique Muscle

1. The patient is supine. Gentle compression is applied to the trochlea with a finger tip, a pencil eraser, or a cotton-tipped applicator **(Figure 15.16)**.
2. Local stretching is done by directing the patient's gaze superiorly and laterally.
3. Myofascial release is directed superiorly to the forehead.
4. There is no muscle play.
5. Therapeutic stretching is the same as local stretching.

Neck Muscles

Sternocleidomastoid Muscle

1. The entire muscle is grasped in a pincer grasp (see Figure 15.5), including both the sternal and clavicular head. Pincer grasp is maintained when performing local compression and local stretch.
2. The pincer grasp is maintained while the muscle is pulled sideways, and the fingers move between the sternocleidomastoid and the scalene muscles **(Figure 15.17)**.
3. The fingers that separate the sternocleidomastoid from the scalene muscles are moved upward and downward between the two muscles.

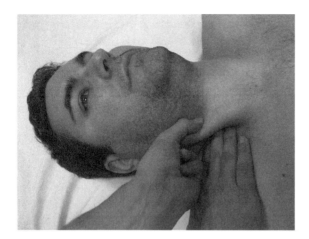

Figure 15.17 Muscle Play Between the Sternocleidomastoid and Scalene Muscles

4. Therapeutic stretching includes ipsilateral head rotation, contralateral side-bending, extension, and chin tuck. These movements are performed simultaneously.

Levator Scapulae Muscle

Upper Division

1. Firm but gentle flat palpation is applied to the muscle in the neck at a point where the muscle is most firm or most tender. Pressure is applied to this zone.
2. Local stretching is performed in an either rostral or caudal direction.
3. There is no muscle play.
4. Myofascial release is done from the neck upward or from the mastoid process insertion downward.
5. Therapeutic stretching is performed by bringing the ipsilateral arm over the head while flexing the neck and turning the face to the contralateral side. The shoulder is depressed.

Lower Division

1. The patient is placed in a side-lying position, with the shoulder to be treated in the superior location.
2. The taut bands are identified by cross-fiber palpation perpendicular to the muscle fibers directed superiorly, almost parallel to the spine.
3. Compression is applied to the muscle just superior and medial to the upper medial border of

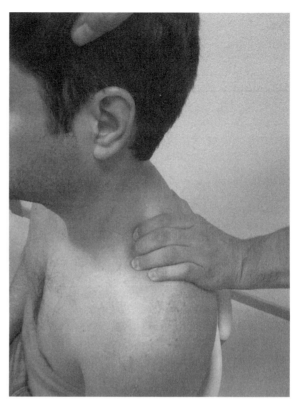

Figure 15.18 Muscle Play Between the Levator Scapulae and Upper Trapezius Muscles

the scapula, rostral to the medial aspect of the scapular spine.
4. Local stretching is directed rostrally.
5. Myofascial release is directed upward, laterally, and over the scapula.
6. Muscle play is performed between the upper trapezius and the underlying levator scapula, at the anterior edge of the trapezius (**Figure 15.18**).
7. Therapeutic stretching is performed by bringing the ipsilateral arm over the head, while flexing the neck and turning the face to the contralateral side. The shoulder is depressed.
8. Home stretching is performed in the same manner as described in step 7, except without shoulder depression.

Splenius Capitis Muscle

1. The patient is placed in either a prone or side-lying position.
2. The muscle is palpated by flat palpation against the occiput.

3. Compression is applied until local and referred pain are gone, and the taut band relaxes.
4. Local stretching is directed from the occiput to the neck.
5. There is no myofascial release because of the hair, and no muscle play.
6. Therapeutic and home stretching both consist of neck flexion with the chin tucked to the contralateral clavicle.

Splenius Cervicis Muscle

1. The patient is placed in either prone or side-lying position.
2. The diagonal muscle fibers are palpated perpendicularly to the inferomedially directed fibers, to identify the trigger zone that is often found at approximately the C5 level, lateral to the midline.
3. Compression is applied until the local and referred pain have diminished and the taut band has softened.
4. Local stretching is directed in either a rostral or caudal direction.
5. Myofascial release is directed rostrally and caudally.
6. There is no muscle play.
7. Therapeutic and home stretching are the same as for the splenius capitis.

Sub-Occipital Muscles: The Oblique Capitis Inferior

1. The patient is placed in either a prone or side-lying position.
2. The muscle is palpated perpendicular to its fiber direction to identify the trigger zone.
3. Compression is followed by local stretching that can be directed toward the C2 posterior process or to the transverse process of C1.
4. Myofascial release is performed over the neck.
5. There is no muscle play.
6. Therapeutic stretching is performed with the patient sitting, by rotation of the head 10° to 15° to the contralateral side. The second cervical vertebra will also rotate, turning the posterior process to the ipsilateral side of the muscle, negating the stretch. Therefore, the clinician stands on the contralateral side of the patient, places one hand on the back of the neck, with the thumb placed against the body of C2 contralateral to the C2

posterior process. This positioning minimizes rotation of C2 when the head is turned. The clinician cradles the patient's head, whose face is nestled between the therapist's arm and chest, with the therapist's hand on the occiput. The therapist then rotates the head to the contralateral side while firmly pushing against the C2 lateral mass.

Semispinalis Muscle

1. The patient is placed in either a prone or side-lying position.
2. The inferolaterally directed fibers are cross-palpated to identify the trigger zone.
3. Compression is followed by local stretching.
4. Myofascial release is performed over the neck.
5. There is no muscle play.
6. Therapeutic and self-stretching are done with the neck flexed and the face turned slightly to the ipsilateral side.

Shoulder Muscles: Trapezius Muscle

1. The patient is placed in a side-lying position.
2. The muscle can be palpated by pincer and flat palpation, depending on the patient's build and the degree of muscle relaxation.
3. The trigger areas are treated with compression until local and referred pain are gone, and the taut bands are relaxed, followed by local stretching.
4. Muscle play is performed as described for the levator scapulae muscle.
5. Myofascial release is directed toward the neck and toward the shoulder.
6. Therapeutic stretching is performed with the patient supine. The therapist stands or sits at the patient's head; holds the head with one hand under the occiput; moves the head in contralaterally side-bent, ipsilateral head rotation, and forward neck flexion; and then stabilizes or depresses the shoulder with the free hand (**Figure 15.19**).
7. Home stretching is done with the patient sitting, with the head rotated to the ipsilateral side, side-bent to the contralateral side, neck flexed, and shoulder stabilized by placing the ipsilateral arm behind the back and holding the wrist with the other hand.

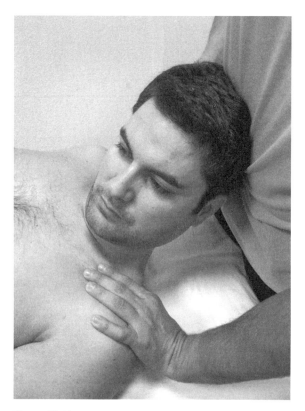

Figure 15.19 Therapeutic Stretching of the Left Upper Trapezius Muscle

CONCLUSIONS

Myofascial trigger points are among the most common causes of musculoskeletal pain, yet can be treated effectively by both noninvasive and invasive means. Noninvasive treatment consists of manual therapy, which has been shown to be effective in eliminating or reducing pain that originates in the TrP. Studies have shown that latent TrPs are active causes of musculoskeletal dysfunction and, therefore, should be treated as well as active TrPs. Taut bands alone may also cause dysfunction and, therefore, are appropriate targets of treatment, although the effect of taut bands has not been as well studied as the effects of latent and active TrPs. Manual techniques can be combined with invasive treatment (needling), as well as performed alone. Inactivation of TrPs by manual techniques should be combined with more global physical therapy rehabilitation programs that include muscle reeducation and strengthening, once pain is reduced.

The results of these approaches can be quite satisfying. Special populations, however, require modifications of the manual approach. In particular, hypermobile individuals should have only local treatment of TrPs and only minimal or no stretching after TrP inactivation.

REFERENCES

Bartsch T, Goadsby PJ. Stimulation of the greater occipital nerve induces increased central excitability of dural afferent input. *Brain* 2002;125:1496–1509.

Calandre EP, Hidalgo J, Garcia-Leiva JM, Rico-Villademoros F. Trigger point evaluation in migraine patients: an indication of peripheral sensitization linked to migraine predisposition? *Eur J Neurol* 2006;13:244–249.

Chaitow L. Integrated neuromuscular inhibition technique. *Br J Osteopathy* 1994;13:17–20.

Chen KH, Hong CZ, Kuo FC, et al. Electrophysiologic effects of a therapeutic laser on myofascial trigger spots of rabbit skeletal muscle. *Am J Phys Med Rehabil* 2008;87:1006–1014.

Chen Q, Bensamoun S, Basford JR, et al. Identification and quantification of myofascial taut bands with magnetic resonance elastography. *Arch Phys Med Rehabil* 2007;88:1658–1661.

Chen Q, Basford JR, An KN. Ability of magnetic resonance elastography to assess taut bands. *Clin Biom* 2008;23:623–629.

D'Ambrogio KJ, Roth GB. *Positional Release Therapy.* St. Louis: Mosby; 1997.

Dundar U, Evcik D, Samli F, et al. The effect of gallium arsenide aluminum laser therapy in the management of cervical myofascial pain syndrome: a double-blind, placebo-controlled study. *Clin Rheumatol* 2007;26:930–934.

Fernández-Carnero J, Ge HY, Kimura Y, et al. Increased spontaneous electrical activity at a latent myofascial trigger point after nociceptive stimulation of another latent trigger point. *Clin J Pain* 2010;26:138–143.

Fernández-de-las-Peñas C. Physical therapy and exercise in headache. *Cephalalgia* 2008;28(suppl 1):36–38.

Fernández-de-las-Peñas C, Cuadrado ML, Pareja JA. Myofascial trigger points, neck mobility and forward head posture in unilateral migraine. *Cephalalgia* 2006a;26:1061–1070.

Fernández-de-las-Peñas C, Cuadrado ML, Gerwin RD, Pareja JA. Myofascial disorders in the trochlear region in unilateral migraine. *Clin J Pain* 2006b;22:548–553.

Fernández-de-las-Peñas C, Alonso-Blanco C, Fernández J, Miangolarra-Page JC. The immediate effect of ischemic compression technique and transverse friction massage on tenderness of active and latent myofascial triggers points: a pilot study. *J Bodyw Mov Ther* 2006c;10:3–9.

Fernández-de-las-Peñas C, Cuadrado ML, Arendt-Nielsen L, et al. Myofascial trigger points and sensitisation: an updated pain model for tension type headache. *Cephalalgia* 2007;27:383–393.

Fernández-de-las-Peñas C, Cuadrado ML, Arendt-Nielsen L, Pareja JA. Side-to-side differences in pressure pain thresholds and pericranial muscle tenderness in strictly unilateral migraine. *Eur J Neurol* 2008;15:162–168.

Fernández-de-las-Peñas C, Galán-del-Río F, Alonso-Blanco C, et al. Referred pain from muscle trigger points in the masticatory and neck–shoulder musculature in women with temporomandibular disorders. *J Pain* 2010a;11:1295–1304.

Fernández-de-las-Peñas C, Madeleine P, Caminero AB, et al. Generalized neck–shoulder hyperalgesia in chronic tension-type headache and unilateral migraine assessed by pressure pain sensitivity topographical maps of the trapezius muscle. *Cephalalgia* 2010b;30:77–86.

Fryer G, Hodgson L. The effect of manual pressure release on myofascial trigger points in the upper trapezius muscle. *J Bodyw Mov Ther* 2005;9:248–255.

Ge HY, Zhang Y, Boudreau S, et al. Induction of muscle cramps by nociceptive stimulation of latent myofascial trigger points. *Exp Brain Res* 2008;187:623–629.

Gemmell H, Miller P, Nordstrom H. Immediate effect of ischaemic compression and trigger point pressure release on neck pain and upper trapezius trigger points: a randomized controlled trial. *Clin Chiropractic* 2008;11:30–36.

Gerwin RD, Dommerholt J, Shah J. An expansion of Simons' integrated hypothesis of trigger point formation. *Curr Pain Headache Rep* 2004;8:468–475.

Giamberardino MA, Tafuri E, Savini A, et al. Contribution of myofascial trigger points to migraine symptoms. *J Pain* 2007;8:869–878.

Gosselin RD, Suter M, Ji R. Decosterd I. Glial cells and chronic pain. *Neuroscientist* 2010;16:519–531.

Gröbli C, Dejung B. Nichtmedikamentöse therapie myofaszialer schmerze. *Schmerz* 2003;17:475–480.

Gröbli C, Dommerholt J. Myofasziale triggerpunkte: pathologie und behandlungsmöglichkeiten. *Manuelle Medizin* 1997;35:295–303.

Gur A, Sarac AJ, Cevik R, et al. Efficacy of 904nm gallium arsenide low level laser therapy in the management of chronic myofascial pain in the neck: a double-blind and randomized-controlled study. *Lasers Surg Med* 2004;35:229–235.

Hodges P, van den Hoorn W, Dawson A, Cholewicki J. Changes in the mechanical properties of the trunk in low back pain may be associated with recurrence. *J Biomech* 2009;42:61–66.

Hoheisel U, Mense S, Simons DG, Yu XM. Appearance of new receptive fields in rat dorsal horn neurons following noxious stimulation of skeletal muscle: a model for referral of muscle pain? *Neurosci Lett* 1993;153:9–12.

Hong CZ, Chen YC, Pon CH, Yu J. Immediate effects of various physical medicine modalities on pain threshold of an active myofascial trigger point. *J Musculoskeletal Pain* 1993;1:37–53.

Hou CR, Tsai LC, Cheng KF, et al. Immediate effects of various physical therapeutic modalities on cervical myofascial pain and trigger-point sensitivity. *Arch Phys Med Rehabil* 2002;83:1406–1414.

Ilbuldu E, Cakmak A, Disci R, Aydin R. Comparison of laser, dry needling, and placebo laser treatments in myofascial pain syndrome. *Photomed Laser Surg* 2004;22:306–311.

Jaeger B, Reeves JL. Quantification of changes in myofascial trigger point sensitivity with the pressure algometer following passive stretch. *Pain* 1986;27:203–210.

Jones LN. *Strain and Counter-strain*. Newark, OH: American Academy of Osteopathy; 1981.

Kuan TS, Hong CZ, Chen JT, et al. The spinal cord connections of the myofascial trigger spots. *Eur J Pain* 2007;11:624–634.

Lewit K. *Manipulative Therapy in Rehabilitation of the Locomotor System*. 3rd ed. Oxford, UK: Butterworth Heinemann; 1999.

Lucas KR, Polus BI, Rich P. Latent myofascial trigger points: their effects on muscle activation and movement efficiency. *J Bodyw Mov Ther* 2004;8:160–166.

McPartland J. Expression of the endocannabinoid system in fibroblasts and myofascial tissues. *J Bodyw Mov Ther* 2008;12:169–182.

Mense S, Gerwin R. *Muscle Pain: Understanding the Mechanisms*. Berlin: Springer-Verlag; 2010.

Nagrale A, Glynn P, Joshi A, Ramteke G. Efficacy of an integrated neuromuscular inhibition technique on upper trapezius trigger points in subjects with non-specific neck pain: a randomized controlled trial. *J Man Manipul Ther* 2010;18:38–44.

Niddam DM, Chan RC, Lee SH, et al. Central modulation of pain evoked from myofascial trigger point. *Clin J Pain* 2007;23:440–448.

O'Callaghan JP, Miller DB. Spinal glia and chronic pain. *Metabolism* 2010;59(suppl 1):S21–S26.

Roth JK, Roth RS, Weintraub JR, Simons DG. Cervicogenic headache caused by myofascial trigger points in the sternocleidomastoid muscle: a case report. *Cephalalgia* 2007;27:375–380.

Shah JP, Phillips TM, Danoff JV, Gerber LH. An in vitro microanalytical technique for measuring the local biochemical milieu of human skeletal muscle. *J Appl Physiol* 2005;99:1977–1984.

Shah JP, Danoff JV, Desai MJ, et al. Biochemicals associated with pain and inflammation are elevated in sites near to and remote from active myofascial trigger points. *Arch Phys Med Rehabil* 2008;89:16–23.

Simons DG. Understanding effective treatments of myofascial trigger points. *J Bodywork Mov Ther* 2002;6:81–88.

Simons DG, Travell JG, Simons LS. *Myofascial Pain and Dysfunction: The Trigger Point Manual*. Vol. 1, 2nd ed. Baltimore: Williams & Wilkins; 1999:69–78.

Sikdar S, Shah JP, Gilliams E, et al. Novel applications of ultrasound technology to visualize and characterize myofascial trigger points and surrounding soft tissue. *Arch Phys Med Rehabil* 2009;90:1829–1838.

Sluka KA, Winter OC, Wemmie JA. Acid-sensing ion channels: a new target for pain and CNS diseases. *Curr Opin Drug Discov Devel* 2009;12:693–704.

Tfelt-Hanson P, Lous I, Olesen J. Prevalence and significance of muscle tenderness during common migraine attacks. *Headache* 1981;21:49–54.

Vernon H, Schneider M. Chiropractic management of myofascial trigger points and myofascial pain syndrome: a systematic review of the literature. *J Manipulative Physiol Ther* 2009;32:14–24.

Wang YH, Ding XL, Zhang Y, et al. Ischemic compression block attenuates mechanical hyperalgesia evoked from latent myofascial trigger points. *Exp Brain Res* 2010;202:265–270.

Xu YM, Ge HY, Arendt-Nielsen L. Sustained nociceptive mechanical stimulation of latent myofascial trigger point induces central sensitization in healthy subjects. *J Pain* 2010;11:1348–1355.

Zhang Y, Ge HY, Yue SW, et al. Attenuated skin blood flow response to nociceptive stimulation of latent myofascial trigger points. *Arch Phys Med Rehabil* 2009;90:325–332.

CHAPTER
16

Muscle Energy Techniques

Gary Fryer, PhD, BSc, ND

INTRODUCTION

Muscle energy technique (MET) is a manual procedure involving the voluntary contraction of skeletal muscle against the controlled resistance of the practitioner (Mitchell & Mitchell, 1995; Greenman, 2003). MET has been claimed to be useful for lengthening a shortened muscle, mobilizing an articulation with restricted mobility, strengthening a physiologically weakened muscle, and reducing localized edema and passive congestion (Mitchell et al., 1979; Bourdillon et al., 1992; Mitchell & Mitchell, 1995; Ehrenfeuchter & Sandhouse, 2003; Chaitow, 2006). This technique can be applied to address dysfunctions of myofascial tissues as well as dysfunctions of the spinal unit and peripheral joints.

Although resisted muscle effort to mobilize the spine has been documented in the osteopathic profession since the early twentieth century (Swart, 1919), MET was developed by osteopathic physician Fred Mitchell, Sr., during the 1950s. The approach was systemized and further developed by Fred Mitchell, Jr., and it has continued to evolve with contributions from many authors. MET was developed through clinical observation and innovation, and was based on a rationale that was consistent with existing knowledge of the time. The evidence underpinning both the biomechanical model on which many of the techniques were based and the rationale for therapeutic action has become dated, however, and alternative approaches and explanations for therapeutic effect have since been offered (Fryer, 2009, 2011).

Although different approaches to the application of MET are possible, post-isometric relaxation (or "contract–relax") is the most widely advocated technique. This technique involves the accurate localization of forces to the joint or muscle barrier (by stretching the shortened tissue), using an isometric contraction (3 to 7 seconds) of the stretched muscle against an unyielding counterforce supplied by the clinician. This contraction is followed by relaxation of the muscle and careful engagement of the new barrier to "take up the slack." Typically, three to five repetitions of the procedure are required (Mitchell et al., 1979; Bourdillon et al., 1992; Mitchell & Mitchell, 1995; Ehrenfeuchter & Sandhouse, 2003; Chaitow, 2006).

Similarities exist between MET and other forms of post-isometric stretching, at least for lengthening the muscles. The most common forms of post-isometric stretching referred to in the research literature are variations of proprioceptive neuromuscular facilitation (PNF) techniques, and include contract–relax (CR; Wallin et al., 1985; Handel et al., 1997; Spernoga et al., 2001), in which the muscle being stretched is contracted, relaxed, and then further stretched; agonist contract–relax (ACR; Osternig et al., 1990; Ferber et al., 2002), in which contraction of the agonist (rather than the muscle being stretched) actively moves the joint through the restrictive barrier for increased range and extensibility; and contract–relax agonist–contract (CRAC; Etnyre & Abraham, 1986; Godges et al., 2003), which is a combination of the CR and ACR methods. Other than when applied to facilitate muscle stretch, the two treatment procedures—MET and PNF—have different approaches and goals. MET was developed to address pelvic, intervertebral, or peripheral joint dysfunction according to biomechanical principles, whereas PNF emphasizes the need to improve rotational trunk stability and generally uses stronger contraction forces (Chaitow, 2006).

Evidence for Effectiveness of Muscle Energy Techniques

No studies for the treatment of migraine using MET exist in the peer-reviewed literature. The primary rationale for using MET for this pain condition is its ability to eliminate cervical triggers of migraine (such as muscle and joint dysfunctions, which are sources of nociceptive pain). In this respect, the rationale for treatment is the same as for other manual techniques, including spinal manipulation/mobilization, which have received more research attention and for which evidence of potential effectiveness for headaches, including migraine, has been reported (Bronfort et al., 2004, 2010). The rationale for the use of MET is also based on evidence (albeit limited) of its effectiveness for improving spinal range of motion, decreasing spinal pain, improving proprioception, and increasing the extensibility of myofascial tissues (Fryer, 2011).

Like many manual therapeutic approaches, the efficacy and effectiveness of MET are as yet under-researched,

and little evidence is available to guide practitioners in the choice of the most useful technique variations (such as the preferred number of repetitions, strength of contraction, or duration of stretch phase), causing frustration for those trying to integrate relevant evidence into practice. MET is commonly used as part of an individualized treatment approach involving different manual therapy techniques, but little evidence supports the clinical effectiveness of this technique when it is used as the primary approach for treatment of patient conditions. As a consequence, inclusion of MET in the therapeutic regimen for migraine is largely based on a theoretical physiological rationale and anecdotal evidence, although a small but growing pool of evidence provides at least preliminary support for its efficacy and effectiveness in this condition (Fryer, 2009, 2011).

Only a few controlled trials have examined MET as the primary technique for the treatment of acute low back pain (LBP) using clinical outcomes (Wilson et al., 2003; Salvador et al., 2005; Selkow et al., 2009). These studies reported decreased pain following treatment with MET, but each study involved relatively small numbers of subjects, and two of the studies (Salvador et al., 2005; Selkow et al., 2009) applied MET only to lengthen hip musculature. In their study, Wilson et al. (2003) assigned 19 patients with acute LBP who had been diagnosed with a segmental lumbar dysfunction to either a MET group or a control group. The MET group received a specific MET for their diagnosed dysfunction, a home exercise program that included a MET self-treatment component, abdominal "drawing in," and progressive strengthening exercises. The control group received a sham treatment and the same home exercise program. Those patients treated with MET showed a significant improvement in Oswestry Disability Index scores relative to the control patients (mean change of 83% for MET versus 65% for controls), and every patient treated with MET had a greater improvement than those in the control group.

The lack of clinically relevant research is not surprising given that MET is typically used in conjunction with other techniques. Several clinical trials investigating osteopathic management have included MET as a treatment component for the management of headaches and neck pain (Fryer et al., 2005; Anderson & Seniscal, 2006; Schwerla et al., 2008) and for LBP (Licciardone et al., 2003, 2010). These studies have reported significantly reduced pain and disability, lending further plausibility to the effectiveness of muscle energy, at least as part of a more comprehensive treatment package.

Although research into MET as the primary treatment involving clinical outcomes is scarce, evidence (drawn largely from studies examining similar PNF techniques) supports the rationale of using MET for treating patients with reduced mobility of the spine and for increasing the extensibility of muscles. Little research has investigated the effect of MET on the muscles of the cervical region, but inferences may be drawn from the considerable body of research examining post-isometric stretching techniques for the extensibility of other muscles, primarily the hamstring muscle group. MET and PNF stretching methods have been shown to bring about greater improvements in joint range of motion and muscle extensibility compared to passive, static stretching, both in the short term and in the long term (Sady et al., 1982; Wallin et al., 1985; Osternig et al., 1990; Magnusson et al., 1996b; Feland et al., 2001; Ferber et al., 2002; Ballantyne et al., 2003). Because of differences in the study designs and measurement methods, it is difficult to pinpoint the most efficacious elements of the various treatment protocols. Nevertheless, it appears that ACR and CRAC methods are more effective for increasing range of motion than CR methods when applied to the hamstring muscles. However, caution must be exercised when attempting to generalize these results from the hamstring muscles to treatment of the cervical musculature, because the neck and shoulder muscles are smaller, less fibrous, and likely to be painful in patients with neck and head pain.

Many authors in the field of MET have emphasized its utility for treating spinal dysfunction (Mitchell et al., 1979; Bourdillon et al., 1992; Mitchell & Mitchell, 1995; Ehrenfeuchter & Sandhouse, 2003; Greenman, 2003; DiGiovanna et al., 2005), and a small number of studies have examined range of motion in the spine following treatment. Schenk et al. (1994) found that MET treatment of asymptomatic subjects with limitations of active motion (10° or more) over a 4-week period achieved significant gains in rotation (approximately 8°), whereas a control group showed little change. Fryer and Ruszkowski (2004) found that MET using a 5-second isometric contraction produced a significantly greater increase in the restricted direction of cervical rotation in volunteers who displayed at least 4° of asymmetry in active atlanto-axial (C1–C2) rotation, compared to a sham-treatment group. The increase in range of motion did not come at the expense of the unrestricted direction, which also demonstrated small mean increases. MET with a 20-second isometric contraction also induced increased range of motion, but appeared to be less effective than the 5-second contraction. Similarly, Burns and Wells (2006) found an immediate increase in active rotation, lateral bending, and overall range of cervical motion (approximately 4°) following the application of MET, compared to a control sham procedure, in an asymptomatic group with multiplanar motion restrictions.

Evidence Recommendation

Although evidence exists to support the use of MET for increasing spinal range of motion and improving pain and disability, this evidence is generally weak on a number of grounds, including methodology, subject numbers, and generalizability to the clinical situation. Further investigation of this approach is needed, including research into the duration of effect and the clinical benefit for symptomatic individuals. Given that no study has examined the treatment of migraine using MET as the primary approach, the evidence level may, therefore, be considered Level 0 (no evidence) (Van Kleef et al., 2009). Nevertheless, evidence showing benefit with low risk when MET is used as a treatment for LBP does exist (Wilson et al., 2003; Salvador et al., 2005; Selkow et al., 2009); moreover, if MET is considered as part of a treatment package (as would usually be the case in practice), there is evidence of its benefit for headaches and neck pain (Fryer et al., 2005; Anderson & Seniscal, 2006; Schwerla et al., 2008) and for LBP (Licciardone et al., 2003, 2010) that may be considered as Level 1B+ evidence. Further research regarding the effectiveness of MET in clinical conditions is needed, but there is sound rationale for this technique's inclusion in a multimodal approach for the treatment of migraines.

Therapeutic Mechanisms

Although the mechanisms by which MET may produce therapeutic benefit are largely speculative, this therapy may have neurologic and biomechanical effects through mechanisms other than those typically described in MET texts (Fryer & Fossum, 2010). Traditionally, MET has been proposed to produce muscle relaxation via Golgi tendon organ and muscle spindle reflexes (Kuchera & Kuchera, 1992; Mitchell & Mitchell, 1995), but this explanation seems unlikely given that studies have reported *increases* in electromyographic activity following post-isometric stretching techniques, rather than decreases (Osternig et al., 1990; Mitchell et al., 2009). MET has also been proposed to reset the neurologic resting length of muscles, but it appears that motor activity does not play a significant role in limiting passive stretch of a muscle, at least in healthy, uninjured subjects (Magnusson et al., 1996a, 1996c).

To produce lasting changes to the extensibility of muscles, MET would likely be required to produce plastic change (micro-tearing and remodeling) to connective tissue elements (Lederman, 2005), but few lasting changes in human muscle properties have been found (Fryer, 2006). Studies measuring pre- and post-force (torque) show little viscoelastic change after passive or isometric stretching; rather, they indicate that the muscle extensibility reflects increased tolerance to an increased stretching force (Magnusson et al, 1996a, 1996c; Ballantyne et al., 2003). Although they represent short- and medium-term applications of stretching, PNF and MET do not appear to affect the biomechanics of healthy muscle, although studies are required to determine whether the same is true for injured and healing muscle tissue.

Increased extensibility of muscles due to an increase in the patient's tolerance to stretching may be a result of a decrease in pain perception (hypoalgesia) following the stimulation of muscle and joint mechanoreceptors, which may activate centrally mediated pathways, such as the periaqueductal gray in the midbrain region and non-opioid serotonergic and noradrenergic descending inhibitory pathways (Souvlis et al., 2004; Fryer & Fossum, 2010). Additionally, MET may produce hypoalgesia via peripheral mechanisms associated with increased fluid drainage. Rhythmic muscle contraction increases muscle blood and lymph flow rates (Coates et al., 1993; Havas et al., 1997), while mechanical forces (such as tissue loading and stretching) may also affect fibroblast mechanical signal transduction processes (Langevin et al., 2004), by changing the interstitial pressure and increasing transcapillary blood flow (Langevin et al., 2005). Through these processes, MET may assist in clearing high concentrations of pro-inflammatory cytokines in the affected tissues, thereby resulting in decreased sensitization of peripheral nociceptors.

In addition to hypoalgesia, MET may work in the neurologic sphere to enhance proprioception and motor control in patients with pain. Patients with spinal pain have decreased awareness of direction of spinal motion and position (Leinonen et al., 2002; Grip et al., 2007; Lee et al., 2008). In addition, research suggests that high-velocity spinal manipulation improves head repositioning in patients with chronic neck pain (Rogers, 1997; Palmgren et al., 2006). Recently gathered evidence suggests that techniques using isometric muscle contraction may improve proprioception (Malstrom et al., 2010; Ryan et al., 2010). Malstrom et al. (2010) reported that a sustained isometric lateral flexion neck muscle contraction (30% of maximal voluntary contraction) increased accuracy of head repositioning ability by reducing overshoot, particularly in the direction of the activated side. Likewise, improvement in medial-lateral postural stability has been reported following CRAC PNF techniques applied to the hamstring, plantar flexor, and hip flexor muscles in healthy individuals compared to a no treatment group (Ryan et al., 2010). Again, there is need for further research in this area, but the studies carried out to date suggest that muscle energy may enhance proprioception, which may potentially improve motor control and stability in the neck.

Principles of Treatment Application

The principles of MET application differ depending on whether this technique is applied to large muscles or segmental joint dysfunctions; these principles are described in more detail in this section. In essence, the aims when applying MET to a muscle are threefold: to lengthen the muscle, to decrease pain, and to deactivate muscle trigger points (TrPs). When MET is applied to spinal joint dysfunctions, the primary goals are to improve range and quality of joint motion, to reduce pain and tenderness, and to improve the palpable tone of the surrounding soft tissues.

The force and duration of isometric contraction during MET can vary, as can the force and the duration of stretch, depending on the tissues targeted. In general, a gentle force of contraction is recommended for MET directed at spinal segments and for muscles containing TrPs, so as to selectively recruit the local segmental muscles or irritable TrP fibers. More moderate stretching and contraction forces are recommended for increasing the extensibility of shortened, painless, and fibrotic muscles, so as to maximize the post-contraction hypoalgesia and create substantial tension on the connective tissue elements for plastic change (Mitchell & Mitchell, 1995; Fryer, 2006).

An Integrated Approach to Muscle Energy

MET was developed by osteopathic physicians and was intended to be applied in a holistic manner consistent with osteopathic philosophy. Osteopathy emphasizes the unity and interconnectedness of the body, the interrelationship of structure and function, and the important influence that the musculoskeletal system may exert on other systems and general health. Thus the MET approach was based on a specific diagnostic model that emphasized a global view of body biomechanics and included screening global posture, movement patterns, and gross and segmental range of motion (Mitchell et al., 1979). For example, in patients presenting with neck and arm pain, the body would be examined from head to toe (posture, static and dynamic symmetry, active and passive range of motion), and treatment would be directed at any or all of the regions believed to be problematic—lower limb, pelvic, lumbar, thoracic, rib cage, neck, head, or upper extremity. Implicit in this approach are the concepts that dysfunction in one region may cause compensation and strain in other regions and that treatment that addresses only the symptomatic site is likely to achieve only short-term relief. In recent years, the remote effects of a manual intervention have received attention from some researchers, resulting in reports of cervical treatment improving shoulder symptoms and hamstring flexibility (Aparicio et al., 2009; McClatchie et al., 2009), and of thoracic treatment improving neck pain (Cleland et al., 2005; González-Iglesias et al., 2009) and shoulder pain and disability (Boyles et al., 2009).

Assessment and treatment of the thorax—including the spinal joints, ribs, and muscles—are extremely important for patients with neck pain and headaches. Treatment of this region should precede treatment of the neck because (in the author's experience) such therapy often produces changes and improvements in both symptoms and physical findings in the neck and related tissues. Due to limitations of space, techniques for the thorax and other parts of the spine will not be described here. The same principles apply to joints in these regions, however, and techniques will be obvious to readers who understand these principles.

MET may be applied in combination with other manual techniques, such as soft-tissue manipulation, passive joint articulation, high-velocity thrust, and gentle indirect techniques like functional techniques and counter-strain (where tissues are held in a position of ease). There is no universal agreement on the criteria for technique selection for a given condition or patient, and probably practitioner and patient preferences are significant determinants in these areas. Techniques may be selected based on their likely therapeutic mechanisms, despite the speculative nature of those mechanisms. For example, MET may be used where fluid drainage and improved proprioception are desired, high-velocity manipulation may be employed where joint end-feel is particularly hard, end-range articulation may be used where joint motion appears restricted by fibrotic changes in periarticular tissues, and indirect approaches may be applied where significant inflammation and pain are present. The integration of these different techniques may involve intuitive cues from palpation and the pragmatic use of alternative techniques when the initial therapeutic choices fail to achieve the intended tissue and motion changes.

Cautions and Contraindications

MET is a safe technique, and the literature does not include any reports of serious adverse reactions with its use. The cautions and contraindications for MET are common to other soft-tissue techniques, and involve care with stretching force when dealing with acute pain conditions and with forces and leverages in the presence of weakened bone. With MET, very light to moderate applications of stretch or isometric contraction are normally performed; thus this method is perceived to be a safe technique with little risk of serious injury. When applied to previously injured, healing tissues, forces of contraction or stretch should be matched to the stage of healing and repair to avoid further tissue damage and promote optimal healing (Lederman, 2005).

Cerebrovascular accidents following high-velocity manipulation of the cervical spine have been reported as unpredictable rare complications (Di Fabio, 1999; Haldeman et al., 2001). Although no such incidents have been reported for MET, care and caution should still be taken when treating the cervical spine. Fortunately, the leverages advocated for MET applied to the cervical spine are generally subtle and minimal, and the avoidance of end-range rotation and extension leverages may reduce risks posed by MET.

MUSCLE ENERGY TECHNIQUES APPLIED TO THE CERVICAL MUSCLES

MET can be applied to muscles and soft tissues of the cervical region to stretch and lengthen these tissues, to deactivate muscle TrPs, and to improve lymphatic drainage. The main principles for application of MET to myofascial structures include the following concepts:

1. Stretch the involved muscle to its "barrier" (sense of palpated resistance or end range).
2. Apply light stretching force to the initial or "first barrier" if the muscle is acutely painful.
3. Apply moderate stretching force to a comfortable sensation of stretch experienced by the patient if the muscle is only mildly painful or not painful.
4. With isometric contraction of the stretched muscle, ask the patient to gently contract the targeted muscle (push away from the barrier) against your controlled, unyielding resistance for 5 to 7 seconds. A light contraction force should be used if the muscle is painful or contains TrPs. If the muscle is relatively pain-free, a moderate contraction force is permitted.
5. For muscle relaxation purposes, the patient should fully relax for several seconds, with the stretch maintained. A deep inhalation or exhalation may assist relaxation. Chaitow

(2006) recommends maintaining this stretch for as long as 60 seconds in the case of chronically shortened muscles (and then removing the muscle from stretch for a rest period); however, a long period of stretch may be inappropriate for small cervical muscles. A stretch maintained for approximately 10 seconds is generally recommended for neck and shoulder muscles that are judged to be shortened, fibrotic, and unprovoked by stretching, whereas a few seconds' duration is appropriate for tender and painful muscles.

6. Reengage the barrier. The "slack" that has developed in the tissues following the contraction and relaxation phases is "taken up," and usually the muscle can be lengthened to a new barrier without using increased force. This process is repeated two to four times, or until a satisfactory change in length and tissue texture is noted.

7. Reassess following treatment.

This section describes techniques for muscles commonly identified as developing TrPs (Simons et al., 1999) and those susceptible to becoming shortened (Greenman, 2003; Chaitow, 2006; Liebenson, 2007). Not all cervical muscles that are claimed to refer pain to the head are covered here, because some of the smaller muscles are difficult to stretch and are more amenable to other therapeutic techniques (e.g., manual pressure release). Additionally, the pectoral muscles are included in this section because shortness in these muscles may profoundly affect cervical posture and produce strain and irritation in headache-producing structures.

For optimal localization or effectiveness, many of the following stretches require subtle "fine-tuning" for each individual patient. Clinicians are encouraged to experiment with small amounts of additional leverage—flexion, rotation, side-bending, and traction—using palpation of tissue stretch and patient feedback to maximize the localization of the techniques.

The stretching techniques described here should be applied slowly and carefully and with a request for patient feedback. If the patient experiences discomfort or sensation other than a pleasant stretching sensation, cease the procedure immediately and reassess the patient. Additionally, if any of the following signs of vertebrobasilar insufficiency appear, the technique should be ceased and the patient reassessed: vertigo, visual disturbances, dysphagia, dysarthria, hoarseness, facial numbness, paraesthesias, confusion, or syncope (drop attacks) (Gibbons & Tehan, 2006).

Upper Trapezius Muscle

The upper trapezius muscle is reported to be frequently beset by TrPs and is a commonly overlooked source of temporal headaches (Simons et al., 1999; Fernández-de-las-Peñas et al., 2007). The levator scapulae muscle, which is reported to produce local pain in the ipsilateral neck, will also be stretched during the treatment of the trapezius muscle.

Procedure

1. The patient is supine, with arms resting by the sides. The therapist stands at the head of the table.

2. Stabilize the shoulder of the treated side with one hand, and contact the occiput, mastoid region, and upper neck with the other hand (**Figure 16.1**, main photo). If the weight of the patient's head is heavy, support and stabilize your hand using support of your abdomen or chest. Alternatively, use a crossed-arm position, where your hands contact and stabilize both of the patient's shoulders and your crossed arms support the upper neck and head (Figure 16.1, inset photo).

3. Fully flex and side-bend the neck away from the involved side until a sense of tissue resistance is palpated, and the patient reports a pleasant stretching sensation.

4. Addition of cervical rotation may selectively stretch particular fibers. Differing views exist regarding the amount and direction of rotation needed to select specific parts of the muscle. Liebenson (2007) advocates contralateral rotation for stretch of the upper trapezius and ipsilateral rotation for the levator scapulae. Chaitow (2006) suggests full contralateral rotation for the posterior fibers of the trapezius, half-rotation for the middle fibers, and slight ipsilateral rotation for the anterior fibers. Subtle fine-tuning of rotation using palpatory and patient feedback to determine the most effective position for each individual is recommended.

5. Request the patient to gently push the head and neck back against the therapist's controlled, unyielding resistance for 5 to 7 seconds. The direction of patient force can be either in extension or side-bending; however, rotation is not recommended because it is more difficult to control and stabilize. Alternatively, shoulder elevation can be requested and resisted.

6. Allow the patient to relax for a few seconds (or more), maintaining the stretch.

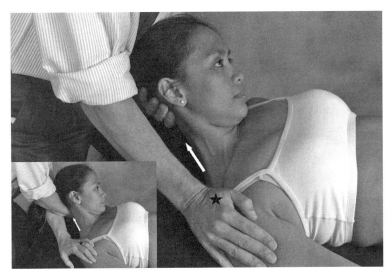

Figure 16.1 MET Applied to the Upper Trapezius and Levator Scapulae Muscles. The primary leverages are cervical flexion and lateral flexion away from the treated side; however, subtle rotation may be introduced to localize particular fibers of the trapezius or levator scapulae muscles (arrow). Note that the shoulder is firmly depressed and stabilized (star). The patient is instructed to gently push his or her head back against the resistance provided by the practitioner, or to elevate the shoulder. An alternative contact can be used with crossed hands (inset photo).

7. Reengage the new barrier by taking up any slack that has developed since the contraction–relaxation phases (the muscle is further lengthened), using shoulder depression.
8. Repeat the procedure two to four times.
9. Reassess the patient after treatment.

Sub-Occipital and Posterior Cervical Muscles

The deep sub-occipital muscles—rectus capitis posterior major and minor and the inferior and superior oblique—have been reported to be a common source of headache (Fernández-de-las-Peñas et al., 2006a), particularly with head pain that is deep and poorly localized that refers from the occiput to the orbit (Simons et al., 1999). The posterior cervical muscles, including the cervical multifidus, semispinalis capitis, longissimus capitis, and the more superficial splenius capitis and cervicis, have all been reported to produce referred pain to the head (Simons et al., 1999). The following stretches should be modified using subtle additions of leverage (flexion, rotation, or side-bending) according to changes in palpated resistance and reports of stretching from the patient so as to localize the stretch to the most involved fibers.

Procedure
1. The patient is supine, arms resting by the sides. The therapist stands at the head of the table.

2. Stabilize the shoulder of the treated side with one hand, and contact the occiput and mastoid region (not the neck) with the other hand. If the weight of the patient's head is heavy, support and stabilize the hand using support of your abdomen or chest (**Figure 16.2**).

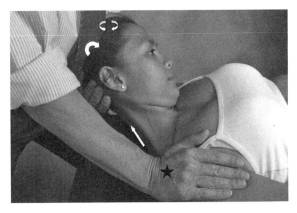

Figure 16.2 MET Applied to the Sub-Occipital and Posterior Cervical Muscles. The neck is flexed and side-bent away from the treated side. The shoulder is firmly depressed and stabilized (star), and then subtle occipital traction and flexion should be introduced to localize the stretch the sub-occipital muscles (arrow). Further modification using occipital rotation and side-bending can be based on palpatory and patient feedback to optimize localization of the stretch (arrows). The patient is instructed to look up at the ceiling and gently press his or her head back against the resistance provided by the clinician.

3. Fully flex the patient's neck, and then side-bend it away from the treated side until a sense of resistance is palpated.

4. Introduce subtle occipital flexion and traction until a sense of resistance is palpated and the patient reports a pleasant stretching sensation in the sub-occipital region. Subtle addition of rotation and side-bending can be made according to changes in palpated resistance and sensation of stretching from the patient so as to localize the stretch to the most involved fibers.

5. Request the patient to look up at the ceiling and gently push the head back against the resistance of the practitioner for 5 to 7 seconds.

6. Allow the patient to relax for a few seconds.

7. Reengage the new barrier by taking up any slack that has developed since the contraction and re-laxation phases (the muscle is further lengthened).

8. Repeat the procedure two to four times.

9. Reassess the patient after treatment.

A variation of this technique that may be more specific to the sub-occipital muscles is as follows (**Figure 16.3**):

1. The patient is supine, arms resting by the sides. The therapist stands at the head of the table.

2. Contact the occiput with the first finger and medial hand, and rest the other hand over the frontal region of the patient's head.

3. Flex the head on the neutral neck using a combination of cephalic traction with the lower hand and caudal pressure with the upper hand until a pleasant stretch is perceived. Subtle addition

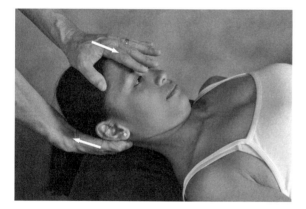

Figure 16.3 MET Applied to the Sub-Occipital Muscles. The neck is in neutral position, and the clinician introduces occipital traction and head flexion (arrows) until resistance or a barrier is palpated. The patient is instructed to nod the head upward against the resistance provided by the practitioner.

of rotation and side-bending can be made as required.

4. Request the patient to nod the head upward against the offered resistance for 5 to 7 seconds.

5. Allow the patient to relax for a few seconds.

6. Reengage the new barrier by taking up any slack that has developed since the contraction and relaxation phases (the muscle is further lengthened).

7. Repeat the procedure two to four times.

8. Reassess the patient after treatment.

Sternocleidomastoid Muscle

The sternocleidomastoid (SCM) muscle has been cited as a frequent cause of atypical facial neuralgia and tension headache (Simons et al., 1999; Fernández-de-las-Peñas et al., 2006b). Referred muscle pain from the sternal division may extend to the vertex, cheek, eye, and throat, whereas referred pain from the clavicular division typically produces frontal headache or earache. The SCM muscle requires careful positioning when treated with MET, because of the potential for strain of related structures—particularly the upper cervical spine—when positioning the patient for an effective stretch. The clavicular division is more amenable to MET stretching than the sternal division, but care is needed to avoid excessive cervical extension and patient discomfort. In the techniques described here, the anterior neck fascia and muscles, such as the digastric and anterior scalene, may also be lengthened, which may contribute to the effectiveness of the techniques.

Upper cervical extension should be avoided or minimized because it can be uncomfortable for the patient, and potentially may irritate the cervical zygapophyseal joints and compress the vertebral artery. The cervical extension required for this technique is minimal, should always be comfortable for the patient, and should be discontinued in the event of any discomfort or signs of vertebrobasilar insufficiency (see above).

The SCM muscle can be treated with MET with the patient either sitting or prone.

Procedure: Seated Patient

1. The patient sits on a low bench or stool. The therapist stands behind the patient.

2. Place your forearm on or under the patient's clavicle on the involved side. It is important that you anchor your hand or forearm into the region by applying a compressive and downward force to take up tissue slack. Inadequate "locking" of

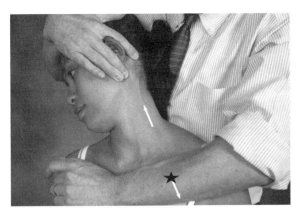

Figure 16.4 MET Applied to the Sternocleidomastoid Muscle (Clavicular Division). The clavicular head and the anterior fascia of the neck can be stretched with the patient sitting by firmly anchoring the fascia around the clavicle (star) and applying the leverages of cervical side-bending, rotation, slight extension, and traction (arrows). The patient is asked to gently push his or her head forward against the resistance of the clinician.

the tissues will result in the need for more cervical leverage to achieve a stretch.

3. Contact both the mastoid process and the anterior ear region with the fingers of one hand. Introduce a small amount of neck rotation and side-bending away from the treated side, with *slight* neck extension (avoid upper neck extension, which will produce a stretching sensation in the suprahyoid region) and slight traction (**Figure 16.4**). The "anchoring" of the clavicular tissues should be maintained during this movement. The patient should report a pleasant stretching sensation over the region of the SCM.
4. Request the patient to push the head forward against your resistance for 5 to 7 seconds.
5. Allow the patient to relax for a few seconds.
6. Reengage the new barrier by taking up any slack that has developed since the contraction and relaxation phases (the muscle is further lengthened) by using traction, side-bending, or slight extension.
7. Repeat the procedure two to four times.
8. Reassess the patient after treatment.

Procedure: Supine Patient

1. The patient is supine, without a pillow, arms resting by the sides. A small folded towel can be placed under the thoracic region (not the shoulders) to accentuate slight cervical extension. The therapist stands at the head of the table.

2. Place your hand on or under the patient's clavicle on the involved side (a small folded towel under the hand may improve patient comfort). It is important that a compressive and downward force is applied to take up tissue slack.
3. Contact the mastoid process and anterior ear region with the fingers, and introduce a small amount of neck rotation and side-bending away from the treated side (**Figure 16.5**). Keep the head in neutral or slight flexion, but avoid head extension. The "anchoring" of the clavicular tissues should be maintained during this movement. The patient should report a pleasant stretching sensation over the region of the SCM.
4. Request the patient to lift the head forward against your resistance for 5 to 7 seconds.
5. Allow the patient to relax for a few seconds.
6. Reengage the new barrier by taking up any slack that has developed since the contraction and relaxation phases (the muscle is further lengthened).
7. Repeat the procedure two to four times.
8. Reassess the patient after treatment.

The sternal division of the SCM is more difficult to stretch than the clavicular division, and direct massage and myofascial release techniques are often more suitable for this region. Although a stretch using ipsilateral rotation would seem logical according to the action of this muscle, such leverages are rarely effective.

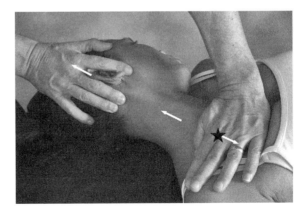

Figure 16.5 MET Applied to the Sternocleidomastoid Muscle. The clavicular head and the anterior fascia of the neck can be stretched with the patient supine by firmly anchoring the fascia around the clavicle (star) and applying the leverages of cervical side-bending, rotation, slight extension, and traction (arrows). The patient is asked to gently lift his or her head from the table against the resistance provided by the practitioner.

Procedure: Sternal Division

1. The patient sits on a low bench or stool. The therapist stands behind the patient.
2. Place your forearm on or under the patient's clavicle on the involved side. It is important that you "anchor" your forearm by applying a compressive and downward force to take up tissue slack. Inadequate "locking" of the tissues will result in the need for more cervical leverage to achieve a stretch.
3. Contact the mastoid process and anterior ear region with the fingers of your hand, and introduce a small amount of neck rotation to the side of the treated muscle (**Figure 16.6**). Following this manipulation, introduce posterior translation of the chin and head (avoid upper cervical extension), followed by side-bending to the *opposite side* and slight extension. "Anchoring" of the clavicular tissues should be maintained during this movement. The patient should report a pleasant stretching sensation over the region of the sternal head of the SCM.
4. Request the patient to push the head forward against your resistance for 5 to 7 seconds.
5. Allow the patient to relax for a few seconds.
6. Reengage the new barrier by taking up any slack that has developed since the contraction

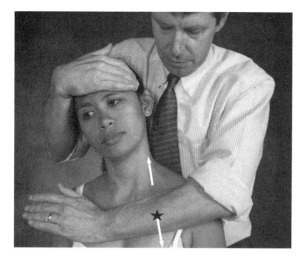

Figure 16.6 MET Applied to the Sternocleidomastoid Muscle (Sternal Division). The sternal head can be stretched by anchoring the tissues around the medial clavicle and sternum (star) and introducing a small amount of neck rotation to the side of the treated muscle, followed by side-bending to the opposite side and slight extension (arrows). The patient is requested to gently push his or her head forward against the resistance of the clinician.

and relaxation phases (the muscle is further lengthened).
7. Repeat the procedure two to four times.
8. Reassess the patient after treatment.

Scalene Muscles

The scalene muscles (anterior, middle, and posterior) are reported to be a commonly overlooked source of back, shoulder, and arm pain, and TrPs in these muscles are claimed to contribute to many patients' symptoms related to cervicogenic headache (Simons et al., 1999). Opinions differ on the degree and direction of rotation required for the stretch of the scalene muscles. Chaitow (2006) recommended slight rotation to the opposite side as a means to localize the anterior scalene, 45% of rotation for the middle scalene, and full rotation for the posterior scalene. Gerwin (2005) advocated ipsilateral rotation, whereas Liebenson (2007) recommended rotation to the involved side for the anterior fibers, no rotation for the middle fibers, and rotation to the opposite direction for the posterior fibers. Experimentation using palpatory and patient feedback is recommended.

Procedure

1. The patient is supine, arms resting by the sides. The therapist stands at the head of the table.
2. Contact the mastoid, lateral occiput, and upper cervical pillars to stabilize the neck and prevent excessive upper cervical lateral flexion. Place your other hand over the patient's shoulder and lateral clavicle region for stabilization. Alternatively, your hand can be placed over the patient's hand with the thenar eminence below the medial clavicle to stabilize the first and second ribs.
3. Place the patient's neck in slight extension (remove pillow), laterally flex the neck away from the treated side, and introduce slight rotation (**Figure 16.7**). Experiment with varying degrees of rotation to find the most effective stretch.
4. Request the patient to gently laterally flex the head against your resistance for 5 to 7 seconds.
5. Allow the patient to relax for a few seconds. A deep inhalation and exhalation may assist with relaxing the scalene muscles.
6. Reengage the new barrier by taking up any slack that has developed since the contraction and relaxation phases (the muscle is further lengthened).
7. Repeat the procedure two to four times.
8. Reassess the patient after treatment.

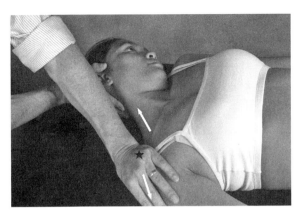

Figure 16.7 MET Applied to the Scalene Muscles. The scalene muscles can be stretched using slight cervical extension (no pillow, hand fixing on the shoulder or first or second ribs [star and arrow]), contralateral lateral flexion, and varying amounts of rotation (arrow). Cervical rotation may be varied so as to stretch different fibers. The patient is instructed to gently laterally flex his or her head and neck against the resistance of the practitioner.

Pectoralis Major Muscle

Although TrPs in the pectoralis major typically refer pain to the chest and arm (Simons et al., 1999), shortened muscles can produce a round-shouldered, head-forward posture that may lead to ongoing strain of the cervical tissues and further contribute to cervicogenic headaches.

The technique described here is not suitable for any patient with an unstable shoulder joint, previous shoulder injury, or limited shoulder movement due to pain. Do not use external rotation as the primary leverage, as this approach will frequently cause pain and discomfort, even in the healthy shoulder joint.

Procedure

1. The patient is supine, arms resting by the sides. The therapist stands at the side of the table, on the side to be treated.
2. Abduct the patient's shoulder to 90° and place it in comfortable external rotation. The amount of arm abduction can be varied to select particular fibers, with decreased abduction (less than 90°) tending to localize the clavicular fibers and increased abduction (more than 90°) localizing the sternal fibers.
3. Anchor the tissues by placing your hand or forearm over the patient's sternum using a light compressive and lateral force away from the treated side. Pre-tension on the fascia will help minimize the amount of leverage necessary on the shoulder.

4. Grasp the patient's arm close to the elbow.
5. Gently apply horizontal extension and traction (down the length of the humerus) to the shoulder, while maintaining the anchoring pressure near the sternum (**Figure 16.8**). The patient should experience a pleasant stretching sensation through the pectoral region. The addition of traction frequently produces a much more effective stretch and will minimize the amount of leverage required on the shoulder.
6. Request the patient to gently push the arm toward the ceiling for 5 to 7 seconds against your resistance. Ensure you are positioned so your applicator arm is straight, and the isometric force is easily resisted against your body weight.
7. Allow the patient to relax for a few seconds.
8. Reengage the new barrier by taking up any slack that has developed since the contraction and relaxation phases (the muscle is further lengthened) by gently increasing the horizontal extension.
9. Repeat the procedure two to four times.
10. Reassess the patient after treatment.

Pectoralis Minor Muscle

The pectoralis minor muscle may refer pain to the anterior deltoid region or the ulnar side of the arm, hand, and fingers, and may entrap the axillary artery and brachial plexus in a manner that mimics cervical radiculopathy (Simons et al., 1999). Like the pectoralis major muscle,

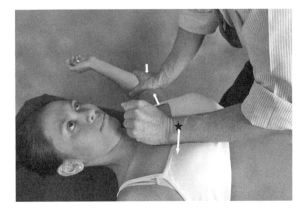

Figure 16.8 MET Applied to the Pectoralis Major Muscle. The pectoralis major muscle is stretched by anchoring the fascia around the chest and sternum (star) and slowly introducing shoulder horizontal extension with traction (arrows). The patient is instructed to gently push his or her arm toward the ceiling against the resistance of the clinician.

a shortened pectoralis minor muscle affects posture through round shoulders and forward head posture, which may contribute to the production of headaches. Several variations for the application of MET to shortened pectoralis minor muscles exist.

Procedure 1

1. The patient is supine, close to the edge of the table so that the involved shoulder slightly overhangs the table. The involved arm hangs comfortably over the edge. The therapist stands at the side of the table on the involved side.
2. Rest your hand or forearm on either the sternum or upper chest, and apply a compressive and lateral force to take up tissue slack in the direction away from the involved muscle.
3. Cup your hand over the patient's anterior shoulder and slowly apply a force in a posterior and lateral direction with a straight arm (the table should be low), while maintaining a firm anchor on the pectoral tissues (Figure 16.9, main photo). A small towel can be folded and placed on the patient's anterior shoulder to cushion the practitioner's hand if the patient experiences discomfort from the pressure. The patient should perceive a pleasant stretching sensation in the pectoral region.

4. The patient is requested to gently push the shoulder in an anterior direction toward the ceiling for 5 to 7 seconds.
5. Allow the patient to relax for a few seconds.
6. Reengage the new barrier by taking up any slack that has developed since the contraction and relaxation phases (the muscle is further lengthened) by gently increasing the posterior and lateral pressure on the shoulder.
7. Repeat the procedure two to four times.
8. Reassess the patient after treatment.

An alternative application for the pectoralis minor muscle that incorporates a modified myofascial release technique is as follows (Figure 16.9, inset photo):

1. The patient is supine, with elbows bent and hands resting on the abdomen (or under the small of the back if the arms tend to move during the treatment). The therapist stands at the side of the table, on the side to be treated. The patient should be warned that the technique may cause discomfort and will be discontinued if discomfort becomes substantial.
2. Slide one hand, with the fingertips together and extended, under the patient's anterior axillary fold. Slowly move medially and superiorly toward the direction of the sternal notch (under

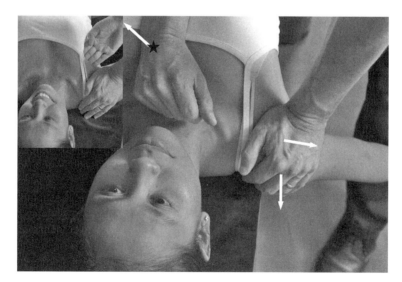

Figure 16.9 MET Applied to the Pectoralis Minor Muscle. The chest and pectoral tissues are anchored by the hand or forearm (star), a posterior and lateral pressure is introduced to the shoulder (arrows), and the patient is instructed to push the shoulder toward the ceiling against the practitioner's resistance (main photo). In an alternative technique (inset photo), the hand and extended fingertips are introduced under the anterior axillary fold and directed medially and superiorly until tissue resistance is palpated. A posterior and lateral pressure is introduced to the shoulder, and the patient is instructed to push the shoulder toward the ceiling against the practitioner's resistance.

the pectoralis major and lateral edge of pectoralis minor) until tissue resistance is palpated.

3. Using your other hand, cup the anterior shoulder and exert a posterior and lateral force (a small folded towel may be placed under the hand), while maintaining the pressure under the axillary fold. The table should be low enough to allow your arm to be straight and resist the contraction force using your body weight.

4. Request the patient to gently push the shoulder in an anterior direction toward the ceiling against the resistance of your hand for 5 to 7 seconds.

5. Allow the patient to relax for a few seconds.

6. Reengage the new barrier by taking up any slack that has developed since the contraction and relaxation phases (the muscle is further lengthened) by gently increasing the posterior and lateral pressure on the shoulder.

7. Repeat the procedure two to four times.

8. Reassess the patient after treatment.

MUSCLE ENERGY TECHNIQUES APPLIED TO THE CERVICAL JOINTS

Although MET can be directed to myofascial structures, the vast majority of descriptions in MET texts relate to its use for intervertebral and pelvic dysfunctions, indicating that MET is considered a "manipulative" procedure as much as a "soft-tissue" technique. MET is offered as a gentle alterative to high-velocity, low-amplitude thrust techniques, and procedures have been described to address specific biomechanical dysfunctions of the spine and pelvis (Mitchell et al., 1979; Bourdillon et al., 1992; Mitchell & Mitchell, 1995; Ehrenfeuchter & Sandhouse, 2003; Greenman, 2003; DiGiovanna et al., 2005).

The traditional paradigm for the application of MET to the spine is primarily mechanical: precise ranges of joint motion loss are determined, and subtle leverage is applied to engage each restrictive barrier so as to increase the joint motion in all restricted planes (Bourdillon et al., 1992; Mitchell & Mitchell, 1995; Ehrenfeuchter & Sandhouse, 2003; Greenman, 2003; DiGiovanna et al., 2005). This biomechanical paradigm is likely to be overly simplistic, however, and alternative explanations for the therapeutic effect have been reviewed.

Principles of Application to Cervical Intervertebral Joints

The application of MET to the intervertebral joints of the spine differs from application of this technique to large muscles in terms of localization, control, and force.

The basic principles of application for intervertebral segments are as follows:

1. *Localization.* Careful attention is required to accurately engage the restricted barrier to the initial sense of increasing resistance to motion ("first" or "feather edge" of the barrier) at the involved level (Mitchell & Mitchell, 1995). The primary plane of motion restriction should be engaged first, and fine-tuning performed using secondary planes of motion restriction (if detected) or translation. It is essential that the patient should be relaxed, so that active muscle contraction does not help or hinder the engagement of the restrictive barrier.

2. *Contraction and control.* The patient is instructed to actively push—using a *very gentle* force—away from the restrictive barrier, against the practitioner's controlled, unyielding counterforce for 3 to 5 seconds. Too strong a contraction will recruit larger, multisegmental muscles, making it more difficult to maintain accurate localization. The practitioner should give clear instructions to the patient, and should be relaxed and well balanced to facilitate patient relaxation.

3. *Relaxation.* The patient should be allowed to relax fully for several seconds.

4. *Reengage the barrier.* Usually the restrictive barrier is perceived to diminish, and the practitioner should "take up the slack" to reengage this barrier.

5. *Repetition.* The procedure is typically performed three to five times.

6. *Reassess.* The practitioner should determine whether the procedure has changed the clinical findings.

Some authors have recommended different durations of isometric contraction for cervical MET, ranging from 2–3 seconds (Mitchell & Mitchell, 1995) to 3–5 seconds (Greenman, 2003; DiGiovanna et al., 2005) to 5–7 seconds (Chaitow, 2006). The research literature provides little guidance as to the most effective application. In the only study found that examined contraction duration of MET applied to the cervical spine, no additional benefits were conferred by use of a 20-second contraction compared to a 5-second contraction (Fryer & Ruszkowski, 2004). The author recommends a 3- to 5-second contraction when MET is applied to spinal joints, whereas a 5- to 7-second contraction is recommended when this technique is applied to larger muscles, as a longer contraction may promote more viscoelastic changes in these structures.

Spinal Coupled Motion

The MET approach for segmental somatic dysfunction has traditionally been based on the biomechanical principles of spinal coupled motion proposed by Harrison Fryette (1954) and the pelvic biomechanical model developed by Mitchell (1958). Coupled motion—the involuntary segmental coupling of one plane of motion with another—has been attributed to a combination of anatomic joint plane, ligamentous tension, and intervertebral disc mechanics. Fryette's model described neutral coupled motion (Type 1), in which lateral flexion in one direction is accompanied by rotation to the opposite direction, and non-neutral coupled motion (Type 2, named because the motion occurred if the segment was hyperflexed or hyperextended), in which lateral flexion and rotation are coupled to the same side. According to this model, only three combinations of multiple-plane motion restrictions are possible: neutral Type 1 dysfunctions (restriction of lateral flexion and rotation to opposite sides) and two non-neutral Type 2 dysfunctions—ERS dysfunction ("extended" segment, being a motion restriction of flexion, side-bending, and rotation to the same side, due possibly to a facet that resists flexion) or FRS dysfunction ("flexed" segment, being a motion restriction of extension, side-bending, and rotation to the opposite side, due possibly to a facet that resists extension).

Further, the Fryette model has been used as a predictive diagnostic model, through which restricted coupled motions are predicted based on apparent neutral or non-neutral spinal posture or involvement of flexion/extension restriction; clinical decisions (specific techniques) are then based on these predictions. This model has been criticized on two bases, however: for its prescriptive diagnostic labeling and for making invalid inferences from static positional assessment (Gibbons & Tehan, 1998; Fryer, 2000). Authors of MET texts commonly advocate the assessment of static positional asymmetry (spinal transverse process or sacral base), and the comparison of such asymmetry with the spine in different positions (neutral, flexion, extension). Based on these findings, inferences are made concerning specific motion restriction combinations, and specific MET applications are generally advocated. For treatment, motion restrictions according to this model will either be coupled in a Type 1 pattern (not involving flexion or extension) or follow a Type 2 pattern (involving either flexion/extension), with no possibility of other combinations (for example, Type 1 with extension). Therefore, no descriptions of techniques for these combinations are found in MET texts.

Assessment of segmental static asymmetry has been advocated to detect segmental rotation and coupled

motion. This assessment has not proved to be reliable (Spring et al., 2001), however, and spinal coupled motion appears to be inconsistent in the lumbar and thoracic regions, with variability between spinal levels and between individuals (Legaspi & Edmond, 2007; Sizer et al., 2007). Legaspi and Edmond (2007) found little agreement on the existence or type of coupled motion and concluded that physical therapists should not rely on presumed coupling for evaluation or treatment. Similarly, Sizer et al. (2007) failed to find any evidence of consistent patterns of motion coupling in the thoracic spine, but concluded that more quality studies are required to confirm spinal coupling patterns in flexed and extended postures.

Cervical spinal kinematics are complex. In addition to coupled rotation and lateral flexion, coupled motions include flexion, extension, and translation. Coupled motion in the typical cervical spine (C2–C7) is claimed to occur only as Type 2 motion in MET texts. Consistent ipsilateral side-bending and rotation have been observed in some studies (Cook et al., 2006; Ishii et al., 2006), whereas other studies have suggested that the amount and direction of these movements may vary, being influenced by gender, age, and cervical posture (Edmondston et al., 2005; Malmstrom et al., 2006). In the upper cervical region, coupled motion appears to be consistent, with opposite side-bending and rotation occurring at the occipito-atlantal and atlanto-axial joints, and coupled extension observed to consistently occur with rotation (Ishii et al., 2004).

Given the variability and complexity of coupled motions in the cervical spine, practitioners are advised to be guided by the motion restrictions that present on palpation (despite the issues of reliability of motion palpation), rather than to administer treatment based on an expectation of what "should be" according to any biomechanical model. In addition, regardless of whether spinal segmental coupling is consistent or variable between individuals, when the primary motion is introduced by the practitioner performing MET, spinal coupling (in whatever direction is normal for that individual) will occur automatically—due to the very nature of conjunct motion—and without the need for its conscious introduction by the practitioner. The pragmatic approach is, therefore, to address the key range(s) of motion restriction; coupled motion will occur without the aid of the practitioner.

Middle and Lower Cervical Spine (C2–C7)

Lateral translation is commonly advocated as the initial diagnostic procedure to identify motion restriction in the cervical spine. It is most analogous to the primary motion of lateral flexion, and side-bending activation force is easily controlled by the practitioner. Many authors recommend introducing either cervical flexion or extension first, and then localizing the lateral flexion (depending on whether lateral translation is most restricted in either of these positions during assessment). This order of motion introduction is easily controlled and localized. Although MET texts traditionally describe only Type 2 multiplanar restrictions (ERS and FRS dysfunctions), procedures may be adapted and applied for restrictions in either a single plane (side-bending, rotation, flexion, or extension) or multiple planes, depending on the individual clinical findings.

Procedure for Restriction of Flexion, Side-Bending, and Rotation at C2–C7

1. The patient is supine. The therapist stands or sits at the head of the table.
2. Place the fingertips (first through third) of both hands on right and left articular pillars of the upper segment (e.g., the C3 pillars for a C3–C4 dysfunction).
3. Flex the neck to the level of dysfunction (**Figure 16.10**). Introduce side-bending or lateral translation until the first barrier at that segment is engaged. Fine-tune the manipulation by applying very subtle additional leverage (rotation, more or less flexion/extension) as required.
4. Request the patient to gently push the head toward the midline (side-bending away from the restrictive barrier) *or* to extend against your resistance for 3 to 5 seconds.

5. Allow the patient to relax for a few seconds.
6. Reengage the new barrier by taking up any slack in side-bending or extension that has developed since the contraction and relaxation phases.
7. Repeat the procedure two to four times.
8. Reassess the patient after treatment.

Procedure for Restriction of Extension, Side-Bending, and Rotation at C2–C7

1. The patient is supine. The therapist stands or sits at the head of the table.
2. Two alternative hand positions are suitable for introducing segmental extension:
   - Place the fingertips (first through third) of both hands on right and left articular pillars of the upper segment (e.g., the C3 pillars for a C3–C4 dysfunction).
   - Place the index and middle finger on one articular pillar and the thumb on the opposite pillar (right and left pillars of the lower segment). The other hand contacts the patient's head. This "pincer" hold is useful for introducing highly localized extension (without the need to extend the neck) and lateral translation and for creating a local fulcrum for lateral flexion (**Figure 16.11**).
3. Extend the segment by lifting the fingertips on the pillars until the extension barrier is palpated. Introduce side-bending (using the cephalic hand

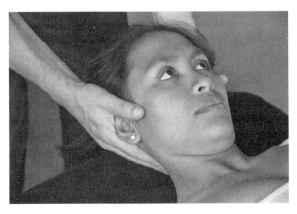

Figure 16.10 Treatment of Dysfunction of C2–C7: Restriction of Flexion, Side-Bending, and Rotation. The practitioner carefully localizes motion to the involved segment and engages each restricted plane. The patient is instructed to gently push back (into either side-bending or extension) against the practitioner's unyielding resistance.

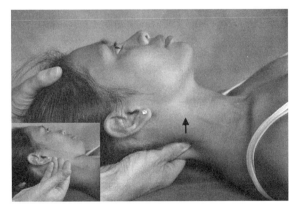

Figure 16.11 Treatment of Dysfunction of C2–C7: Restriction of Extension, Side-Bending, and Rotation. The "pincer" hold is used for contact on articular pillars to introduce localized segmental extension and translation (arrow, main photo; hand position, inset photo). The practitioner carefully engages extension at the involved segment, followed by side-bending and subtle rotation. The patient is instructed to gently push back (side-bending or flexion) against the practitioner's resistance (main photo).

to introduce motion and either the fingers or thumb of the pincer hand as a fulcrum) or introduce lateral translation (using the pincer contact) of the segment until the barrier is engaged. Fine-tune the manipulation by applying very subtle additional leverage (rotation, more or less flexion or extension) as required.

4. Request the patient to gently push the head toward the midline (side-bending away from the restrictive barrier) *or* to flex against your resistance for 3 to 5 seconds.
5. Allow the patient to relax for a few seconds.
6. Reengage the new barrier by taking up any slack in side-bending or extension that has developed since the contraction and relaxation phases.
7. Repeat the procedure two to four times.
8. Reassess the patient after treatment.

Atlanto-Axial Junction (C1–C2)

The primary movement at the C1–C2 segment is rotation. Although some sources advocate addressing additional planes (Mitchell & Mitchell, 1995), the author's experience suggests that the engagement of C1–C2 rotation as the primary plane is highly effective. The neck is placed in flexion, which relatively "locks" the lower cervical joint segments and localizes the rotation to the C1–C2 segment (Ogince et al., 2007).

Procedure

1. The patient is supine. The therapist stands or sits at the head of the table.
2. The fingertips of both hands are placed on the articular pillars of the upper segment, with palms cradling the head. Your chest or abdomen can also be used to support your hands.
3. Flex the patient's neck fully (until a sense of resistance) to relatively "lock" the middle and lower cervical spine (**Figure 16.12**). Maintain the flexion and rotate the neck until the barrier of restricted rotation is engaged. Fine-tune the manipulation by applying additional leverages (side-bending, flexion, extension) as determined with palpation.
4. Request the patient to gently rotate the head toward the midline (rotate away from the restrictive barrier) against your unyielding resistance for 3 to 5 seconds.
5. Allow the patient to relax for a few seconds.

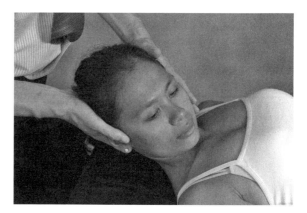

Figure 16.12 Treatment of the Atlanto-Axial (C1–C2) Junction. The practitioner flexes the neck to produce relative locking to minimize rotation below C1, and rotates the head to the restrictive barrier. The patient is instructed to gently rotate toward the midline against the practitioner's resistance.

6. Reengage the new barrier by taking up any slack in rotation that has developed since the contraction and relaxation phases.
7. Repeat the procedure three to five times.
8. Reassess the patient after treatment.

Occipito-Atlantal Junction (C0–C1)

The primary movements at the C0–C1 joint are flexion and extension, but examination and treatment of the restricted side-bending and rotation components also appear to be clinically rewarding. Techniques can be used to address a single plane (usually either flexion/extension) or multiple planes (contralateral side-bending and rotation, with flexion or extension).

Procedure for Single-Plane Restriction of Either Flexion or Extension

1. The patient is supine. The therapist stands or sits at the head of the table.
2. Place one hand under the occiput with the fingertips palpating the sub-occipital tissues close to the C0–C1 joint line, and the other hand resting on the patient's forehead.
3. Gently flex (**Figure 16.13**, main photo), or extend (Figure 16.13, inset photo), the head without engaging movement in the cervical spine until the initial sense of barrier at C0–C1 is palpated.
4. Request the patient to gently extend (or flex) the head using the instruction to "Nod the head upward" or "Look upward" (or downward) against your unyielding resistance for 3 to 5 seconds.

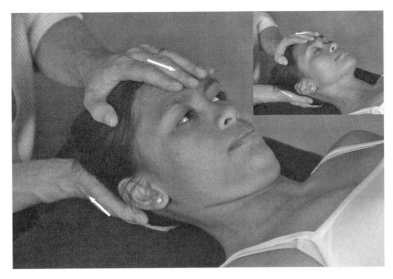

Figure 16.13 Treatment of the Occipito-Atlantal (C0–C1) Junction. Single-plane restriction, flexion (main photo): The practitioner carefully flexes the head to the barrier (arrows), and the patient is requested to gently extend the head against the practitioner's resistance. Single-plane restriction, extension (inset photo): The practitioner carefully extends the head to the barrier (arrows), and the patient is requested to gently flex the head against the practitioner's resistance.

5. Allow the patient to relax for several seconds.
6. Reengage the new barrier by taking up any slack in flexion (or extension) that has developed since the contraction and relaxation phases.
7. Repeat the procedure two to four times.
8. Reassess the patient after treatment.

Procedure for Multiple-Plane Restriction of Flexion (or Extension), Contralateral Side-Bending, and Rotation

1. The patient is supine. The therapist stands or sits at the head of the table.
2. Cradle the occiput and head using both hands, with the fingertips palpating the sub-occipital muscles near the C0–C1 joint line.
3. Gently flex (or extend) the head until the initial sense of barrier is palpated (**Figure 16.14**).
4. Introduce side-bending through a combination of gentle side-bending and lateral translation of the head on the neck until the barrier is engaged. Fine-tune the manipulation by applying subtle contralateral rotation, if required.
5. Request the patient to gently push the head toward the midline (side-bending away from the restrictive barrier) against your unyielding resistance for 3 to 5 seconds. Alternatively, a flexion (or extension) activating force can be used.

6. Allow the patient to relax for several seconds.
7. Reengage the new barrier by taking up any slack in flexion (or extension) or side-bending that has developed since the contraction and relaxation phases.
8. Repeat the procedure two to four times.
9. Reassess the patient after treatment.

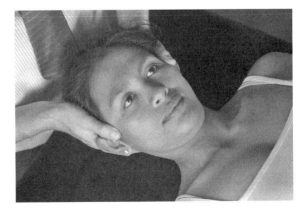

Figure 16.14 Treatment of the Occipito-Atlantal (C0–C1) Junction. Multiple-plane restriction, involving flexion or extension, side-bending, and rotation: The practitioner carefully flexes (or extends) the head to the barrier, and then introduces lateral translation, with further subtle side-bending or rotation as required. The patient is requested to gently push in either a side-bending or flexion/extension direction against the practitioner's resistance.

ACKNOWLEDGMENTS

The author expresses gratitude to Rolena Stephenson for her contribution as model and Deborah Goggin, MA, Scientific Writer, A. T. Still Research Institute, A. T. Still University, for reviewing this manuscript.

This chapter is based on the following source: Fryer G, Fossum C. Muscle energy techniques. In: Fernández-de-las-Peñas C, Arendt-Nielsen L, Gerwin RD, eds. *Tension-Type and Cervicogenic Headache: Pathophysiology, Diagnosis, and Management.* Sudbury, MA: Jones & Bartlett Learning; 2010:309–326.

REFERENCES

Anderson RE, Seniscal C. A comparison of selected osteopathic treatment and relaxation for tension-type headaches. *Headache* 2006;46:1273–1280.

Aparicio ÉQ, Quirante LB, Blanco CR, Sendín FA. Immediate effects of the suboccipital muscle inhibition technique in subjects with short hamstring syndrome. *J Manipulative Physiol Ther* 2009;32:262–269.

Ballantyne F, Fryer G, McLaughlin P. The effect of muscle energy technique on hamstring extensibility: the mechanism of altered flexibility. *J Osteopath Med* 2003;6:59–63.

Bourdillon JF, Day EA, Bookhout MR. *Spinal Manipulation.* 5th ed. Oxford, UK: Butterworth-Heinemann; 1992.

Boyles RE, Ritland BM, Miracle BM, et al. The short-term effects of thoracic spine thrust manipulation on patients with shoulder impingement syndrome. *Man Ther* 2009;14:375–380.

Bronfort G, Nilsson N, Haas M, et al. Non-invasive physical treatments for chronic/recurrent headache. *Cochrane Database Syst Rev* 2004;3:CD001878.

Bronfort G, Haas M, Evans R, et al. Effectiveness of manual therapies: the UK evidence report. *Chiropr Osteopat* 2010;18:3.

Burns DK, Wells MR. Gross range of motion in the cervical spine: the effects of osteopathic muscle energy technique in asymptomatic subjects. *J Am Osteopath Assoc* 2006;106:137–142.

Chaitow L. *Muscle Energy Techniques.* 3rd ed. Edinburgh: Churchill Livingstone; 2006.

Cleland JA, Childs MJD, McRae M, et al. Immediate effects of thoracic manipulation in patients with neck pain: a randomized clinical trial. *Man Ther* 2005;10:127–135.

Coates G, O'Brodovich H, Goeree G. Hindlimb and lung lymph flows during prolonged exercise. *J Appl Physiol* 1993;75:633–638.

Cook C, Hegedus E, Showalter C, Sizer PS Jr. Coupling behavior of the cervical spine: a systematic review of the literature. *J Manipulative Physiol Ther* 2006;29:570–575.

Di Fabio RP. Manipulation of the cervical spine: risks and benefits. *Phys Ther* 1999;79:50–65.

DiGiovanna EL, Schiowitz S, Dowling DJ. *An Osteopathic Approach to Diagnosis and Treatment.* 3rd ed. Philadelphia: Lippincott William & Wilkins; 2005.

Edmondston SJ, Henne SE, Loh W, Ostvold E. Influence of cranio-cervical posture on three-dimensional motion of the cervical spine. *Man Ther* 2005;10:44–51.

Ehrenfeuchter WC, Sandhouse M. Muscle energy techniques. In: Ward RC, ed. *Foundations for Osteopathic Medicine.* 2nd ed. Philadelphia: Lippincott William & Wilkins; 2003:881–907.

Etnyre BR, Abraham LD. Gains in range of ankle dorsi-flexion using three popular stretching techniques. *Am J Phys Med* 1986;65:189–196.

Feland JB, Myrer JW, Schulthies SS, et al. The effect of duration of stretching of the hamstring muscle group for increasing range of motion in people aged 65 years or older. *Phys Ther* 2001;81:1100–1117.

Ferber R, Osternig LR, Gravelle DC. Effect of PNF stretch techniques on knee flexor muscle EMG activity in older adults. *J Electrom Kinesiol* 2002;12:391–397.

Fernández-de-las-Peñas C, Alonso-Blanco C, Cuadrado ML, et al. Trigger points in the suboccipital muscles and forward head posture in tension type headache. *Headache* 2006a;46:454–460.

Fernández-de-las-Peñas C, Alonso-Blanco C, Cuadrado ML, et al. Myofascial trigger points and their relationship to headache clinical parameters in chronic tension type headache. *Headache* 2006b;46:1264–1272.

Fernández-de-las-Peñas C, Ge HY, Arendt-Nielsen L, et al. Referred pain from trapezius muscle trigger point shares similar characteristics with chronic tension type headache. *Eur J Pain* 2007;11:475–482.

Fryer G. Muscle energy concepts: a need for change. *J Osteopath Med* 2000;3:54–59.

Fryer G. Muscle energy technique: research and efficacy. In: Chaitow L, ed. *Muscle Energy Techniques.* 3rd ed. Edinburgh: Churchill Livingstone; 2006:109–132.

Fryer G. Research-informed muscle energy concepts and practice. In: Franke H, ed. *Muscle Energy Technique: History–Model–Research* (monograph). Ammersestr: Jolandos; 2009:57–62.

Fryer G. Muscle energy technique: an evidence-informed approach. *Int J Osteopath Med* 2011;14:3–9.

Fryer G, Fossum C. Therapeutic mechanisms underlying muscle energy approaches. In: Fernández-de-las-Peñas C, Arendt-Nielsen L, Gerwin RD, eds. *Tension-Type and Cervicogenic Headache: Pathophysiology, Diagnosis, and Management.* Sudbury, MA: Jones & Bartlett Learning; 2010:221–229.

Fryer G, Ruszkowski W. The influence of contraction duration in muscle energy technique applied to the atlanto-axial joint. *J Osteopath Med* 2004;7:79–84.

Fryer G, Alivizatos J, Lamaro J. The effect of osteopathic treatment on people with chronic and sub-chronic neck pain: a pilot study. *Int J Osteopath Med* 2005;8:41–48.

Fryette H. *Principles of Osteopathic Technique.* Newark, OH: American Academy of Osteopathy; 1954.

Gerwin R. Headache. In: Ferguson LW, Gerwin R, eds. *Clinical Mastery in the Treatment of Myofascial Pain.* Baltimore: Lippincott Williams & Wilkins; 2005:1–29.

Gibbons P, Tehan P. Muscle energy concepts and coupled motion of the spine. *Man Ther* 1998;3:95–101.

Gibbons P, Tehan P. *Manipulation of the Spine, Thorax and Pelvis: An Osteopathic Perspective.* 2nd ed. London: Churchill Livingstone; 2006.

Godges JJ, Mattson-Bell M, Thorpe D, Shah D. The immediate effects of soft tissue mobilization with proprioceptive neuromuscular facilitation on gleno-humeral external rotation and overhead reach. *J Orthop Sports Phys Ther* 2003;33:713–718.

González-Iglesias J, Fernández-de-las-Peñas C, Cleland JA, et al. Inclusion of thoracic spine thrust manipulation into an electro-therapy/thermal program for the management of patients with acute mechanical neck pain: a randomized clinical trial. *Man Ther* 2009;14:306–313.

Greenman PE. *Principles of Manual Medicine.* 3rd ed. Philadelphia: Lippincott William & Wilkins; 2003.

Grip H, Sundelin G, Gerdle B, Karlsson JS. Variations in the axis of motion during head repositioning: a comparison of subjects with whiplash-associated disorders or non-specific neck pain and healthy controls. *Clin Biomech* 2007;22:865–873.

Haldeman S, Kohlbeck FJ, McGregor M. Unpredictability of cerebro-vascular ischemia associated with cervical spine manipulation therapy: a review of sixty-four cases after cervical spine manipulation. *Spine* 2001;27:49–55.

Handel M, Horstmann T, Dickhuth HH, Gulch RW. Effects of contract–relax stretching training on muscle performance in athletes. *Eur J Appl Physiol Occup Physiol* 1997;76:400–408.

Havas E, Parviainen T, Vuorela J, et al. Lymph flow dynamics in exercising human skeletal muscle as detected by scintography. *J Physiol* 1997;504:233–239.

Ishii T, Mukai Y, Hosono N, et al. Kinematics of the upper cervical spine in rotation: in vivo three-dimensional analysis. *Spine* 2004;29:E139–E144.

Ishii T, Mukai Y, Hosono N, et al. Kinematics of the cervical spine in lateral bending: in vivo three-dimensional analysis. *Spine* 2006;31:155–160.

Kuchera WA, Kuchera ML. *Osteopathic Principles in Practice.* Kirksville, MO: Kirksville College of Osteopathic Medicine Press; 1992.

Langevin HM, Cornbrooks CJ, Taatjes DJ. Fibroblasts form a body-wide cellular network. *Histochem Cell Biol* 2004;122:7–15.

Langevin HM, Bouffard NA, Badger GJ, et al. Dynamic fibroblast cytoskeletal response to subcutaneous tissue stretch ex vivo and in vivo. *Am J Physiol Cell Physiol* 2005;288:C747–756.

Lederman E. *The Science and Practice of Manual Therapy.* 2nd ed. Edinburgh: Elsevier Churchill Livingstone; 2005.

Lee HY, Wang JD, Yao G, Wang SF. Association between cervicocephalic kinesthetic sensibility and frequency of subclinical neck pain. *Man Ther* 2008;13:419–425.

Legaspi O, Edmond SL. Does the evidence support the existence of lumbar spine coupled motion? A critical review of the literature. *J Orthop Sports Phys Ther* 2007;37:169–178.

Leinonen V, Maatta S, Taimela S, et al. Impaired lumbar movement perception in association with postural stability and motor- and somatosensory-evoked potentials in lumbar spinal stenosis. *Spine* 2002;27:975–983.

Licciardone JC, Stoll ST, Fulda KG, et al. Osteopathic manipulative treatment for chronic low back pain: a randomized controlled trial. *Spine* 2003;28:1355–1362.

Licciardone JC, Buchanan S, Hensel KL, et al. Osteopathic manipulative treatment of back pain and related symptoms during pregnancy: a randomized controlled trial. *Am J Obstet Gynecol* 2010;202:1–8.

Liebenson C, Tunnell P, Murphy DR, Gluck-Bergman N. Manual resistance techniques. In: Liebenson C, ed. *Rehabilitation of the Spine: A Practitioner's Manual.* 2nd ed. Baltimore: Lippincott Williams & Wilkins; 2007:407–459.

Magnusson M, Simonsen EB, Aagaard P, et al. A mechanism for altered flexibility in human skeletal muscle. *J Physiol* 1996a;497:293–298.

Magnusson SP, Simonsen EB, Aagaard P, et al. Mechanical and physical responses to stretching with and without pre-isometric contraction in human skeletal muscle. *Arch Phys Med Rehabil* 1996b;77:373–378.

Magnusson M, Simonsen EB, Dyhre-Poulsen P, et al. Viscoelastic stress relaxation during static stretch in human skeletal muscle in the absence of EMG activity. *Scand J Med Sci Sports* 1996c;6:323–328.

Malmstrom E, Karlberg M, Fransson PA, et al. Primary and coupled cervical movements: the effect of age, gender, and body mass index: a 3-dimensional movement analysis of a population without symptoms of neck disorders. *Spine* 2006;31:E44–E50.

Malmstrom EM, Karlberg M, Holmstrom E, et al. Influence of prolonged unilateral cervical muscle contraction on head repositioning: decreased overshoot after a 5-min static muscle contraction task. *Man Ther* 2010;15:229–234.

McClatchie L, Laprade J, Martin S, et al. Mobilizations of the asymptomatic cervical spine can reduce signs of shoulder dysfunction in adults. *Man Ther* 2009;14:369–374.

Mitchell FL Jr, Mitchell PKG. *The Muscle Energy Manual.* Vol. 1. East Lansing, MI: MET Press; 1995.

Mitchell FL Jr, Moran PS, Pruzzo NA. *An Evaluation and Treatment Manual of Osteopathic Muscle Energy Procedures.* Valley Park, MO: Mitchell, Moran and Pruzzo; 1979.

Mitchell FL Sr. Structural pelvic function. Kirksville: *Academy of Applied Osteopathy Yearbook.* 1958:71–90.

Mitchell UH, Myrer J, Hopkins J, et al. Neurophysiological reflex mechanisms' lack of contribution to the success of PNF stretches. *J Sport Rehabil* 2009;18:343–357.

Ogince M, Hall T, Robinson K, Blackmore AM. The diagnostic validity of the cervical flexion–rotation test in C1/2-related cervicogenic headache. *Man Ther* 2007;12:256–262.

Osternig LR, Robertson RN, Troxel RK, Hansen, P. Differential responses to proprioceptive neuromuscular facilitation (PNF) stretch techniques. *Med Sci Sports Exerc* 1990;22:106–111.

Palmgren PJ, Sandstrom PJ, Lundqvist FJ, Heikkila H. Improvement after chiropractic care in cervicocephalic kinesthetic sensibility and subjective pain intensity in patients with nontraumatic chronic neck pain. *J Manipulative Physiol Ther* 2006;29:100–106.

Rogers RG. The effects of spinal manipulation on cervical kinesthesia in patients with chronic neck pain: a pilot study. *J Manipulative Physiol Ther* 1997;20:80–85.

Ryan EE, Rossi MD, Lopez R. The effects of the contract–relax–antagonist–contract form of proprioceptive

neuromuscular facilitation stretching on postural stability. *J Strength Cond Res* 2010;24:1888–1894.

Sady SP, Wortman M, Blanke D. Flexibility training: ballistic, static or proprioceptive neuromuscular facilitation? *Arch Phys Med Rehabil* 1982;63:261–263.

Salvador D, Neto PED, Ferrari FP. Application of muscle energy technique in garbage collectors with acute mechanical lumbar pain. *Fisioterapia e Pesquisa* 2005;12:20–27.

Schenk RJ, Adelman K, Rousselle J. The effects of muscle energy technique on cervical range of motion. *J Man Manip Ther* 1994;2:149–155.

Schwerla F, Bischoff A, Nurnberger A, et al. Osteopathic treatment of patients with chronic non-specific neck pain: a randomised controlled trial of efficacy. *Forsch Komplementmed* 2008;15:138–145.

Selkow NM, Grindstaff TL, Cross KM, et al. Short-term effect of muscle energy technique on pain in individuals with non-specific lumbopelvic pain: a pilot study. *J Man Manip Ther* 2009;17:E14–E18.

Simons DG, Travell JG, Simons LS. *Myofascial Pain and Dysfunction: The Trigger Point Manual.* Vol. 1. 2nd ed. Baltimore: William & Wilkins; 1999.

Sizer PS Jr, Brismee JM, Cook C. Coupling behavior of the thoracic spine: a systematic review of the literature. *J Manipulative Physiol Ther* 2007;30:390–399.

Souvalis T, Vicenzino B, Wright A. Neurophysiological effects of spinal manual therapy. In: Boyling JD, Jull GA, eds. *Grieve's Modern Manual Therapy: The Vertebral Column.* 3rd ed. Edinburgh: Elsevier Churchill Livingstone; 2004:367–380.

Spernoga SG, Uhl TL, Arnold BL, Gansneder BM. Duration of maintained hamstring flexibility after a one-time, modified hold–relax stretching protocol. *J Athl Train* 2001;36:44–48.

Spring F, Gibbons P, Tehan P. Intra-examiner and inter-examiner reliability of a positional diagnostic screen for the lumbar spine. *J Osteopath Med* 2001;4:47–55.

Swart J. *Osteopathic Strap Technic.* Kansas City: Joseph Swart; 1919.

Van Kleef M, Mekhail N, van Zundert J. Evidence-based guidelines for interventional pain medicine according to clinical diagnoses. *Pain Pract* 2009;9:247–251.

Wallin D, Ekblom B, Grahn R, Nordenborg T. Improvement of muscle flexibility: a comparison between two techniques. *Am J Sports Med* 1985;13:263–268.

Wilson E, Payton O, Donegan-Shoaf L, Dec K. Muscle energy technique in patients with acute low back pain: a pilot clinical trial. *J Orthop Sports Phys Ther* 2003;33:502–512.

Neuromuscular Therapies in Treatment of Migraine

Leon Chaitow, ND, DO

INTRODUCTION TO NEUROMUSCULAR THERAPY

Neuromuscular therapy (NMT), as presented in this chapter, is defined as a therapeutic initiative incorporating an eclectic selection of manual soft-tissue and movement therapies, suitable for addressing structural and functional features that may be contributing to migraine and other headaches, usually as an adjunctive approach to other therapeutic methods. In the context of migraine, the choice to use NMT might be based on an assessment or evaluation that indicates a possible involvement of muscle and/or articular (e.g., cervical spine, cranial) structures as contributory or maintaining features of an individual's head pain or because of expressed patient preference. Neuromuscular therapy considers both local and global causes of pain and dysfunction, as well as perpetuating factors that affect the musculoskeletal system in general, and peripheral and central sensitization processes in particular.

Objectives of NMT

The objectives of NMT include alteration of the ground substance of connective tissue (Pohl, 2010), deactivation of myofascial trigger points, reduction of ischemic states, and assessment and beneficial modification of postural alignment, musculoskeletal dysfunction, and neural entrapment (Chaitow & DeLany, 2003).

Bialosky et al. (2009) noted that mechanical soft-tissue treatments (like those used in NMT) initiate neurophysiological responses, both peripheral and central. As a consequence, manual therapy, as used in NMT, might produce the following clinical outcomes:

- Changes of blood levels of β-endorphin serotonin (Degenhardt et al., 2011)
- Production of endogenous cannabinoids (McPartland et al., 2005; Greco et al., 2010)
- Improved circulation and drainage
- Decreased muscle spasm
- Relaxation
- Realignment of soft tissues
- Breaking of adhesions
- Increased range of motion
- Removal of cellular exudates

Prevention and Modulating Objectives

In line with the guidelines offered by the U.S. Headache Consortium, in relation to treatment of migraine by means of physical treatment, prevention—rather than symptom alleviation—is usually the primary objective of such approaches. While physical modalities such as NMT may at times be used alone, in treating patients with chronic migraine, such methods are far more commonly used in conjunction with more traditional (mainstream) forms of migraine management, as part of an integrated protocol. Objectives may include reducing both the frequency and the severity of migraines, while simultaneously reducing use of medication (Goslin et al., 1999; Campbell et al., 2010).

Patient Preferences

It is well documented that some headache sufferers prefer nonstandard, nonpharmacological, treatment of their problem. Additionally, not all patients respond well to drug therapies. Moreover, some pharmacological treatments are unsuitable for some patients, particularly in individuals with specific coexisting conditions or during pregnancy. As a result, many patients express a preference for nonstandard therapeutic methods to help manage (or prevent) their migraine symptoms (Nies, 1990; Astin, 1998).

In this chapter, NMT is not presented as a panacea for migraine, but rather cast as a noninvasive, potentially effective tool for modifying tissue status, when it can be shown to be dysfunctional and contributing to sensitization, possibly resulting in migraine (Chaitow, 2008; Chaitow & DeLany, 2008).

Etiological Features of Migraine

The etiology of one individual's migraine may differ markedly from that of another person's condition. In many cases of chronic migraine, a biomechanical element is suspected to exist, possibly involving the trigeminal nerve as one of the prime generators of head pain (Trescot, 2000; Young, 2007). Another biomechanical source of migraine pain may be the presence of active muscle trigger points (Giamberardino et al., 2007). These possibilities are explored further later in this chapter and in other chapters of this textbook.

Establishing a Case for NMT

The case for the use of manual therapy modalities, such as NMT, in the context of the treatment of migraine depends on establishing an etiological connection between tissues and structures that can be influenced by such treatment, and linking these structures to the generation or maintenance of headaches in general and migraines in particular. This chapter therefore focuses on two key features:

- Evidence of possible biomechanical associations with the evolution or maintenance of migraine, involving postural, functional, and localized structural features, any of which may contribute to evolution and maintenance of central sensitization
- Description of, and evidence for, the possible value in treatment (or prevention) of migraine, employing methods that are incorporated into an eclectic selection of modalities that fall under the umbrella term "neuromuscular therapies" (NMT)

CENTRAL SENSITIZATION: ITS BIOMECHANICAL CORRELATES AND CONTRIBUTION TO MIGRAINE

Central sensitization is defined as "an augmentation of responsiveness of central pain-signaling neurons to input from low-threshold mechanoreceptors" (Nijs & Van Houdenhove, 2009). The evolution of chronic migraine has been shown to have a strong association with the process of central sensitization, in which an individual experiences enhanced sensitivity to various modes of painful and nonpainful stimuli (Buchgreitz et al., 2006). For example, Burstein et al. (2000) demonstrated that a subset of migraine patients experience peri-orbital cutaneous allodynia when non-noxious stimuli are applied. Allodynia, in such individuals, frequently extends into the ipsilateral head and arm. The inference drawn by Burstein et al. (2000) was that these phenomena represented evidence of hyperexcitability of spinal and supraspinal pain pathways, a characteristic of central sensitization.

Staud (2006) has described the ways in which peripheral pain impulses can lead to central sensitization. In many chronic pain states, including chronic migraine, irritable bowel syndrome, and fibromyalgia syndrome, repetitive, persistent, or recurrent peripheral nociceptive features can lead to neuroplastic changes in the spinal cord and brain, which in turn results in central sensitization and consequent pain. As Xu et al. (2010) explain, even the nociceptive input from latent trigger points can contribute to central sensitization, such that only minimal nociceptive input (resulting from touch, pressure, or heat) may be required to maintain the chronic pain state once central sensitization has evolved.

Widespread and generalized central sensitization has been identified as operating in fibromyalgia syndrome (Bradley, 2005; Vierck, 2006), which is a common accompanying diagnosis in patients with chronic headache

(de Tommaso et al., 2002) and—mainly in females—in patients with migraine (Ifergane et al., 2006). Yunus (2007a) has described the overlap of a number of chronic pain conditions, including chronic migraine, as central sensitivity syndromes. This author asserts that in such conditions, hyperexcitability of central neurons results from the influence of various neurotransmitter and neurochemical activities, with the central sensitization itself being contingent on abnormal or continued peripheral inputs for its development and maintenance. Readers are referred to Chapters 6 and 8 for more information on central sensitization.

Background to Sensitization: Adaptation and Local and Global Dysfunction

Selye (1984) defined both the general adaptation syndrome (GAS), which affects the individual as a whole, and the local adaptation syndrome (LAS), which affects a local area of the body that is subjected to stressors demanding adaptation. The GAS and LAS models explain how adaptation progresses over time, with modifications to function occurring, adaptive capacity eventually becoming exhausted, and symptoms ultimately emerging. The neuromusculoskeletal adaptive changes involved in such processes can be seen to represent a record of the body's attempts to adapt and adjust to the multiple and varied stresses that have been imposed upon it over time. The results of repeated postural and traumatic insults over a lifetime, combined with the somatic effects of emotional and psychological origin, will often present a confusing pattern of tense, shortened, bunched, fatigued, and, ultimately, fibrous soft tissues.

The many forms of biomechanical stressors that affect the body include the following factors (Vleeming et al., 1990; Simons et al., 1999; Liebenson, 2007; Lewit, 2009):

- Congenital and inborn factors, such as a short or long leg, small hemi-pelvis, or fascial influences (Simons et al., 1999)
- Overuse, misuse, and abuse factors, such as injury, or inappropriate or repetitive patterns of use involved in work, sport, or activities of daily life (Schamberger, 2002)
- Immobilization or disuse (irreversible changes can occur after 8 weeks) (Cramer et al., 2010)
- Postural stress patterns (Haugstadt et al., 2006)
- Inappropriate breathing patterns (O'Sullivan & Beales, 2007)
- Chronic negative emotional states such as depression or anxiety (Galletti et al., 2009)
- Reflexive influences (trigger points, facilitated spinal regions) (Giamberardino et al., 2007)

Adaptation Implications

When widespread functional changes develop—for example, affecting respiratory function and posture—they have implications for the total economy of the body (Timmons & Ley, 1994). In the presence of a constant neurologic feedback of impulses from neural reporting stations to the brain, levels of psychological arousal will increase and the ability of the individual, or local hypertonic tissues, to relax effectively will decrease, with consequent reinforcement of hypertonicity and inevitably relative ischemia—an environment ideal for myofascial trigger point evolution (Shah et al., 2005; Simons, 2008). Functional patterns of use, of a biologically unsustainable nature, are likely to evolve in such a scenario, leading to chronic musculoskeletal problems and pain (Crockett et al., 2002). At this stage, restoration of normal function would require therapeutic input to address both the multiple changes that have occurred. In addition, the individual would likely need reeducation on how to use the body, how to breathe, and how to display posture in more sustainable ways.

Soft-Tissue Changes

Soft-tissue changes involving pain, hypertonicity or hypotonicity, joint dysfunction, antagonist muscle imbalances, and overactive synergist muscles may lead to localized areas of hyperreactivity, in the form of myofascial trigger points and neural entrapment (Moore, 2004; Lewit, 2009). Additionally, pain due to damage or inflammation of peripheral tissues is clearly capable of causing chronic widespread pain (Clauw, 2007). Another example of a local musculoskeletal disorder associated with chronic pain—and one that is frequently seen in manual therapy practice—is arthritis, which may potentially cause continuous activation of local nociceptors that initiate or sustain central sensitization.

The broad description of evolving adaptive processes, which are associated with multiple stressor features, is clearly recognizable as outlining the evolution of central sensitization (Woolf, 2011). It has long been established that subgroups of migraine (Burnstein et al., 2000; Weissman-Fogel et al., 2003) can be viewed as central sensitivity syndromes.

Reducing the Nociceptive Barrage

Yunus (2007a) has suggested that effective manual therapy in subacute cases of musculoskeletal dysfunction should be capable of limiting the afferent barrage of noxious input to the central nervous system, thereby preventing chronicity. Nijs et al. (2009) go even further, affirming the importance of decreasing the afferent nociceptive influence of trigger points, by means of soft-tissue mobilization, as part of comprehensive care of patients of chronic pain. NMT aims to reduce the effects of adaptation/compensation by enhancing musculoskeletal function—including improved posture, respiratory function, and general mobility and stability, and by reducing noxious inputs resulting from the active presence of, for example, myofascial trigger points.

When Is a Headache a Migraine?

It might be useful to explore the possibility that a patient suffering from headache, whether diagnosed as migraine or not, may benefit from appropriate treatment of the neck muscles and joints. Such treatment might involve mobilization or manipulation of restricted joints (Chapter 14), release of excessive tension in muscles (Chapters 15 and 16), or deactivation of trigger points (Chapter 15) that are capable of feeding pain into the head and neck region (Edeling, 1997; Zwart, 1997; Herzog, 1999; Simons et al., 1999).

Pearce (1995) noted that in 1860 Hilton described the concept of headaches originating from the cervical spine, while in 1983 Sjaastad et al. (1990) introduced the term "cervicogenic headache" (CGH). Diagnostic criteria have been established by several expert groups in recognition of the fact that CGHs originate in the neck or occipital region, and are associated with tenderness of cervical paraspinal tissues. Prevalence estimates range from 0.4% to 2.5% of the general population, up to 15% to 20% of patients with chronic headaches. CGH affects patients with a mean age of 42.9 years, has a 4:1 female disposition, and tends to be chronic. Almost any pathology affecting the cervical spine has been implicated in headache genesis from the cervical structures within the spinal nucleus of the trigeminal nerve. The main differential diagnoses are tension-type headache and migraine headache, which demonstrate considerable overlap in their symptoms and findings. No specific pathology has been noted on imaging or diagnostic studies that correlates with CGH, however (Haldeman & Dagenais, 2001). Readers are referred to Fernández-de-las-Peñas et al.'s (2010a) textbook for information on CGH and tension-type headache management.

Nevertheless, although they may be associated with many of the same symptoms as true migraine (such as nausea, vomiting, and sensitivity to light), many headaches are not migraines at all, but rather arise from neural irritation, or trigger point activity in the neck (Fernández-de-las-Peñas et al., 2010a). In addition, many individuals suffer both migraine headaches and severe headaches that derive from the neck (Sjaastad et al., 1990; Bono et al., 1998). One study of patients with neck injuries reported that 35% suffered from headaches deriving from their necks, while another 11% experienced both neck-related headaches and migraines (Bono et al., 2000).

Different causes of headache may require different treatment approaches. Some will require a focus on posture, some on neck restrictions (Quinn et al., 2002), some on trigger points, and others on imbalances affecting the temporomandibular joint (Dworkin & LeResche, 1991).

Recognizing Central Sensitization in Patients

Nijls et al. (2010) summarized the many features associated with central sensitization: hypersensitivity to bright light, touch, noise, pesticides, mechanical pressure, medication, and temperature (high and low). The presence of some or all of these symptoms, together with information gathered during the history taking and the diagnosis, as well as confirmatory results from the assessments listed below, can help in identifying central sensitization in a specific patient. The following tests have been suggested (Yunus, 2007b):

- Assessment of pressure pain thresholds at sites remote from the symptomatic site
- Assessment of sensitivity to touch during manual palpation at sites remote from the symptomatic site
- Assessment of sensitivity to vibration at sites remote from the symptomatic site
- Assessment of sensitivity to heat at sites remote from the symptomatic site
- Assessment of sensitivity to cold at sites remote from the symptomatic site
- Assessment of pressure pain thresholds during and following exercise
- Assessment of joint end-feel
- Brachial plexus provocation tests

Symptom exacerbation, at both symptomatic and distant sites, indicates central sensitization. Note, however, that a variety of other indications may also suggest this condition, including increased pain during or following exercise.

Fundamental Principle

A fundamental principle emerges from the current understanding of the sensitization process: therapeutic strategies that reduce the overall stress burden, whether they relate to biomechanics, biochemistry, or psychosocial features, will reduce central sensitization. There is now evidence of the validity of this principle, as discussed later in the chapter (Affaitati et al., 2011; Wolff, 2011). In relation to migraine, this understanding strongly suggests that treatment methods that are noninvasive and nonstressful—such as those employed in NMT—should contribute to lowered adaptation demands, reduced sensitization, and less pain.

METHODS TO REDUCE PERIPHERAL AND CENTRAL SENSITIZATION

Basic soft-tissue modalities, clustered under a heading of NMT, have been shown to offer benefits in cases of chronic migraine, and to represent realistic noninvasive alternatives to pharmacological interventions (Lawler & Cameron, 2006). Other biomechanically related therapeutic objectives that may reduce local and central sensitization, and therefore the onset or symptoms of migraine, may include enhanced posture, improved ergonomics (discussed later in this section), improved balance (migraine-associated dizziness), and elimination of hyperventilation (Furman & Jacob, 2001; Haugstadt et al., 2006; Wiltink et al., 2009; Yamada et al., 2011). Our contention is that NMT interventions that focus on improved biomechanics and function offer an appropriate means of reducing biomechanically related peripheral inputs to the process of central sensitization and, therefore, migraine.

NMT: Therapeutic Options

NMT recognizes that recovery from, or modulation of, both general and local adaptive changes requires focus on both the stressors and the stressed (whether the whole person or a local area), such that the obstacles impeding homeostatic, self-regulatory tendencies toward recovery are eliminated. The effects of therapeutic modalities and methods that aim to reduce the effects of adaptation—including the methods and modalities that make up NMT—can be summarized under three broad subheadings: reducing adaptive load, improving functionality, and relieving symptoms.

Reducing Adaptive Load

The adaptation burden can be eased if habits of daily life (whether dietary, psychological, physical, or other) are modified to become more physiologically acceptable patterns. Some examples include improved posture, optimal exercise, better dietary and sleep habits, improved breathing function, and more effective stress management.

Improving Functionality

Adaptation represents the interaction between stress load (psychosocial, biochemical, biomechanical) and the recipient of that load. Reduction in load (as discussed earlier) focuses on one part of that equation, whereas enhanced functionality addresses the other. Some examples include restoration of mobility, motor control, balance, stability, strength and endurance in biomechanical features, aerobic status, improved circulation, lymph drainage, assimilation, and elimination.

Relieving Symptoms

Ideally, the focus on symptom relief should have a secondary intent—namely, to not increase already exhausted adaptation demands. Examples of these outcomes include soft-tissue or osseous mobilization, trigger point inactivation, improved movement potential, and reduced pain. Various strategies have been suggested as being capable of reducing ongoing peripheral nociceptive input that contributes to central sensitization. Indeed, the feature that is most relevant to this chapter's discussion relates to removal or reduction of biomechanically induced peripheral features that may be contributing to the sensitization process.

Neuromuscular Therapies

For the sake of clarity, it is important to make the distinction between *neuromuscular therapies*—which are the focus of this chapter in terms of their application to migraine headaches—and *neuromuscular technique* (also known by the acronym NMT)—which is only one of the manual therapy methods that make up the tools of neuromuscular therapy.

NMT comprises an eclectic selection of soft-tissue manipulation and associated methods that focus attention on assessment and/or treatment of somatic dysfunction. The modalities and methods used in NMT derive from a variety of therapeutic realms, including osteopathy, chiropractic, physical therapy, manual medicine, massage therapy, and naturopathic medicine (Chaitow, 2008; Chaitow & DeLany, 2008). Some of these methods are described elsewhere in this book, such as trigger point release (Chapter 15), myofascial release

(Chapter 15), muscle energy technique (Chapter 16), and cranial manipulation (Chapter 20). Those modalities will, therefore, not be discussed in any detail in this chapter, even though they represent integral aspects of NMT. Note that both European and American forms of NMT incorporate assessment and treatment features simultaneously, with one informing the other, as well as accepted orthopaedic assessment methods. Additionally, both forms of NMT incorporate both moving and stationary pressures applied to tissues, using variable pressures to achieve objectives, including inhibitory (ischemic) compression, cross-fiber friction, and gliding and stretching methods.

Physiological Effects of NMT

Despite its predominantly physical/biomechanical approach to treatment of pain and dysfunction, NMT has a broader perspective. For example, in conditions such as migraine, clinical attention is given to modifying the effects of adaptation demands resulting from a wide variety of stressor influences, including the following factors:

- Biomechanical: congenital, overuse, misuse, trauma, and disuse features, affecting both local and global structures and functions
- Biochemical: toxicity, endocrine factors, imbalance, nutritional imbalance and/or deficiencies, ischemia, and inflammation
- Psychosocial: "stress," anxiety, depression, unresolved emotional states, and somatization

In reality, of course, all of these influences are inseparable. For example, mood is altered by physical activity as well as by manual therapy (Pluess et al., 2009). Likewise, the biochemical effects of bodywork can be profound (Bender et al., 2007), as evidenced by up-regulation of substances capable of inducing analgesia and euphoria, such as endorphins and endocannabinoids, following exercise or manual treatment (McPartland et al., 2005). Greco et al. (2010) reported that "available results strongly suggest that activation of endocannabinoids can represent a promising therapeutical tool for reducing both the physiological and inflammatory components of pain that are likely involved in migraine attacks" (p. 85).

NMT interventions have been shown to be effective in addressing muscular, myofascial, and joint dysfunction. These widespread effects suggest that appropriate use of NMT modalities, in treatment of identified local dysfunction, is likely to be of benefit in patients with migraine-related central sensitization.

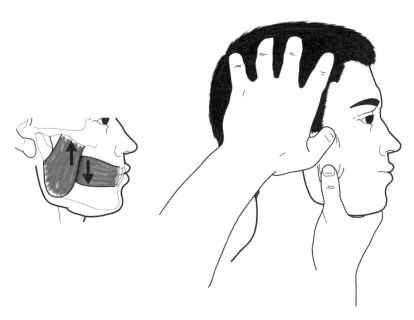

Figure 17.1 An S-Shaped Stretch is Induced Via Thumbs Holding Hypertonic Tissues at, or Toward, their Restriction Barriers, Until Release/Relaxation Occurs

Examples of NMT Modalities in Treatment of Muscular, Myofascial, and Joint Dysfunction

Muscle Energy Technique

MET (see Chapter 16) has been shown to improve range of motion, including within spinal joints (Kamani, 2000; Lenehan et al., 2003), and to improve muscle extensibility more effectively than passive, static stretching, both in the short term and in the long term (Feland et al., 2001; Ferber et al., 2002). In addition, studies offer support for the hypoalgesic effects of MET—for example, in relation to spinal pain (Cassidy et al., 1992; Wilson et al., 2003).

Myofascial Release

Robb and Pajaczkowski (2009) applied myofascial release to the adductor muscle complex in individuals who had painfully strained these structures during athletic activity (ice hockey). Use of the technique resulted in a significant reduction in perceived pain and as well as an increase in tolerance to applied manual pressure. **Figure 17.1** illustrates the myofascial release technique applied to the masseter muscle.

Positional Release Technique (Strain/ Counter-Strain)

Gentle, noninvasive methods such as positional release technique (PRT) and strain/counter-strain (SCS) have been shown to relieve local myofascial pain in the upper trapezius muscles (Atienza-Meseguer et al., 2006), as well as low back pain (Lewis & Flynn, 2001) and general myofascial pain conditions (Dardzinski et al., 2000). **Figure 17.2** illustrates the application of SCS to the temporalis muscle.

Examples of Neuromuscular Technique

Studies validating NMT demonstrated that this technique is associated with a significant increase in cervical range of motion (Patel, 2002), a significant increase in strength of the quadriceps (Palmer, 2002), a significant increase in passive ankle dorsiflexion range of motion (Tomlinson, 2002), and an increase in cervical range of motion following application of NMT to the diaphragm (Rice, 2002).

Integrated Neuromuscular Inhibition Technique

The integrated neuromuscular inhibition technique (INIT) is an evolution of NMT that combines various other

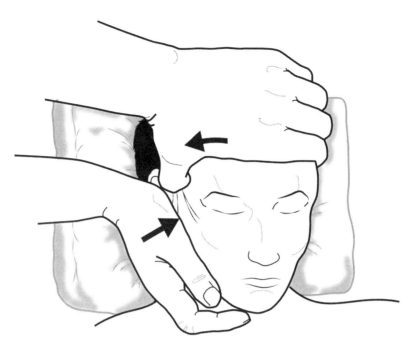

Figure 17.2 A tender point on the temporalis muscle is lightly compressed to induce a degree of discomfort. The other hand introduces a light degree of force that "crowds" the palpated tissues, until the discomfort is markedly reduced. This "position of ease" is held for up to 90 seconds.

modalities (Chaitow, 1994). Nagrale et al. (2010) have confirmed the efficacy of INIT in patients with nonspecific neck pain resulting from the presence of trigger points in the upper trapezius muscle.

DYSFUNCTIONAL PERIPHERAL FEATURES CONTRIBUTING TO CENTRAL SENSITIZATION

The peripheral features that may contribute to central sensitization and that are briefly examined in this chapter include muscle and joint dysfunction, myofascial trigger points, poor posture, and neural impingement or entrapment.

Muscle and Joint Pain and Sensitization

Affaitati et al. (2011) showed in a randomized, placebo-controlled trial that both local muscle and joint pains have a direct impact on increased central sensitization, and that the systematic identification and subsequent treatment of these local conditions can lead to reduced central sensitization in patients with fibromyalgia syndrome. This study examined contributing features of central sensitization in relation to a diagnosis of fibromyalgia (not migraine); nevertheless, it is the etiology of sensitization (not fibromyalgia) that is of interest in this chapter. Findings from this study are of profound importance in understanding the rationale for use of methods such as NMT in treatment of any pain-related condition—whether that be fibromyalgia or migraine. First, the results of the study show that, in fibromyalgia patients with concurrent myofascial pain syndromes, due to either trigger points or focal joint pain from osteoarthritis or microtraumas, local treatment of the peripheral muscle/joint sources not only relieved local symptoms, but also significantly improved the widespread symptoms in terms of reduction of both spontaneous diffuse pain and tenderness at all tender point sites. Second, the results indicate that local treatment is able to encourage general desensitization.

Giamberardino et al. (2007) insisted that "Cervical trigger points with referred areas in migraine sites contribute substantially to migraine symptoms, the peripheral nociceptive input from trigger points probably enhancing the sensitization level of central sensory neurons" (p.869). Strategies to reduce nociceptive input might involve inactivation of myofascial trigger points (as discussed in Chapter 15 and in the next subsection), mobilization of restricted articular structures (discussed in Chapters 14, 16, and 18), or release/relaxation of tissues that might be impinging on neural structures (discussed in Chapter 19 and later in this chapter) via interventions involving physical therapy, muscle relaxants, muscle injections, and anti-inflammatory analgesics (Staud, 2006). As an example, Moore (2004) showed that correcting posture-related muscular imbalance, as well as vertebral restrictions, appears to increase the effectiveness of associated treatment for cervicogenic headache.

Trigger Points and Migraine

Trigger points are described in Chapter 15; however, because these pain-generators are a major focus for NMT, a brief summary is called for in this chapter. Trigger points are localized areas of deep tenderness and increased resistance; digital pressure on such trigger will often produce twitching and fasciculation. Pressure maintained on such a point will produce referred pain. If a number of active trigger points exist, the reference areas may overlap, creating a myofascial pattern of pain. Srbely et al. (2010) report that myofascial pain is the most common form of musculoskeletal pain. Dommerholt (2010) has described myofascial trigger points (TrP) as "hyperirritable spots in skeletal muscle that are associated with hypersensitive palpable nodules in a taut band. An individual, active, trigger point is painful on compression and gives rise to characteristic referred pain, referred tenderness, motor dysfunction, and autonomic phenomena" (p. 131).

According to these authors, a minimal criterion for diagnosis of a trigger point is spot tenderness in a palpable band, with subject recognition of the pain as being "familiar" and replicating symptoms (Simons et al., 1999). When the TrP is provoked by means of compression, needling, or some other method, the individual's recognition of a previously experienced pain complaint indicates an active TrP, whereas recognition of an unfamiliar pain indicates a latent TrP. Additionally, painful limits to full range of motion, local twitch response, altered sensation in the target (referral) zone, EMG evidence of spontaneous electrical activity (SEA), the muscle being painful upon contraction, and the muscle testing as weak all serve as confirmatory signs that a trigger point is present (Simons et al., 1999). In addition, altered cutaneous humidity (usually increased), altered cutaneous temperature (increased or decreased), altered cutaneous texture (sandpaper-like quality, roughness), and a "jump" sign (i.e., an exclamation by the patient due to extreme tenderness of the palpated point) may be observed (Chaitow & DeLany, 2008; Lewit, 2009).

One of the main objectives in NMT is removal of these features of somatic dysfunction and their causes, which requires an appreciation of possible activating features that result in the presence of myofascial trigger points (e.g.,

poor posture, overuse, trauma). Such an appreciation offers indications as to therapeutic choices (Chaitow, 1994).

Examples of Primary Trigger Point–Activating Factors

A number of these factors have been identified (Travell & Simons, 1992; Simons et al., 1999; Simons, 2008):

- Persistent or repetitive muscular contraction, due to strain or overuse
- Trauma and consequent local inflammatory reaction (Lavelle et al., 2007)
- Adverse environmental conditions (e.g., cold, heat, damp, draughts)
- Prolonged immobility
- Febrile illness
- Systemic biochemical imbalance (e.g., hormonal, nutritional)

Examples of Secondary Trigger Point–Activating Factors

These factors include the following issues (Simons et al., 1999; Mense et al., 2001; Baldry, 2005):

- Compensating synergist and antagonist muscles to those housing trigger points, which may also develop trigger points
- Satellite trigger points that evolve in referral pain zones (from key triggers or visceral disease referral, such as myocardial infarct)
- Infection
- Allergy (food and other)
- Nutritional deficiencies (especially C, B-complex, and iron) (Simons et al., 1999)
- Hormonal imbalances (thyroid, in particular)
- Low oxygenation of tissues

NMT Modalities and Trigger Points

The modalities encompassed with the NMT category include MET; PRT, including SCS; myofascial release; trigger point release; connective tissue massage (CTM); INIT; scar-tissue release; and many more variations on the theme of soft-tissue manipulation. In the examples of treatment aimed at trigger point deactivation described here, one or combinations of these methods were employed. These examples need to be considered in the context of peripheral nociceptive features that contribute to central sensitization, with migraine a possible feature of that. As Giamberardino et al. (2007) have reported, myofascial trigger point activity frequently makes a profound contribution to migraine symptoms.

- A case study and retrospective review examined 20 patients with chronic myofascial pain (pain deriving from the presence of active trigger points), lasting for an average of 2.7 years, who were treated with SCS (Dardzinski et al., 2000). For all these patients, medical treatment had failed to provide pain relief or return of function. A reduction in pain and an increase in function of 50% to 100% occurred in 19 of 20 patients immediately after SCS therapy, with partial improvement maintained for 6 months in 11 of 20 patients, at which time 4 were still pain free (Dardzinski et al., 2000).
- Ibáñez-García et al. (2009) reported that SCS was as effective as neuromuscular technique (trigger point release method) in deactivating trigger points in the masseter muscle. Rodriguez-Blanco et al. (2006) demonstrated immediate functional improvements in terms of changes in active mouth-opening ability, following a single treatment of latent trigger points in the masseter muscle involving either MET or SCS.
- Seventy-two patients with chronic pelvic pain (CPP) were randomized to a manual therapy group whose members received CTM applied to the abdominal wall, back, buttocks, and thighs, as well as internal pelvic muscles in which connective tissue abnormalities were identified (FitzGerald et al., 2009). Treatment included either of two trigger point release methods: MET or MFR. Comparison was made between these forms of myofascial therapy and traditional external global therapeutic massage. The myofascial therapy group had a response rate of 57%, significantly higher than the 21% response rate found in the global therapeutic massage treatment group (P = 0.03). The overall response rate of 57% in the myofascial therapy group suggests that this approach represents a clinically meaningful treatment option for peripheral pain conditions (FitzGerald et al., 2009). Given the existence of such evidence, it is not surprising that the European Association of Urology has published guidelines suggesting that trigger points should be considered in the treatment of CPP (Fall et al., 2010)
- Nagrale et al. (2010) treated 60 patients with nonspecific neck pain relating to upper trapezius trigger points, using a combination of manual

modalities in the sequence known as Integrated Neuromuscular Inhibition Technique, or INIT (Chaitow, 1994). Results revealed large pre–post-effect sizes within the INIT group (Cohen's d: 0.97, 0.94, and 0.97). Additionally, significantly greater improvements in pain and neck disability and lateral cervical flexion ROM were detected in favor of the INIT group (0.29–0.57, 0.57–1.12, and 0.29–0.57) at a 95% CI, respectively.

Posture as an Etiological Feature in the Sensitization Process

Standing or sitting with the head forward relative to the body, in a slouched posture, puts a great deal of stress on the muscles and joints of the upper back and neck; over time, this stance can lead to formation of trigger points, nerve irritation, and headaches (Simons et al., 1999; Haugstadt et al., 2006). Forward head posture often accompanies temporomandibular disorders (TMD) and related myofascial dysfunctions, including the evolution of trigger points. An association has been identified between neck pain and TMD (Ciancaglini et al., 1999). Related to headaches, Fernández-de-las-Peñas et al. (2006a) found a correlation between forward head posture and trigger points in the sub-occipital muscles in patients with chronic tension-type headache. **Figure 17.3** illustrates sub-occipital release, as applied in NMT.

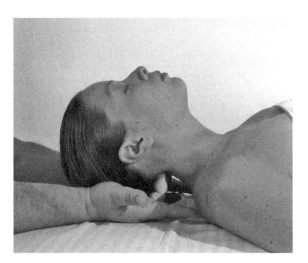

Figure 17.3 The patient's head rests on the practitioner's vertically inclined digits. The weight of the head gradually (over several minutes) causes the induced pressure onto the fingers to relax the sub-occipital muscles. Very light degrees of stretch are introduced, by means of digital flexion/traction applied to the occipital bone.

Examining for anterior head position has been noted by Simons et al. (1999) to be "the single most useful postural parameter" related to head and neck pain. These authors note that a forward head position occurs with rounded shoulders and results in sub-occipital, posterior cervical, upper trapezius, and splenius capitis shortening—commonly leading to loss of cervical lordosis. Such postural changes may overload sternocleidomastoid and splenius cervicis muscles, placing extension strain on the occipito-atlantal joint, and increasing the chance of compression pathologies. This outcome is extremely pertinent to migraine because sensory information from the cervical spine converges with trigeminal afferents within the spinal tract of the trigeminal nucleus, while fibers arriving in the subnucleus caudalis descend to C2–C3 and even C6 (Xiong & Matsushita, 2000).

Restricted spinal segments in the cervical region (especially at the C0–C3 levels) as well as trigger points in the sternocleidomastoid and upper trapezius muscles have been found to be significantly more common in patients with TMD (Fernández-de-las-Peñas et al., 2010b), with unilateral migraine (Fernández-de-las-Peñas et al., 2006b), and with bilateral migraine (Calandre et al., 2006). Diverse musculoskeletal disorders, such as chronic neck pain (Curatolo et al., 2001; Sterling et al., 2004; Freeman et al., 2009), disc herniation (O'Neill et al., 2007), shoulder impingement syndrome (Hidalgo-Lozano et al., 2010), and epicondylalgia (Fernandez-Carnero et al., 2009) all have been shown to encourage pain sensitivity involving deep uninvolved tissues, in turn leading to central sensitization and progression toward chronicity of headache and migraine (Filatova et al., 2008).

Correcting posture takes time, and requires regular exercising of taught postural correction procedures, so that what feels uncomfortable at first (such as holding the head closer to its anatomic position) gradually becomes comfortable and starts to "feel right." Teachers of the Alexander technique have perfected a gradual rehabilitation program that should ideally be accompanied by treatment (and self-treatment) aimed at stretching and releasing restricted muscles and joints, and at toning and balancing the body as a whole (Dommerholt, 2000; Wilson, 2002).

Neural Impingement/Entrapment and Migraine

A major etiological feature in extracranial causes of headache can be observed in examples of neural entrapment. Trescot (2000) has explained the manner in which entrapments involving the trigeminal nerve may result in unilateral or bilateral throbbing headaches. The initial trigger might have involved trauma such as that experienced when the face or head receives a blow or strikes another object. In due course, if subsequent scar tissue tightens, it may cause entrapment followed by symptoms such as auras, unilateral or bilateral throbbing, photophobia, hyperacusis, nausea, and vomiting. Trescot (2000) notes that "such headaches meet all the International Headache Society (IHS) criteria for migraine" (p. 197). Trescot (2000) also observes that "[physicians] treating headache patients are beginning to realize that the symptomatic diagnosis of migraines (unilateral throbbing headache associated with photophobia, phonophobia and emesis) does not distinguish between intracranial and extra-cranial causes of headaches" (p. 197). Young (2007) reports that "since the trigeminal nerve innervates the sinuses, face, and neck regions and is thought to be involved with migraines, if one successfully treats the... sites (involved with the trigeminal nerve), it is not infrequent to dramatically diminish the migraine onset" (p. 150).

Migraine-type headaches resulting from extracranial sources offer the opportunity for NMT, or other approaches (such as acupuncture or dry needling), to influence the condition by means of scar-tissue release, myofascial release, and other neuromuscular techniques (Ward, 1993; Lewit & Olasnka, 2004; Chaitow & DeLany, 2008; Valouchová & Lewit, 2009). Examples of NMT strategies for modification of neural entrapments, are described later in this chapter.

Examples of neural dysfunction/entrapment contributing to migraine include the following:

- *Supra-orbital neuralgia.* Entrapments of the first division of the trigeminal nerve can cause headaches that may be mistaken for frontal sinusitis, with or without aura. These headaches often occur just before menses, and may be triggered by bright lights that cause squinting.

- *Infra-orbital neuralgia.* Headaches, sometimes diagnosed as migraine, may derive from the second division of the trigeminal nerve, and possibly be misdiagnosed as maxillary sinusitis. Just as in the case of entrapment of the supra-orbital nerve, prior injury may have initiated this condition. Menstrual influences are also apparent in many cases.

- *Auriculo-temporal nerve.* Entrapment of the auriculo-temporal nerve—a third-division trigeminal nerve that leaves the foramen ovale and then travels anteriorly to the temporomandibular joint (TMJ)—may produce severe throbbing headaches (due to the proximity to the temporal artery) located largely in the temporal regions. This nerve pierces the temporalis muscle and can be aggravated by bruxism and so-called TMJ dysfunction (Ismail et al., 2007). It has been proposed (Yin et al., 2007) that therapies targeting the masticatory system, including occlusal splints, masticatory muscle work, lifestyle intervention of oral habits, myofascial therapy, cranial manipulation, and acupuncture, might significantly influence neurologic activity via sensorimotor integration between the brainstem, subcortical and cortical centers, the cervical region, proprioception, and body posture.

- *Posterior auricular nerve.* Ear pain and parietal headaches can be caused by entrapment of the posterior auricular nerve by the sternocleidomastoid muscle. This effect can occur during flexion/extension injuries, especially if the head was turned at impact.

- *Greater and lesser occipital nerve.* The occipital nerve is made up of the dorsal rami of C2 and C3 (Bogduk, 1981). Classic occipital neuralgia causes pain in the back of the head; however, because the ganglion interconnects with the trigeminal ganglion in the brainstem (Kerr, 1981), occipital neuralgia may refer to any of the branches of the trigeminal nerves, especially the retro-orbital area. These nerves pierce the nuchal fascia at the base of the skull and, therefore, are prone to trauma from flexion/extension injuries, as well as entrapment by spasm of the trapezius muscle.

Bogduk and Govind (2009) confirmed the results of laboratory and clinical studies showing that pain from upper cervical joints and muscles can be referred to the head; however, these authors categorically state that clinical diagnostic criteria are unreliable, and that a cervical source of pain can be established only by use of fluoroscopically guided, controlled, diagnostic nerve blocks. A counter-argument suggests that another way of establishing such a connection would be to remove the symptoms by appropriate noninvasive manual methods, such as those employed in NMT. These techniques include specific scar-release methods (Lewit & Olsanska, 2004; Valouchová & Lewit, 2009).

Zito et al. (2006) have suggested means of distinguishing cervicogenic headache sufferers from those with migraine, although the reliability of these discriminatory signs remains to be confirmed. In the Zito et al. study, persons with cervicogenic headache presented with restrictions in cervical motion, a higher frequency of muscle tightness, and poorer (albeit nonsignificant) performance on the craniocervical flexion test. These indicators of musculoskeletal dysfunction were not apparent in the group with migraine with aura.

Neural Entrapment as a Pain-Generator

Peripheral nerve entrapments of the extremities are common, and can occur anywhere along the course of a peripheral nerve. The onset of such entrapment typically follows either traumatic (acute) injury or an evolving chronic process. The pathophysiology is similar in all cases, involving local ischemia due to mechanical pressure (McKinnon, 2002; Pham & Gupta, 2009). Recent literature confirms the value of deep soft-tissue mobilization methods, including NMT techniques such as myofascial release and neurodynamic therapy (Hyde & Gengenbach, 2007).

NMT Treatment of Scars

A scar is considered to be "active" (i.e., symptom producing) if at least one of its structural layers does not move in harmony with the rest—in other words, if resistance to passive movement in at least one direction can be palpated (Lewit & Olsanska, 2004). Active scars (e.g., abdominal scars) can restrict normal functional movement, which the patient then feels as low back pain. Such effects can be relieved by treatment of scars on the abdomen and below the symphysis (Kobesova et al., 2007).

Palpation may reveal areas of restricted (elastically) hyperalgesic scar tissue that harbor active trigger points. These areas can often be inactivated by performing mini-myofascial release stretches (or acupuncture). Valouchová and Lewit (2009) report that very light sustained myofascial stretching effectively normalizes such restrictions, as demonstrated by altered surface electromyography (SEMG) evidence and symptomatic improvement.

In summary, migraine is commonly associated with central sensitization. Further, peripheral nociceptive features, including joint restrictions, myofascial trigger points, postural imbalances, neural impingement, and scar tissue, can increase or maintain central sensitization. Soft-tissue manipulation methods, clustered under the umbrella term NMT, can normalize many peripheral contributory features, such as myofascial trigger points. Reduced central sensitization may, in turn, reduce the intensity and frequency of migraines.

EXAMPLES OF NMT

To employ NMT as a treatment modality requires a sound understanding of musculoskeletal anatomy and physiology, as well as good palpation and general manual skills. The examples given here are provided for informational purposes only, as the acquisition of NMT skills requires supervised training and cannot be acquired from the written word alone.

NMT in Palpation and Treatment of Myofascial Trigger Points

The discussion in this section is modified from the work Chaitow and DeLany (2008).

Central Trigger Point Palpation and Treatment

Recent advances in imaging technology have allowed trigger points to be observed as areas of "denser" tissue within myofascial structures (Sikdar et al., 2008). The localized areas of dense tissue are discussed at greater length in Chapter 15 of this textbook.

- When assessing tissues for central trigger points or to treat a central trigger point that is not associated with an inflamed attachment site, the tissue is placed in a relaxed position by slightly (passively) approximating its ends. For example, the forearm would be passively supinated and the elbow slightly flexed for biceps brachii.
- The approximate center of the fibers should be located with a thumb or finger contact.
- Tendons should be ignored. Only the length of the fibers is considered when locating their center, which is also the endplate zone of most muscles, and a common location of central trigger points (Simons et al., 1999).
- Digital pressure (flat or pincer compression) should be applied to the center of taut muscle fibers where trigger point nodules are found.
- The tissue may be treated in this position, or a slight stretch may be added to increase the palpation level of the taut band and nodule.
- As the tension becomes palpable, pressure should be increased into the tissues to meet and match it.
- The fingers should then slide longitudinally along the taut band, near mid-fiber, to assess for a palpable nodule or thickening of the associated myofascial tissue.

- An exquisite degree of spot tenderness is usually reported near or at trigger point sites.
- Sometimes stimulation from the examination may produce a local twitch response, especially when a transverse snapping palpation is used. When present, the local twitch response serves as a confirmation that a trigger point has been encountered.
- When pressure is increased (gradually) into the core of the nodule, the tissue may refer sensations— usually pain—to either the surrounding tissue or distant tissues, which the person either may recognize as being familiar (if it is an active trigger point) or may not report as being familiar (in which case it is a latent trigger point). Sensations may also include tingling, numbness, itching, burning, or paresthesia, although pain is the most common referral.
- The degree of pressure should be adjusted so that the person reports a mid-range number between 5 and 7 on his or her discomfort scale, as the pressure is maintained. (Alternative protocols for application of pressure to trigger points are described in the discussion of INIT later in this chapter.)
- Because the tenderness of the tissue will vary from person to person, and even from tissue to tissue in the same person, the pressure applied may range from less than a few grams (an ounce) to a kilogram (2 pounds). Whatever the pressure used, it should always register no more than 5 to 7 on the patient's discomfort scale when the correct pressure is used.
- The practitioner should feel the tissues "melting and softening" under the sustained pressure. The patient frequently reports a perception that the practitioner is reducing the pressure on the tissue, even though it is being sustained at the same level.
- Pressure can be mildly increased as tissue relaxes and tension releases, provided the discomfort scale is respected.
- The length of time for which pressure is maintained will vary, but tension should ease within 8 to 12 seconds, and the patient's discomfort level should drop.
- If the area does not begin to respond within 8 to 12 seconds, the amount of pressure should be adjusted accordingly (usually lessened), the angle of pressure altered, or a more precise location sought.
- Because the tissues are being deprived of normal blood flow while pressure is being applied to them (blanching), clinical experience suggests that 20 seconds is the maximum length of time to hold the pressure.

Chapter 15 details other soft-tissue therapies targeted at inactivating trigger points.

Adding Stretch to the Palpation

Slightly stretching the muscle tissue often makes the taut fibers much easier to palpate. Caution should be exercised, however, if movement produces pain or if palpation of the attachment sites reveals excessive tenderness that may represent an attachment trigger point and inflammation. Placing more tension on these already distressed tissues may provoke an inflammatory response. Additionally, care must be taken to avoid aggressive applications (e.g., friction) while the tissue is being stretched, as injury is more likely to occur when tissue is in a stretched position. A proper sequence is as follows:

1. Manually commence a process of slowly elongating the muscle fibers (stretching the muscle slowly by separating the ends) while palpating at mid-fiber level for the first sign of tissue resistance (tension).
2. As the muscle fibers are stretched, the first fibers to become taut may be shortened fibers that may house trigger points.
3. As the tissue tension reduces, the tissue may be further stretched, until more taut fibers are felt.
4. The same procedure is used to release these fibers until either the full range of motion is restored or a barrier is met that does not respond to this procedure.

Other Trigger Point Treatment Considerations

- Trigger points frequently occur in "nests." In such cases, three or four repetitions of the protocol may need to be applied to the same area.
- Each time that digital pressure is released, blood flushes into the tissue; this flow brings with it nutrients and oxygen, while removing metabolic waste (Simons et al., 1999).
- The treatment as described in the preceding section is usually followed with several passive elongations (stretches) of the tissue to that tissue's range of motion barrier, unless the attachments present with signs of inflammation.
- The person is then asked to perform at least three or four active repetitions of the stretch, which the patient should be encouraged to continue to do as "homework."

- It is important to avoid excessive treatment at any one session, as a degree of micro-trauma may be inherent in the processes described.
- Residual discomfort, as well as the adaptive demands that this form of therapy imposes on repair functions, calls for treatment to be tailored to the individual's ability to respond—a judgment that the practitioner needs to make. If in doubt, it is better to provide less therapy at one time, even though this approach may slow progress, than to overwhelm the tissues or the person.
- Treatment of the point directly, as described in the preceding subsection, should be followed by range of motion work, as well as by one or more forms of hydrotherapy, such as heat (unless inflamed), ice, contrast hydrotherapy, or a combination of mild heat to the belly and ice to the tendons. Stretches should be performed before any prolonged applications of cold, as the fascia elongates best when warm and more liquid. When cold, the elastic components of muscle and fascia are less pliable and less easily stretched (Klingler, 2011). If tissues are cold, it is helpful to rewarm the area with a hot pack or mild movement therapy before stretches are applied to reduce the patient's perception of pain (Green, 2004).

This description relates to trigger points associated with the center of muscles. A different protocol is used for trigger points close to attachments due to risk of enthesitis if these tissues are irritated.

Summary of NMT (American Version) Application

- A gliding stroke offers feedback and helps to identify local dense tissue that might possibly house a trigger point.
- Assess these tissues for taut bands using pincer compression techniques.
- Assess attachment sites for tenderness, especially where taut bands attach.
- Return to the taut band and find central nodules or localized spot tenderness.
- Elongate the tissue slightly if attachment sites indicate this is appropriate; alternatively, tissue may be placed in neutral or approximated position.
- Compress central trigger points for 8 to 12 seconds (using pincer compression techniques or flat palpation).

- The patient is instructed to exhale as pressure is applied, which often augments the release of the contracture.
- Appropriate pressure should elicit a discomfort scale response in the range of 5 to 7.
- If a response in the tissue begins within 8 to 12 seconds, it can be held for up to 20 seconds.
- Allow the tissue to rest for a brief time.
- Adjust pressure and repeat this process, including application to other taut fibers.
- Passively elongate the fibers.
- Actively stretch the fibers, if appropriate.
- Appropriate hydrotherapies may accompany the procedure.
- Advise the patient about specific procedures that can be used at home to maintain the effects of therapy.

Example of NMT for Temporalis Muscle

The following treatments, whose description is modified from Chaitow (2005), should not be performed if temporal arteritis is suspected. The patient is placed in a supine or side-lying position, and the practitioner uses the first two fingers to apply transverse friction to the entire temporal fossa, a small portion at a time. The fingers begin cephalad to the zygomatic arch and on the most anterior aspect of the rather large tendon of temporalis.

The fingers are moved cephalad to address the most anterior fibers of temporalis. Transverse friction is applied while applying sufficient pressure to feel the vertical fibers or to produce a mid-range discomfort level. The fibers are examined along their entire length to the upper edge of the temporal fossa. Taut fibers identified in association with central and attachment trigger points are treated with static pressure.

The fingers are moved posteriorly over a fingertip width and placed once again on the tendon just above the zygomatic arch. The examination now addresses the next group of fibers in a similar manner. This process is continued throughout the temporal fossa. Because this muscle is fan shaped, the middle fibers lie on a diagonal, while the most posterior fibers are oriented anteroposteriorly over the ear.

The portion of the tendon that lies above the zygomatic arch can be assessed by using transverse friction while the mouth is open or closed. An open-mouth treatment stretches the tendon and requires less pressure than its closed-mouth counterpart. The tendon may also be pressed as the patient actively and slowly shortens and lengthens the tissues under pressure.

With the patient's mouth still open, the practitioner locates the coronoid process, which is the first bone encountered (besides teeth) when moving the finger from the corner of the mouth toward the top of the ear. The mouth is opened as far as possible, which will lower the coronoid process to below the zygomatic arch (unless depression of the mandible is restricted) and make the temporalis tendon available to palpation. Caution must be exercised along the anterior aspect of the coronoid process to avoid compressing the parotid duct against the anterior aspect of the bony surface. This duct may be palpated on most people by using a light cranial/caudal friction approximately midway along the anterior aspect of the coronoid process. Once it is located, the palpating finger is placed cephalad to the parotid duct, so as to avoid contact with it during treatment.

The palpating finger needs to be placed so that it is completely anterior to the masseter and does not press through masseter fibers, as this effect could be wrongly interpreted as temporalis tenderness. Additionally, the practitioner's index finger rests below the zygomatic arch, with its lateral edge touching the inferior surface of the arch and the palpating finger pad "hooked" onto the anterior surface of the coronoid process. The fingernail faces toward the ceiling when the finger is properly placed on the supine patient's face. When the tendon attachment is located, it is often found to be exquisitely tender, such that pressure may need to be reduced significantly. Static pressure may be used or, if the tendon attachment is not too tender, light friction may be applied.

INIT Hypothesis

Clinical experience indicates that by combining the methods of direct inhibition (pressure mildly applied, either continuously or in a make-and-break pattern) (Nimmo, 1992) with the concept of SCS and MET, a specific targeting of dysfunctional soft tissues should be achieved (Chaitow & DeLany, 2003). The INIT hypothesis (Chaitow, 1994) includes the following stages:

- The trigger point is identified by palpation, after which ischemic compression is applied, sufficient for the patient to be able to report that the referred pattern of pain is being activated.
- The preferred sequence after this identification is for that same degree of pressure to be maintained for 5 to 6 seconds, followed by 2 to 3 seconds of release of pressure.
- This pattern is repeated for as long as 2 minutes, or until the patient reports either that the local or

referred symptoms (pain) have been reduced or that the pain has increased; the latter is a rare but significant event sufficient to warrant ceasing application of pressure. See the note later in this section about modification of INIT, in cases of extreme sensitivity (Nimmo, 1992; Schneider, 2001).

- Upon reapplication of pressure during this make-and-break sequence, if reported pain decreases or increases (or if 2 minutes elapses with neither of these changes being reported), the ischemic compression aspect of the INIT treatment ceases.
- A moderate degree of pressure is then reintroduced and whatever level of pain is noted is ascribed a value of 10. The patient is asked to offer feedback information in the form of pain "scores," relative to the reference value of 10, as the area is repositioned according to the guidelines of positional release methodology. A position is sought that reduces reported pain to a score of 3 or less (Rodriguez-Blanco et al., 2006).
- This "position of ease" is held for not less than 20 seconds to allow for (it is presumed) neurologic resetting, reduction in nociceptor activity, and enhanced local circulatory interchange (Chaitow & DeLany, 2003).
- The position of ease will effectively have "folded" the tissues surrounding the trigger point, such that an isometric contraction introduced into these tissues will target the very fibers that subsequently require lengthening. After maintaining the ease position for 20 seconds, an isometric contraction, focused on the musculature around the trigger point, is initiated.
- Next, the tissues are stretched both locally and, where possible, in a manner that involves the whole muscle (usually after a second isometric contraction involving the entire muscle) (Nagrale et al., 2010).
- It is then useful to add a reeducational activation of antagonists to the muscle housing the

trigger point, possibly using Ruddy's rhythmic pulsing methods to complete the treatment (Ruddy, 1961).

Modification

In cases of extreme sensitivity, where central sensitization prevails, the procedure should be modified to eliminate the ischemic compression sequence, and begin instead with the assignment of pain score values.

Summary of INIT Sequence

1. Locate the trigger point.
2. Apply ischemic compression until the level of pain changes.
3. Perform positional release of trigger point tissues.
4. Provide local *focused* isometric contraction of these tissues.
5. Perform local stretching.
6. Contract the whole muscle isometrically.
7. Stretch the whole muscle.
8. Facilitate antagonists.

CONCLUSIONS

Migraine is commonly a result of chronic central sensitization, which is itself encouraged and maintained by areas of peripheral sensitization. Reduction in peripheral sensitized features, such as local instances of painful soft-tissue and articular dysfunction that are feeding into the central pattern, offers the possibility of a degree of desensitization, with the objective being a reduction in symptoms such as those associated with migraine. NMT incorporating a variety of modalities that have been well studied (e.g., muscle energy techniques, neuromuscular technique, positional release technique, myofascial release technique, trigger point release) may be employed as part of a comprehensive protocol to achieve this end.

REFERENCES

Affaitati G, Costantini R, Fabrizio A, et al. Effects of treatment of peripheral pain generators in fibromyalgia patients. *Eur J Pain* 2011;15:61–69.

Astin J. Why patients use alternative medicine: results of a national study. *JAMA* 1998;279:1548–1553.

Atienza-Meseguer A, Fernández-de-las-Peñas C, Navarro-Poza JL, et al. Immediate effects of the strain/counter-strain

technique in local pain evoked by tender points in the upper trapezius muscle. *Clin Chirop* 2006;9:112–118.

Baldry PE. *Acupuncture, Trigger Points and Musculoskeletal Pain.* 3rd ed. Edinburgh: Elsevier-Churchill Livingstone; 2005.

Bender T, Nagy G, Barna I, et al. The effect of physical therapy on beta-endorphin levels. *Eur J Appl Physiol* 2007;100:371–382.

Bialosky J, Bishop M, Price D, et al. The mechanisms of manual therapy in the treatment of musculoskeletal pain: a comprehensive model. *Man Ther* 2009;14:531–538.

Bogduk N. The anatomy of occipital neuralgia. *Clin Exp Neurol* 1981;44:202–208.

Bogduk N, Govind J. Cervicogenic headache: an assessment of the evidence on clinical diagnosis, invasive tests, and treatment. *Lancet Neurol* 2009;8:959–968.

Bono G, Antonaci F, Ghirmai S, et al. The clinical profile of cervicogenic headache as it emerges from a study based on the early diagnostic criteria. *Funct Neurol* 1998;13:75–77.

Bono G, Antonaci F, Ghirmai S, et al. Whiplash injuries: clinical picture and diagnostic work-up. *Clin Exp Rheumatol* 2000;18:S23–S28.

Bradley L. Psychiatric co-morbidity in fibromyalgia. *Curr Pain Headache Rep* 2005;9:79–86.

Buchgreitz L, Lyngberg L, Bendtsen A, et al. Frequency of headache is related to sensitization: a population study. *Pain* 2006;123:19–27.

Burstein R, Yarnitsky D, Goor-Aryeh I, et al. An association between migraine and cutaneous allodynia. *Ann Neurol* 2000;47:614–624.

Calandre EP, Hidalgo J, Garcia-Leiva JM, Rico-Villademoros F. Trigger point evaluation in migraine patients: an indication of peripheral sensitization linked to migraine predisposition? *Eur J Neurol* 2006;13:244–249.

Campbell J, Penzien D, Wall E. Evidenced-based guidelines for migraine headache: behavioral and physical treatments. American Academy of Neurology; 2010. Available at: http://www.siumed.edu/neuro/AAA2010/documents/68.pdf.

Cassidy JD, Lopes AA, Yong-Hink K. The immediate effect of manipulation versus mobilization on pain and range of motion in the cervical spine: a randomized controlled trial. *J Manipulative Physiol Ther* 1992;15:570–575.

Chaitow L. Integrated neuromuscular inhibition technique. *Br J Osteopathy* 1994;13:17–20.

Chaitow L. *Cranial Manipulation: Theory and Practice.* 2nd ed. Edinburgh: Elsevier; 2005.

Chaitow L, ed. *Naturopathic Physical Medicine: Theory and Practice for Manual Therapists and Naturopaths.* Edinburgh: Churchill Livingstone; 2008.

Chaitow L, DeLany J. Neuromuscular techniques in orthopaedics. *Techn Orthopaed* 2003;18:74–86.

Chaitow L, DeLany J. *Clinical Applications of Neuromuscular Techniques. Vol. 1: Upper Body.* 2nd ed. Edinburgh: Churchill Livingstone; 2008.

Ciancaglini R, Testa M, Radaelli G. Association of neck pain with symptoms of temporomandibular dysfunction in the general adult population. *Scand J Rehabil Med* 1999;31:17–22.

Clauw D. Fibromyalgia: update on mechanisms and management. *J Clin Rheumatol* 2007;13:102–109.

Cramer GD, Henderson CN, Little JW, et al. Zygapophyseal joint adhesions after induced hypomobility. *J Manipulative Physiol Ther* 2010;33:508–518.

Crockett HC, Gross LB, Wilk KE, et al. Osseous adaptation and range of motion at the gleno-humeral joint in professional baseball pitchers. *Am J Sports Med* 2002;30:20–26.

Curatolo M, Petersen-Felix S, Arendt-Nielsen L, et al. Central hypersensitivity in chronic pain after whiplash injury. *Clin J Pain* 2001;17:306–315.

Dardzinski JA, Ostrov BE, Hamann LS. Myofascial pain unresponsive to standard treatment: successful use of a strain and counter-strain technique with physical therapy. *J Clin Rheumatol* 2000;6:169–174.

Degenhardt B, Nissar A, Johnson J, Towns L. Role of osteopathic manipulative treatment in altering pain biomarkers: a pilot study. *J Am Osteopath Assoc* 2011;107:387–400.

de Tommaso M, Guido M, Libro G, et al. Abnormal brain processing of cutaneous pain in migraine patients during the attack. *Neurosci Lett* 2002;333:29–32.

Dommerholt J. Posture. In: Tubiana R, Amadio P, eds. *Medical Problems of the Instrumentalist Musician.* London: Martin Dunitz; 2000:399–419.

Dommerholt J. Performing arts medicine – Instrumentalist musicians: part III – Case histories. *J Bodywork Mov Ther* 2010;14:127–138.

Dworkin S, LeResche L. Assessing clinical signs of temporomandibular disorders. *J Prosthet Dent* 1991;63:574–579.

Edeling J. Manual therapy rounds: cervicogenic, tension-type headache with migraine: a case study. *J Man Manipulative Ther* 1997;5:33–38.

Fall M, Baranowski AP, Elneil S, et al. EAU guidelines on chronic pelvic pain. *Eur Urol* 2010;57:35–48.

Feland JB, Myrer JW, Schulthies SS, et al. The effect of duration of stretching of the hamstring muscle group for increasing range of motion in people aged 65 years or older. *Phys Ther* 2001;81:1100–1117.

Ferber R, Osternig LR, Gravelle DC. Effect of PNF stretch techniques on knee flexor muscle EMG activity in older adults. *J Electrom Kinesiol* 2002;12:391–397.

Fernandez-Carnero J, Fernández-de-Las-Peñas C, de la Llave-Rincon AI, et al. Widespread mechanical pain hypersensitivity as sign of central sensitization in unilateral epicondylalgia: a blinded, controlled study. *Clin J Pain* 2009;25:555–561.

Fernández-de-las-Peñas C, Alonso-Blanco C, Cuadrado ML, et al. Trigger points in the suboccipital muscles and forward head posture in tension type headache. *Headache* 2006a;46:454–460.

Fernández-de-las-Peñas C, Cuadrado ML, Pareja JA. Myofascial trigger points, neck mobility and forward head posture in unilateral migraine. *Cephalalgia* 2006b;26:1061–1070.

Fernández-de-las-Peñas C, Arendt-Nielsen L, Gerwin RD, eds. *Tension Type and Cervicogenic Headache: Patho-physiology, Diagnosis and Treatment.* Sudbury, MA: Jones & Bartlett Learning; 2010a.

Fernández-de-las-Peñas C, Galán-del-Río F, Alonso-Blanco C, et al. Referred pain from muscle trigger points in the masticatory and neck–shoulder musculature in women with temporomandibular disorders. *J Pain* 2010b;11:1295–1304.

Filatova E, Latysheva N, Kurenkov A. Evidence of persistent central sensitization in chronic headaches: a multi-method study. *J Headache Pain* 2008;9:295–300.

FitzGerald MP, Anderson RU, Potts J, et al. Randomized multicenter feasibility trial of myofascial physical therapy for the treatment of urological chronic pelvic pain syndromes. *J Urology* 2009;82:570–580.

Freeman MD, Nystrom A, Centeno C. Chronic whiplash and central sensitization: an evaluation of the role of a myofascial trigger points in pain modulation. *J Brachial Plex Peripher Nerve Inj* 2009;4:2.

Furman J, Jacob R. A clinical taxonomy of dizziness and anxiety in the oto-neurological setting. *J Anxiety Disord* 2001;15:9–26.

Galletti F, Cupini LM, Corbelli I, et al. Pathophysiological basis of migraine prophylaxis. *Prog Neurobiol* 2009;89:176–192.

Giamberardino MA, Tafuri E, Savini A, et al. Contribution of myofascial trigger points to migraine symptoms. *J Pain* 2007;8:869–878.

Goslin RE, Gray RN, McCrory DCD, et al. Behavioral and physical treatments for migraine headache. *Tech Rev* 1999;2:2.

Greco R, Gasperi V, Maccarrone M, et al. The endocannabinoid system and migraine. *Exp Neurol* 2010;224:85–91.

Green BG. Temperature perception and nociception. *J Neurobiol* 2004;61:13–29.

Haldeman S, Dagenais S. Cervicogenic headaches. *Spine* 2001;1:31–46.

Haugstadt GK, Haugstad TS, Kirste UM. Posture, movement patterns, and body awareness in women with chronic pelvic pain. *J Psychosom Res* 2006;61:637–644.

Herzog J. Use of cervical spine manipulation under anesthesia for management of cervical disk herniation, cervical radiculopathy, and associated cervicogenic headache syndrome. *J Manipulative Physiol Ther* 1999;22:166–170.

Hidalgo-Lozano A, Fernández-de-las-Peñas C, Alonso-Blanco C, et al. Muscle trigger points and pressure pain hyperalgesia in the shoulder muscles in patients with unilateral shoulder impingement: a blinded, controlled study. *Exp Brain Res* 2010;202:915–925.

Hyde T, Gengenbach M. *Conservative Management of Sports Injuries.* Sudbury, MA: Jones and Bartlett; 2007.

Ibáñez-García J, Alburquerque-Sendín F, Rodríguez-Blanco C, et al. Changes in masseter muscle trigger points following strain-counter/strain or neuro-muscular technique. *J Bodywork Mov Ther* 2009;13:2–10.

Ifergane G, Buskila D, Simiseshvely N, et al. Prevalence of fibromyalgia syndrome in migraine patients. *Cephalalgia* 2006;26:451–456.

Ismail F, Demling A, Hessling K, et al. Short-term efficacy of physical therapy compared to splint therapy in treatment of arthrogenous TMD. *J Oral Rehabil* 2007;34:807–813.

Kamani H, Walters N. Muscle energy technique. The effect on joint mobility and agonist/antagonist muscle activity. Presented at the 2nd International Conference on Advances in Osteopathic Research (ICAOR); The Law Society, London; 2000.

Klingler W. Temperature effects on fascia. In: Schleip R, Huijing P, Findley T, Chaitow L, eds. *Fascia in Manual and Movement Therapies.* London: Elsevier; in press.

Kobesova A, Morris CE, Lewit K, et al. 20-year-old pathogenic "active" postsurgical scar: a case study of a patient with persistent right lower quadrant pain. *J Manipulative Physiol Ther* 2007;30:234–238.

Lavelle ED, Lavelle W, Smith H. Trigger points. *Med Clin North Am* 2007;91:353–361.

Lawler S, Cameron L. A randomized, controlled trial of massage therapy as a treatment for migraine. *Ann Behav Med* 2006;32:50–59.

Lenehan K, Fryer G, McLaughlin P. Effect of MET on gross trunk range of motion. *J Osteopathic Med* 2003;6:13–18.

Lewis T, Flynn C. Use of strain–counter-strain in treatment of patients with low back pain. *J Man Manipul Ther* 2001; 9:92–98.

Lewit K. *Manipulative Therapy: Musculoskeletal Medicine.* Edinburgh: Churchill Livingstone; 2009.

Lewit K, Olsanska S. Clinical importance of active scars: abnormal scars as a cause of myofascial pain. *J Manipulative Physiol Ther* 2004;27:399–402.

Liebenson C. *Rehabilitation of the Spine: A Practitioner's Manual.* 2nd ed. Philadelphia: Lippincott Williams & Wilkins; 2007.

McKinnon S. Pathophysiology of nerve compression. *Hand Clin* 2002;18:231–241.

McPartland JM, Giuffrida A, King J, et al. Cannabimimetic effects of osteopathic manipulative treatment. *J Am Osteopath Assoc* 2005;105:283–291.

Mense S, Simons DG, Russell IJ. *Muscle Pain: Understanding Its Nature, Diagnosis, and Treatment.* Baltimore: Lippincott Williams & Wilkins; 2001.

Moore M. Upper crossed syndrome and its relationship to cervicogenic headache. *J Manipulative Physiol Ther* 2004; 27:414–420.

Nagrale A, Glynn P, Joshi A, Ramteke G. Efficacy of an integrated neuromuscular inhibition technique on upper trapezius trigger points in subjects with non-specific neck pain: a randomized controlled trial. *J Man Manipul Ther* 2010;18:38–44.

Nies A. Principles of therapeutics. In: Gilman AG, Rall TW, Nies AS, Taylor P, eds. *Goodman and Gilman's: The Pharmacological Basis of Therapeutics.* 8th ed. New York: Pergamon Press; 1990:62–83.

Nijs J, Van Houdenhove B. From acute musculoskeletal pain to chronic widespread pain and fibromyalgia: application of pain neurophysiology in manual therapy practice. *Man Ther* 2009;14:3–12.

Nijs J, Van Houdenhove B, Oostendorp R. Recognition of central sensitization in patients with musculoskeletal pain: application of pain neurophysiology in manual therapy practice. *Man Ther* 2010;15:135–141.

Nimmo RL. *The Receptor–Tonus Method.* Pasedena, TX: Texas Chiropractic College; 1992.

O'Neill S, Manniche C, Graven-Nielsen T, Arendt-Nielsen L. Generalized deep tissue hyperalgesia in patients with chronic low-back pain. *Eur J Pain* 2007;11:415–420.

O'Sullivan P, Beales D. Changes in pelvic floor and diaphragm kinematics and respiratory patterns in subjects with sacroiliac joint pain following a motor learning intervention: a case series. *Man Ther* 2007;12:209–218.

Palmer D. Comparison of a muscle energy technique and neuro-muscular technique on quadriceps muscle strength. 2002. Available at: http://www.osteopathic-research.com/cgi-bin/or/Search1.pl?show_one=30704.

Patel P. Comparison of neuromuscular technique and a muscle energy technique on cervical range of motion. 2002. Available at: http://www.osteopathic-research.com/cgi-bin/or/Search1.pl?show_one=30175.

Pearce J. Cervicogenic headache: an early description. *J Neurol Neurosurg Psych* 1995;58:698.

Pham K, Gupta R. Understanding the mechanisms of entrapment neuropathies. *Neurosurg* 2009;26:E7.

Pluess M, Conrad A, Wilhelm FH. Muscle tension in generalized anxiety disorder: a critical review of the literature. *J Anxiety Dis* 2009;23:1–11.

Pohl H. Changes in structure of collagen distribution in the skin caused by a manual technique. *J Bodywork Mov Ther* 2010;14:27–34.

Quinn C, Chandler C, Moraska A. Massage therapy and frequency of chronic tension headaches. *Am J Public Health* 2002;92:1657–1661.

Rice G. The effect of a NMT to the diaphragm on cervical range of motion. 2002. Available at: http://www.osteopathic-research.com/cgi-bin/or/Search1.pl?show_one=30707.

Robb A, Pajaczkowski J. Prospective investigation on hip adductor strains using myofascial release. In: Huijing PA, Hollander P, Findley TW, Schleip R, eds. *Fascia Research II*. Munich: Elsevier; 2009:96.

Rodriguez-Blanco C, Fernández-de-las-Peñas C, Xumet J, et al. Changes in active mouth opening following a single treatment of latent myofascial trigger points in the masseter muscle involving post-isometric relaxation or strain/counter-strain. *J Bodywork Mov Ther* 2006;10:197–205.

Ruddy T. Osteopathic rhythmic resistive duction therapy. In: *Yearbook of Academy of Applied Osteopathy 1961*. Indianapolis, IN: Academy of Applied Osteopathy; 1961:58.

Schamberger W. *The Malalignment Syndrome*. Edinburgh; Churchill Livingstone; 2002.

Schneider M. *The Collected Writings of Nimmo and Vannerson: Pioneers of Chiropractic Trigger Point Therapy*. Pittsburgh, PA: Michael Schneider; 2001.

Selye H. *The Stress of Life*. New York: McGraw-Hill; 1984.

Shah JP, Phillips TM, Danoff JV, Gerber LH. An in vivo microanalytical technique for measuring the local biochemical milieu of human skeletal muscle. *J Appl Physiol* 2005;99:1977–1984.

Sikdar S, Shah J, Gilliams E, et al. Assessment of myofascial trigger points (MTrP): a new application of ultrasound imaging and vibration sonoelastography. 30th Annual International IEEE EMBS Conference; Vancouver, Canada; 2008.

Simons D. New views of myofascial trigger points: etiology and diagnosis. *Arch Phys Med Rehabil* 2008;89:157–159.

Simons D, Travell J, Simons L. *Myofascial Pain and Dysfunction: The Trigger Point Manual*. Vol 1. 2nd ed. Baltimore, MD: Williams & Wilkins; 1999.

Sjaastad O, Fredriksen TA, Pfaffenrath V. Cervicogenic headache: diagnostic criteria. *Headache* 1990;301:725–726.

Srbely J, Dickey J, Bent L, et al. Capsaicin-induced central sensitization evokes segmental increases in trigger point sensitivity in humans. *J Pain* 2010;11:636–643.

Staud R. Biology and therapy of fibromyalgia: pain in fibromyalgia syndrome. *Arthritis Res Ther* 2006;8:208.

Sterling M, Jull G, Vicenzino B, Kenardy J. Characterization of acute whiplash associated disorders. *Spine* 2004;29:182–188.

Timmons B, Ley R, eds. *Behavioral and Psychological Approaches to Breathing Disorders*. New York: Plenum Press; 1994.

Tomlinson K. Comparison of neuromuscular technique and muscle energy technique on dorsiflexion range of motion. 2002. Available at: http://www.osteopathic-research.com/cgibin/or/Search1.pl?show_one=30795.

Travell JG, Simons DG. *Myofascial Pain and Dysfunction: The Trigger Point Manual*. Vol. 1. Baltimore: Williams and Wilkins; 1992.

Trescot A. Headache management in an interventional pain practice. *Pain Phys* 2000;3:197–200.

Valouchová P, Lewit K. Surface electromyography of abdominal and back muscles in patients with active scar. *J Bodywork Mov Ther* 2009;13:262–267.

Vierck C Jr. Mechanisms underlying development of spatially distributed chronic pain (fibromyalgia). *Pain* 2006;124:242–263.

Vleeming A, Volkers ACW, Snijders C, Stoeckart R. Relation between form and function in the sacroiliac joint. Part 2: biomechanical aspects. *Spine* 1990;15:133–136.

Ward RC. Myofascial release concepts. In: Basmajian JV, Nyberg R, eds. *Rational Manual Therapy*. Baltimore: Williams and Wilkins; 1993:223–242.

Weissman-Fogel I, Sprecher E, Granovsky Y, et al. Repeated noxious stimulation of the skin enhances cutaneous perception of migraine patients in-between attacks: clinical evidence for cutaneous sub-threshold increase in membrane excitability of central, trigeminovascular neurons. *Pain* 2003;104:693–700.

Wilson A. *Effective Management of Musculoskeletal Injury*. Edinburgh: Churchill Livingstone; 2002.

Wilson E, Payton O, Donegan-Shoaf L, Dec K. Muscle energy technique in patients with acute low back pain: a pilot clinical trial. *J Orthop Sports Phys Ther* 2003;33:502–512.

Wiltink J, Tschan R, Michal M, et al. Dizziness: anxiety, health care utilization and health behavior. *J Psychosom Res* 2009;66:417–424.

Woolf CJ. Central sensitization: implications for the diagnosis and treatment of pain. *Pain* 2011;152:S2–S15.

Xiong G, Matsushita M. Upper cervical afferents to the motor trigeminal nucleus and the subnucleus oralis of the spinal trigeminal nucleus in the rat: an anterograde and retrograde tracing study. *Neurosci Lett* 2000;286:127–130.

Xu YM, Ge HY, Arendt-Nielsen. Sustained nociceptive mechanical stimulation of latent myofascial trigger point induces central sensitization in healthy subjects. *J Pain* 2010;11:1348–1355.

Yamada K, Moriwaki K, Oiso H. High prevalence of comorbidity of migraine in outpatients with panic disorder and effectiveness of psychopharmacotherapy for both disorders: a retrospective open label study. *Psychiatry Res* 2011;185:145–148.

Yin CS, Lee YJ, Lee YJ. Neurological influences of the temporomandibular joint. *J Bodywork Mov Ther* 2007;11:285–294.

Young J. Pain and traumatic brain injury. *Med Rehabil Clin N Am* 2007;18:145–163.

Yunus M. Fibromyalgia and overlapping disorders: the unifying concept of central sensitivity syndromes. *Semin Arthritis Rheum* 2007a;36:330–356.

Yunus MB. Role of central sensitization in symptoms beyond muscle pain, and the evaluation of a patient with widespread pain. *Best Pract Res Clin Rheumatol* 2007b;21:481–497.

Zito G, Jull G, Story I. Clinical tests of musculoskeletal dysfunction in the diagnosis of cervicogenic headache. *Man Ther* 2006;11:118–129.

Zwart J. Neck mobility in different headache disorders. *Headache* 1997;37:6–11.

Neuromusculoskeletal Assessment and Management in Pediatric Migraine

Michiel Trouw, PT, MT (OMT), and Harry Von Piekartz, PT, MSc, PhD

INTRODUCTION

The incidence of headache that may be classified under the label "pediatric migraine" is increasing (Abu-Arefeh & Russel, 1994; Göbel, 2004) and appears to have a significant influence on the quality of life of children, as is the case with such chronic complaints as arthritis and cancer (Hershey, 2010). Nonetheless, pediatric migraine is a specific form of migraine that is studied much less frequently than migraine in the adult population. Bigal and Arruda (2010) concluded that pediatric migraine occurs in the various age phases in children, and not just after puberty. In addition to the significant inconvenience to the child experiencing the headache, this condition often has a marked influence on the family of the child in question (Menkes, 1974; Galli et al., 2009). It would appear useful to view such an illness as migraine in the group of children in which it begins at an early age, as this perspective might possibly yield more information about the pathobiological mechanism of the condition (Bigal & Arruda, 2010). Recent studies have shown that early recognition and treatment of children with primary headache is useful and may prevent the condition from becoming chronic (Fendrich et al., 2007; Hershey, 2010).

EPIDEMIOLOGY

The average age for the onset of pediatric migraine is 7 years in boys and 11 year in girls (Lewis, 2004). The prevalence of this condition increases as children grow older. In a recent epidemiologic study in Turkey involving 2,669 children, 46.2% of the children between 5 and 13 years of age stated that headache caused significant daily limitations. According to the criteria established in the *International Classification of Headache Disorders* of 2004 (ICHD-II), 3.4% of these children had migraine and another 8.7% had probable migraine (Isik et al., 2009). An Italian study showed that 40% of 4,836 children in an 11- to 15-year-old age cohort had headache at least once a week (Santinello et al., 2009). Hershey (2010) arrived at much the same figures by examining various epidemiologic studies carried out in Thailand, Germany, and Taiwan. Readers are referred to Chapter 13 for more data on this topic.

CLASSIFICATION

As a rule, the diagnosis of migraine is mainly established based on the subjective examination (Lee & Olness, 1997; Virtanen et al., 2007) and against the background of ICHD-II, which is the most commonly used classification. This classification differentiates between primary and secondary forms of headache and has a hierarchical structure. In ICHD-II, migraine is subdivided into different subgroups. In the context of this chapter, we will not discuss these divisions further (see Chapter 13 of this textbook for more information). At the classification of 2004, the International Headache Society (IHS) considered the specific picture of pediatric migraine by adapting a number of factors to it (**Table 18.1**).

The greatest difference between the ICHD-II criteria for children and those for adults is the minimal duration of an attack—1 hour for children and 4 hours or longer in adults. The supplementary memo to ICHD-II also states that migraine is often bilateral in children, and is usually localized frontotemporally with photophobia and phonophobia. These classification criteria mean that a population of children is most likely being excluded from epidemiologic studies due to the fact that attacks lasting less than 1 hour (when untreated) are not included. In children who, at the time of history taking, have not yet had five attacks consistent with the described criteria, the type of headache is classified as probable migraine (Göbel, 2004). Therefore, the numbers of children who have migraine may have been significantly underestimated by adhering to the criteria in the ICHD-II (Bigal & Arruda, 2010).

The ICHD-II has a better sensitivity than its predecessor criteria (ICHD-I), but was revealed to have moderate specificity (53% to 77%) in a study with children and adults

Table 18.1 Criteria for Migraine Without Aura and Pediatric Migraine Without Aura

1.1 Migraine Without Aura	1.1 Pediatric Migraine Without Aura
A. At least five attacks fulfilling criteria B–D	
B. Headache attacks lasting 4–72 hours (untreated or unsuccessfully treated)	Attacks may last 1–72 hours.
C. Headache has at least two of the following characteristics: 1. Unilateral location 2. Pulsating quality 3. Moderate or severe pain intensity 4. Aggravation by or causing avoidance of routine physical activity (e.g., walking or climbing stairs)	Migraine headache is commonly bilateral in young children; the adult pattern of unilateral pain usually emerges in late adolescence or early adult life.
D. During headache at least one of the following: 1. Nausea and/or vomiting 2. Photophobia and phonophobia	In young children, photophobia and phonophobia may be inferred from their behavior.
E. Not attributed to another disorder	

Source: ICHD-II, 2004.

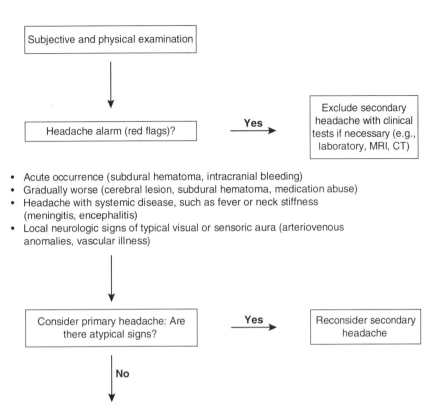

Figure 18.1 Pediatric Headache and Red Flags Algorithm

with migraine (Lima et al., 2005). These criteria have, indeed, been adapted for children, but the system still raises questions because classification does not seem to screen all pediatric migrainous headaches. The question, therefore, is whether the known pathophysiological models for migraine and the possible contributing factors in pediatric headache are always as clear as described in the literature. According to Hershey (2010), more investigation is necessary to arrive at better markers for the recognition of pediatric migraine because the symptoms are often so variable, and because contributing factors frequently play a role in recurrent pediatric migraine. **Figure 18.1** shows an algorithm for the diagnosis of pediatric headache.

CLINICAL PRESENTATION OF PEDIATRIC MIGRAINE WITH OVERLAPPING SECONDARY HEADACHE FORMS

As previously stated, symptoms of pediatric migraine are not always as clear-cut as the ICHD-II has described. Often, the patient experiences a mixture of the primary headache (classic pediatric headache) and the secondary

forms that are determined, for example, by an indirect cause or an indirect mechanism triggering the headache (Überall, 1999). Thus these forms are more difficult to classify with the ICHD-II.

Frequently, children who are diagnosed as having pediatric migraine are also known to have a previous history of other complaints (Pothmann et al., 1994; Biedermann, 2004). The clinician may observe that other complaints—such as otitis media, sinusitis maxillaris, and dysfunctions of the masticatory system and the craniocervical region—can influence symptoms of migraine or other forms of headache. These dysfunctions can be a contributing factor in the occurrence or the continuation of the recurrent pediatric headache.

We can hypothesize that headache in children often comprises a mixture of primary and secondary headaches, and that the functional complaints may not all be accounted within the ICHD-II. The clinician must understand that the etiology is frequently not 100% clear and must assume a multicausal model. With this background, pain and its behavior can be pinpointed more clearly and be given a place in the context of the child.

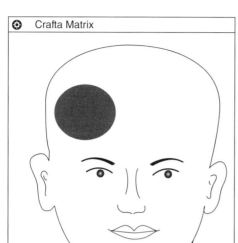
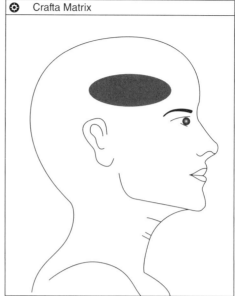

Figure 18.2 Bodychart of the Head for Assessing Headache Pain Pattern (Crafta©)

The most important characteristic of this mixed headache form is its recurrent nature. Although pain can vary considerably in terms of character, most of the attacks are between 1 and 6 hours in duration (Rothner, 2001). A typical location for the headache is frontal and temporal (**Figure 18.2**), although children younger than age 5 years sometimes report their headache to be in the abdominal region (McGrath, 2001; Von Piekartz, 2005). Those younger than 12 to 14 years often describe the pain as pressure, whereas after this age pain is usually described as pulsating (Lütschg, 2009). Other qualities and localizations are also conceivable.

Caution is necessary in these patients owing to the frequent similarities in pain symptoms for the various forms of headache (migraine versus tension-type headache). The clinician must differentiate any "red flags," as they may indicate serious pathology, before proceeding further with the neuromusculoskeletal examination (**Table 18.2**).

CONTRIBUTING FACTORS

Based on the current literature, one may cautiously conclude that most headaches in children are diagnosed as pediatric migraine and treated with medication. The percentage of chronification of diagnosed migraine is high; thus it appears that medication alone does not always prove to be successful treatment (Rothner, 2001). Contributing

factors may potentially play a role in the increasing chronification of pediatric headache (**Table 18.3**). The literature indicates that a connection may exist among genetic, emotional, psychological, hormonal, and environmental factors in the development of pediatric headache. Moreover, neuromusculoskeletal changes have been cited by several authors in connection with migraine (Vernon et al., 1992; Watson & Trott, 1993; Marcus et al., 1999; Fernández-de-las-Peñas et al., 2006; Von Piekartz et al., 2007).

Table 18.2 Red Flags for Pediatric Headache

Red Flag	Possible Pathology
Sudden onset	• Subdural hematoma • Intracranial bleeding
Gradual worsening	• Cerebral lesion • Subdural hematoma • Medicine abuse
Headache with general signs of illness such as: • Fever • Neck stiffness	• Meningitis • Encephalitis
Local neurologic signs or typical visual/sensory aura	• Arteriovenous anomalies • Vascular disease

Source: Based on Lewis, 2004.

Table 18.3 Possible Contributing Factors to Pediatric Headache

Past history
Emotional and psychological factors
Acquired factors
Lifestyle
Factors from the locomotor system
Growth

Source: Based on Von Piekartz, 2007.

Past History

Children with parents who have recurrent headache appear to have a greater chance of developing headache themselves. If only one parent has headache, the prevalence of pediatric headache rises to 64%; if both parents have this condition, however, pediatric prevalence is reported to be 98% (Messinger et al., 1991). Additionally, sleeping problems, poor general health, and metabolic problems will result in a higher chance of developing headache (Aromaa et al., 1998).

Emotional and Psychological Influences

An increased stress or fear condition, irritation, and perfectionism can play a role in the emotional and psychological side of the child (Andrasik et al., 1998). In addition, a school situation where a great deal of pressure or stress is experienced may be a contributing factor (Pothmann et al., 1994).

Acquired Factors

Acquired factors encompass those factors related to a certain environment and family composition. Thus they might include the quality of the air in a room, the food, as well as the relationships within a family (Joffe et al., 1983; Andrasik et al., 1998; Überall, 1999).

Lifestyle

Factors such as little sleep, brief sleepiness during the day, and restless sleeping can be contributing or maintaining factors for headache in both adults and children (Bruni et al., 1997; Paiva et al., 1997; Feikema, 1999). Parafunctions in the orofacial area, such as tongue biting, cheek biting, lip sucking, nail biting, or tooth grinding and clamping may also be contributing factors in children with headache (Molina et al., 2001). In addition, drinking little or too much coffee or cola has been suggested by Feikema (1999) as a possible factor in the development of headache.

Factors Related to the Musculoskeletal System

Based on the literature and our own clinical experiences, it appears that the musculoskeletal system can be a contributing factor in recurrent pediatric headache (Biedermann, 1999; Von Piekartz et al., 2007). It is, however, important that all such identified dysfunctions be assessed in relation to the pain symptoms of the child. The symptoms and dysfunctions must have a clear connection with the complaints reported by the child (as discussed later in this chapter).

Growth

Two contributing factors are mentioned in the context of growth. First, juvenile headaches, especially migraine, can be accompanied by growth-dependent changes within the neurobiological process in the brain. This effect becomes apparent if the response to a repeated stimulus is too strong or lasts for too long. Habituation is protection from overstimulation of the brain, but often does not act adequately in children and may produce (vascular) headache (Siniatchin et al., 2000). Second, reduced brain expansion, increased intracranial volume, and increased intracranial pressure can be caused by a (minimal) deformed skull or cranio-synosthosis (Agrawal et al., 1992). Researchers have reported that the first symptoms of minimal long-term increased brain pressure are headache, sensorimotor deficits, and intellectual retardation, which are usually reversible if treated (Biedermann, 2004; Von Piekartz et al., 2007).

WHY NEUROMUSCULOSKELETAL EXAMINATION IS USEFUL IN PEDIATRIC MIGRAINE

Experimental and neurobiological studies of the last decade confirm the hypothesis that the trigeminal nucleus caudalis plays a significant role in the physiology and blood supply of the head (see Chapter 5). The expression of pain in primary headaches is associated with activity in intracranial perivascular sensory nerve fibers, which originate in the trigeminal ganglion and project to the trigeminocervical complex in the brainstem (Liu et al., 2009). The trigeminal nucleus caudalis is the region of the brainstem where the pars caudalis of the trigeminal nerve connects to the gray matter of the spinal marrow.

Here, the trigeminal nerve tracks have an anatomic connection with the upper three cervical spinal nerves. The transition of the trigeminal nerve nucleus spinalis to the gray matter of the spinal marrow is so strong that no differentiation can be made based on cell structure (Bogduk, 1988). The nucleus proprius of the cervical gray matter and the trigeminal nucleus found in this location serve as the main centers for the transmission of nociceptive information (Bogduk, 1988). As shown by Busch et al. (2006), reduction of sensory input from the cervical region in humans inhibits the nociceptive transmission in the ophthalmic nerve. After a blockade in the greater occipital nerve, for instance, the nociceptive blink reflex is decreased (Busch et al., 2006). These findings support the hypothesis proposing the existence of functional connectivity between trigeminal and upper cervical afferent pathways in humans (Liu et al., 2009).

Thus a strong connection links the trigeminal nerve with the highest three spinal nerves that innervate the upper cervical spinal column. In particular, the ophthalmic nerve is strongly represented in this trigeminal nucleus caudalis. This concept fits with the frequently mentioned clinical picture of a cervical headache (Hall et al., 2010) but also represents the region where migrainous headache, with the secondary-order neurons, via convergence of afferent signals at this level, can pass on information from both the trigeminal nerve and the upper three peripheral nerves to the third-order neurons in the hypothalamus and thalamus. Subcortical nuclei, such as those found in the thalamus, hypothalamus, and amygdala, have a strong neuro-vegetative function (blood flow regulation), but also play a significant role in pain modulation through an inhibitory and excitatory regulatory system via the production of serotonin (Nelson, 1994; Holland., 2009).

We propose that because of the strong neural innervation, the influence upon the autonomic nervous system, the connection with the trigeminocervical nucleus caudalis, and the craniofacial region including the dura mater and the connective tissue membrane falx cerebelli and tentorium cerebelli of the still-growing child (Shah & Kalra, 2009), there are many good reasons to carry out a neuromusculoskeletal examination in a child suspected of having migraine. Furthermore, it is useful to pay attention to these regions during such an examination, with the underlying thought of reducing the (long-term) nociceptive influence that may be a contributing factor in children with a diagnosis of migraine.

In fact, studies looking at changes in the neuromusculoskeletal system in headache in general and in migraine confirm this hypothesis. Watson and Trott (1993), for example, were able to reproduce signs and symptoms of headache during passive intervertebral movements in the upper cervical spine in a headache population, but not in healthy subjects. Fernández-de-las-Peñas et al. (2006) found that active trigger points in the craniofacial musculature can also play a role in the occurrence of migraine. A recent study revealed that trigger points in the cranium and in the cervical spinal column are strongly related to migraine symptoms (Giamberardino et al., 2007).

The craniofacial structures can be deformed through stress and have a strong innervation and a significant projection onto the somatosensory cortex (Levine et al., 1998). The reaction to this deformation through external force has been established as being able to cause increased nociception (Heisley & Adams, 1993; Oleski et al., 2002). In clinical practice, the pattern of (minimal) skull deformities in the growth phase associated with headache and neuromuscu-loskeletal dysfunctions is not uncommon (Koenen, 2009).

Certainly in children, in whom the cranium adjusts very significantly during the growth phase, it is quite conceivable that this process might influence, among other things, the dura and the cranium (Levine et al., 1998). This supposition has not been scientifically confirmed, however.

NEUROMUSCULOSKELETAL EXAMINATION IN PEDIATRIC MIGRAINE

Most outcome instruments are not adequate for the assessment of the neuromusculoskeletal system. Nonetheless, based on the recognition of the clinical pattern and the inventory of any associated factors, the systematic use of such instruments before, during, and after treatment can be a significant tool for making clinical decisions. This section describes the main outcome instruments and neuro-orthopaedic tests that can be easily used in daily clinical practice to obtain an impression of the pediatric patient with headache.

Colored Analogue Scale

The colored analogue scale (CAS; **Figure 18.3**) can be easily used to measure pain in children (McGrath & Koster, 2001). McGrath et al. (1996) indicated that the visual analogue scale (VAS) is also valid and reliable for the measurement of pain in children. These researchers were able to show that the facial affective scale (FAS) and CAS have similar characteristics as the VAS. Hicks et al. (2001) showed that there is a strong positive correlation in terms of validity for the FAS ($r = 0.93$) with the VAS for children between 5 and 12 years of age and the CAS. The VAS is a responsive instrument that can measure the change in time as well (Carlsson, 1983). The minimal clinically significant difference (MCSD) was

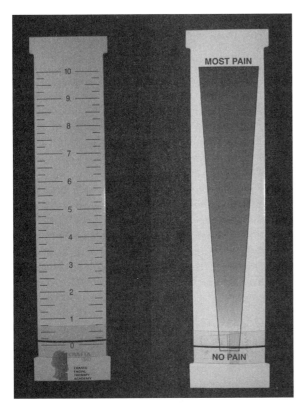

Figure 18.3 Numerical Analogue Scale (left) and Colored Analogue Scale (right) for Assessing the Intensity of Headache

found to be 10 mm (95% CI: 7–12 mm) for children with acute pain on the VAS (Powell et al., 2001).

In a study by Mönch-Tegeder and Von Piekartz (in press), pain intensity was assessed by a CAS in children with migraine (as classified by the ICHD-II guideline; $n = 32$) in comparison to a control group ($n = 45$). A significant difference ($P = 0.026$) was observed between CAS scores for the migraine group (mean: 3.25; SD: 1.27) and the control group (mean: 1.75; SD: 1.27).

Algometer

The algometer allows the clinician to easily establish the pressure-pain threshold and tolerance of different tissues of the head-neck region. The child is asked to indicate to the clinician when the pressure, which gradually increases, is experienced as pain. It is important to clearly explain to the child what level of pain is wanted. This instrument has been extensively used in studies involving headache patients (Jensen et al., 1988; Sandrini et al., 1994; Fernández-de-las-Peñas et al., 2010). It has reasonable inter-tester and good intra-tester reliability when applied to individuals with orofacial pain (Farella et al., 2000; Chaves et al., 2007). When Mönch-Tegeder and Von Piekartz (in press) assessed pressure-pain thresholds in 32 children with migraine, they found that children with pediatric migraine exhibited lower pressure-pain thresholds in the upper trapezius muscles (left: $P = 0.034$; right: $P = 0.027$) as compared to healthy children (**Table 18.4**).

The Craniocervical Angle

Postural changes occur more frequently in people with headache (Marcus et al., 1999) and they can play a role in the maintenance of symptoms. The craniocervical angle is the most commonly used method of assessing forward head posture (**Figure 18.4**). It is measured by drawing a line from the tragus of the ear to the dorsal aspect of the spinous process of C7 vertebra, and then measuring this line in terms of an angle with the horizontal line (Raine & Twomey, 1997). This can be done in the classic manner by measuring with a goniometer on a printed photo with specified reference points; alternatively, the clinician can use the Crafta clinimetry program, whereby the photo is measured in a clinimetry computer program. The reliability of the classic assessment of the craniocervical angle (Watson & Trott, 1993) is as high as the reliability

Table 18.4 Pressure-Pain Thresholds in Children with Migraine

Muscle	Children with Migraine	Control Group	P Value
Upper trapezius left	2.5 (0.75)	3.7 (0.65)	0.021
Upper trapezius right	2.5 (0.61)	3.6 (0.45)	0.033
Rectus capitis left	3.1 (0.85)	3.2 (0.72)	0.223
Rectus capitis right	3.2 (0.90)	3.3 (0.54)	0.532
Temporalis left	3.8 (0.85)	4.3 (0.42)	0.032
Temporalis right	3.6 (0.76)	4.6 (0.34)	0.039
Masseter left	2.3 (0.58)	3.9 (0.45)	0.013
Masseter right	2.3 (0.53)	3.8 (0.54)	0.026

Source: Mönch-Tegeder & Von Piekartz, in press.

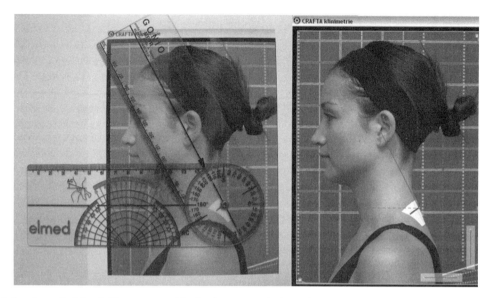

Figure 18.4 Craniocervical Angle Measurement Via Goniometer and Via Crafta© Clinimetry Program

of assessment with the Crafta clinimetric program (Knust et al., in press). A lower craniocervical angle suggests a greater forward head posture, which has been associated with an increased activity of deep-dorsal muscles and inhibition of the deep flexors (Briggs et al., 2004), and with lower pressure-pain thresholds (La Touche et al., 2011).

Watson and Trott (1993) and Fernández-de-las-Peñas et al. (2006) found a connection between migraine and a smaller craniocervical angle. In a recent study by Mönch-Tegeder and Von Piekartz (in press), it was demonstrated that in a sample of children with migraine (*n* = 32) the craniocervical angle was clearly steeper than in the studies conducted by Watson and Trott (1993) and Fernández-de-las-Peñas et al. (2006) in adults. **Table 18.5** shows an overview of the craniocervical angle in different headaches and at various ages.

Cervical Range of Motion

Cervical mobility can be measured with a goniometer that assesses cervical range of motion (CROM).

This device typically consists of a head-mounted set of glasses with one gravity-based inclinometer in front to measure lateral flexion, and another at the side to measure flexion-extension. An added goniometer with a compass point is used for rotation by placing magnets (north–south) on the patients' neck and clavicles. This applies for flexion-extension, lateral flexion, and rotation in both directions. The CROM instrument has been reported to have excellent validity for cervical flexion-extension, lateral flexion, and rotation measurements (Tousignant et al., 2002). In Tousignant et al.'s study, the results of the CROM measurements were compared with X-ray data referenced as the gold standard. The results of both measurements had a strong correlation. In addition, an angle change of 5° to 10° indicates that there is change in mobility in the cervical spine (Fletcher & Bandy, 2008).

Mönch-Tegeder and Von Piekartz (in press) observed that children with migraine exhibited restricted cervical range of motion in five of the six movements assessed as part of CROM as compared to healthy children (**Table 18.6**). The inclusion criteria for pediatric migraine

Table 18.5 Overview of the Craniocervical Angle in Different Headaches and at Various Ages

	Age	Headache Group	Healthy Control	Mean Difference
Watson & Trott (1993)	25–40 years	44.5° (cervical headache)	49.1°	4.6°
Fernández-de-las-Peñas et al. (2006)	18–57 years	44.7° (migraine)	53.7°	9°
Mönch-Tegeder & Von Piekartz (2011)	8–16 years	51.2° (pediatric migraine)	55.5°	4.3°

Table 18.6 Cervical Range of Motion in Children with Pediatric Migraine and Healthy Children

	Migraine Group (n = 32)	Control Group (n = 45)	Significance (P)
Flexion	59.58° ± 7.82°	62.25° ± 5.50°	0.266
Extension	80.83° ± 6.69°	82.75° ± 6.17°	0.416
Lateral flexion left	46.25° ± 5.28°	45.00° ± 6.07°	0.559
Lateral flexion right	43.33° ± 3.89°	44.75° ± 4.72°	0.389
Rotation left	78.33° ± 4.92°	79.25° ± 5.20°	0.626
Rotation right	79.17° ± 5.14°	81.25° ± 4.55°	0.242

Source: Mönch-Tegeder & Von Piekartz, in press.

in their study were consistent with the guidelines of the ICDH-II. Similar results were also found by Lynch-Caris et al. (2008).

A generalized restricted CROM may potentially be associated with a craniocervical dysfunction; however, no study has been conducted to investigate this relationship. Intervertebral passive movements of the upper cervical spine may support this clinical finding.

Neurodynamic Long Sitting Slump Test

The Long Sitting Slump (LSS) is a modification of the standard slump test that purports to examine mobility of the longitudinal part of the nervous system (see also Chapter 19). The sensory response, flexibility of the trunk, and craniocervical flexion can be measured by this means. The starting posture consists of extension of both legs and dorsiflexion of the feet and ankles. From there, the examiner moves the trunk to flexion, and then the craniocervical region into flexion (see Figure 19.2). The assessment involves measuring neck flexion in degrees with the CROM and the sensory response with an analogue scale.

Von Piekartz et al. (2007) compared the sensory responses during the LSS in a sample of children with migraine (n = 31), children with headache with cervical dysfunctions (n = 32), and a control group (n = 45). Eighty-one percent of the children showed an increase in sensory response with the addition of dorsiflexion of the feet and ankles to the LSS, with the children from the migraine group reporting the most sensory responses in the legs (intensity: 5.5; SD: 1.7) (Von Piekartz et al., 2007). This response discriminated the pediatric migraine group from the cervical headache group, which showed sensory reactions in the column (80%) with an intensity of 5.4 (SD: 2.3). Finally, within the control group, 36% had a sensory response in the legs, similar to the

pediatric migraine group, but with a clearly lower intensity (mean: 0.9, SD: 0.85).

Range of motion of craniocervical flexion during the LSS was also clearly striking, particularly when the sum was calculated with and without extension of the knees. The sum of neck flexion with extension of the knees, NF (a), and in knee flexion, NF (b), was 16.6 (SD: 5.7) for the control group, 17.8 (SD: 8.6) for the migraine group, and 5.6 (SD: 4.7) for the cervical headache group (P < 0.001).

Vestibular System: Dix-Hallpike Maneuver and Balance

Many migraine patients also suffer from dizziness (Neuheuser et al., 2001), and patients with dizziness tend to have more migraines (Riina et al., 2005). Uneri and Turkdogan (2003) proposed that "vestibular instability" has a strong influence on the mechanism of equilibrium, such that complaints of dizziness can occur, although this concept also challenges the notion of a strong autonomic reaction with great influence upon cranial vascularization. A possible secondary symptom of migraine that occurs quite early in life is benign paroxysmal position dizziness (BPPD) in children (Drigo et al., 2001). This vestibular disorder is coupled with episodic attacks of dizziness. Such complaints may begin between the second and fourth years of life, and often stop spontaneously within a few months; nevertheless, a group of these patients develops migraine later on. In a study of 19 children with migraine, Drigo et al. (2001) found a connection between their headache and BPPD. In another study, which included 125 children with complaints of dizziness, children who were dizzy also suffered from migraine more frequently (Lipa et al., 2008). Marcelli et al. (2010) observed that vestibular disorders are not always clinically manifested; in their study, children with migraine, although they had a positive otolaryngological examination indicating an overstimulation of the vestibular system, did not present with clear otolaryngological symptoms.

The Dix-Hallpike test can be used as clinical examination of the vestibular system (Von Brevern & Lempert, 2002). In this test, the patient is positioned into cervical rotation of 45°, and then passively moved rapidly from a sitting position to a supine position with extension of the craniocervical region. Dix and Hallpike (1952) describe the test as positive if nystagmus occurs within a small number of seconds. Although the standardization of this test is not perfect (Fife et al., 2008), it is considered by several authors to be the gold standard test for BPPD (Von Brevern & Lempert, 2002; Cohen, 2004). Chapter 22 of this book provides more information on this test.

Our clinical experience has shown that this test can be used in children with headache, because they often have slight dizziness or balance disorders. A positive test in this context does not suggest a diagnosis of BPPD, but rather an imbalance within the vestibular system. Experience also shows that in children with migraine, the test often has a latency time of a few minutes. In the study by Mönch-Tegeder and Von Piekartz (in press) it was seen that, of the 32 children diagnosed with migraine, 2 children immediately responded after the Dix-Hallpike maneuver and 13 had an increase in dizziness and complaints (including pressure in the head) within 2 minutes. Four children still had mild complaints 10 minutes after the maneuver.

For balance assessment of a child with headache, the Movement Assessment Battery for Children (Movement ABC) can be used (Von Piekartz, 2007). This test can differentiate, per age period (4–6 years; 7–8 years; 9–10 years; and 10–12 + years), how, among other things, the balance of a child is in a static and dynamic sense. This can give a good impression of the motor capacity of the child. In particular, this instrument can be used as a reassessment tool after therapy in children with headache.

Craniofacial Assessment

In connection with the craniofacial growth of school-aged children—which often runs closely with increased headache, followed by migraine and secondary factors such as otitis media, chronic sinusitis, and orofacial and craniocervical dysfunctions—a systematic screening of the facial skeleton is an important part of the examination of children with pediatric headache. Craniofacial dysfunctions can lead to decreasing orofacial functions through an increase in (unnecessary) nociception that can contribute to the complaints of the child (Chaitow,

2005; Von Piekartz, 2007). For detailed information about craniofacial assessment and its influence upon structures and neuromodulation, see Chapter 20.

TREATMENT AND MANAGEMENT: CASE REPORTS

Before the treatment begins, any possible "red flags" must first be ruled out. As stated in the introduction to this chapter, neuromusculoskeletal dysfunctions that are found during examination may be a possible contributing factor in the child with pediatric migraine. During a brief number of sessions (three to six), the clinician must determine whether such dysfunctions are relevant to the child's complaints. A systematic evaluation of the complaints (in consultation with the child's parents or guardians) and an assessment of neuromusculoskeletal function may lead to a fundamental overview of possible treatments. The two case reports presented here provide some treatment suggestions, including neuromusculoskeletal treatments. Such treatment is naturally augmented with support and advice for the parents and the child.

Case 1

A child ("M") with a diagnosis of migraine without aura was referred to the clinician at the age of 11 by his pediatrician. During history taking, he reported suffering from a strong frontal headache on the right side for approximately 3 months. The attacks lasted 4 to 6 hours and occurred weekly. Occasionally, attacks were accompanied by vomiting. The child missed school during the serious attacks and was often tired. There was no recognizable cause for the complaint. He had been treated by different health-care professionals, including a family practitioner, who had prescribed paracetamol; a physical therapist, who treated the cervical spine with mobilization, exercise therapy, and massage; and the pediatrician, who made the diagnosis of migraine and had prescribed Sandomigran (pizotifen). There was, however, no clear improvement.

When we asked specifically about oral habits, the child appeared to mostly chew on the right side. Due to his complaints, he missed at least 1 day per week from school. He also said that he had no energy and did not much enjoy football and playing. His parents confirmed this decrease in activity energy.

Neuromusculoskeletal Examination

The neuromusculoskeletal examination was done according to the Crafta protocol and focused on the presence of dysfunctions that have a correlation with the right frontal headache. The emphasis was on the head, neck, and jaw area.

M estimated the intensity of his headaches over the last 5 days as 78 mm on the CAS. A myofascial trigger point (Simons et al., 1999) in the right masseter muscle (0.5 cm ventral to the mandible angle) and referred pain to the right frontal area were observed at a pressure of 0.58 kg/cm². This point was extremely painful as compared to the left masseter muscle (only locally painful at a pressure of 1.55 kg/cm²). Rotation of the cervical spine was 55° to the left and 75° to the right, whereby the rotation C0–C2 left was limited (–50% in comparison with the other side). Assessment of general craniofacial region by occiput-frontal techniques (see Chapter 20) were stiff in the frontal-diagonal direction and gave the patient his familiar symptom of the right frontal headache.

Which Structure Has Priority?

It is possible that the trigger point within the right masseter muscle played a role due to the high tone and the possibility of referred pain in the frontal region of the head (Simons et al., 1999) and the low pressure-pain threshold. In fact, the referred pain from the trigger point within the masseter muscle reproduced the frontal headache experienced by the child.

The craniofacial region (occiput-frontal movements) was further considered given that its movement assessment also reproduced the headache, although the patient's history did not include any indication of craniofacial morphological adaptations. Finally, craniocervical dysfunctions could also have played a role; because these had been treated without significant improvement, however, they were relegated to a lower level on the list.

Proposed Treatment

Inactivation of the trigger point within the right masseter, normal function of the mandibular elevators, and improvement of the compliance of the occiput-frontal region through passive movements were components of the treatment. The total treatment consisted of seven sessions in 5 months. The first four were given once a week over 4 consecutive weeks; the fifth treatment was 2 weeks later; the sixth a month later; and the last treatment 2 months later.

The patient reacted well to an intra-oral stretch technique of the masseter muscle. The therapist moved the mandible with the left hand in depression and laterotrusion to the left, while simultaneously using the right index finger to place sustained local diagonal pressure on

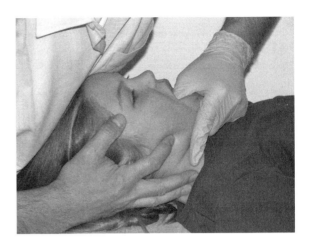

Figure 18.5 Transversal Movement on the Right Masseter Muscle Trigger Point

the trigger point within the right masseter (Von Piekartz, 2007). This intra-oral technique was chosen due to the good grip afforded with this method, which allowed the stretch to be intensive (**Figure 18.5**).

Additionally, a compression technique on the right occipital-frontal diagonal was used in three series of 20 repetitions of 2 seconds (**Figure 18.6**). Both techniques were carried out with the patient in a supine position and were well tolerated by the child, although they did at times produce a sensory response in the form of local pain in the masseter muscle.

Course of Treatment

The pressure-pain threshold over the masseter muscle and the cervical range of motion on left rotation were

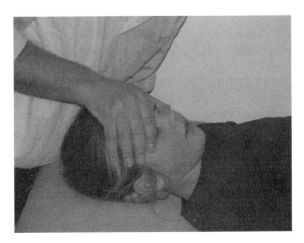

Figure 18.6 Occipital-Frontal Technique

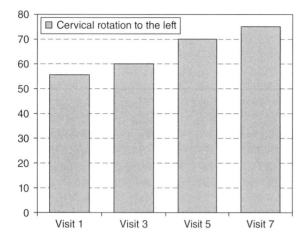

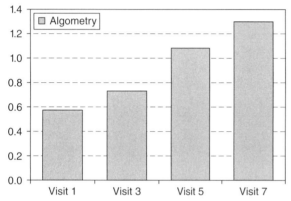

Figure 18.7 Evolution of Pressure-Pain Thresholds Over Masseter Muscle Trigger Point (Bottom) and Cervical Range of Motion for Left Rotation (Top)

reassessed in the first, third, fifth, and seventh treatment sessions (**Figure 18.7**), whereas the CAS (pain) was assessed in the first, third, and fifth treatments, and 2 months after the last treatment. After the second treatment, the patient reported that he no longer took the Sandomigran.

Six months after the last treatment, M was completely pain free without further headache. He no longer missed school, and he experienced no pain or limitations. He was playing football again without any problems. During the time that he was undergoing treatment, he very quickly decreased his Sandomigran use and even his use of paracetamol, which was needed only very occasionally.

Criteria of the ICHD-II (2004) in terms of migraine without aura under point D were not clearly present in this case, and it appeared that other structures were involved (category E, ICDH-II). Therefore, this situation probably involved headache associated with cranium or cranio-mandibular dysfunction.

Case 2

"H" was a 9-year-old boy who had experienced unilateral headache around his right eye since his sixth year of life. Because the headache occurred at the same time as the child started his new school, the family practitioner and the parents assumed that it was associated with a stress situation and would clear up on its own. After 6 months, the headache increased and the practitioner prescribed medication, without significant relief. The neurologist then diagnosed "pediatric migraine" and prescribed Imigran (triptan). Headache attacks were clearly less in the first 6 months after this therapy was prescribed (decreasing from five times to one or two times per month), but came back more intensely around the patient's eighth birthday. The neurologist increased the dosage with the same medicine and stated that this headache would probably decrease on its own when H reached 12 years of age.

H's school performance was also affected. Each month, he missed an average of 8 days of school due to his headache attacks, giving him a learning deficit for which he had to compensate on his good days. Additionally, he was often tired and had difficulties in physical exercise at school and playing football due to poor balance. A pediatric physiotherapist exercised with him for 6 months in an attempt to restore his "onshore" equilibrium but no clear improvement was observed.

H had had a wry-neck as a baby that the pediatrician diagnosed as "myogenic torticollis." At 4 years old, a persistent otitis media (9 months) that responded well to antibiotics was diagnosed.

Neuromusculoskeletal Examination

During the first examination, H reported a score of 4.2 on the CAS when asked how limiting his headache had been over the last 5 days. He had no headache at the time of examination. During the examination, a postural deviation of his head (lateral flexion and rotation to the right), a decreased left facial region with mild scoliosis (right convex), and a "floppy" posture were observed. The general equilibrium and balance tests, such as standing on one leg for 10 seconds (particularly on the right), were not possible. Cervical flexion (32°), left lateral flexion (24°), and right rotation (51°) were significantly limited as compared to cervical extension (76°), right lateral flexion (41°), and left rotation (76°).

Passive intervertebral segmental motion assessment confirmed that a movement dysfunction at the C1–C2 and C2–C3 segments was present on the right side. During the craniofacial examination, among other things, the right diagonal occiput and the left frontal assessment were clearly decreased in compliance; after seven repetitions, this test reproduced H's headache, albeit in a mild version (CAS 2.3). Examination of the occiput region in combination with temporal and sphenoidal techniques (Chapter 20) also indicated clear answers in terms of less compliance, increased resistance, and increased sensory response (headache) in comparison with the other side (for more information see Chapter 20; Chaitow, 2005; Von Piekartz, 2007).

The LSS test demonstrated a limitation in sitting (angle sacrum-bench 63°) and marked neck flexion limitation (32°), whereby the sum with and without flexion of the knees was 5°. A sensory response in the legs with an intensity of 7.7 on the CAS was noted. During the Dix-Hallpike maneuver, no dizziness or nystagmus was observed, but standing on one leg was noticeably improved (equilibrium tests were done immediately before the Dix-Hallpike maneuver). Based on the first examination, it was concluded that marked dysfunctions may have been influencing the patient's symptoms, which could in turn have a significant effect on his quality of life. After screening for red and yellow flags, it was decided to start treatment with the initial focus on the craniocervical and facial regions.

Proposed Treatment

Passive mobilization with slow continuing techniques without pain was carried out over the C1–C2 and C2–C3 segments. Immediately after mobilization, a reassessment of other dysfunctions that were found was conducted to determine any change observed. This also applied to the treatment of the occipital-sphenoidal-temporal region which was performed during the second and third treatments.

During the fourth and fifth treatments, based on the improvement of the headache and the decrease in neuromusculoskeletal dysfunctions, cautious LSS neural mobilization and the Dix-Hallpike maneuver were added as exercises. During the fifth treatment (after 8 weeks), it was observed that H's posture was less "floppy"; the craniocervical angle had improved; H's head was less deviated; and his cervical range of motion had improved—to flexion of 43°, left lateral flexion of 45°, and right rotation of 63°, as confirmed by intervertebral/segmental movements. Moreover, the compliance of the occipital-sphenoidal passive motions was increased without provoking pain. On the LSS, the sacrum-bench angle had remained

the same but the neck flexion (48°) and the sum of the neck flexion during the flexion-extension excursion of the legs was noticeably improved (11°) and the sensory response in the legs was 2.3 on the CAS. Finally, balance reactions and standing on one leg were improved.

Course of Treatment

According to H, his headache attacks had occurred only once over the last month, and they were less intense than before. The score on the CAS over the last 5 days was 0.8. The postural and movement coordination observed by his teacher and pediatric physiotherapist was "average" for his age. H also played outside with his friends more often and, according to his parents, he was enjoying it more. The use of Imigran was decreased (over the last month, only one administration at the prescribed dosage was necessary).

During a follow-up appointment 4 months after treatment, it was observed that H's headache attacks and activity levels had remained stable. The headache attacks occurred only twice, possibly due to other contributing factors such as influenza and too little sleep.

On the basis of these two cases, it can be reasoned that the observed neuromusculoskeletal dysfunctions should be treated systematically on the basis of the severity of their presence and the past history. In the case studies presented here, treatment was guided through continuous assessment and reassessment of other dysfunctions and the complaints of the two patients. This process confirmed the existing clinical pattern of the neuromusculoskeletal dysfunctions in pediatric migraine.

CONCLUSIONS

Pediatric migraine as an isolated diagnosis may be insufficient in some cases, as it can be related to a lack of adequate classification and multiple contributing factors. Neuromusculoskeletal dysfunctions can be relevant contributing factors in the clinical evolution of pediatric migraine. Such dysfunctions, particularly when substantiated with external evidence, can be easily examined using pain outcomes, the craniocervical angle, cervical range of motion, pain threshold measurements, neurodynamic testing, and vestibular equilibrium and balance testing. Treatment of neuromusculoskeletal dysfunctions must be supported by fundamental clinical reasoning strategies, whereby clinical evidence of the dysfunctions of the individual pediatric patient is centralized.

REFERENCES

Abu-Arefeh I, Russel G. Prevalence of headache and migraine in schoolchildren. *BMJ* 1994;309:765–769.

Agrawal K, Karoon A, Mishra S, Panda K. Intracranial pressure and intracranial volume in children with craniosynostosis. *Plastic & Reconstructive Surg* 1992;90:394–398.

Andrasik F, Kabela E, Quinn S, et al. Psychological function of children who have recurrent migraine. *Pain* 1998; 34:43–52.

Aromaa M, Sillanpää ML, Rautava P, Helenius H. Childhood headache at school entry: a controlled clinical study. *Neurology* 1998;50:1729–1736.

Biedermann H. Biomechanische besonderheiten des occipito-cervicalen überganges bei kindern. In: Biedermann H, ed. *Manualtherapie bei Kindern*. Stuttgart: Enke; 1999.

Biedermann H. *Manual Therapy in Children*. Edinburgh: Churchill & Livingstone; 2004.

Bigal ME, Arruda MA. Migraine in the pediatric population: evolving concepts. *Headache* 2010;50:1130–1143.

Bogduk N. Hoofdpijn en duizeligheid bij cervicale afwijkingen. In: Grieve P, ed. *Moderne Manuele Therapie van de Wervelkolom*. Lochem: De Tijdstroom; 1988.

Briggs A, Straker L, Grieg A. Upper quadrant postural changes of schoolchildren in response to interaction with different information technologies. *Ergonomics* 2004; 47;790–819.

Bruni O, Fabrizi P, Ottaviano S, Cortesi F. Prevalence of sleep disorders in childhood and adolescence with headache: a case-control study. *Cephalalgia* 1997;17:492–498.

Busch V, Jakob W, Juergens T, et al. Functional connectivity between trigeminal and occipital nerves revealed by occipital nerve blockade and nociceptive blink reflexes. *Cephalalgia* 2006;26:50–55.

Carlsson AM. Assessment of chronic pain: aspects of the reliability and validity of the visual analogue scale. *Pain* 1983;16:87–101.

Chaitow L. *Cranial Manipulation: Theory and Practice.* 2nd ed. Edinburgh: Churchill Livingstone; 2005.

Chaves T, Nagamine H, de Sousa L. Intra and inter-rater agreement of pressure pain threshold for masticatory structures in children reporting orofacial pain related to temporomandibular disorders and symptom free children. *J Orofac Pain* 2007;21:133–142 .

Cohen H. Side-lying as an alternative to the Dix-Hallpike test of the posterior canal. *Otol Neurotol* 2004;25:130–134.

Dix M, Hallpike C. The pathology, symptomatology and diagnosis of certain common disorders of the vestibular system. *Proc Royal Soc Med* 1952;45:341–345.

Drigo P, Carli G, Laverda A. Benign paroxysmal vertigo of childhood. *Brain Develop* 2001;23:38–41.

Farella M, Michelotti A, Steenks M, et al. The diagnostic value of pressure algometry in myofascial pain of jaw muscles. *J Oral Rehabil* 2000;27:9–14.

Feikema WJ. Hoofdpijn en chronisch slaaptekort: een vaak miskende relatie bij kinderen en volwassenen. *Nederlands Tijdschrift voor Geneeskunde* 1999;138:1897–1900.

Fendrich K, Vennemann M, Pfaffenrath V, et al. Headache prevalence among adolescents: the German DMKG headache study. *Cephalalgia* 2007;27:347–354.

Fernández-de-las-Peñas C, Cuadrado M, Pareja JA. Myofacial trigger points, neck mobility and forward head posture in unilateral migraine. *Cephalalgia* 2006;26:1061–1070.

Fernández-de-las-Peñas C, Fernández-Mayoralas DM, Ortega-Santiago R, et al. Bilateral widespread mechanical pain sensitivity in children with frequent episodic tension type headache suggesting impairment in central nociceptive processing. *Cephalalgia* 2010;30:1049–1055.

Fife T, Iverson D, Lempert T, et al. Practice parameter: therapies for benign paroxysmal positional vertigo (an evidence-based review). *Neurology* 2008;70:2067–2074.

Fletcher J, Bandy W. Intrarater reliability of CROM measurement of cervical spine active range of motion in persons with and without neck pain. *J Orthop Sports Phys Ther* 2008;38:640–645.

Galli F, Canzano L, Scalisi TG, Guidetti V. Psychiatric disorders and headache familial recurrence: a study on 200 children and their parents. *J Headache Pain* 2009;10:187–197.

Giamberardino M, Tafuri E, Savini A, et al. Contribution of myofascial trigger points to migraine symptoms. *J Pain* 2007;8:869–878.

Göbel H. *Die Kopfschmerzen. 2. Auflage.* Berlin: Springer Verlag; 2004.

Hall T, Briffa K, Hopper D, Robinson K. Reliability of manual examination and frequency of symptomatic cervical motion segment dysfunction in cervicogenic headache. *Man Ther* 2010;15:542–546.

Heisley S, Adams T. Role of cranial bone mobility in cranial compliance. *Neurosurgery* 1993;33:869–877.

Hershey AD. Current approaches to the diagnosis and management of paediatric migraine. *Lancet Neurol* 2010;9: 190–204.

Hicks CL, Von Baeyer CL, Spafford PA, et al. The Faces Pain Scale—Revised: toward a common metric in pediatric pain measurement. *Pain* 2001;93:173–182.

Holland PR. Modulation of trigemino-vascular processing: novel insights into primary headache disorders. *Cephalalgia* 2009;29(suppl 3):1–6.

ICHD-II: Headache Classification Committee of the International Headache Society. The International Classification of Headache Disorders (2nd edition). *Cephalalgia* 2004;24(suppl 1): 1–160.

Isik U, Topuzoglu A, Ay P, et al. The prevalence of headache and its association with socioeconomic status among schoolchildren in Istanbul, Turkey. *Headache* 2009;49: 697–703.

Jensen K, Tuxen C, Olesen J. Pericranial muscle tenderness and pressure-pain threshold in the temporal region during common migraine. *Pain* 1988;35:65–70.

Joffe R, Bakal DA, Kaganov J. A self-observation study of headache symptoms in children. *Headache* 1983; 23:20–25.

Knust M, Trouw M, Von Piekartz H. Kopfhaltung und kraniomandibuläre dysfunktionen. *Publikation.* In press.

Koenen W. Sensomotorische dyskybernese im vorschul- und schulalter. In: Coenben W, ed. *Manuelle Medizin bei Sauglingen und Kindern.* Heidelberg: Springer; 2009: 123–139.

La Touche R, París-Alemany A, Von Piekartz H, et al. The influence of cranio-cervical posture on maximal mouth opening and pressure pain threshold in patients with myofascial temporomandibular pain disorders. *Clin J Pain* 2011;27:48–55.

Lee L, Olness K. Clinical and demographic characteristics of migraine in urban children. *Headache* 1997;37:269–276.

Levine JP, Bradley JP, Roth DA, et al. Studies in cranial suture biology: regional dura mater determines overlying suture biology. *Plast Reconstr Surg* 1998;101:1441–1447.

Lewis D. Toward the definition of childhood migraine. *Curr Opin Ped* 2004;16:628–636.

Lima MM, Padula NA, Santos LC, et al. Critical analysis of the International Classification of Headache Disorders diagnostic criteria (ICHD I-1988) and (ICHD II-2004) for migraine in children and adolescents. *Cephalalgia* 2005;25:1042–1047.

Lipa R, Varela A, Santos Perez S, et al. Alterations of balance in patients under 16 years of age distributed by age groups. *Acta Otorrinolaringol Esp* 2008;59:455–462.

Liu Y, Broman J, Zhang M, Edvinsson L. Brainstem and thalamic projections from a cranio-vascular sensory nervous centre in the rostral cervical spinal dorsal horn of rats. *Cephalalgia* 2009;29:935–948.

Lütschg J. Kopfschmerzen in kindesalter. *Pädiatrie* 2009; 3:7–12.

Lynch-Caris T, Majeske K, Brelin-Fornaric J, Nashid S. Establishing reference values for cervical spine range of motion in pre-pubescent children. *J Biomech* 2008;41:2714–2719.

Marcelli V, Furia T, Marciano E. Vestibular pathways involvement in children with migraine: a neuro-otological study. *Headache* 2010;50:71–76.

Marcus D, Scharff L, Mercer S, Turk D. Musculoskeletal abnormalities in chronic headache: a controlled comparison of headache diagnostic groups. *Headache* 1999;39:21–27.

McGrath P. Headache in children: the nature of the problem. In: McGrath P, Hillier L, eds. *The Child with Headache: Diagnosis and Treatment. Progress in Pain Research and Management, Vol. 19*. Seattle: IASP Press; 2001:1–27.

McGrath P, Koster A. Headache measures for children: a practical approach. In: McGrath P, Hillier L, eds. *The Child with Headache: Diagnosis and Treatment. Progress in Pain Research and Management, Vol. 19*. Seattle: IASP Press; 2001:29–56.

McGrath P, Seifert CE, Speechley KN, et al. A new analogue scale for assessing children's pain: an initial validation study. *Pain* 1996;64:435–443.

Menkes MM. Personality characteristics and family roles of children with migraine. *Pediatrics* 1974;53:560–564.

Messinger HB, Spierings EL, Vincent AJ. Overlap of migraine and tension type headache in the International Headache Society classification. *Cephalalgia* 1991;11:233–237.

Molina OM, Santos Dos J, Mazzetto M, et al. Oral jaw behaviors in TMD and bruxism: a comparison study by severity and bruxism. *J Craniom Practice* 2001;19:114–123.

Mönch-Tegeder I, Von Piekartz HJM. Neuromusculoskeletal qualities in pediatric migraine: a cross section study. *J Mandibular Function*. In press.

Nelson CF. The tension headache. Migraine headache continuum: a hypothesis. *J Manipulative Physiol Ther* 1994;17:156–167.

Neuheuser H, Leopold M, Von Brevern M, et al. The interrelations of migraine, vertigo and migrainous vertigo. *Neurology* 2001;56:684–686.

Oleski SL, Smitj GH, Crow WT. Radiographic evidence of cranial bone mobility. *Cranio* 2002;20:34–38.

Paiva T, Farinha A, Martins A, et al. Chronic headaches and sleep disorders. *Arch Int Med* 1997;157:1701–1705.

Pothmann R, Von Frankenberg S, Müller B, et al. Epidemiology of headache in children and adolescents: evidence of high prevalence of migraine among girls under 10. *Int J Behavior Med* 1994;1:76–89.

Powell CV, Kelly A, Williams A. Determining the minimum clinically significant difference in visual analogue pain score for children. *Ann Emerg Med* 2001;37:28–31.

Raine S, Twomey L. Head and shoulder posture variations in 160 asymptotic women and men. *Arch Phys Med Rehabil* 1997;78:1215–1223.

Riina N, Ilmari P, Kentala E. Vertigo and imbalance in children: a retrospective study in a Helsinki University otorhinolaryngology clinic. *Arch Otolaryngo Head Neck Surg* 2005;113:996–1000.

Rothner A. Differential diagnosis of headache in children and adolescents. In: McGrath P, Hillier L, eds. *The Child with Headache: Diagnosis and Treatment. Progress in Pain Research and Management, Vol. 19*. Seattle: IASP Press; 2001:57–76.

Sandrini G, Antonaci F, Bono G, Nappi G. Comparative study with EMG, pressure algometry and manual palpation in tension-type headache and migraine. *Cephalalgia* 1994;14:451–457.

Santinello M, Vieno A, De Vogli R. Primary headache in Italian early adolescents: the role of perceived teacher unfairness. *Headache* 2009;49:366–374.

Shah UH, Kalra V. Pediatric migraine. *Int J Pediatr* 2009:424192.

Simons D, Travell J, Simons L. *Myofascial Pain and Dysfunction: The Trigger Point Manual. Vol. 1: Upper Half of the Body*. Baltimore: Williams & Wilkins; 1999.

Siniatchkin M, Kropp MP, Gerber WD, Stephani U. Migraine in childhood: are periodically occurring migraine attacks related to dynamic changes of cortical information processing? *Neurosci Lett* 2000;279:1–4.

Tousignant M, Duclos E, Laflèche S, et al. Validity study for the cervical range of motion device used for lateral flexion in patients with neck pain. *Spine* 2002;15:812–817.

Überall MA. Pharmakologische akuttherapie der migraine bei kindern. *Der Schmerz* 1999;13(suppl 1):37–38.

Uneri A, Turkdogan D. Evaluation of vestibular functions in children with vertigo attacks. *Arch Dis Child* 2003;88:510–511.

Vernon H, Steinmann I, Hagino C. Cervicogenic dysfunction in muscle contraction headache and migraine: a descriptive study. *J Manipulative Physiol Ther* 1992;15:418–429.

Virtanen R, Aromaa M, Rautava P, et al. Changing headache from preschool age to puberty: a controlled study. *Cephalalgia* 2007;27:294–303.

Von Brevern M, Lempert T. Benigner paroxysmaler lagerungsschwindel: rasch erkennen, erfolgreich behandeln. *Hals Nase und Ohr* 2002;50:671–681.

Von Piekartz HJM. *Kiefer, Gesichts- und Zervikalregion, Neuromusckuloskeletale Untersuchung, Therapie und Management.* Stuttgart: Georg Thieme Verlag; 2005:451–457.

Von Piekartz H. *Craniofacial Pain: Neuromusculoskeletal Assessment, Treatment and Management.* Philadelphia: Butterworth Heinemann Elsevier; 2007.

Von Piekartz HJM, Schouten S, Aufdemkampe G. Neurodynamic responses in children with migraine or cervicogenic headache versus a control group: a comparative study. *Man Ther* 2007;12:153–160.

Watson D, Trott P. Cervical headache: an investigation of natural head posture and upper cervical flexor muscle performance. *Cephalalgia* 1993;13:272–284.

Neurodynamic Approach for Migraines

Emilio Puentedura, PT, DPT, PhD,OCS, GDMT, CSMT, FAAOMPT,
Adriaan Louw, PT, MAppSc, GCRM, CSMT, Paul Mintken, PT, DPT,
OCS, FAAOMPT, and Ina Diener, PT, BAppSc, PhD

INTRODUCTION

Several authors in the current textbook as well as numerous published articles have alluded to the fact that migraines are complex and poorly understood (Burstein, 2001; Silberstein, 2004; Goadsby, 2005; Fernández-de-las-Peñas et al., 2009; Varkey et al., 2009; Saracco et al., 2010). There is continued debate regarding the exact etiology of migraines, triggers causing migraine, and treatments for the migraine sufferer (Burstein, 2001; Parsons & Strijbos, 2003; Goadsby, 2005). Writing a chapter on the use of neurodynamic tests in the evaluation and treatment of migraine sufferers is, therefore, quite a daunting task. To date, no randomized controlled trials (RCT) have been conducted to assess the direct effect of neural tissue mobilization techniques compared to other treatment interventions for headache patients, let alone migraine-specific studies. Moreover, considering the difficulty of classifying headaches and determining where a tension-type headache (TTH) or a cervicogenic headache (CeH) stops and a migraine starts, evaluation and management of purely migraine headaches become problematic. Finally, considering the significant suffering of the migraine patient with "additional" symptoms, such as nausea, vomiting, aura, light sensitivity, and more, it would even be understandable that some might question the use of a movement-based treatment of the neuromeningeal structures in patients who are so severely afflicted.

This chapter, which is dedicated to the consideration of neurodynamics for migraine headaches, primarily views migraines from a neural tissue perspective. It focuses on five areas: (1) the definition of a migraine;

(2) the role of neural sensitivity in headache; (3) assessment of neurodynamics in headache; (4) treatment of neurodynamic dysfunction; and (5) the effects of exercise, blood flow, and nerves in migraine headache.

WHAT IS A MIGRAINE?

When reviewing the diagnostic criteria presented by the International Headache Society (2004) for the various headache types, considerable overlap of symptoms is apparent. CeH shares similar characteristics with TTH and migraine without aura (D'Amico et al., 1994; Leone et al., 1995; Fishbain et al., 2003), and neck pain is a symptom frequently reported in patients with TTH and migraine (Solomon, 1997; Fishbain et al., 2001; Bartsch & Goadsby, 2003b). None of the criteria for diagnosing CeH put forth by Sjaastad et al. (1998) are, in isolation, exclusive to CeH. Several authors have reported that pain with neck movement is characteristic of CeH (Sjaastad et al., 1998; Hall & Robinson, 2004; Ogince et al., 2007), whereas others have noted that neck pain is common in patients with migraine, TTH, and CeH (Bansevicius et al., 1999; Jull et al., 2007; Ogince et al., 2007).

This overlap is most likely due to the convergence of afferents in the trigeminocervical nucleus (Kerr & Olafson, 1961; Bartsch & Goadsby, 2002, 2003b; Cady, 2007). Considering the complex intricacy of the nervous system and the significant overlap between symptoms associated with TTH, CeH, and migraine, it has been proposed that clinicians view migraines and TTH not as two separate entities, but rather as part of a continuum (Cady et al., 2002; Vargas, 2008). The continuum approach implies that patients with TTH may develop migraines and, conversely, patients with migraine may develop TTH. Additionally, adoption of the continuum approach toward TTH and migraine suggests that treatments aimed at alleviating TTH may help patients with migraines and may even be effective in preventing the development of a migraine attack. Nevertheless, some critics have argued that the continuum view of headaches may not be valid (Rasmussen, 1996) owing to the aforementioned difficulty in diagnosing and classifying headaches in the first place.

Many of the headache classifications were developed by neurologists, who might potentially overlook important musculoskeletal impairments that may be identified by movement-based specialists, such as physical therapists. Therapists who do not adhere to the continuum view of TTH and migraine may wish to view headaches as either vascular or musculoskeletal in nature. Conditions affecting both of these systems can

be exacerbated by stress and tension. Both the vascular and musculoskeletal systems can provide a nociceptive input to the trigeminocervical complex, resulting in a headache. Neurons in the trigeminocervical complex are the major relay neurons for nociceptive afferent input from vascular structures, the meninges, and cervical structures; consequently, they are the neural substrates of all head pain (Bartsch & Goadsby, 2003b).

Some primary headaches appear to have a referred pain component, frequently involving structures in the neck (Bogduk, 2001; Fernández-de-las-Peñas et al., 2007). The neurophysiological mechanism behind this referral from the head into the neck also lies in the convergence of afferent fibers from the trigeminal nerve and the upper three cervical nerve roots in the trigeminocervical nucleus (Bartsch & Goadsby, 2003a; Bogduk, 2004b). The spinal nucleus of the trigeminal nerve extends caudally to the dorsal horn of the upper three cervical spinal segments (Narouze, 2007). Kerr and Olafson (1961) demonstrated that afferents from the trigeminal nerve and the upper three cervical roots converge in the trigeminocervical nucleus caudalis in the upper cervical cord. The trigeminocervical nucleus resides in the upper part of the cervical spinal cord, where descending sensory fibers from the trigeminal nerve converge with sensory fibers from the upper cervical nerve roots (Shevel & Spierings, 2004). The convergence of these fibers suggests a mechanism by which pain may "'spread'" from the cervical region to the trigeminal area, and vice versa—a concept often referred to as the Kerr principle (Kerr, 1961; Fredriksen & Sjaastad, 2000).

Bartsch and Goadsby (2002) demonstrated, in a rat model, that a significant percentage of neurons in the trigeminocervical nucleus show convergent afferent input from the dura, skin, and muscles of the upper cervical spine. As a result, nociceptive input from structures innervated by the upper three cervical nerve roots—including the joints, muscles, dura mater, nerves, bones, and vascular structures—may lead to the onset of headache (Bogduk, 2004a). This convergence of neural tissue in the trigeminocervical nucleus allows for multiple tissues to become generators of head pain (**Figure 19.1**). Chapter 5 provides more information on the trigeminocervical nucleus caudalis.

In chronic headache, the up-regulation of the neural system via central sensitization further complicates the diagnosis of headache. It has long been believed that migraines are purely vascular in nature, yet a growing body of evidence has recently begun implicating central sensitization of the nervous system in chronic headache (Burstein, 2001; Parsons & Strijbos, 2003;

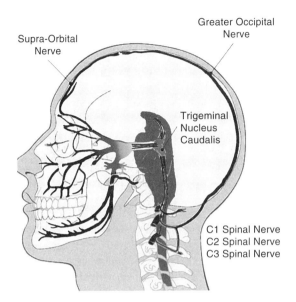

Figure 19.1 The Trigeminocervical Complex Demonstrating the Convergence of Sensory Input to the Trigeminal Nucleus Caudalis Neurons from the Upper Three Cervical Nerve Roots

Goadsby, 2005). Many patients with headache disorders have had symptoms for a long time and may display signs of central sensitization, adding yet another layer to the complexity of the clinical problem solving. "Central sensitization" is defined as a condition in which peripheral noxious inputs into the central nervous system lead to an increased excitability, whereby the response to normal inputs is greatly enhanced (Woolf, 2007). It has been proposed that central sensitization in migraines is induced by afferent input from the dura mater traveling on the trigeminovascular pain pathway (Malick & Burstein, 2000). The convergence of differing afferent signals in the trigeminal nucleus might then sensitize second-order neurons (Malick & Burstein, 2000; Cady, 2007). Repeated noxious stimuli may cause low-threshold neurons with very large receptive fields to depolarize with the presentation of even innocuous mechanical stimuli (Woolf, 2007). Injured neural tissue may actually alter its chemical makeup and reorganize synaptic contacts in the spinal cord such that innocuous inputs are directed to cells that normally receive only noxious inputs (Woolf, 2000).

The central nervous system becomes "hyperexcitable" due to a combination of increased responsiveness and decreased inhibition (Woolf, 2000). This situation is analogous to the volume being turned up on the system such that normally innocuous stimuli generate painful sensations, and noxious stimuli cause an exaggerated pain

response. Central sensitization has been described as a change in both the software and the hardware of the central nervous system (Woolf, 2000) such that the cellular depolarization threshold is reduced (Shevel & Spierings, 2004). Cellular activity continues after peripheral nociception stops, and spreads to other neighboring cells (Woolf & Salter, 2000). In a person with headaches, nociceptive specific cells in the trigeminal nucleus may begin to depolarize with input from primary afferent mechanoreceptors that normally have a low threshold (Woolf et al., 1994). Pain is then perceived in the presence of afferent input that is usually not perceived as noxious. In the "centrally sensitized" patient with chronic headaches, this phenomenon may lead to the onset of a headache, even in the presence of normal stimuli such as movement or pressure. Chapter 6 provides in-depth information on central sensitization mechanisms in migraine.

THE BIOLOGICAL PLAUSIBILITY OF A NEURODYNAMIC MECHANISM IN HEADACHE

Although it is not the purpose of this chapter to delve into the different hypotheses and pathophysiological mechanisms related to the development of a migraine headache, it is important to consider how clinicians interested in neurodynamics for migraine patients might view the physical properties of the nervous system in these patients. The nervous system can be affected by pathology either inside the nervous tissue itself or in the tissues in which it resides and functions, and signs and symptoms may originate from both local and distant neural and non-neural sources (Slater et al., 1994). Neural tissue may become sensitive to movement, thereby becoming a pain generator in patients with headaches following trauma, postural changes, compression, or inflammation (Hall & Elvey, 1999; Chen et al., 2004; Dilley et al., 2005; Greening et al., 2005). Numerous neural structures in the head and upper cervical spine have the potential to cause head pain, including the dura mater, the greater occipital nerve, the upper cervical nerves, and the dorsal root ganglion (Alix & Bates, 1999; Jansen, 1999; Thakur et al., 2002; Bogduk, 2004b).

Few studies have been published on the presence of neural tissue sensitivity in patients with headache. Researchers have reported that 7.4% to 10% of subjects with CeH exhibit neural mechano-sensitivity (Jull et al., 2002; Jull & Niere, 2004; Zito et al., 2006). In these investigations, mechano-sensitivity of neural tissues was assessed maintaining the upper cervical spine in flexion while tensioning neural tissues in the upper and lower extremities via the brachial plexus provocation test (Jull et al., 2002) and the straight leg raise test (Zito et al., 2006). A positive test was defined as a perceived change in tissue resistance with provocation of neck pain or headache with the added movements.

A more recent study investigated the difference in cervical flexion and sensory responses (intensity and location) during a modified Long Sitting Slump (LSS) test (**Figure 19.2**) in 123 children aged 6 to 12 years (Von Piekartz et al., 2007). In this investigation, the test was performed on children with migraine, those with CeH, and a control group. The results indicated that the intensities of the sensory response rate were highest in the migraine and CeH groups compared to controls. The children with migraines predominantly had a sensory response in the legs (81.9%), whereas the CeH group had a sensory response in the spine (80%). A total of 18% of the test subjects felt their responses in the head, including 5 patients in the migraine group and 7 patients in the CeH group. The children with CeH showed cervical flexion ranges that differed significantly ($P < 0.001$) from those of both the control group and the migraine headache group. This finding may lend credence to Breig's "tissue-borrowing" phenomena (Breig, 1960, 1978). The reproducibility of the modified LSS test in the study by Von Piekartz et al. (2007) was ICC 0.96 (95% CI: 0.89–0.99).

Most studies on CeH have focused on the joints of the upper cervical spine (Bogduk, 2004a) and muscle dysfunction (Jull et al., 1999; Petersen, 2003; Jull & Niere, 2004; Zito et al., 2006; Jull et al., 2007). Little is known about the role of the nervous system in CeH (Jull, 1994). Any discussion of the potential influence of the nervous system on CeH, however, requires a knowledge of normal nerve movement or "neurodynamics" (Shacklock, 2005a). One of the main roles of the nervous system is electrochemical communication (Butler, 2000). The nervous system needs to perform these complex signaling processes while simultaneously dealing with movement issues (lengthening, sliding) (Coppieters & Butler, 2008), pressure (tunnels, pinch, surrounding tissues) (Breig, 1978; Butler, 1991, 2000; Shacklock, 2005a), and blood flow changes (increased and/or decreased blood flow, blood pressure changes) (Breig, 1978; Butler, 1991, 2000; Shacklock, 2005a).

Clinicians and researchers have begun investigating the physical properties of nerves, examination procedures aimed at detecting "normal" and "abnormal" movement of neural tissue, and potential treatment strategies to improve neural tissue movement impairments (Butler, 1991, 2000; Elvey, 1997; Greening et al., 1999; Shacklock, 2005a). Neurodynamics is best described as the systematic assessment of the mechanics and physiology of a part of the nervous system (Shacklock, 2005).

Dura Mater Sensitivity

The upper cervical dura mater may be a potential headache generator, as it has innervation from ventral rami of the upper three cervical nerves. The ligamentum nuchae and the rectus capitus posterior minor muscle both have fibrous connections to the dura in this region (Hack et al., 1995; Mitchell et al., 1998; Bogduk, 2001, 2004a). The dura has also been shown to attach to the back of the

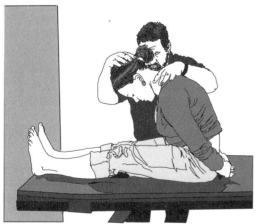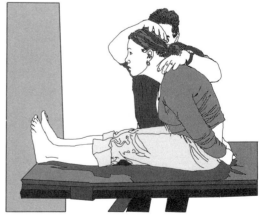

Figure 19.2 **The Modified Long Sitting Slump (Lss) Test May be Used as a Neurodynamic Treatment Technique for Patients with Migraine Headaches.** The patient is placed in the long sitting position with feet held in dorsiflexion by a wall and the trunk is slumped, hips slightly flexed and cervical spine is flexed to onset of a sensory response. The therapist can then gently assist as the patient performs oscillatory upper cervical extension and flexion movements as a means to mobilize neural structures presumed to be contributing to the headache experience.

body of the C2 vertebra and the cranial fossa (Hack et al., 1995). Flexion of the upper cervical spine is, therefore, important in structural differentiation and is used in provocation tests assessing the potential for contribution of upper cervical neural tissues in a patient with headache (Jull, 1997; Jull & Niere, 2004; Von Piekartz et al., 2007). Based on animal studies and research into mechanisms of nociception and neurogenic inflammation, it is thought that the movement of the dura may evoke pain, and a neurogenically inflamed (craniocervical) dura may lead to changes in the contractile state of the blood vessels in the head leading to migraine (Groen et al., 1988; Moskowitz & Macfarlane, 1993; Bove & Moskowitz, 1997).

Many authors have implicated the dura mater as a potential source of headaches, including migraine (Butler, 2000; Bartsch & Goadsby, 2002, 2003a; Bogduk, 2004a; Jull & Niere, 2004; Shacklock, 2005a). Three meninges surround the brain and spinal cord—the pia mater, the arachnoid, and the dura mater. The pia and arachnoid mater most likely have little to no mechanical properties and purportedly control fluid and ion-channel flow (Haines et al., 1993). In comparison, the dura mater seems to have unique features emphasizing potential adaptations that allow for movement. The cranial and spinal dura are continuous and are made up of both elastin and collagen fibers. The ventral dura is thinner than the dorsal dura. Furthermore, the ventral dura contains 7% elastin fibers, whereas the dorsal dura has about twice this amount (Nakagawa et al., 1994). The elastin content allows the cord and meninges to lengthen and remain functional during an almost 30% increase in spinal canal length from spinal extension to spinal flexion (Troup, 1986) (**Figure 19.3**).

As stated earlier, the dura mater of the upper cervical cord and the posterior cranial fossa are connected and receive innervation from branches of the upper three cervical nerves; as such, they are capable of being one of the causes of CeH (Bogduk, 2004a). The fact that the dura is so richly innervated may make the best case for its potential role in headaches, particularly in CeH, TTH, or migraine (Moskowitz, 1993; Hu et al., 1995; Malick & Burstein, 2000; Turnbull & Shepherd, 2003). Another example of this etiology occurs in post–dural puncture headaches. During an epidural steroid injection (ESI), the dura may be punctured. With the dural puncture, leakage of cerebrospinal fluid (CSF) changes the overall pressure of the CSF. It is believed that this decreased pressure causes a downward pull on the cranial dura, which, due to its innervation, then produces a headache (Turnbull & Shepherd, 2003). These headaches have been shown to be posture dependent. That is, when a patient lies down, the headache is eased by virtue of the decreased CSF pressure. When the patient sits upright, a drop in CSF pressure causes the downward (and thus potentially painful) pull of the spinal and cranial dura (Turnbull & Shepherd, 2003). Such post–dural puncture headaches are often relieved with the delivery of a blood patch (Hess, 1991). The seal eliminates the CSF pressure change, thus decreasing the downward pull on the dura.

Based on research investigating post-epidural headaches, it seems plausible that any condition that causes a similar downward pull on the dura may also create such a "dural headache." Thus the dura may be implicated in the pathogenesis of several types of headache as it has

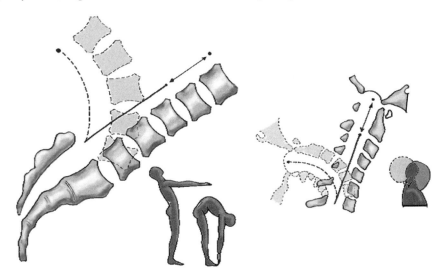

Figure 19.3 Change in Length of the Spinal Canal (and thus its Contents) from Flexion to Extension: Images taken Tracing of X-Rays

the potential, via afferent input into the trigeminal nerve in the trigeminocervical nucleus (Bartsch & Goadsby, 2003b; Bogduk, 2004a), to cause symptoms associated with many primary and secondary headaches (Bogduk, 2004a, 2005).

Greater Occipital Nerve Sensitivity

Some sections of this chapter are painted with a broad brush—including many headache issues related to TTH, CeH, and migraine. One area that has been looked at more specifically for the treatment of migraines, and that warrants specific discussion here, is the greater occipital nerve. Numerous studies have implicated the greater occipital nerve in the development of migraines (Ward, 2003; Magnoux, 2004; Ashkenazi & Young, 2005; Leinisch-Dahlke et al., 2005; Han et al., 2006; Ashkenazi & Levin, 2007; Rozen, 2007; Ashkenazi et al., 2008; Cooper, 2008; Di Stani et al., 2008; Matute et al., 2008; Selekler, 2008; Young, 2008; Young et al., 2008; Baykal, 2009; Selekler et al., 2009; Baron et al., 2010; Saracco et al., 2010). The greater occipital nerve is currently the subject of many studies, mainly aimed at therapeutic injections (greater occipital nerve block [GONB]; **Figure 19.4**) to decrease nociception

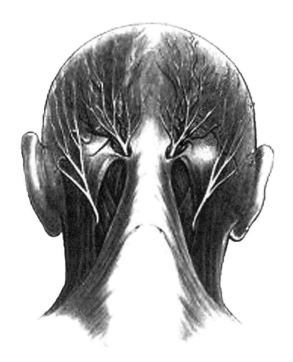

Figure 19.4 The Greater Occipital Nerve Block (GONB) is performed by accessing the greater occipital nerve as it exits the sub-Occipital triangle bounded by the rectus capitis posterior major, oblique capitis lateralis and oblique capitis inferior

(Young, 2008; Young et al., 2008; Krolikowski & Weatherby, 2010; Saracco et al., 2010; Weibelt et al., 2010; Young, 2010). Considering that the greater occipital nerve is a peripheral nerve, it has certain movement requirements—that is, *space, movement,* and need for adequate *blood* supply. This concept will be discussed again later in the chapter.

Two cadaver studies have highlighted the mechanical characteristics of the greater occipital nerve (Mosser et al., 2004; Janis et al., 2010). These studies describe in detail the concern of space issues around the greater occipital nerve and discuss the ways in which the limited space around the nerve might contribute to migraines. Limited space, it would seem, has the potential to inhibit the normal movement and blood supply to the greater occipital nerve, which in turn may lead to increased sensitivity of the nerve. The subsequent rationale for using GONB in the treatment of migraines is strengthened by the fact that there is a convergence of sensory input to trigeminal nucleus caudalis neurons from both cervical and trigeminal fibers (Ashkenazi & Levin, 2007).

The path of the greater occipital nerve can be addressed with invasive procedures such as chemodenervation of the semispinalis capitis muscle, corrugator resection during endoscopic brow lift, injection of botulinum A toxin, and trigger point injections (Mosser et al., 2004). The study by Janis et al. (2010) provides information on potential barriers to movement along the mechanical path of the greater occipital nerve. In this study, the authors dissected the posterior neck and scalp of 25 fresh cadaveric heads and revealed six major compression points along its course. The deepest (most proximal) point was between semispinalis and obliquus capitis inferior, near the spinous process. The second point was at its entrance into semispinalis. The previously described "intermediate" point was at the nerve's exit from semispinalis. A fourth point was located at the entrance of the nerve into the trapezius muscle. The fifth point of compression was where the nerve exits the trapezius fascia insertion into the nuchal line. The occipital artery often crosses the greater occipital nerve, especially in this distal region of the trapezius fascia, which is the final point of potential compression (Janis et al., 2010).

Although no studies have evaluated the effect of neural mobilization techniques on the greater occipital nerve or in migraine patients in general, it is plausible, based on the anatomic and physiological requirements of the greater occipital nerve, that movement-based techniques aimed at restoring proper movement and blood flow to the greater occipital nerve may be of benefit to the migraine patient. Additionally, therapists who treat patients with a multimodal approach including neurodynamics would most likely incorporate joint mobilization and manipulation, soft-tissue mobilization, and exercise and postural strategies into the treatment plan; all of these therapies may positively affect the tissues surrounding the greater occipital nerve, thereby addressing the "container" of the greater occipital nerve (Fernández-de-las-Peñas et al., 2006a, 2006b; Fernández-de-las-Peñas, 2008).

Post-Traumatic Headache and Neural Sensitivity

Recent research into whiplash-associated disorder (WAD) has shown that patients with WAD have restricted mobility and increased pain with upper limb neurodynamic tests, compared to asymptomatic subjects (Sterling et al., 2002). Additionally, decreased knee extension and ankle dorsiflexion range of motion were observed during slump testing in patients with WAD compared to asymptomatic subjects (Yeung et al., 1997). These two whiplash studies suggest that neck trauma may lead to altered movement capabilities of the nervous system distant to the area of injury. Following Breig's "tissue-borrowing" concept (Breig, 1960, 1978), the opposite might also be true: trauma, pain, or altered movement in the periphery and other spinal regions may lead to mechanical changes in the pull on the cervical and cranial dura, which, if sensitized, may contribute to the development of a headache.

More research is needed to further explore the movement properties of the nervous system in regard to headaches. Even the innervation of the meninges is designed for movement (Butler, 2000). Terminals are twisted and in coiled bundles (Groen et al., 1988), meaning that when a healthy, nonsensitized dura is stretched, minimal forces are placed on the mechano-sensitive nerve endings. This anatomic design feature further underscores the dura's movement capabilities in healthy individuals. One might then extrapolate that when this normal movement is altered, the tissues may become sensitized to movement and serve as a potential pain generator in patients with headache.

ASSESSMENT OF NEURODYNAMICS IN HEADACHE PATIENTS

The challenge for the clinician is to differentially diagnose the cause of the patient's symptoms and provide the patient with an effective treatment based on current best evidence. This task can be difficult, especially for the migraine patient, as he or she may report different triggers for the migraine. If a physical examination

demonstrated neurodynamic impairments, however, addressing these deficits may influence the headache.

Research by Breig (1978) and others has demonstrated that flexion of the cervical spine leads to tension in the dura and spinal cord, resulting in a cephalad movement of the cauda equina. This factor ultimately limits the available mobility of the sciatic nerve (Breig, 1960, 1978; Reid, 1960; Breig & Marions, 1963; Breig & el-Nadi, 1966; Breig & Troup, 1979; Johnson & Chiarello, 1997). If a headache patient displays sensitivity to neural tissue movement tests, then it could be argued that assessment and treatment (including neural mobilization) should address this issue.

Studies comparing the range of motion for CeH patient groups and non-headache groups have shown a significant decrease in cervical spine mobility in the former, in terms of rotation, extension, and flexion (Zwart, 1997; Ogince et al., 2007; Von Piekartz et al., 2007). It is also important to consider the attachment of surrounding tissues that might potentially affect normal physiological dural movement. As noted earlier, cadaveric studies have confirmed the existence of a fibrous connection between the rectus capitus posterior minor (RCPM) muscle and the cervical dura (Hack et al., 1995). This pull on the dura may be further enhanced by the connection of the ligamentum nuchae and the posterior spinal dura at the C1 and C2 spinal levels (Mitchell et al., 1998). Changes in the length and pull of these tissues may, therefore, produce a potential painful reaction in the dura, as in post–dural puncture headache. Doursounian et al. (1989) demonstrated that neck/head flexion results in an increased tension in the tissues of the brainstem, cord, cranial nerves, and layers of the dura. Given this relationship, upper cervical flexion should be carefully examined prior to assessing the strength of the deep neck flexors. Anatomically, the CCFT tests upper cervical flexion, which may cause a downward pull on the dura. If the dura and other upper cervical spine neural structures are mechano-sensitive, it is plausible that this sensitization may, via the trigemino-cervical complex, initiate headache symptoms.

Although most of the original "movement studies" were performed on cadavers, newer research using real-time ultrasound indicates that nerves have not only longitudinal movement, but also significant lateral movement capabilities (Wiesler et al., 2006a, 2006b; Coppieters & Alshami, 2007; Dilley et al., 2007). Furthermore, these ultrasound studies reveal that, compared to normal populations, patients with pathology have decreased neural tissue movement (Wiesler et al., 2006a, 2006b; Coppieters & Alshami, 2007; Dilley et al., 2007). The concept of neural tissue movement disorders has led to the development of structured neurodynamic tests to assess the movement capabilities of a specific nerve branch (Elvey, 1979; Butler, 1991, 2000; Shacklock, 2005a). These tests are designed to identify physical dysfunction of the nervous system.

TREATMENT OF NEURODYNAMIC DYSFUNCTION

Neurodynamic interventions aimed at maintaining or increasing the normal movement properties of the dura and other neural structures may be potentially beneficial for patients with headaches (Rumore, 1989; Butler, 2000; Shacklock, 2005a). From an anatomic and physiological perspective, neural tissue has three important requirements—space, movement, and adequate blood supply (Butler, 1991, 2000). If any or all of these requirements are compromised, it may lead to clinical signs and symptoms.

Space

An easy way for clinicians to view the nervous system is that the delicate nerves, spinal cord, and meninges all travel within containers or passage ways. For nerves to properly function, they need to have the ability to "slide" and "glide" unhindered through different areas of the body (Butler, 2000; Shacklock, 2005a; Coppieters & Butler, 2007). As nerves travel through the body, they encounter many surrounding tissues including muscle, bone, ligaments, and fascia (Breig, 1978; Butler, 1991, 2000; Shacklock, 2005a). Numerous studies have shown that if the interface, or "container," is injured or damaged, that condition may have repercussions for the adjacent neural tissues. Examples include damage to the cubital tunnel (Coppieters et al., 2004), carpal tunnel (Mackinnon, 1992; Nakamichi & Tachibana, 1995; Byl & Melnick, 1997; Coveney et al., 1997; Rozmaryn et al., 1998; Greening et al., 1999), intervertebral foramen (de Peretti et al., 1989; Fritz et al., 1998; Chang et al., 2006; Siddiqui et al., 2006), spinal canal (Fritz et al., 1998; Chang et al., 2006), and piriformis (Kuncewicz et al., 2006). When these spaces are compromised and nerves sustain unwanted pressure or irritation, it may lead to the onset of symptoms.

Movement

Closely linked to the issue of the space requirements of the nervous system is the nervous system's ability to perform complex signaling processes during physiological movement. Under normal conditions, nerves move quite well (Beith et al., 1995; Greening et al., 1999; Wright et al., 2001; Dilley et al., 2003; Shacklock, 2005a; Coppieters & Butler, 2007). Indeed, early cadaver studies showed that the nervous system is extremely well designed to handle movement. When the body shifts from a cervical spine neutral position to cervical spine flexion, the spinal cord lengthens approximately 10% (Marguilies et al., 1992; Yuan et al., 1998); when the body goes from cervical spine extension to cervical spine flexion, the cervical cord lengthens approximately 20% (Breig, 1960). It has also been shown that the spinal canal (the "container") can lengthen approximately 30% upon making the transition from spinal extension to spinal flexion (Troup, 1986).

Studies have shown that neural tissue mobilization is effective in the treatment of hamstring injuries (Kornberg & Lew, 1989), lateral epicondylitis (Drechsler et al., 1997), cervico-brachial neurogenic disorders (Coppieters et al., 2003a), hand pain (Sweeney & Harms, 1996), carpal tunnel syndrome (Rozmaryn et al., 1998; Coppieters & Alshami, 2007), cubital tunnel syndrome (Coppieters et al., 2004), and ulnar nerve transposition (Weirich et al., 1998). After the development and refinement of neurodynamic tests, clinicians began to utilize these tools in various forms of treatment, in essence trying to restore and maintain the normal anatomic and physiological requirements of the nervous system (Shacklock, 2005b; Coppieters & Butler, 2007). As this realm is an emerging science, however, only a limited number of research studies on neural tissue mobilization have been published to date.

Blood Flow

Neural tissue is extremely "blood-thirsty." The brain and spinal cord are estimated to account for only 2% of the total body mass, yet they consume 20% to 25% of the available oxygen in the circulating blood (Dommisse, 1994). Moreover, if a nerve is "stretched" by more than 6% to 8% of its normal length, blood flow in the peripheral nerve will slow (Lundborg & Rydevik, 1973; Ogata & Naito, 1986). If the nerve is elongated by approximately 15%, blood flow may be completely occluded (Ogata & Naito, 1986). Adequate blood flow, nutrition, and movement are, therefore, interdependent.

The application of significant, sustained pressure to a nerve may lead to its demyelination (Dyck et al., 1990), which in turn may lead to "peripheral sensitization" such that responses to mechanical, chemical, or thermal stimuli become exaggerated (Asbury & Fields, 1984; Devor & Seltzer, 1999; Hall & Elvey, 1999; Woolf & Mannion, 1999). If blood flow to neural tissue is interrupted, it can result in a hypoxic state, which may in turn lead to an ischemic-based pain state. Ischemic pain is a class of nociceptive pain in which lack of movement, sustained posturing, or decreased circulation creates an acidic environment (lower pH); such an imbalance has been linked to pain (Butler, 2000). From the basic science literature, it seems that treatment techniques aimed at restoring movement, and thus blood flow, have the potential to decrease ischemic-based pain states, as does maintaining normal movement and function of the nervous system (Rozmaryn et al., 1998; Coppieters & Butler, 2007).

Habitual postures of increased forward head with excessive upper cervical spine extension have been identified in office workers with neck pain (Watson & Trott, 1993; Grimmer, 1997; Szeto et al., 2002). In these forward head postures, the posterior neck musculature, such as the RCPM, may undergo adaptive shortening. Attempts at postural correction (e.g., verbal cues or exercises) may lead to a direct pull on the dura, which may contribute to the development of a headache. Clinicians should be aware of this close relationship between the dura, the RCPM muscle, and ligamentum nuchae, as it may have treatment implications. Caution is warranted, as even gentle movement on sensitized neural tissue may potentially lead to the development or exacerbation of a headache. In summary, a valid case can be made for the inclusion of neurodynamic tests and potential neural tissue mobilization in all headache patients.

EXERCISE, BLOOD FLOW, AND NERVES IN MIGRAINE HEADACHE

Although the focus of this chapter is the discussion of neurodynamics in treating migraine headaches, another important consideration regarding nerves and migraines needs to be mentioned that fits within the discussion in this chapter regarding blood flow to nerves. There is mounting interest in exercise—especially aerobic exercise—as a means of managing patients with migraine (Stoica & Enulescu, 1994; Narin et al., 2003; Busch & Gaul, 2008a, 2008b; Dittrich et al., 2008; Varkey et al., 2009; Sahin et al., 2010). The majority of the studies on this topic explain the effect of aerobic exercises on a vascular and chemical level (Stoica & Enulescu, 1994; Narin et al., 2003; Busch & Gaul, 2008a, 2008b; Dittrich et al., 2008; Varkey et al., 2009; Sahin et al., 2010). Although this rationale is not disputed, it should be acknowledged that aerobic exercise will not only increase overall blood flow to the body and neural tissue, but also precipitate movement of the neuromeningeal structures during the exercise-related movement (Dommisse, 1994).

Considering that the nervous system requires approximately 25% of the cardiac output, it can be argued that the optimization of blood flow to the nervous system may also contribute to the possible mechanism behind the positive treatment effects of aerobic exercise for migraine. Additionally, some evidence indicates that aerobic exercise is helpful in easing neuropathic pain (Carmody & Cooper, 1987; Kemppainen et al., 1998; O'Connor & Cook, 1999; Koltyn, 2000; Quintero et al., 2000; Hoffman et al., 2005; Kuphal et al., 2007).

Considering the aforementioned discussion of irritation of various nervous system structures, especially the greater occipital nerve, practitioners of physical therapy that utilizes movement-based treatment should be aware of this possible treatment effect. Considering that neurodynamic techniques have evolved to less sustained techniques and more gentle "sliding" techniques, neural mobilization may be considered beneficial for migraines on a circulatory level. Mechano-sensitive neural tissues within patients may be treated with specific controlled movements of the spine and extremities that move or slide the neural tissues relative to the surrounding tissues (Shacklock, 1995; Elvey, 1997; Hall & Elvey, 1999; Shacklock, 2005a; Coppieters & Butler, 2008). The effect of these treatments has not been investigated in patients with headache, except for a single case report (Rumore, 1989), but many clinicians, including the authors, have utilized these techniques successfully in patients with headaches.

CONCLUSIONS

Very little is known about the role of neurodynamics in headaches, particularly in migraines. No randomized controlled trials have been performed investigating the effects of neurodynamic treatments in patients with headaches, although an emerging base of evidence has demonstrated the efficacy of such techniques in other musculoskeletal conditions. The basic science evidence (anatomy and physiology) would imply that the nervous system, especially the dura and greater occipital nerve, may have a potential role in the development of migraine. Spinal manipulation and mobilization, in combination with exercise, represents the current best practice for the conservative management of patients with cervicogenic headaches (Jull et al., 2002, 2007). The mechanisms behind these beneficial interventions remain unclear, but they are often explained in terms of their effects on local joints and muscles. Although none of these claims is disputed, it could be argued that these techniques may also have a direct or indirect effect on the neural structures responsible for causing headaches.

In any event, if migraines are to be viewed from this perspective or as part of a broader musculoskeletal/vascular approach, neural mobilization should at least be considered in the management of a migraine patient. This understanding reflects the growing evidence base that points to the efficacy of neural mobilization in other spinal and orthopaedic disorders (Kornberg & Lew, 1989; Kornberg & McCarthy, 1992; Sweeney & Harms, 1996; Drechsler et al., 1997; Rozmaryn et al., 1998; Weirich et al., 1998; Coppieters & Butler, 2001; Akalin et al., 2002; Coppieters et al., 2003b, 2004, 2009; Wehbe & Schlegel, 2004; Pinar et al., 2005; Nee & Butler, 2006; Brininger et al., 2007; Coppieters & Alshami, 2007; Oskay et al., 2010) and suggests that the use of neural tissue mobilization may be beneficial in headache patients (Rumore, 1989; Butler, 1991, 2000; Shacklock, 2005a; Von Piekartz et al., 2007; Louw et al., 2009).

This chapter should be seen as a first attempt at addressing a neurophysiological link between the physical properties of the nervous system and headaches, particularly migraine. The field of neurodynamics also encompasses pain science and neuroscience, including ion-channel expression (Devor & Seltzer, 1999), central sensitization (Butler, 2000; Woolf, 2007), and changes in the central nervous system, including the brain—particularly in chronic pain states. These aspects were not discussed within this chapter but are certainly important as we consider altering pain states and neural tissue sensitivity in patients with headache. Might we be able to change the "software" of the central nervous system via the gentle introduction of movement through the neural tissues, thereby inducing a permanent change in this central pain state in patients with headache? This remains to be seen, and future research may give us some of these answers.

REFERENCES

Akalin E, El O, Peker O, et al. Treatment of carpal tunnel syndrome with nerve and tendon gliding exercises. *Am J Phys Med Rehabil* 2002;81:108–113.

Alix ME, Bates DK. A proposed etiology of cervicogenic headache: the neurophysiologic basis and anatomic relationship between the dura mater and the rectus posterior capitis minor muscle. *J Manipul Physiol Ther* 1999;22:534–539.

Asbury AK, Fields HL. Pain due to peripheral nerve damage: an hypothesis. *Neurology* 1984;34:1587–1590.

Ashkenazi A, Levin M. Greater occipital nerve block for migraine and other headaches: is it useful? *Curr Pain Headache Rep* 2007;11:231–235.

Ashkenazi A, Young WB. The effects of greater occipital nerve block and trigger point injection on brush allodynia and pain in migraine. *Headache* 2005;45:350–354.

Ashkenazi A, Matro R, Shaw J, et al. Greater occipital nerve block using local anaesthetics alone or with triamcinolone for transformed migraine: a randomised comparative study. *J Neurol Neurosurg Psychiatry* 2008;79:415–417.

Bansevicius D, Westgaard RH, Sjaastad, OM. Tension-type headache: pain, fatigue, tension, and EMG responses to mental activation. *Headache* 1999;39:417–425.

Baron EP, Tepper SJ, Mays M, et al. Acute treatment of basilar-type migraine with greater occipital nerve blockade. *Headache* 2010;50:1057–1059.

Bartsch T, Goadsby PJ. Stimulation of the greater occipital nerve induces increased central excitability of dural afferent input. *Brain* 2002;125:1496–1509.

Bartsch T, Goadsby PJ. Increased responses in trigeminocervical nociceptive neurons to cervical input after stimulation of the dura mater. *Brain* 2003a;126:1801–1813.

Bartsch T, Goadsby PJ. The trigeminocervical complex and migraine: current concepts and synthesis. *Curr Pain Head Reports* 2003b;7:371–376.

Baykal M. Greater occipital nerve block in migraine headache. *Agri* 2009;21:83.

Beith ID, Robins EJ, Richards PR. An assessment of the adaptive mechanisms within and surrounding the peripheral nervous system, during changes in nerve bed length resulting from underlying joint movement. In: Shacklock MO, ed. *Moving in on Pain*. Australia: Butterworth-Heinemann; 1995.

Bogduk N. Cervicogenic headache: anatomic basis and pathophysiologic mechanisms. *Curr Pain Head Reports* 2001;5:382–386.

Bogduk N. The neck and headaches. *Neurol Clin* 2004a; 22:151–171, vii.

Bogduk N. Role of anesthesiologic blockade in headache management. *Curr Pain Head Reports* 2004b;8:399–403.

Bogduk N. Distinguishing primary headache disorders from cervicogenic headache: clinical and therapeutic implications. *Headache Currents* 2005;2:27–36.

Bove GM, Moskowitz MA. Primary afferent neurons innervating guinea pig dura. *J Neurophysiol* 1997;77:299–308.

Breig A. *Biomechanics of the Central Nervous System*. Stockholm: Almqvist and Wiksell; 1960.

Breig A. *Adverse Mechanical Tension in the Central Nervous System*. Stockholm: Almqvist and Wiksell; 1978.

Breig A, el-Nadi AF. Biomechanics of the cervical spinal cord: relief of contact pressure on and overstretching of the spinal cord. *Acta Radiol Diagn (Stockh)* 1966;4:602–624.

Breig A, Marions O. Biomechanics of the lumbosacral nerve roots. *Acta Radiol Diagn (Stockh)* 1963;1:1141–1160.

Breig A, Troup JD. Biomechanical considerations in the straight-leg-raising test: cadaveric and clinical studies of the effects of medial hip rotation. *Spine* 1979;4:242–250.

Brininger TL, Rogers JC, Holm M, et al. Efficacy of a fabricated customized splint and tendon and nerve gliding exercises for the treatment of carpal tunnel syndrome: a randomized controlled trial. *Arch Phys Med Rehabil* 2007;88:1429–1435.

Burstein R. Deconstructing migraine headache into peripheral and central sensitization. *Pain* 2001;89:107–110.

Busch V, Gaul C. Exercise in migraine therapy: is there any evidence for efficacy? A critical review. *Headache* 2008a;48:890–899.

Busch V, Gaul C. Exercise in migraine treatment: review and discussion of clinical trials and implications for further trials. *Schmerz* 2008b;22:137–147.

Butler DS. *Mobilisation of the Nervous System.* London: Churchill Livingstone; 1991.

Butler DS. *The Sensitive Nervous System.* Adelaide: Noigroup Publications; 2000.

Byl NN, Melnick M. The neural consequences of repetition: clinical implications of a learning hypothesis. *J Hand Therapy* 1997;10:160–174.

Cady RK. The convergence hypothesis. *Headache* 2007;47:S44–S51.

Cady R, Schreiber C, Farmer K, et al. Primary headaches: a convergence hypothesis. *Headache* 2002;42:204–216.

Carmody J, Cooper K. Swim stress reduces chronic pain in mice through an opioid mechanism. *Neurosci Lett* 1987; 74:358–363.

Chang SB, Lee SH, Ahn Y, et al. Risk factor for unsatisfactory outcome after lumbar foraminal and far lateral microdecompression. *Spine* 2006;31:1163–1167.

Chen C, Cavanaugh JM, Song Z, et al. Effects of nucleus pulposus on nerve root neural activity, mechanosensitivity, axonal morphology, and sodium channel expression. *Spine* 2004;29:17–25.

Cooper W. Images from headache: resolution of trigeminal mediated nasal edema following greater occipital nerve blockade. *Headache* 2008;48:278–279.

Coppieters MW, Alshami AM. Longitudinal excursion and strain in the median nerve during novel nerve gliding exercises for carpal tunnel syndrome. *J Orthop Res* 2007; 25:972–980.

Coppieters MW, Butler DS. In defense of neural mobilization. *J Orthop Sports Phys Ther* 2001;31:520–521; author reply 522.

Coppieters MW, Butler DS. Do "sliders" slide and "tensioners" tension? An analysis of neurodynamic techniques and considerations regarding their application. *Man Ther* 2007. doi:10.1016/j.math.2006.12.008.

Coppieters MW, Butler DS. Do "sliders" slide and "tensioners" tension? An analysis of neurodynamic techniques and considerations regarding their application. *Man Ther* 2008;13:213–221.

Coppieters MW, Stappaerts KH, Karel H, et al. Aberrant protective force generation during neural provocation testing and the effect of treatment in patients with neurogenic cervicobrachial pain. *J Manipulative Physiol Therapeutics* 2003a; 26:99–106.

Coppieters MW, Stappaerts KH, Wouters LL, et al. The immediate effects of a cervical lateral glide treatment technique in patients with neurogenic cervicobrachial pain. *J Orthop Sports Phys Ther* 2003b;33:369–378.

Coppieters MW, Bartholomeeusen KE, Katrien E, et al. Incorporating nerve-gliding techniques in the conservative treatment of cubital tunnel syndrome. *J Manipulative Physiol Therapeutics* 2004;27:560–568.

Coppieters MW, Hough AD, Dilley A. Different nerve-gliding exercises induce different magnitudes of median nerve longitudinal excursion: an in vivo study using dynamic ultrasound imaging. *J Orthop Sports Phys Ther* 2009;39:164–171.

Coveney B, Trott P, Grimmer KA. The upper limb tension test in a group of subjects with a clinical presentation of carpal tunnel syndrome. Tenth Biennial Conference: Manipulative Physiotherapists Association of Australia; Melbourne; 1997.

D'Amico D, Leone M, Bussone G. Side-locked unilaterality and pain localization in long-lasting headaches: migraine, tension-type headache, and cervicogenic headache. *Headache* 1994;34:526–530.

de Peretti F, Micalef JP, Bourgeon A, et al.. Biomechanics of the lumbar spinal nerve roots and the first sacral root within the intervertebral foramina. *Surg Radiol Anatomy* 1989;11:221–225.

Devor M, Seltzer Z. Pathophysiology of damaged nerves in relation to chronic pain. In: Wall PD, Melzack R, eds. *Textbook of Pain.* Edinburgh: Churchill Livingstone; 1999.

Dilley A, Lynn B, Greening J, et al. Quantitative in vivo studies of median nerve sliding in response to wrist, elbow, shoulder and neck movements. *Clin Biomechanics* 2003;18:899–907.

Dilley A, Lynn B, Pang SJ. Pressure and stretch mechanosensitivity of peripheral nerve fibres following local inflammation of the nerve trunk. *Pain* 2005;117:462–472.

Dilley A, Odeyinde S, Greening J, et al. Longitudinal sliding of the median nerve in patients with non-specific arm pain. *Man Ther* 2007. doi:10.1016/j.math.2007.07.004.

Di Stani F, Piovesan EJ, Scattoni L, et al. Occipital neuroma triggered cluster headache responding to greater occipital nerve blockade. *Arq Neuropsiquiatr* 2008;66:74–76.

Dittrich SM, Gunther V, Franz G, et al. Aerobic exercise with relaxation: influence on pain and psychological well-being in female migraine patients. *Clin J Sport Med* 2008;18:363–365.

Dommisse GF. The blood supply of the spinal cord and the consequences of failure. In: Boyling J, Palastanga N, eds. *Grieve's Modern Manual Therapy.* Edinburgh: Churchill Livingstone; 1994.

Doursounian L, Alfonso JM, Iba-Zizen, MT, et al. Dynamics of the junction between the medulla and the cervical spinal cord: an in vivo study in the sagittal plane by magnetic resonance imaging. *Surg Radiol Anatomy* 1989;11:313–322.

Drechsler WI, Knarr JF, Snyder-Mackler L. A comparison of two treatment regimens for lateral epicondylitis: a randomized trial of clinical interventions. *J Sport Rehabil* 1997;6:226–234.

Dyck PJ, Lais AC, Giannini C, et al. Structural alterations of nerve during cuff compression. *Proc Natl Acad Sci* 1990;87:9828–9832.

Elvey R. Brachial plexus tension test and the pathoanatomical origin of arm pain. In: Glasgow E, Twomey L, eds. *Aspects of Manipulative Therapy.* Lincoln: Institute of Health Sciences; 1979:105–110.

Elvey RL. Physical evaluation of the peripheral nervous system in disorders of pain and dysfunction. *J Hand Ther* 1997;10:122–129.

Fernández-de-las-Peñas C. Physical therapy and exercise in headache. *Cephalalgia* 2008;28:36–38.

Fernández-de-las-Peñas C, Alonso-Blanco C, Cuadrado ML, et al. Are manual therapies effective in reducing pain from tension-type headache? A systematic review. *Clin J Pain* 2006a;22:278–285.

Fernández-de-las-Peñas C, Cuadrado ML, Gerwin RD, et al. Myofascial disorders in the trochlear region in unilateral migraine: a possible initiating or perpetuating factor. *Clin J Pain* 2006b;22:548–553.

Fernández-de-las-Peñas C, Simons D, Cuadrado ML, et al. The role of myofascial trigger points in musculoskeletal pain syndromes of the head and neck. *Curr Pain Headache Reports* 2007;11:365–372.

Fernández-de-las-Peñas C, Madeleine P, Caminero A, et al. Generalized neck-shoulder hyperalgesia in chronic tension-type headache and unilateral migraine assessed by pressure pain sensitivity topographical maps of the trapezius muscle. *Cephalalgia* 2010; 30:77–86.

Fishbain DA, Cutler R, Cole B, et al. International Headache Society headache diagnostic patterns in pain facility patients. *Clin J Pain* 2001;17:78–93.

Fishbain DA, Lewis J, Cole B, et al. Do the proposed cervicogenic headache diagnostic criteria demonstrate specificity in terms of separating cervicogenic headache from migraine? *Curr Pain Headache Reports* 2003;7:387–394.

Fredriksen TA, Sjaastad O. Cervicogenic headache: current concepts of pathogenesis related to anatomical structure. *Clin Experimental Rheumatol* 2000;18:S16–S18.

Fritz JM, Delitto A, Welch WC, et al. Lumbar spinal stenosis: a review of current concepts in evaluation, management, and outcome measurements. *Arch Physical Med Rehabil* 1998;79:700–708.

Goadsby PJ. Migraine pathophysiology. *Headache* 2005; 45:S14–S24.

Greening J, Smart S, Leary R, et al. Reduced movement of median nerve in carpal tunnel during wrist flexion in patients with non-specific arm pain. *Lancet* 1999;354: 217–218.

Greening J, Dilley A, Lynn B. In vivo study of nerve movement and mechanosensitivity of the median nerve in whiplash and non-specific arm pain patients. *Pain* 2005;115:248–253.

Grimmer K. An investigation of poor cervical resting posture. *Australian J Physiother* 1997;43:7–16.

Groen GJ, Baljet B, Drukker J. The innervation of the spinal dura mater: anatomy and clinical implications. *Acta Neurochirurgica* 1988;92:39–46.

Hack GD, Koritzer RT, Robinson WL, et al. Anatomic relation between the rectus capitis posterior minor muscle and the dura mater. *Spine* 1995;20:2484–2486.

Haines DE, Harkey HL, Mefty O. The "subdural" space: a new look at an outdated concept. *Neurosurgery* 1993;32: 111–120.

Hall TM, Elvey RL. Nerve trunk pain: physical diagnosis and treatment. *Man Ther* 1999;4:63–73.

Hall T, Robinson K. The flexion–rotation test and active cervical mobility: a comparative measurement study in cervicogenic headache. *Man Ther* 2004;9:197–202.

Han DW, Koo BN, Chung WY, et al. Preoperative greater occipital nerve block in total thyroidectomy patients can reduce postoperative occipital headache and posterior neck pain. *Thyroid* 2006;16:599–603.

Hess JH. Postdural puncture headache: a literature review. *Am Assoc Nurse Anesthestists J* 1991;59:549–555.

Hoffman MD, Shepanski BA, Mackenzie SP, et al. Experimentally induced pain perception is acutely reduced by aerobic exercise in people with chronic low back pain. *J Rehabil Res Dev* 2005;42:183–190.

Hu JW, Vernon H, Tatourian I. Changes in neck electromyography associated with meningeal noxious stimulation. *J Manipulative Physiol Therapeutics* 1995;18:577–581.

International Headache Society. ICHD-II: The International Classification of Headache Disorders: 2nd edition. *Cephalalgia* 2004;24(suppl 1):9–160.

Janis JE, Hatef DA, Ducic I, et al. The anatomy of the greater occipital nerve: part II. Compression point topography. *Plast Reconstr Surg* 2010;126:1563–1572.

Jansen J. Laminoplasty: a possible treatment for cervicogenic headache? Some ideas on the trigger mechanism of CeH. *Functional Neurol* 1999;14:163–165.

Johnson EK, Chiarello CM. The slump test: the effects of head and lower extremity position on knee extension. *J Orthop Sports Phys Ther* 1997;26:310–317.

Jull G. Headaches of cervical origin. In Grant R, ed. *Physical Therapy of the Cervical and Thoracic Spine.* New York: Churchill Livingstone; 1994:261–285.

Jull G. Management of cervical headache. *Man Ther* 1997;2: 182–190.

Jull G, Niere K. The cervical spine and headache. In Boyling J, Jull GA, eds. *Grieve's Modern Manual Therapy: The Vertebral Column.* London: Churchill Livingstone; 2004.

Jull G, Barrett C, Magee R, et al. Further clinical clarification of the muscle dysfunction in cervical headache. *Cephalalgia* 1999;19:179–185.

Jull G, Trott P, Zito G, et al. A randomized controlled trial of exercise and manipulative therapy for cervicogenic headache. *Spine* 2002;27:1835–1843; discussion 1843.

Jull G, Amiri M, Bullock-Saxon J, et al. Cervical musculoskeletal impairment in frequent intermittent headache. Part 1: subjects with single headaches. *Cephalalgia* 2007;27:793–802.

Kemppainen P, Hamalainen O, Kononen M. Different effects of physical exercise on cold pain sensitivity in fighter pilots with and without the history of acute in-flight neck pain attacks. *Med Sci Sports Exerc* 1998;30:577–582.

Kerr RW. A mechanism to account for frontal headache in cases of posterior-fossa tumors. *J Neurosurg* 1961;18: 605–609.

Kerr RW, Olafson RA. Trigeminal and cervical volleys: convergence on single units in the spinal gray at C-1 and C-2. *Arch Neurol* 1961;5:171–178.

Koltyn KF. Analgesia following exercise: a review. *Sports Med* 2000;29:85–98.

Kornberg C, Lew P. The effect of stretching neural structures on grade one hamstring injuries. *J Orthop Sports Phys Ther* 1989;10:481–487.

Kornberg C, McCarthy T. The effect of neural stretching technique on sympathetic outflow to the lower limbs. *J Orthop Sports Phys Ther* 1992;16:269–274.

Krolikowski K, Weatherby S. POH06 Headache management: greater occipital nerve injection as part of clinical practice. *J Neurol Neurosurg Psychiatry* 2010;81:e52.

Kuncewicz E, Gajewska K, Sobieska M, et al. Piriformis muscle syndrome. *Annales Academiae Medicae Stetinensis* 2006; 52:99–101; discussion 101.

Kuphal KE, Fibuch E, Taylor BK. Extended swimming exercise reduces inflammatory and peripheral neuropathic pain in rodents. *J Pain* 2007;8:989–997.

Leinisch-Dahlke E, Jurgens T, Bogdahn U, et al. Greater occipital nerve block is ineffective in chronic tension type headache. *Cephalalgia* 2005;25:704–708.

Leone M, D'Amico D, Moschiano F, et al. Possible identification of cervicogenic headache among patients with migraine: an analysis of 374 headaches. *Headache* 1995;35: 461–464.

Louw A, Mintken P, Puentedura E. Neuophysiologic effects of neural mobilization maneuvers. In: Fernández-de-las-Peñas C, Arendt-Nielsen L, Gerwin RD, eds. *Tension-Type and Cervicogenic Headache.* Sudbury, MA: Jones and Bartlett; 2009:231–245.

Lundborg G, Rydevik B. Effects of stretching the tibial nerve of the rabbit: a preliminary study of the intraneural circulation and the barrier function of the perineurium. *J Bone Joint Surg (Brit)* 1973;55:390–401.

Mackinnon SE. Double and multiple "crush" syndromes: double and multiple entrapment neuropathies. *Hand Clinics* 1992;8:369–390.

Magnoux E. Greater occipital nerve blockade for cluster headache. *Cephalalgia* 2004;24:239.

Malick A, Burstein R. Peripheral and central sensitization during migraine. *Functional Neurol* 2000;15:28–35.

Marguilies SS, Meandey DF, Bilston LB. In vivo motion of the human spinal cord in extension and flexion. Proceedings of the International Conference on the Biomechanics of Impacts; Verona, Italy; 1992.

Matute E, Bonilla S, Girones A, et al. Bilateral greater occipital nerve block for post-dural puncture headache. *Anaesthesia* 2008;63:557–558.

Mitchell BS, Humphreys BK, O'Sullovan E. Attachments of the ligamentum nuchae to cervical posterior spinal dura and the lateral part of the occipital bone. *J Manipulative Physiol Therapeutics* 1998;21:145–148.

Moskowitz MA. Neurogenic inflammation in the pathophysiology and treatment of migraine. *Neurology* 1993;43: S16–S20.

Moskowitz MA, Macfarlane R. Neurovascular and molecular mechanisms in migraine headaches. *Cerebrovasc Brain Metabol Rev* 1993;5:159–177.

Mosser SW, Guyuron B, Janis JE, et al. The anatomy of the greater occipital nerve: implications for the etiology of migraine headaches. *Plast Reconstr Surg* 2004;113: 693–697; discussion 698–700.

Nakagawa H, Mikawa Y, Watanabe R. Elastin in the human posterior longitudinal ligament and spinal dura: a histologic and biochemical study. *Spine* 1994;19:2164–2169.

Nakamichi K, Tachibana S. Restricted motion of the median nerve in carpal tunnel syndrome. *J Hand Surg (Brit)* 1995; 20:460–464.

Narin SO, Pinar L, Erbas D, et al. The effects of exercise and exercise-related changes in blood nitric oxide level on migraine headache. *Clin Rehabil* 2003;17:624–630.

Narouze S. *Cervicogenic Headache: Diagnosis and Treatment.* ASA Refresher Courses in Anesthesiology; 2007.

Nee RJ, Butler DS. Management of peripheral neuropathic pain: integrating neurobiology, neurodynamics, and clinical evidence. *Physical Ther Sport* 2006;7:36–49.

O'Connor PJ, Cook DB. Exercise and pain: the neurobiology, measurement, and laboratory study of pain in relation to exercise in humans. *Exerc Sport Sci Rev* 1999;27:119–166.

Ogata K, Naito M. Blood flow of peripheral nerve: effects of dissection, stretching and compression. *J Hand Surg (Am)* 1986;11:10–14.

Ogince M, Hall T, Robinson K, et al. The diagnostic validity of the cervical flexion–rotation test in C1/2–related cervicogenic headache. *Man Ther* 2007;12:256–262.

Oskay D, Meric A, Kirdi N, et al. Neurodynamic mobilization in the conservative treatment of cubital tunnel syndrome: long-term follow-up of 7 cases. *J Manipulative Physiol Ther* 2010;33:156–163.

Parsons AA, Strijbos PJ. The neuronal versus vascular hypothesis of migraine and cortical spreading depression. *Curr Opin Pharmacol* 2003;3:73–77.

Petersen SM. Articular and muscular impairments in cervicogenic headache: a case report. *J Orthop Sports Phys Ther* 2003;33:21–30; discussion 30–32.

Pinar L, Enhos A, Ada S, et al. Can we use nerve gliding exercises in women with carpal tunnel syndrome? *Adv Ther* 2005;22:467–475.

Quintero L, Moreno M, Avila C, et al. Long-lasting delayed hyperalgesia after subchronic swim stress. *Pharmacol Biochem Behav* 2000;67:449–458.

Rasmussen BK. Migraine and tension-type headache are separate disorders. *Cephalalgia* 1996;16:217–220; discussion 223.

Reid JD. Effects of flexion–extension movements of the head and spine upon the spinal cord and nerve roots. *J Neurol Neurosurg Psychiatry* 1960;23:214–221.

Rozen T. Cessation of hemiplegic migraine auras with greater occipital nerve blockade. *Headache* 2007;47:917–919.

Rozmaryn LM, Dovelle S, Rothman ER, et al. Nerve and tendon gliding exercises and the conservative management of carpal tunnel syndrome. *J Hand Ther* 1998;11:171–179.

Rumore AJ. Slump examination and treatment in a patient suffering headache. *J Physiother* 1989;35:262–263.

Sahin S, Cinar N, Benli Aksungar F, et al. Attenuated lactate response to ischemic exercise in migraine. *Med Sci Monit* 2010;16:CR378–CR382.

Saracco MG, Valfre W, Valfre W, et al. Greater occipital nerve block in chronic migraine. *Neurol Sci* 2010;31:S179–S180.

Selekler MH. Greater occipital nerve blockade: trigeminicervical system and clinical applications in primary headaches. *Agri* 2008;20:6–13.

Selekler M, Kutlu A, Dundar G.. Orgasmic headache responsive to greater occipital nerve blockade. *Headache* 2009;49:130–131.

Shacklock M. Neurodynamics. *Physiotherapy* 1995;81:9–16.

Shacklock M. *Clinical Neurodynamics.* Edinburgh: Elsevier; 2005a.

Shacklock M. Improving application of neurodynamic (neural tension) testing and treatments: a message to researchers and clinicians. *Man Ther* 2005b;10:175–179.

Shevel E, Spierings EH. Role of the extracranial arteries in migraine headache: a review. *Cranio* 2004;22:132–136.

Siddiqui M, Karadimas E, Nicol M, et al. Influence of X Stop on neural foramina and spinal canal area in spinal stenosis. *Spine* 2006;31:2958–2962.

Silberstein SD. Migraine pathophysiology and its clinical implications. *Cephalalgia* 2004;24:2–7.

Sjaastad O, Fredriksen TA, Pfaffenrath V. Cervicogenic headache: diagnostic criteria. The Cervicogenic Headache International Study Group. *Headache* 1998;38:442–445.

Slater E, Butler DS, Shacklock M. The dynamic central nervous system: examination and assessment using tension tests. In: Boyling J, Palastanga N, eds. *Grieve's Modern Manual Therapy: The Vertebral Column.* Edinburgh: Churchill Livingstone; 1994: 587–606.

Solomon S. Diagnosis of primary headache disorders: validity of the International Headache Society criteria in clinical practice. *Neurol Clin* 1997;15:15–26.

Sterling M, Treleaven J, Jull G. Responses to a clinical test of mechanical provocation of nerve tissue in whiplash associated disorder. *Man Ther* 2002;7:89–94.

Stoica E, Enulescu O. Catecholamine response to exercise in migraine. *Rom J Neurol Psychiatry* 1994;32:21–27.

Sweeney J, Harms A. Persistent mechanical allodynia following injury of the hand: treatment through mobilization of the nervous system. *J Hand Ther* 1996;9:328–338.

Szeto GP, Straker L, Raine S. A field comparison of neck and shoulder postures in symptomatic and asymptomatic office workers. *Applied Ergonomics* 2002;33:75–84.

Thakur R, Hogan LA, Pannella-Vaughn J. Tension and cervicogenic headaches. *Consultant* 2002;42:1512–1515.

Troup JDG. Biomechanics of the lumbar spinal canal. *Clin Biomechanics* 1986;1:31–43.

Turnbull DK, Shepherd DB. Post–dural puncture headache: pathogenesis, prevention and treatment. *Brit J Anaesthesia* 2003;91:718–729.

Vargas BB. Tension-type headache and migraine: two points on a continuum? *Curr Pain Headache Rep* 2008;12:433–436.

Varkey E, Cider A, Carlsson J, et al. A study to evaluate the feasibility of an aerobic exercise program in patients with migraine. *Headache* 2009;49:563–570.

Von Piekartz HJ, Schouten S, Aufdemkampe G. Neurodynamic responses in children with migraine or cervicogenic headache versus a control group: a comparative study. *Man Ther* 2007;12:153–160.

Ward JB. Greater occipital nerve block. *Semin Neurol* 2003;23:59–62.

Watson DH, Trott PH. Cervical headache: an investigation of natural head posture and upper cervical flexor muscle performance. *Cephalalgia* 1993;13:272–284; discussion 232.

Wehbe MA, Schlegel JM. Nerve gliding exercises for thoracic outlet syndrome. *Hand Clin* 2004;20:51–55, vi.

Weibelt S, Andress-Rothrock D, King W, et al. Suboccipital nerve blocks for suppression of chronic migraine: safety, efficacy, and predictors of outcome. *Headache* 2010;50:1041–1044.

Weirich SD, Gelberman RH, Best SA, et al. Rehabilitation after subcutaneous transposition of the ulnar nerve: immediate versus delayed mobilization. *J Shoulder Elbow Surg* 1998;7:244–249.

Wiesler ER, Chloros GD, et al. Ultrasound in the diagnosis of ulnar neuropathy at the cubital tunnel. *J Hand Surg (Am)* 2006a;31:1088–1093.

Wiesler ER, Chloros GD, Cartwright MS, et al. The use of diagnostic ultrasound in carpal tunnel syndrome. *J Hand Surg (Am)* 2006b;31:726–732.

Woolf CJ. Pain. *Neurobiol Dis* 2000;7:504–510.

Woolf CJ. Central sensitization: uncovering the relation between pain and plasticity. *Anesthesiology* 2007;106:864–867.

Woolf CJ, Mannion RJ. Neuropathic pain: aetiology, symptoms, mechanisms, and management. *Lancet* 1999;353:1959–1964.

Woolf CJ, Salter MW. Neuronal plasticity: increasing the gain in pain. *Science* 2000;288:1765–1769.

Woolf CJ, Shortland P, Sivilotti LG. Sensitization of high mechanothreshold superficial dorsal horn and flexor motor neurones following chemosensitive primary afferent activation. *Pain* 1994;58:141–155.

Wright TW, Glowczewskie F Jr, Cowin D, et al. Ulnar nerve excursion and strain at the elbow and wrist associated with upper extremity motion. *J Hand Surg (Am)* 2001;26:655–662.

Yeung E, Jones M, Hall B. The response to the slump test in a group of female whiplash patients. *Aust J Physiother* 1997;43:245–252.

Young WB. Cessation of hemiplegic migraine auras with greater occipital nerve blockade: a comment. *Headache* 2008;48:481.

Young WB. Blocking the greater occipital nerve: utility in headache management. *Curr Pain Headache Reports* 2010;14:404–408.

Young W, Cook B, Malik S, et al. The first 5 minutes after greater occipital nerve block. *Headache* 2008;48:1126–1128.

Yuan Q, Dougherty L, Marguiles SS. In vivo human cervical spinal cord deformation and displacement in flexion. *Spine* 1998;23:1677–1683.

Zito G, Jull G, Story I. Clinical tests of musculoskeletal dysfunction in the diagnosis of cervicogenic headache. *Man Ther* 2006;11:118–129.

Zwart JA. Neck mobility in different headache disorders. *Headache* 1997;37:6–11.

Manual Therapy in the Cranial Region

César Fernández-de-las-Peñas, PT, DO, PhD, Javier González-Iglesias, PT, DO, PhD, Harry Von Piekartz, PT, MSc, PhD, and Graham Gard, DO

PERSPECTIVES ON THE MANAGEMENT OF THE CRANIUM

A variety of approaches are employed for the management of the cranium. This chapter discusses the current status of manual therapy used to influence the craniofacial region. Several scientific studies support manual therapy as treatment for the cranium, and a clinical integration of different hypotheses should be considered as a basis for clinical practice.

Cranial–Sacral Therapy

The therapeutic intervention to the skull that is most extensively used on a worldwide basis is cranial–sacral therapy (CST). This nonpharmacological clinical approach has been proposed as a technique for the management of migraine. Scientific evidence of its efficacy, however, remains limited (Mann et al., 2008). CST appears to be a very safe treatment method, but side effects can arise from its use (McPartland, 1996), probably due to poor application (Upledger, 1996). The proposed goals of CST are to release articular and membranous cranial restrictions, reduce neural entrapments related to the skull, enhance the rate and amplitude of the cranial rhythmic pulse, and reduce venous congestion (Greenman, 1996). Nevertheless, no definitive scientific evidence supports these outcome-related assumptions.

According to current osteopathic visions of CST, intrinsic rhythmic movements of the brain cause rhythmic fluctuations of cerebrospinal fluid, and specific relational changes among dural membranes, cranial bones, and the sacrum (McPartland & Skinner, 2005; Hartman, 2006). This procedure, which is called "the primary respiratory mechanism," is based on the following hypotheses: (1) inherent rhythmic motility of the brain and spinal cord; (2) rhythmic fluctuation of cerebrospinal fluid; (3) articular mobility of the cranial bones; (4) mobility of intracranial and intraspinal dural membranes; and (5) mobility of the sacrum between the iliac bones. The primary respiratory mechanism concept assumes the presence of a rhythmic involuntary motion of the sacrum related to the involuntary motion of the occiput, which can in turn be perceived by the therapist. McPartland and Mein (1997) have suggested that palpation of this mechanism yields a harmonic signal from several senses, including temperature receptors, mechanoreceptors, and proprioceptors. However, inter-examiner reliability for simultaneous palpation at the occiput and the sacrum has been found to be poor (ICCs: −0.09 to 0.31) (Moran & Gibbons, 2001). In addition, no evidence has been found

that different clinicians perceive this phenomenon or even that the perceived phenomenon is real (Hartman & Norton, 2002).

The primary respiratory mechanism is poorly understood, and its origin remains unknown, although a number of hypotheses have been proposed to explain it (Nelson et al., 2001). The most widely accepted theory suggests that CTS is based on inherent mobility of the nervous system and fluctuation of cerebrospinal fluid resulting in a rhythmic pulsation, which is then translated through the dural membranes to the cranial bones (Brooks, 2000). Green et al. (1999) concluded that there is evidence for cerebrospinal fluid pulsation as measured by magnetic resonance imaging, encephalography, and myelography monitoring. However, this hypothesis has been questioned (Hartman, 2006). Others have theorized a harmonic effect of vascular and neurologic processes as the origin of the primary respiratory mechanism (Moskalenko et al., 1999, 2001).

Gard (2009) proposed a more complex hypothesis based on the venous system of the brain. This broad theory differs from those mentioned previously in that the cerebrospinal fluid is perceived as simply a fluid acting under pressure in a semi-sealed container (i.e., the skull and spinal column). The brain, connective tissue, and the cerebrospinal fluid are of relatively fixed volume. Although the cerebrospinal fluid is replaced every 4 to 6 hours, its volume does not change instantaneously, so none of these factors will directly influence intracranial pressure in the short term. Blood volume inside the skull, however, varies constantly depending on flow. Therefore, controlling this flow offers a mechanism for management of pressure. The vascular anatomy inside the skull presents a complete system for management of intracranial pressure and makes the following assumptions:

1. The cavernous sinuses control venous outflow through the spinal venous network.
2. The internal and external vertebral venous plexus system allows for a controlled release of venous blood out of the internal spinal/skull vault, as well as a reversible flow of blood back into the cavity when there is a sharp drop in intracranial pressure.
3. A ball valve system operates in the great cerebral vein and cavernous sinus, where the cerebrospinal fluid–filled arachnoid granulations swell to reduce venous blood flow when the cerebrospinal fluid pressure increases (Gard, 2009).

This model would explain the mechanisms of an involuntary movement originating within the cranium and spine. The techniques altering cranial bone function within this model are similar to those posited by the other theories, but the intention is always to encourage continuous expansion of the surrounding bones from an arbitrary point at the center of the skull, depending on the bony anatomy (Gard, 2009).

The pain and aura of migraine can be explained in this model as follows: A stable skull rests at its maximum available expansion. Mechanical restriction through the skull and upper neck will distort the skull vault in a way that reduces its internal volume. The resultant increase in intracranial pressure causes the cerebrospinal fluid–filled arachnoid granulations to expand into their relevant blood vessels. In the cavernous sinuses, they shut off blood flow from the venous sinuses in the skull to the veins of the spinal column, forcing more blood out of the jugular vein. The cerebrospinal fluid can drain into the vacant space within the spinal column, thereby reducing the intracranial pressure. In the great cerebral vein, the blood supply to the choroid plexuses, where the cerebrospinal fluid is produced, is restricted. The net effect is an instantaneous reduction in the intracranial blood volume and a reduction in the cerebrospinal fluid volume over a period of hours. If either of these processes is compromised and the mechanics of the skull are restricted so as to reduce intracranial volume, intracranial pressure would be increased with no mechanism for its release, thereby engorging the cavernous sinuses and compressing the cranial nerves passing adjacent to them. Combining these neurologic symptoms with symptoms from localized C0–C1 joints can explain the symptoms of migraine (Gard, 2009).

Cranium–Facial Tissue Therapy Based on the Stress-Transducer Mechanism

Experimental studies in cranial growth, orthodontics, and cranial plastic surgery have shown that cranial growth, function, and dentition are sensitive parameters that strongly influence one another (Oudhof, 2000; Zöller et al., 2005). The main mechanism behind this phenomenon is interactive bone tension (the stress-transducer mechanism). It is necessary for normal growth and function of the organs of the head and face, such as the mouth, ears, eyes, and the position of the atlas upon the occiput bone (Rocabado & Iglash, 1991; Von Piekartz, 2007). It can also change afferences or nociception, facilitating motor dysfunction. For instance, facial asymmetry caused by unilateral maxillary sinusitis can lead to an abnormal stress-transducer effect on facial and neurocranial tissue, leading to abnormal growth

(Linder-Aronson & Woodside, 2000). This development may be expressed as abnormal motor responses of both the sternocleidomastoid and masseter muscles (Palazzi et al., 1996).

Postural changes or prolonged incorrect mouth-breathing habits can change the external functional pressure on the cranium, facilitating abnormal interactive bone tissue tension (stress-transduction) (Enlow & Han, 1996). This phenomenon can encourage (abnormal) craniofacial growth, which may influence the deep cervical or masticatory muscles, thereby leading to abnormal afferent input or nociception (Von Piekartz, 2007).

Long-term minimal external pressure on specific parts of the skull can influence the shape of the neuro- and viscero-cranium, and indirectly affect the function of dentition. Nevertheless, the actual mechanism underlying different craniofacial growth models is not completely clear. Manual techniques to influence cranial passive accessory movements (passive movements on the cranium that cannot be actively performed by the patient), as described in this chapter, have the potential to influence stress-transducer mechanisms of the craniofacial region, thereby affecting cranial–facial morphology. They can also reduce motor activity and pain (Hu et al., 1995; Von Piekartz, 2007). For a comprehensive overview of different theories of cranial manual therapy, readers are referred to Chaitow (2005).

BASIC SCIENCES SUPPORTING THE MANAGEMENT OF THE CRANIUM

This section highlights several studies from basic sciences that either support or refute the main premises on which the treatment of the cranium is based. It also discusses various therapeutic approaches focused on the biomechanical and biochemical paradigms.

Can the Cranial Bones Move?

One of the most important assumptions for the management of the region of the cranium is the existence of mobility between the cranial bones. Motion of the cranial bones is intrinsically related to the cranial sutures (the fibrous tissues linking the cranial bones), which are the major sites of bone growth along the leading margins of the cranial bones during craniofacial development (Opperman, 2000).

The neurosurgical literature has provided preliminary evidence of cranial bone mobility. Heifetz and Weiss (1981) demonstrated a movement of the skull tongs and an expansion of the cranial vault when intracranial pressure was increased between 15 and 20 mm Hg. Other studies have corroborated the existence of skull expansion based on the role that the sutures have in intracranial compliance (Pitlyk et al., 1985; Heisey & Adams, 1993). Adams et al. (1992) found that the parietal bones of adult cats moved between 17 and 70 microns in response to lateral compression forces and to changes in intracranial pressure induced by artificial cerebrospinal fluid injection into the subarachnoid space. Rogers and Witt (1997), however, in a critical review of the literature, found inconclusive evidence for cranial bone mobility. Conversely, a recent study by Crow et al. (2009) found that calvarial structures may move independently of any external or internal force (change of 122 mm²) in normal human subjects due to bone compliance, viscoelastic properties of the bone, and motion around cranial sutures.

Does the Dura Have Any Role in Mobility of the Cranial Bones?

The dura mater provides the molecular blueprints (e.g., the soluble growth factors) for guiding the fate of the pluripotent osteogenic fronts (Warren et al., 2001, 2003). In fact, morphogenesis of the cranial bones and their sutures depends on tissue interactions with the dura, which control the size and shape of bones as well as sutural patency (Gagan et al., 2007; Heller et al., 2007). The cranial dura interacts with overlying tissues of the cranial vault by providing intercellular and mechanical signals, as well as cells (Hajihosseini et al., 2004; Ogle et al., 2004).

Bradley et al. (1997) found that the "regional" posterior frontal dura determines suture fusion. These authors suggested that the molecular mechanisms behind this process involve inductive tissue interactions of the dural cells with the suture cells by means of growth factor–mediated signal pathways (Bradley et al., 1997). In fact, it seems that intercellular signaling mechanisms play a greater role for morphogenesis of the calvaria than biomechanical forces (Opperman et al., 1995).

Can the Cranial Dura or Cranial Sutures Be a Source of Nociception?

It is well accepted that afferent input from dural structures is the neural substrate of primary headache syndromes (Goadsby & Oshinsky, 2007), as early neurosurgical studies demonstrated that stimulation of trigeminal intracranial structures—particularly the supratentorial dura mater and cranial vessels—evoked painful head

sensations (Penfield & McNaughton, 1940; Ray & Wolff, 1940; Feindel et al., 1960).

The nociceptive input from the dura mater to the first synapse in the brainstem is transmitted via Aδ and C fibers in the ophthalmic division of the trigeminal nerve via the trigeminal ganglion to nociceptive second-order neurons in the superficial and deep layers of the medullary dorsal horn of the trigeminocervical complex (Burstein et al., 1998; Schepelmann et al., 1999; Bartsch & Goadsby, 2002; Levy & Strassman, 2002). In fact, these dural-sensitive trigeminal neurons show a high degree of convergent input from other afferent structures, as they typically incorporate facial and corneal receptive fields (Burstein et al., 1998; Schepelmann et al., 1999). Chapter 5 provides a deeper understanding of the cranial dura, as do other texts (Goadsby & Bartsch, 2010)

As previously mentioned, the cranial dura tissue is highly innervated by Aδ and C fibers, and it readily adapts to physiological movements of the cervical spine and other body regions (Kumar et al., 1995). Less adaptation to movement of the dura—for example, in the case of neck and head injuries, or during growth spurts—may contribute to a greater nociceptive barrage directed toward the trigeminal nucleus, which in turn may lead to (head)ache; it can also influence intercellular and mechanical signaling directed at cranial bone tissues (Hajihosseini et al., 2004; Ogle et al., 2004).

In contrast, the role of the cranial sutures in nociception is not clear. Only one study indirectly supports the possibility of nociception in the cranial sutures. Warren et al. (2008) investigated the collagen of sutures in infants with and without ossification, reporting that collagen architecture was similar in sutures with and without fusion. These authors hypothesized that the extracellular matrix, via integrins and the discoid domain receptors, plays an important role in maintaining the balance between suture fusion and patency (Warren et al., 2008). Given that mechanical impulses (forces applied to the collagen tissue) are transmitted from the extracellular matrix through the cellular membrane via integrins (Hu et al., 2003), we can hypothesize that tension within the cranial sutures might induce changes in these processes of cellular transduction. As yet, however, no scientific study has confirmed this hypothesis.

In addition, some authors have suggested that the dura should be considered as a connective tissue structure. In such a scenario, Han (2009) has proposed the connective tissue theory. According to this hypothesis, the signaling present in the loose connective tissue may be capable of transmitting noxious stimuli from the surface to muscles or other deep structures (dura) through the cells of the vascular and neural systems. As a consequence, the excitation of any structure can be perceived in the dura with subsequent activation of dura receptors.

Scientific Evidence for Treatment of the Craniofacial Tissue

Osteopathic medicine has a long tradition of incorporating cranial manipulation techniques, which may explain why most studies on CST have been performed by osteopaths. An overview of the effects of CST based on these findings is presented here.

Although CST is commonly used by therapists in clinical practice, scientific evidence supporting its efficacy remains controversial. Attlee (1994) suggested that a variety of common childhood conditions (e.g., colic, poor sleep, recurrent ear infection, glue ear, regurgitation, poor feeding, and inconsolable screaming) may be treated with CST.

Hanten et al. (1999) investigated the effects of the CV-4 craniosacral technique in patients with tension-type headache and noted a significant positive effect (0.84) on pain intensity as compared to a reference group (protraction–retraction neck exercises) and a control group (no treatment). In fact, a systematic review determined that the quality of this study was high (Fernández-de-las-Peñas et al., 2006a).

There are no published studies investigating the effects of CST on migraine (Mann et al., 2008). A narrative review of the literature found evidence supporting a theoretical link between dysfunction of the craniosacral system and vertigo; however, no clinical trials showing that CST is effective for the treatment of vertigo have been published (Christine, 2009).

There are few studies related to CST and other pain conditions. Ventegodt et al. (2004) did not find any clinical effect of CST in individuals with whiplash-associated disorders. Matarán-Peñarrocha et al. (2010) recently demonstrated that CST contributes to improving anxiety and quality of life in fibromyalgia syndrome. Duncan et al. (2008) demonstrated that a series of treatments using osteopathy in the cranial field, myofascial release, or both improved motor function in children with moderate to severe spastic cerebral palsy.

Randomized clinical trials are clearly needed to demonstrate the effectiveness of CST in the management of patients with chronic pain, particularly headaches. Only when such evidence becomes available can the effectiveness of such therapy be definitively stated.

BASIC ANATOMY OF THE BONES OF THE CRANIUM RELEVANT TO MIGRAINE

This section presents the basic anatomy of the cranial bones that appear to be clinically relevant for the management of migraine. Note that the bones are not classified here as in traditional anatomy, but rather mentioned on the basis of current (patho-) biological and anatomic knowledge on migraine.

Occiput Bone

The occiput (**Figure 20.1**, item A, and **Figure 20.2**, item A) is the main bone of the posterior cranial fossa; it is related to several cranial bones, muscles, and dura structures. The squama of the occiput forms the posterior border of the foramen magnum, and the condyles form the lateral borders. On its anterior aspect, the basiocciput forms the spheno-basilar synchondrosis with the sphenoid bone (Figure 20.2, item B). Additionally, the parietal (lambdoidal suture) and temporal bones (occipito-mastoid suture) are linked to the occiput (Figure 20.1, items B and C). The occiput bone plays an important role in the biomechanics of the upper cervical spine through its relationship with the C1 vertebra (Martin et al., 2010).

Several head, neck and shoulder muscles attach to the occiput bone: rectus capitis posterior minor and major, obliquus capitis superior, rectus capitis anterior and

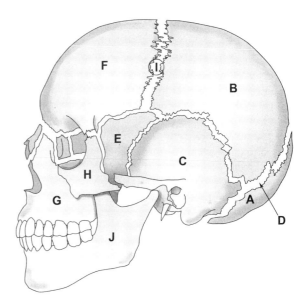

Figure 20.1 Lateral View of the Skull. (A) Occiput bone; (B) parietal bone; (C) temporal bone; (D) lambdoid suture; (E) sphenoid bone; (F) frontal bone; (G) maxillae bone; (H) zygomae bone; (I) bregmatic suture; (J) mandible.

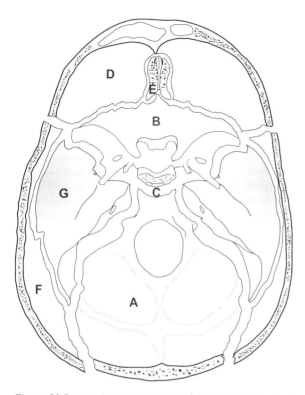

Figure 20.2 Superior Internal View of the Skull. (A) Occiput bone; (B) sphenoid bone; (C) spheno-basilar synchondrosis; (D) frontal bone; (E) ethmoid bone; (F) parietal bone; (G) temporal bone.

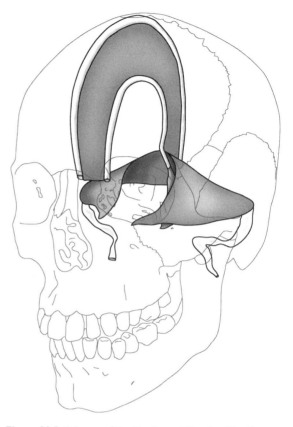

Figure 20.3 Scheme of the Reciprocal Tension Membranes: Falx Cerebri, Falx Cerebelli, and Tentorium Cerebelli

lateralis, longus capitis, upper trapezius, splenius capitis, and semispinalis capitis muscles.

The concept of "mobility" at the spheno-basilar synchondrosis in adults remains questionable (Cook, 2005); however, a slight degree of pliability between the different sutural junctions of the occiput, parietal, and temporal bones is accepted. This pliability is important for permitting the adaptation of the falx cerebri and the tentorium cerebelli, both of which are attached to the occiput (**Figure 20.3**). Nevertheless, a study conducted by Sabini and Elkowitz (2006) found that the lambdoid suture (Figure 20.1, item D) shows a prolonged patency, probably due to external forces originating from occipital muscles.

The occiput bone may be clinically affected by any dysfunction within the upper cervical spine or the parietal, temporal, and sphenoid bones. This dysfunction may induce mechanical tension on any suture: spheno-occipital, anterior/posterior intra-occipital synchondrosis, petro-occipital, and occipito-mastoid synchondrosis (Slater et al., 2008; Choudhary et al., 2010). Furthermore, due to the anatomic relationships between the dura and

the occiput (Figure 20.3), the cranial internal drainage may be altered by changes affecting reciprocal tension membranes due to the complex circulatory system (Couture et al., 2001). The occiput can also change its shape due to long-term (abnormal) stress in the skull itself or to external factors (e.g., long-term pressure from the atlas on the occiput). This stress can influence the localization or the diameter of the foramen jugularis (IX, X, and XI cranial nerves).

Sphenoid Bone

The sphenoid (Figure 20.1, item E), which is situated at the center of the cranium, serves as a biomechanical connection between the posterior part of the fossa and the anterior part of the face (the spheno-basilar synchondrosis; Figure 20.2, item C). The external surface of the two great wings of the sphenoid bone forms the temples, whereas the anterior surfaces form the eye socket in combination with the anterior surface of the lesser wings. The "Turkish saddle," which houses the pituitary gland, is located over the sphenoid bone.

The sphenoid articulates with many other bones in the skull: the occiput (spheno-basilar synchondrosis), temporal, parietals (pterion), frontal, ethmoid, vomer, palatine, and zygoma bones. Furthermore, several head muscles attach to the sphenoid bone: temporalis, medial and lateral pterygoids, buccinators, and the small muscles relating to eye movements. Again, the falx cerebri and tentorium cerebelli are attached to the sphenoid bone (Figure 20.3).

Dysfunctions of the sphenoid bone may excite mechanoreceptors of different cranial sutures: coronal, fronto-sphenoidal, or petrous-sphenoidal. Additionally, owing to the anatomic relationship between the sphenoid bone, the Turkish saddle, and the dura, internal drainage may be altered by changes affecting the reciprocal tension membranes.

Frontal Bone

The frontal bone (Figure 20.1, item F, and Figure 20.2, item D) is the main bone of the anterior cranial region and forms the forehead. It has a central metopic suture, which is generally fused, on the inside of which lie the attachments for the bifurcated falx cerebri (superior sagittal sinus) (Figure 20.3). The inferior part of the frontal bone constitutes the eye socket. The frontal is related to the parietals (coronal suture), sphenoid (eye socket), ethmoid (Figure 20.2, item E), lacrimal, nasal, maxilla (Figure 20.1, item G), and zygoma (Figure 20.1, item H) bones. Several head and face muscles attach to the frontal bone: temporalis, occipito-frontalis, corrugator supercilii, orbicularis oculi, and procerus.

Dysfunctions within the frontal bone may excite mechanoreceptors of cranial sutures related to the eyes and sinuses. Additionally, internal drainage may be altered by changes affecting the reciprocal tension membranes, particularly by congestion of the superior sagittal sinus. Fujimi et al. (2006) identified a convergence of inputs from the superior sagittal sinus and tooth pulp afferents on C1 neurons, which suggests that nociceptive afferent inputs from the superior sagittal sinus may refer pain to the neck.

Parietal Bone

The parietal bones (Figure 20.1, item B, and Figure 20.2, item F) form the roof of the skull. They create the sagittal (coronal) suture over which each side the falx cerebri is attached (superior sagittal sinus) (Figure 20.3). Parietals are related to the frontal (bregma; Figure 20.1, item I), occiput (lambda), temporal, and sphenoid bones.

Attached to the parietal bone are the temporalis, occipito-frontalis, and auricularis superior muscles. Dysfunctions within the parietal bones may excite mechanoreceptors of cranial sutures related to them. Furthermore, longitudinal internal drainage may be altered by changes affecting the reciprocal tension membranes.

Temporal Bone

The temporal bones (Figure 20.1, item C, and Figure 20.2, item G) constitute the lateral part of the skull and are formed by the squama, the zygomatic process, the mastoid process, and the petrous portion. Temporals are related to the parietal, occiput (lambda), sphenoid, zygoma, and mandible bones. In addition, the tentorium cerebelli forms on the petrous portion (Figure 20.3) of the petrosal sinus. The sternocleidomastoid, temporalis, longissimus capitis and splenius capitis muscles attach to the temporal. Christine (2009), in a narrative review of the literature, suggested that temporal bone misalignment and motion asymmetry may cause vertigo, although no clinical trials support this hypothesis.

Ethmoid Bone

The ethmoid bone (Figure 20.2, item E) is formed by the cribriform plate and the crista galli; it contains the air sinuses. In addition, the ethmoid forms the medial part of the eye socket and the nasal septum. It is related to the sphenoid, palatines, nasal, maxilla, and frontal bones, and to the extension of the vomer bone. The falx cerebri attaches to the crista galli (Figure 20.3). There is no direct muscle attachment to this bone.

Maxilla Bone

The maxilla bones (Figure 20.1, item G), which form the superior part of the mouth, articulate with the palatines, zygoma, ethmoid, vomer, nasal, and frontal bones. In addition, these bones house the upper portion of the teeth. Several muscles of facial expression attach to the maxilla: medial pterygoid, masseter, buccinators, risorius, orbicularis oculi, levator labii superioris, nasalis, depressor septim, and levator anguli oris. There are no reciprocal tension-membrane relationships to the maxilla bones. One important and relevant connection is the neural structures from the second division of the trigeminal nerve (V2) that pass through the maxilla before arriving at the teeth; these structures are vulnerable to trauma, particularly during odontological procedures.

Mandible

The mandible (Figure 20.1, item J) has one horizontal portion forming the symphysis menti, and two vertical rami with the coronoid process and the condyle. The condyle of the mandible and the temporal bone forms the temporomandibular joint. This joint receives several orofacial muscles: temporalis, masseter, medial and lateral pterygoid, digastric, cervical platysma, mylohyoid, and geniohyoid. Stuginski-Barbosa et al. (2010) recently demonstrated that patients with migraine are more likely to have tenderness at the temporomandibular joint and on the masticatory muscles as compared to those persons without migraine.

BASIC ANATOMY OF THE CRANIAL NERVES RELEVANT FOR MIGRAINE

This section presents the basic anatomy of the cranial nerves that appear to be clinically relevant for the management of migraine (Von Piekartz, 2007).

Trigeminal Nerve (V)

The trigeminal nerve, which is the biggest sensory nerve of the cranium, is divided into three main branches: ophthalmic (V1), maxillary (V2), and mandibular (V3). This nerve arises from the cranio-ventral part of the pons, including the Gasser's ganglion located in the Meckel's cavity within the temporal bone (**Figure 20.4**, item A).

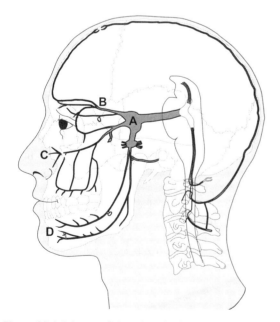

Figure 20.4 Scheme of the Trigeminal Nerve. (A) Gasser's ganglion located in the Meckel's cavity; (B) ophthalmic nerve (V1); (C) maxillary nerve (V2); (D) mandibular nerve (V3).

Thalakoti et al. (2007) found that activation of trigeminal ganglion neurons leads to changes in adjacent glia neurons involving communication through gap junctions and paracrine signaling. Their research suggests that this process may be involved in peripheral sensitization of the trigeminal ganglion, thereby playing an important role in the initiation of migraine.

The ophthalmic nerve (V1) is the most cranial sensory branch of the trigeminal nerve (Figure 20.4, item B). It enters the cavernous sinus laterally and the superior orbital fissure, splitting into three main nerves: frontal, lacrimal, and nasociliary. The supra-orbital and supratrochlear nerves, which innervate the skin of the forehead and the medial corner of the eye, are the terminal branches of the frontal nerve. Some studies have found increased mechanical pain sensitivity over the supra-orbital nerve in patients with chronic tension-type headache (Fernández-de-las-Peñas et al., 2008) and unilateral migraine (Fernández-de-las-Peñas et al., 2009a). The infra-trochlear nerve innervates the skin close to the medial corner of the eye and is the terminal branch of the nasociliary nerve.

The maxillary nerve (V2) is the middle sensory branch of the trigeminal nerve (Figure 20.4, item C). This branch enters the cavernous sinus, reaching the pterygopalatine fossa through the round foramen. Like the ophthalmic nerve, it then splits into three main nerves: infra-orbital, zygomatic, and nasopalatine. The infra-orbital nerve innervates the skin between the upper lip and the lower eyelid and teeth in the maxilla. Fernández-de-las-Peñas et al. (2009b) showed that women with temporomandibular pain had pressure-pain hypersensitivity over the infra-orbital nerve; Fernández-Mayoralas et al. (2010) reported similar results in children with frequent episodic tension-type headache. The zygomatic nerve splits into the zygomatico-temporal and zygomatico-facial branches, which innervate the skin of the upper part of the cheek and the temple. Totonchi et al. (2005) provided an excellent anatomic description of this nerve, allowing for a better management of migraine pain triggered from this region. Finally, the naso-palatine nerve innervates taste sensors and glands at the palate, nose, and pharynx (pterygopalatine ganglion).

The mandibular nerve (V3) is the inferior motor branch of the trigeminal nerve (Figure 20.4, item D). This branch passes the oval foramen of the greater wing of the sphenoid bone and provides the motor innervation for the masticatory muscles: masseter, temporalis, and medial and lateral pterygoid muscles. The mandibular nerve also has sensory and mixed nerves: auriculo-temporal nerve (innervates the skin of the temple, the ear canal, and the tympanic membrane), lingual nerve (innervates the ventral two-thirds of the tongue and the floor of the mouth), inferior alveolar nerve (innervates the teeth of the lower jaw), and buccal nerve (innervates the inner lateral side of the mouth as well as the skin of the lower half of the cheek). The terminal branch of the inferior alveolar nerve is the mental nerve that leaves the mandible through the mental foramen and innervates the skin of the lower lip and chin, as well as the mandibular body. This terminal branch has been found to be hypersensitive in women with temporomandibular pain (Fernández-de-las-Peñas et al., 2009b) and in children with headache (Fernández-Mayorales et al., 2010). Readers are referred to Von Piekartz's (2007) book for a deeper clinical description of the terminal branches of the trigeminal nerve.

Facial Nerve (VII)

The facial nerve is the main motor nerve of the head and face and innervates the mimic muscles. This nerve emerges just under the pons, and then enters into the internal acoustic pore and into the facial canal within the petrous portion of the temporal bone. Once inside the facial canal, it divides into three main nerves: the greater superficial petrous, the chorda tympani, and the stapedius nerves.

The greater superficial petrous nerve passes the lacerated foramen to unite with the deeper petrous nerve in the Vidian's canal. After redistribution of the fibers in the pterygopalatine ganglion, the greater superficial petrous nerve joins with branches of the maxillary nerve (V2).

The chorda tympani nerve returns to the facial canal, penetrates the petrous bone, and passes through the acoustic bones in the middle. It joins the lingular nerve of the mandibular nerve (V3) and is responsible for the taste receptors of the ventral two-thirds of the tongue.

The stapedius nerve innervates the musculature that regulates the vibration of the stapes.

An interaction between the sensory parts of the trigeminal and facial nerves has recently been demonstrated (Sanders, 2010). In fact, electrophysiological studies reveal that the trigeminal nerve, which innervates somatosensation on the tongue, modulates the gustatory (taste) neurons arising from the cranial nerve at the level of the solitary nucleus (medulla and lower pons) (Felizardo et al., 2009; Hummel et al., 2009).

Trochlear (IV) and Abducens (VI) Nerves

The trochlear nerve is a sensory nerve that originates at the dorsal side of the brainstem. It penetrates the dura close to the ophthalmic nerve and enters into the cavernous sinus, reaching the orbit through the superior orbital fissure to innervate the superior oblique muscle. In 2004, Yangüela et al. (2004) described primary trochlear headache, whose pathogenic mechanisms include friction, traction, and microvascular, compressive, neural trauma to the supra-orbital and/or supra-trochlear nerves. In addition, the relevance of the superior oblique muscle has been noted in studies examining tension-type headache (Fernández-de-las-Peñas et al., 2005) and migraine (Fernández-de-las-Peñas et al., 2006b).

Pareja and Sánchez-del-Río (2006) have postulated that nociceptive afferents from the inner part of the orbit may sustain the activation of trigeminal-nucleus neurons, thereby exacerbating migraine. Decreasing the wind-up induced from this nociceptive afferent stimulation may be effective in controlling headache (Pareja & Sánchez-del-Río, 2006).

The abducens nerve is a motor nerve that originates between the pons and the medulla oblongata at the ventral side of the brainstem. It penetrates the dura dorso-caudal of the Turkish saddle, reaches the cavernous sinus after passing through the inferior petrous sinus, and passes through the superior orbital fissure to innervate the lateral rectus muscle on the posterior third (Zhang et al., 2010). In fact, reports have recently described the presence of referred pain from manual exploration of the lateral rectus muscle in patients with chronic tension-type headache (Fernández-de-las-Peñas et al., 2009c).

Vagus Nerve (X)

The vagus nerve innervates parts of the head, but it provides the most important parasympathetic inputs for the thorax and abdomen (Gillig & Sanders, 2010). It starts dorsal of the olive of the medulla oblongata, passes through the jugular foramen (with the glossopharyngeal and accessory nerves), and descends between the internal carotid artery and the external jugular vein. Some research has suggested that vagus nerve stimulation may be effective for migraine, although further trials of this therapy are needed to establish its utility (Hord et al., 2003; Mauskop, 2005).

Accessory Nerve (XI)

Although the accessory nerve is considered a cranial nerve, the cell bodies of this nerve actually reside in the spinal cord at the C1–C5 levels (Gillig & Sanders, 2010).

This nerve crosses the jugular foramen (with the vagus and glossopharyngeal nerves), enters into the sternocleidomastoid muscle, and ends within the upper trapezius muscle.

Sphenopalatine Ganglion

The sphenopalatine ganglion is a parasympathetic cranial ganglion found at the pterygopalatine fossa in the sphenoid bone. It originates from the parasympathetic nerve roots in the maxilla (V2) and facial (VII) nerves and from sympathetic roots in the superior cervical ganglion. This ganglion innervates the lacrimal gland, paranasal sinuses, glands of the mucosa of the nasal cavity and pharynx, gingiva, and mucous membranes and glands of the hard palate.

Ganglia are extremely sensitive to mechanical and adrenal (stress) stimulation and can flow with abnormal spontaneous impulses when they are active (Devor & Seltzer, 1999). Therefore, excitation of the sphenopalatine ganglion may be one source of persistent headache (Quevedo et al., 2005).

MANUAL THERAPY INTERVENTIONS FOR THE CRANIUM

Cranial Dysfunctions and Cranial Therapy Clinical Approach

Cranial dysfunctions may involve both intracranial membranes and cranial articulations. In fact, it has been proposed that cranial strains and stresses may influence the biomechanical behavior of the tissues as well as the local cell biology (Gregersen et al., 2000).

The tissue most affected by cranial dysfunctions is the dura. Henderson et al. (2005a) demonstrated that extracranial tensions to the dura (mean tensile force: 4.96 ± 1.54%) induce greater tensile strains than intracranial pressure originating in the sutures (tensile force: 0.0020% to 0.0410%). Further, tensile strains present in the cranial dura are age dependent (Henderson et al., 2005b). Therefore, based on the mechano-sensitivity and osteogenic nature of the dura and the fact that the dura is integrated into the fibrous tissue at the cranial sutures, tensile strains in the cranial dura may promote osteogenic signaling from the dura at the site of its attachment to the sutures inducing cranial dura restrictions (Sergueef, 2007).

When clinicians decide to treat the cranium, it is important to understand that the pain evoked/induced by the therapist does not necessarily arise from the tissue under the hands (i.e., input-based versus pain-processing mechanisms). Based on the clinical pain pattern and the behavior of symptoms, the therapist can hypothesize which structure is primarily responsible in a particular patient. For example, when local pain in the face is provoked by the therapist with a mobilization, the pain probably comes from strain/compression of bony face tissue. When a global neurocranium technique, such as bilateral compression of the temporal bones, slowly decreases the headache, changes on tension of the intradural membranes can be hypothesized.

Based in clinical experience, therapists can use two different approaches for the management of the cranial region/area: cranial-bone tissue mobilizations and techniques influencing the intracranial dura membrane. Cranial-bone tissue techniques seek to facilitate the stress-transducer function of the cranium by mobilizing the cranial bones related to that suture. Nevertheless, it is a misconception to assume that such mobilization influences only the sutures; rather, the key factor is the transformation of tension movement into the bones where sutures are also involved (Oudhof, 2000). The intracranial dura membrane approaches are targeted to release intracranial soft-tissue structures, particularly the dura, by applying slight compression with the hands. In a practical sense, active combinations of the two stresses are usually involved, so both approaches should be applied before any neurodynamic technique of the cranial nerves is applied.

Cranial-Bone Tissue Techniques

The principles for cranial-bone mobilization techniques are similar to those for mobilization applied over any joint. Maitland et al. (2005) usually perform treatment techniques in an oscillatory manner. These oscillations can be performed with different amplitudes in different positions in the range of movement. Maitland et al. (2005) have described four standard oscillatory grades of movement (**Figure 20.5**): grades I and II are typically used in dysfunctions where the pain is more important than resistance, whereas grades III and IV are usually applied in dysfunctions where the resistance is more relevant than pain (Maitland et al., 2005).

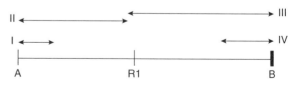

Figure 20.5 Grades of Passive Movement for Mobilization According to Maitland et al (2005)

When selecting the intensity (grade) of the mobilization, clinicians must decide whether they will seek to produce/reproduce the patient's symptoms or whether it is necessary to mobilize the patient's structures into resistance. Further, capitalizing on the stress-transducer qualities of cranial-bone tissue-sustained pressure in a rhythmic way for 2 to 5 seconds is suggested. In this way, the clinician may easily regulate the compliance qualities of cranial-bone tissue. Readers are referred to Von Piekartz's (2007) book for a deeper discussion of the terminology of mobilization. In this chapter, we describe those techniques which we believe more appropriate for the management of the cranium in patients with migraine.

Gard has developed a different methodology of treatment based on his theory of involuntary cranial bone movement. The aim of this therapy is to remove the stresses preventing the expansion of the bones, usually in the upper spinal region (and hence expansion of the skeleton as a whole), and then to encourage the expansion by recreating the natural direction of movement of bones as they are influenced by the intracranial pressure. Treatment originates with a gentle traction pressure to C0–C1, followed by techniques to expand the skull, with the bones being steered outward from the notional center. Oscillation is not necessary in this method. However, grading as described previously also fits this model, as encouraging relaxation of stressed soft tissues is the initial aim, followed by active bony realignment, where some discomfort is acceptable.

Technique to Mobilize the Occiput in All Ranges

Treatment to mobilize the occiput aims to decompress the cranial base, with primary influence upon occipital mobility. Freed from the need to maintain any rhythmic changes through the skull, the practitioner's intention is to optimize C0–C1 movement in all ranges, and then

facilitate expansion of the cranial bones surrounding the occiput through constant directed pressure. The contact-point pressure is maintained just below the symptomatic level that desensitizes the contact area, thereby allowing for stronger cranial bone realignment.

With this technique, the patient is positioned supine, head straight with the practitioner at the head of the table, and forearms resting. Both hands of the therapist cup the skull, with the index fingers immediately posterior to the C0–C1 facet joints (**Figure 20.6**). The intention of force is to move the atlas forward relative to the skull. As soft-tissue tone releases, the therapist directs the fingers to the mastoid processes, for tractioning the lateral aspects of the atlas from the mastoid processes. Although the occiput bone is not directly palpated, the traction to its surrounding bones allows it to be expanded downward relative to the cranial vault. At this point, the middle fingers should be positioned as posterior/medial to the mastoids as possible. The thumbs, placed on the pterion, have the option of moving the sphenoid downward from this point, or the frontal, maxilla, and zygomatic arch bones forward.

These three aspects of movement can be achieved by pivoting the hands around the index finger in such a way that they form a thumbs-up shape with the thumbs pointing toward the chest. Individual techniques can be used as required beyond this point. Maintaining the skull's maximum volume is hypothesized to mitigate the effects of poorly regulated cerebrospinal fluid pressure by allowing for greater asymptomatic engorgement of the cavernous sinuses.

Mobilization of the Temporal and Parietal Bones (Temporo-Parietal Suture)

In mobilization of the temporal and parietal bones, the patient is positioned supine with the head rotated to one side, and the practitioner sits at the head of the patient.

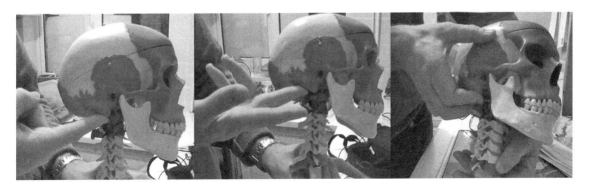

Figure 20.6 Technique to Mobilize the Occiput in all Ranges

The index–middle finger pads of one hand are placed on the parietal bone, above the temporo-parietal suture. The middle finger is placed one finger width above the helix of the ear, on the parietal bone. The index–middle fingers of the other hand are placed superior to the zygomatic area, around the area of the external auditory meatus. The technique consists of mobilizing the temporal and parietal bones around the temporo-parietal suture (**Figure 20.7**).

Mobilization of the Temporal and Occiput Bones (Occipito-Mastoid Suture)

The occipito-mastoid suture is very important for the cranium, as its dysfunction affects the content of the jugular foramen, resulting in changes in the cranial internal drainage (Couture et al., 2001). For this mobilization technique, the patient is positioned supine, and the clinician sits at the head of the table. The therapist applies, with one hand, the "five-finger contact" over the temporal bone: the middle finger is placed in the external auditory canal; the thumb and index fingers are placed superior and inferior to the zygomatic process;

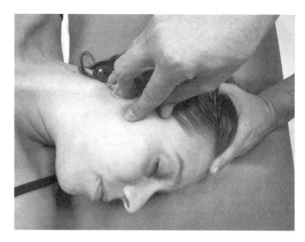

Figure 20.8 "Five-Finger Contact" over the Temporal Bone

and the little–ring fingers are placed over the mastoid (**Figure 20.8**).

The other hand is placed palm up, transversely oriented beneath the occiput bone, with the tips of the index and middle fingers contacting the squamous portion of the occipital squama, immediately medial to the occipito-mastoid suture. The technique consists of mobilizing (over a transverse axis) and distracting the temporal bone in relation to the occiput (**Figure 20.9**).

Bilateral Mobilization of the Temporal Bones

The patient is positioned supine, with the clinician seated at the head of the table. The therapist applies the "five-finger contact" bilaterally over the temporal and induces a bilateral mobilization (over a transverse axis) of both bones (**Figure 20.10**).

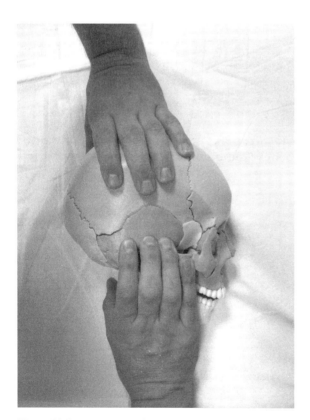

Figure 20.7 Mobilization of the Temporal and Parietal Bones (Temporo-Parietal Suture)

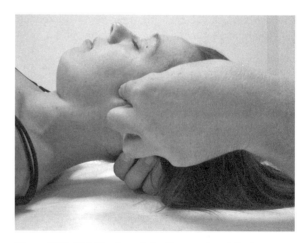

Figure 20.9 Mobilization of the Temporal and Occiput Bones (Occipito-Mastoid Suture)

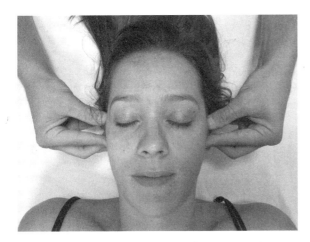

Figure 20.10 Bilateral Mobilization of the Temporal Bones

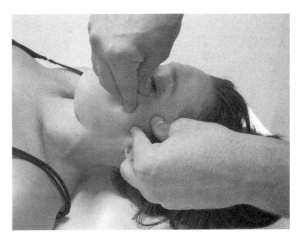

Figure 20.11 Mobilization of the Temporal and Zygoma Bones (Temporo-Zygomatic Suture)

Mobilization of the Temporal and Zygoma Bones (Temporo-Zygomatic Suture)

The patient is positioned supine, and the clinician sits at the head of the table. One hand is placed over the temporal bone with the "five-finger contact," and the other hand holds the zygomatic bone between the index–thumb fingers (**Figure 20.11**). This therapeutic technique consists of mobilizing (over a transverse axis) the temporal bone and distracting the zygoma bone.

Mobilization of the Zygoma Bone

The patient is positioned supine, and the clinician stands in front of the table. One hand grapes the frontal bone between the thumb–index fingers; the thumb and index

fingers of the other hand hold the zygoma bone with an intra-oral contact (**Figure 20.12**). This technique consists of mobilizing the zygoma bone in different directions around those related bones (frontal, maxilla, and temporal).

Mobilization of the Frontal Bone

Mobilization of the frontal bone can be extremely useful in patients who are suffering from frontal headache of vascular origin, as the superior sagittal sinus is located over the bifurcated falx cerebri. For that purpose, the patient is positioned supine, and the therapist sits at the head of the table. The therapist interlaces the fingers so that the hypothenar eminences rest on the lateral

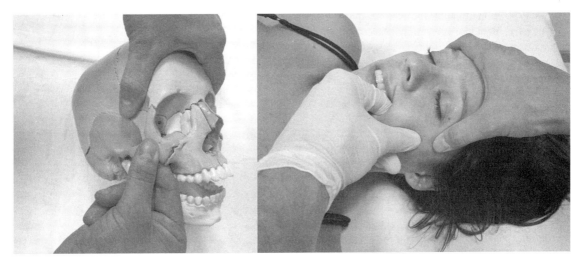

Figure 20.12 Mobilization of the Zygoma Bone

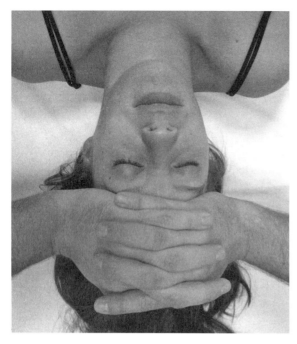

Figure 20.13 Mobilization of the Frontal Bone

angles of the frontal bones, with the fingers covering the metopic suture. The mobilization technique consists of exerting a light compressive force via the hypothenar eminences (i.e., bringing them toward each other) and lifting the frontal bone upward (slightly cephalad and toward the ceiling; **Figure 20.13**). The technique should be applied rhythmically.

Bilateral Mobilization of the Maxilla Bones (Inter-Maxilla Suture)

The patient is positioned supine, and the therapist stands in front of the table. One hand grasps the frontal bone between the thumb–index fingers; the index and middle fingers make intra-oral contact with both sides of the palate (**Figure 20.14**). This technique consists of mobilizing both maxilla bones in different directions around those related bones (frontal, temporal, and zygoma).

Unilateral Mobilization of the Maxilla Bone

The patient is positioned supine, and the therapist stands in front of the table. One hand places the thumb on the vertical branch of the maxilla bone, just on the fronto-maxilla suture; the thumb and index finger of the other hand make intra-oral contact with the maxilla (**Figure 20.15**). This technique consists of mobilizing the maxilla bone in an anterior-to-posterior direction.

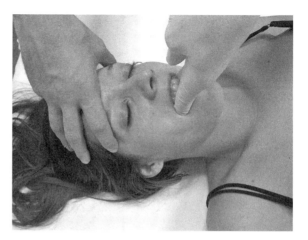

Figure 20.14 Bilateral Mobilization of the Maxilla Bones (Inter-Maxilla Suture)

Intracranial Dura Membrane Techniques

Dura membranous strain causes restriction of normal membranous functioning, altering cerebrospinal fluid motion, physiology of arterial and venous blood flow, and lymphatic flow of the cranium region. When Timoshkin and Sandhouse (2008) investigated the prevalence of the various cranial strain patterns, they found that torsion and side-bending rotation were the most frequently encountered (72%). Additionally, cranial strain patterns showed the highest intra-observer reliability (kappa: 0.67), particularly in patients with asthma or headache (Halma et al., 2008).

Sutherland and Wales (1990) proposed that treating reciprocal tension membranes with different techniques might balance the tension in strained fibers of the dura.

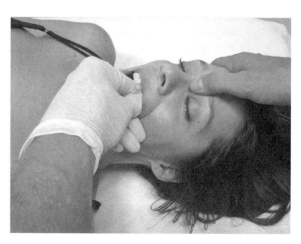

Figure 20.15 Unilateral Mobilization of the Maxilla Bone

These authors suggested that a low degree of pressure should be applied when therapists use an intracranial dura membrane technique. The fingers of the clinician should adapt to the contour of the area to treat. In addition, when palpating the bone, the slight degree of motion that may be noted should be assessed with no preconceptions as to what may be driving it (Chaitow, 2005).

Kostopoulos and Keramidas (1992) examined the changes in elongation of falx cerebri during the application of some craniosacral techniques to the skulls of embalmed cadavers and found the following relative elongation of the falx cerebri: 1.44 mm during frontal lift; 1.08 mm for the parietal lift; 0.28 mm for the sphenobasilar decompression; and inconclusive results for ear pull. Nevertheless, in a more recent study, Downey et al. (2006) reported that low loads of force, similar to those used in clinical practice (in this study, simulating a frontal lift technique), resulted in no significant changes in coronal suture movement or intracranial pressure in rabbits. New studies are urgently needed to further elucidate the mechanisms of the techniques used in clinical practice. In this subsection, we describe intracranial dura membrane techniques claimed to reduce dura tension.

Connective Tissue Bridge at the Sub-Occipital Region

Before beginning the treatment of the cranium, it is necessary to release the sub-occipital muscle area. Thus the aim of this technique is to release restrictions located in the connective tissue bridge between the rectus capitis posterior minor muscle and the dura (Hack et al., 1995).

The patient is positioned supine, and the therapist sits at the head of the table, with forearms firmly over its surface. The therapist puts his or her fingers under the patient's head such that the fingertips of the index–middle fingers are placed at the C5–C6 level. From this position, the fingers are flexed in a cranial direction until they reach the occipital bone. The therapist's contact point should be adjusted until it fills the space between the occipital bone and C1–C2 vertebrae. Once the therapist has located at this point, the metacarpophalangeal joints are flexed 90° and the interphalangeal joints are extended (**Figure 20.16**). This position may induce a constant pressure over the connective tissue bridge between the rectus capitis posterior minor muscle and the dura (Pilat, 2010).

Occipital Condylar Decompression

The patient is positioned supine, and the therapist sits at the head of the table. The therapist cradles the occiput

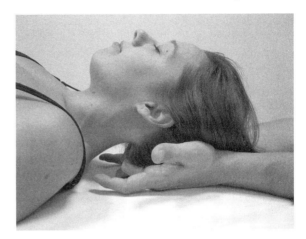

Figure 20.16 Connective Tissue Bridge at the Sub-Occipital Region

in both hands, with the tips of the middle finger contacting the most inferior aspect of the occiput in the midline, the index fingers toward the occipital condyle, and the thumbs on the mastoid processes (**Figure 20.17**). This technique consists of applying postero-superior traction of the occiput bone to slightly adjust the level of cranial tension.

Sphenoid–Occipital Hold Technique

The patient is positioned supine, and the clinician sits at the head of the table. One hand transversally cradles the occiput bone. The other hand is positioned so as to place the thumb on one of the great wings of the sphenoid, and the tip of the index finger on the other great wing

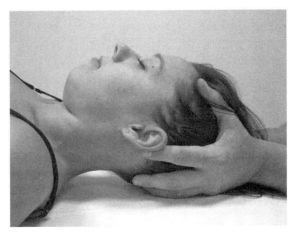

Figure 20.17 Occipital Condylar Decompression

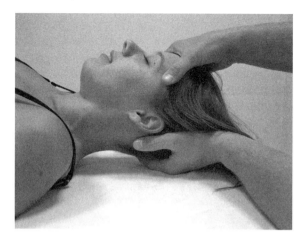

Figure 20.18 Sphenoid-Occipital hold Technique

(**Figure 20.18**). This technique consists of equilibrating the sphenoid and occiput bones by applying slight pressure (grams) in the appropriate direction.

Bilateral Longitudinal Movement of the Temporal Bone

The patient is positioned supine, and the therapist sits at the head of the table, with the forearms resting on the table. The hands of the therapist are placed as follows: thumbs are interlocked over the sagittal suture; the index fingers rest on the greater wings of the sphenoid bone; the middle fingers are anterior to the ear and rest on the pterion; the ring fingers are on the temporal bones behind the external auditory meatus near the asterion; and the little fingers rest on the occipital squama (**Figure. 20.19** and **Figure 20.20**).

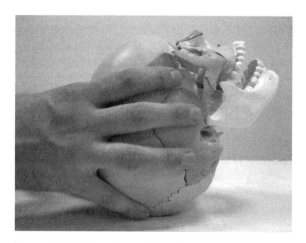

Figure 20.19 Bilateral Longitudinal Movement of the Temporal Bone over a Skull

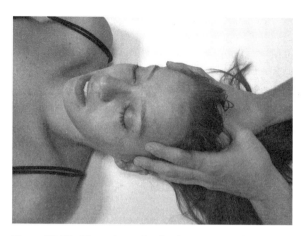

Figure 20.20 Bilateral Longitudinal Movement of the Temporal Bone over a Patient

Indirect Ethmoid Bone Mobilization

The ethmoid bone plays a relevant role in various disease processes such as sinusitis, rhinitis, or functional nasal airway obstruction, which may be related to frontal migraine headaches. In this mobilization technique, the patient is positioned supine, and the clinician sits at the side of the head of the table. The cephalic hand is placed on the frontal bone, with the thumb and index fingers on either side of the nasal notch. The thumb of the caudal hand is placed in intra-oral contact with the vomer, whereas the index finger is placed over the nasal bones (**Figure 20.21**).

Occiput Compression with Posterior–Anterior Movement of the Sphenoid

This technique is one of the main intracranial dura membrane techniques, as it is targeted to one of the most

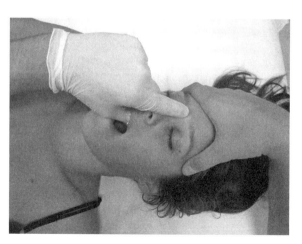

Figure 20.21 Indirect Ethmoid Bone Mobilization

pathogenic cranial dysfunctions: the sphenoid compression. It is also called the sphenoid lift technique (Chaitow, 2005). The aim of this technique is to release the tentorium cerebelli. Although no scientific evidence has been published to support this dysfunction, its relief is clinically seen as having a beneficial effect in migraine and headache patients.

The patient is positioned supine, and the therapist sits at the head of the table, with the forearms resting on the table. The therapist cradles the patient's head so that the fingers grasp the occiput, and the thumbs rest on the great wings of the sphenoid bone (**Figure 20.22**). The technique consists of initially pushing the thumbs toward the floor, which (theoretically) compresses the sphenoid (spheno-basilar junction). After some seconds, the thumbs push toward the ceiling, with the aim of decompressing the sphenoid on the occiput. It is important to note that the pressure applied should be approximately no more than 5 pounds (Upledger & Vredevoogd, 1983).

Distraction of the Frontal Bone (Frontal Lift)

The frontal technique emphasizes the treatment of the falx cerebri, the eyes, and the nasal cavities (Chaitow, 2005; Sergueef, 2007). The clinical experience of patients is that this technique relieves dull headaches, reduces frontal sinus pain often independent of the diagnosis, and causes a general relaxed feeling (Von Piekartz, 2007). For that purpose, the patient is positioned supine, and the therapist sits at the head of the table, with the forearms resting on the table. The therapist places both hands in contact with the frontal bone such that the tips of the index fingers are aligned on either side of the

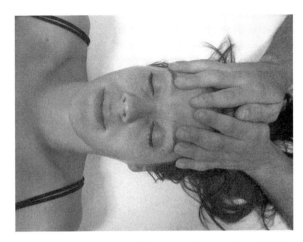

Figure 20.23 Distraction of the Frontal Bone (Frontal Lift)

metopic suture, and the middle, ring, and little fingers rest laterally on the frontal bone (**Figure 20.23**). The technique consists of "lifting" the frontal bone by pushing toward the ceiling with the aim of decompressing the frontal bone.

Distraction of the Parietal Bones (Parietal Lift)

Parietal lift is an effective technique for treating congestive dysfunction of the superior sagittal sinus (Sergueef, 2007). The patient is positioned supine, and the therapist sits at the head of the table, with the forearms resting on the table. The therapist places both hands in contact with the parietal bones so that the index fingers are posterior to the coronal suture and above the spheno-parietal suture, the middle and ring fingers are separated above the temporo-parietal

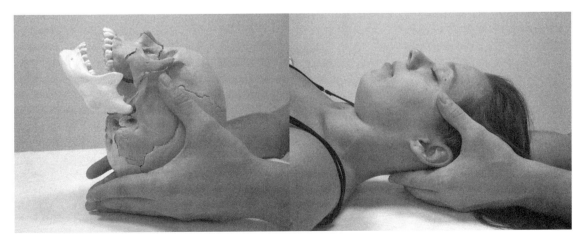

Figure 20.22 Occiput Compression with Posterior-Anterior Movement of the Sphenoid

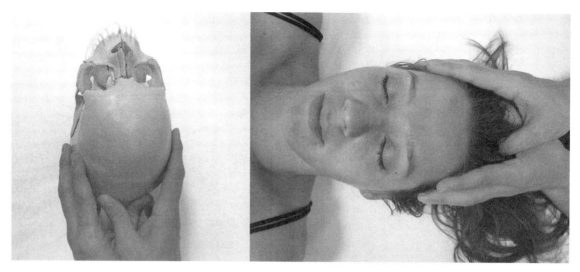

Figure 20.24 Distraction of the Parietal Bones (Parietal Lift)

suture, and the little fingers rest anterior and superior to the lambdoid suture (close to the asterion). The thumbs are crossed above the sagittal suture, acting as a fulcrum, without any direct contact (**Figure 20.24**). Contact with the temporal bones should be avoided during the technique. The technique consists of "lifting" the parietal bones by pushing toward the ceiling with the finger pads.

Bilateral Compression of the Occiput (CV-4 Technique)

Bilateral compression of the occiput, also known as CV-4, is a cranial treatment procedure that has been used by practitioners of cranial manipulation for more than 60 years (King & Lay, 2003). This technique is believed to induce various changes throughout the body, possibly via periaqueductal gray (PAG) substance, which surrounds the fourth ventricle (King & Lay, 2003).

Milnes and Moran (2007) demonstrated that the application of the CV-4 technique had minimal physiological effects in terms of heart rate variability, respiration rate, galvanic skin resistance, and skin temperature in asymptomatic individuals. Conversely, Nelson et al. (2006) found that the CV-4 technique altered the TH frequency component of blood flow velocity. Cutler et al. (2005) reported that sleep latency and muscle sympathetic nerve activity were significantly decreased during the CV-4–induced still point of the cranial rhythmic impulse. Nevertheless, these studies were done on asymptomatic individuals.

Future studies should investigate the effects of CV-4 on individuals with pain symptoms. In fact, Hanten et al. (1999) examined the effects of this technique in patients

with tension-type headache and observed a large effect (0.84) on pain intensity as compared to a reference group (protraction–retraction neck exercises) and a control group (no treatment).

For this technique, the patient lies supine, and the therapist sits at the head of the table, with the forearms resting on the table. The therapist's hands are placed palms up beneath the head of the patient, with one hand resting in the palm of the other, in such a manner that the thenar eminences are parallel and contacting the lateral angles of the occiput medial to the occipito-mastoid suture (**Figure 20.25**).

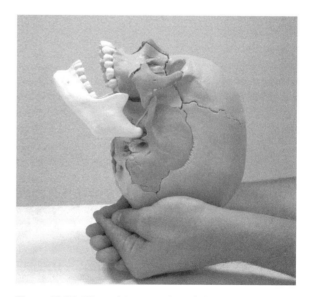

Figure 20.25 Bilateral Compression of the Occiput (CV-4 Technique)

CONCLUSIONS

The anatomy of the cranium and several studies suggest that CST may be an effective complementary approach for neuromusculoskeletal manual approaches for the management of individuals with migraine. In fact, clinicians can use two different approaches for manual management of the cranium area individually or in combination: direct cranial tissue mobilizations and techniques that emphasize mobilization of intra-cranial dural membranes. Although little published scientific evidence supports their use, clinical effects seen in patients support CST. Nevertheless, well-designed studies are urgently needed to clearly define the role of cranial therapy in the management of head pain disorders.

REFERENCES

Adams T, Heisey RS, Smith MC, Briner BJ. Parietal bone mobility in the anesthetized cat. *J Am Osteopath Assoc* 1992;92:599–622.

Attlee T. Cranio-sacral therapy and the treatment of common childhood conditions. *Health Visit* 1994;67:232–234.

Bartsch T, Goadsby PJ. Stimulation of the greater occipital nerve induces increased central excitability of dural afferent input. *Brain* 2002;125:1496–1509.

Bradley JP, Levine JP, McCarthy JG, Longaker MT. Studies in cranial suture biology: regional dura mater determines in vitro cranial suture fusion. *Plast Reconstr Surg* 1997;100:1091–1099.

Brooks RE. Osteopathy in the cranial field: the approach of WG Sutherland, D.O. *Phys Med Rehabil State Art Rev* 2000;14:107–123.

Burstein R, Yamamura H, Malick A, Strassman AM. Chemical stimulation of the intra-cranial dura induces enhanced responses to facial stimulation in brain stem trigeminal neurons. *J Neurophysiol* 1998;79:964–982.

Chaitow L. *Cranial Manipulation: Theory and Practice.* 2nd ed. Edinburgh: Churchill Livingstone; 2005.

Choudhary AK, Jha B, Boal DK, Dias M. Occipital sutures and its variations: the value of 3D-CT and how to differentiate it from fractures using 3D-CT? *Surg Radiol Anat* 2010;32:807–816.

Christine DC. Temporal bone misalignment and motion asymmetry as a cause of vertigo: the craniosacral model. *Altern Ther Health Med* 2009;15:38–42.

Cook A. The mechanics of cranial motion: the spheno-basilar synchondrosis (SBS) revisited. *J Bodywork Mov Ther* 2005;9: 177–188.

Couture A, Veyrac C, Baud C, et al. Advanced cranial ultrasound: transfontanellar Doppler imaging in neonates. *Eur Radiol* 2001;11:2399–2410.

Crow WT, King HH, Patterson RM, Giuliano V. Assessment of calvarial structure motion by MRI. *Osteopath Med Prim Care* 2009;3:8.

Cutler MJ, Holland S, Stupski BA, et al. Cranial manipulation can alter sleep latency and sympathetic nerve activity in humans: a pilot study. *J Altern Complement Med* 2005;11: 103–108.

Devor M, Seltzer Z. Patho-physiology of damaged nerves in relation to chronic pain. In: Wall P, Melzack R, eds. *Textbook of Pain.* 4th ed. Edinburgh: Churchill Livingstone; 1999:129–164.

Downey PA, Barbano T, Kapur-Wadhwa R, et al. Craniosacral therapy: the effects of cranial manipulation on intracranial pressure and cranial bone movement. *J Orthop Sports Phys Ther* 2006;36:845–853.

Duncan B, McDonough-Means S, Worden K, et al. Effectiveness of osteopathy in the cranial field and myofascial release versus acupuncture as complementary treatment for children with spastic cerebral palsy: a pilot study. *J Am Osteopath Assoc* 2008;108:559–570.

Enlow D, Hans M. *Essentials of Facial Growth.* Philadelphia: Saunders; 1996.

Feindel W, Penfield W, McNaughton F. The tentorial nerves and localization of intra-cranial pain in man. *Neurology* 1960;10:555–563.

Felizardo R, Boucher Y, Braud A, et al. Trigeminal projections on gustatory neurons of the nucleus of the solitary tract: a double-label strategy using electrical stimulation of the chorda tympani and tracer injection in the lingual nerve. *Brain Res* 2009;1288:60–68.

Fernández-de-las-Peñas C, Cuadrado ML, Gerwin RD, Pareja JA. Referred pain from the trochlear region in tension-type headache: a myofascial trigger point from the superior oblique muscle. *Headache* 2005;45:731–737.

Fernández-de-las-Peñas C, Alonso-Blanco C, Cuadrado ML, et al. Are manual therapies effective in reducing pain from tension-type headache? A systematic review. *Clin J Pain* 2006a;22:278–285.

Fernández-de-las-Peñas C, Cuadrado ML, Gerwin RD, Pareja JA. Myofascial disorders in the trochlear region in unilateral migraine: a possible initiating or perpetuating factor. *Clin J Pain* 2006b;22:548–553.

Fernández-de-las-Peñas C, Coppieters MW, Cuadrado ML, Pareja JA. Patients with chronic tension type headache demonstrate increased mechano-sensitivity of the supra-orbital nerve. *Headache* 2008;48:570–577.

Fernández-de-las-Peñas C, Arendt-Nielsen L, Cuadrado ML, Pareja JA. Generalized mechanical pain sensitivity over nerve tissues in patients with strictly unilateral migraine. *Clin J Pain* 2009a;25:401–406.

Fernández-de-las-Peñas C, Galán-del-Río F, Fernández-Carnero J, et al. Bilateral widespread mechanical pain sensitivity in myofascial temporomandibular disorder: evidence of impairment in central nociceptive processing. *J Pain* 2009b;10:1170–1178.

Fernández-de-las-Peñas C, Cuadrado ML, Gerwin RD, Pareja JA. Referred pain elicited by manual exploration of the lateral rectus muscle in chronic tension type headache. *Pain Med* 2009c;10:43–48.

Fernández-Mayoralas D, Fernández-de-las-Peñas C, Ortega-Santiago R, et al. Generalized mechanical nerve pain hypersensitivity in children with frequent episodic tension type headache. *Pediatrics* 2010;126:187–194.

Fujimi Y, Takeda M, Tanimoto T, Matsumoto S. *N*-methyl-d-aspartate (NMDA) and non-NMDA receptor antagonists suppress the superior sagittal sinus-evoked activity of C1 spinal neurons responding to tooth pulp electrical stimulation in rats. *Odontology* 2006;94:22–28.

Gagan JR, Tholpady SS, Ogle RC. Cellular dynamics and tissue interactions of the dura mater during head development. *Birth Defects Res C Embryo Today* 2007;81:297–304.

Gard G. An investigation into the regulation of intra-cranial pressure and its influence upon the surrounding cranial bones. *J Bodywork Mov Ther* 2009;13:246–254.

Gillig PM, Sanders RD. Cranial nerves IX, X, XI, and XII. *Psychiatry (Edgmont)* 2010;7:37–41.

Goadsby PJ, Bartsch T. The anatomy and physiology of the trigeminocervical complex. In: Fernández-de-las-Peñas C, Arendt-Nielsen L, Gerwin R, eds. *Tension Type and Cervicogenic Headache: Patho-physiology, Diagnosis and Treatment.* Sudbury, MA: Jones and Bartlett; 2010; 109–116.

Goadsby PJ, Oshinsky M. The patho-physiology of migraine. In: Silberstein SD, Lipton RB, Dodick D, eds. *Wolff's Headache and Other Head Pain.* 8th ed. New York: Oxford; 2007.

Green C, Martin CW, Bassett K, Kazanjian A. A systematic review of craniosacral therapy: biological plausibility, assessment reliability and clinical effectiveness. *Complement Ther Med* 1999;7:201–207.

Greenman P. *Principles of Manual Medicine.* Baltimore, MD: Williams & Wilkins; 1996.

Gregersen H, Kassab GS, Fung YC. The zero-stress state of the gastrointestinal tract: biomechanical and functional implications. *Dig Dis Sci* 2000;45:2271–2281.

Hack GD, Koritzer RT, Robinson WL, et al. Anatomic relation between the rectus capitis posterior minor muscle and the dura mater. *Spine* 1995;20:2484–2486.

Hajihosseini MK, Lalioti MD, Arthaud S, et al. Skeletal development is regulated by fibroblast growth factor receptor 1 signalling dynamics. *Development* 2004;131:325–335.

Halma KD, Degenhardt BF, Snider KT, et al. Intraobserver reliability of cranial strain patterns as evaluated by osteopathic physicians: a pilot study. *J Am Osteopath Assoc* 2008;108:493–502.

Han DG. The other mechanism of muscular referred pain: the "connective tissue" theory. *Med Hypotheses* 2009;73:292–295.

Hanten WP, Olson SL, Hodson JL, et al. The effectiveness of CV-4 and resting position techniques on subjects with tension-type headaches. *J Man Manipulative Ther* 1999;7:64–70.

Hartman SE. Cranial osteopathy: its fate seems clear. *Chiropractic & Osteopathy* 2006;14:10.

Hartman SE, Norton JM. Inter-examiner reliability and cranial osteopathy. *Sci Rev Altern Med* 2002;6:23–34.

Heifetz MD, Weiss M. Detection of skull expansion with increased intracranial pressure. *J Neurosurg* 1981;55:811–812.

Heisey SR, Adams T. Role of cranial bone mobility in cranial compliance. *Neurosurgery* 1993;33:869–876.

Heller JB, Gabbay JS, Wasson K, et al. Cranial suture response to stress: expression patterns of Noggin and Runx2. *Plast Reconstr Surg* 2007;119:2037–2045.

Henderson JH, Chang LY, Song HM, et al. Age-dependent properties and quasistatic strain in the rat sagittal suture. *J Biomech* 2005a;38:2294–2301.

Henderson JH, Nacamuli RP, Zhao B, et al. Age-dependent residual tensile strains are present in the dura mater of rats. *J R Soc Interface* 2005b;2:159–167.

Hord ED, Evans MS, Mueed S, et al. The effect of vagus nerve stimulation on migraines. *J Pain* 2003;4:530–534.

Hu JW, Vernon H, Tatourian I. Changes in neck electromyography associated with meningeal noxious stimulation. *J Manipul Physiol Ther* 1995;18:577–587.

Hu S, Chen J, Fabry B, et al. Intracellular stress tomography reveals stress focusing and structural anisotropy in cytoskeleton of living cells. *Am J Cell Physiol* 2003;285:1082–1090.

Hummel T, Iannilli E, Frasnelli J, et al. Central processing of trigeminal activation in humans. *Ann NY Acad Sci* 2009;1170:190–195.

King HH, Lay E. Osteopathy in the cranial field. In: Ward RC, ed. *Foundations for Osteopathic Medicine.* 2nd ed. Baltimore, MD: Lippincott Williams and Wilkins; 2003:985–1001.

Kostopoulos DC, Keramidas G. Changes in elongation of falx cerebri during craniosacral therapy techniques applied on the skull of an embalmed cadaver. *Cranio* 1992;10:9–12.

Kumar R, Berger RJ, Dunsker SB, Keller JT. Innervation of the spinal dura: myth or reality? *Spine* 1995;20:18–26.

Levy D, Strassman A. Mechanical response properties of A and C primary afferent neurons innervating the rat intracranial dura. *J Neurophysiol* 2002;88:3020–3031.

Linder-Aronson S, Woodside DG. *Excess Face Height Malocclusion: Etiology, Diagnosis and Treatment.* Chicago: Quintessence; 2000.

Maitland GD, Hengeveld E, Banks K, English K. *Maitland's Vertebral Manipulation.* 7th ed. London: Elsevier Health Sciences; 2005.

Mann JD, Faurot KR, Wilkinson L, et al. Craniosacral therapy for migraine: protocol development for an exploratory controlled clinical trial. *BMC Complement Altern Med* 2008;8:28.

Martin MD, Bruner HJ, Maiman D. Anatomic and biomechanical considerations of the cranio-vertebral junction. *Neurosurgery* 2010;66(suppl 3):2–6.

Matarán-Peñarrocha GA, Castro-Sánchez AM, García GC, et al. Influence of cranio-sacral therapy on anxiety, depression and quality of life in patients with fibromyalgia. *Evid Based Complement Alternat Med.* 2011;ID 178769.

Mauskop A. Vagus nerve stimulation relieves chronic refractory migraine and cluster headaches. *Cephalalgia* 2005;25:82–86.

McPartland JM. Cranio-sacral iatrogenesis: side-effects from cranial-sacral treatment: case reports and commentary. *J Bodywork Mov Ther* 1996;1:2–5.

McPartland JM, Mein EA. Entrainment and the cranial rhythmic impulse. *Altern Ther Health Med* 1997;3:40–44.

McPartland J, Skinner E. The biodynamic model of osteopathy in the cranial field. *Explore* 2005;1:20–30.

Milnes K, Moran RW. Physiological effects of a CV4 cranial osteopathic technique on autonomic nervous system function: a preliminary investigation. *Int J Osteop Med* 2007;10:8–17.

Moran RW, Gibbons P. Intraexaminer and interexaminer reliability for palpation of the cranial rhythmic impulse at the head and sacrum. *J Manipulative Physiol Ther* 2001;24:183–190.

Moskalenko YE, Kravchenko TI, Gaidar BV, et al. Periodic mobility of cranial bones in humans. *Hum Physiol* 1999; 25:51–58.

Moskalenko YE, Frymann VM, Weinstein GB, et al. Slow rhythmic oscillations within the human cranium: phenomenology, origin, and informational significance. *Hum Physiol* 2001;27:171–178.

Nelson KE, Sergueef N, Lipinski CL, et al. The cranial rhythmic impulse related to the Traube-Hering-Mayer oscillation: comparing laser–Doppler flowmetry and palpation. *J Am Osteopath Assoc* 2001;101:163–173.

Nelson KE, Sergueef N, Glonek T. The effect of an alternative medical procedure upon low-frequency oscillations in cutaneous blood flow velocity. *J Manipulative Physiol Ther* 2006;29:626–636.

Ogle RC, Tholpady SS, McGlynn KA, Ogle RA. Regulation of cranial suture morphogenesis. *Cells Tissues Organs* 2004;176:54–66.

Opperman LA. Cranial sutures as intramembranous bone growth sites. *Dev Dyn* 2000;209:472–485.

Opperman LA, Passarelli RW, Morgan EP, et al. Cranial sutures require tissue interactions with dura mater to resist osseous obliteration in vitro. *J Bone Miner Res* 1995;10:1978–1987.

Oudhof P. In: Von Piekartz H, Bryden L, eds. *The Cranio-cervical and Cranio-facial Regions in Craniofacial Dysfunction and Pain: Manual Therapy, Assessment and Management.* Oxford, UK: Butterworth-Heinemann; 2000.

Palazzi C, Miralles R, Soto M, et al. Body position effects on EMG activity of sternocleidomastoid and masseter muscle in patients with myogenic cranio-cervical-mandibular dysfunction. *Cranio* 1996;14:200–207.

Pareja JA, Sánchez-del-Río M. Primary trochlear headache and other trochlear painful disorders. *Curr Pain Headache Rep* 2006;10:316–320.

Penfield W, McNaughton FL. Dural headache and the innervation of the dura mater. *Arch Neurol Psychiatry* 1940;44:43–75.

Pilat A. Myofascial induction approaches for headache. In: Fernández-de-las-Peñas C, Arendt-Nielsen L, Gerwin RD, eds. *Tension Type and Cervicogenic Headache: Pathophysiology, Diagnosis and Treatment.* Sudbury, MA: Jones and Bartlett; 2010; 339–367.

Pitlyk PJ, Piantanida TP, Ploeger DW. Noninvasive intracranial pressure monitoring. *Neurosurgery* 1985;17:581–584.

Quevedo JP, Purgavie K, Platt H, Strax TE. Complex regional pain syndrome involving the lower extremity: a report of 2 cases of sphenopalatine block as a treatment option. *Arch Phys Med Rehabil* 2005;86:335–337.

Ray BS, Wolff HG. Experimental studies on headache: pain sensitive structures of the head and their significance in headache. *Arch Surg* 1940;41:813–856.

Rocabado M, Iglash Z. *Musculoskeletal Approach to Maxillofacial Pain.* Baltimore: Lippincott Williams & Wilkins; 1991.

Rogers JS, Witt PL. The controversy of cranial bone motion. *J Orthop Sports Phys Ther* 1997;26:95–103.

Sabini RC, Elkowitz DE. Significance of differences in patency among cranial sutures. *J Am Osteopath Assoc* 2006;106:600–604.

Sanders RD. The trigeminal (V) and facial (VII) cranial nerves: head and face sensation and movement. *Psychiatry (Edgmont)* 2010;7:13–16.

Schepelmann K, Ebersberger A, Pawlak M, et al. Response properties of trigeminal brain stem neurons with input from dura mater encephali in the rat. *Neuroscience* 1999;90:543–554.

Sergueef N. *Cranial Osteopathy for Infants, Children and Adolescents.* London: Churchill Livingston, Elsevier; 2007.

Slater BJ, Lenton KA, Kwan MD, et al. Cranial sutures: a brief review. *Plast Reconstr Surg* 2008;120:170–178.

Stuginski-Barbosa J, Macedo HR, Bigal ME, Speciali JG. Signs of temporomandibular disorders in migraine patients: a prospective, controlled study. *Clin J Pain* 2010;26:418–420.

Sutherland W, Wales A, ed. *Teachings in the Science of Osteopathy.* Portland, OR: Rudra Press; 1990.

Thalakoti S, Patil VV, Damodaram S, et al. Neuron–glia signaling in trigeminal ganglion: implications for migraine pathology. *Headache* 2007;47:1008–1023.

Timoshkin EM, Sandhouse M. Retrospective study of cranial strain pattern: prevalence in a healthy population. *J Am Osteopath Assoc* 2008;108:652–656.

Totonchi A, Pashmini N, Guyuron B. The zygomaticotemporal branch of the trigeminal nerve: an anatomical study. *Plast Reconstr Surg* 2005;115:273–277.

Upledger JE. Cranio-sacral iatrogenesis. *J Bodywork Mov Ther* 1996;1:6–8.

Upledger J, Vredevoogd J. *Craniosacral Therapy.* Seattle: Eastland Press; 1983.

Ventegodt S, Merrick J, Andersen NJ, Bendix T. A combination of gestalt therapy, Rosen body work, and cranio sacral therapy did not help in chronic whiplash-associated disorders (WAD): results of a randomized clinical trial. *Sci World J* 2004;4:1055–1068.

Von Piekartz H. *Craniofacial Pain: Neuromusculoskeletal Assessment, Treatment and Management.* Philadelphia: Butterworth Heinemann Elsevier; 2007.

Warren SM, Greenwald JA, Spector JA, et al. New developments in cranial suture research. *Plast Reconstr Surg* 2001;107:523–540.

Warren SM, Greenwald JA, Nacamuli RP, et al. Regional dura mater differentially regulates osteoblast gene expression. *J Craniofac Surg* 2003;14:363–370.

Warren SM, Walder B, Dec W, et al. Confocal laser scanning microscopic analysis of collagen scaffolding patterns in cranial sutures. *J Craniofac Surg* 2008;19:198–203.

Yangüela J, Sánchez del Río M, Bueno A, et al. Primary trochlear headache: a new cephalalgia generated and modulated on the trochlear region. *Neurology* 2004;62:1134–1140.

Zhang Y, Liu H, Liu EZ, et al. Microsurgical anatomy of the ocular motor nerves. *Surg Radiol Anat* 2010; 32(7):623–628.

Zöller JE, Küber A, Lorber W, Mühling JH. Kraniosynoshosen in kraniofaziale chirurgie. diagnostik und therapie kraniofazialer fehlbildung. *Thieme Stuttgart* 2005;3:25.

Trigger Point Dry Needling

Jan Dommerholt, PT, DPT, MPS, Johnson McEvoy, BSc, MSc, DPT, MISCP, MCSP, PT, and Christian Gröbli, PT

INTRODUCTION

Trigger point dry needling (TrP-DN) is an invasive treatment for myofascial trigger points (TrPs), which is always administered as part of a comprehensive treatment approach to this condition. TrP-DN consists of the insertion of a solid filament needle into the skin, fascia, and /or muscle. Broadly speaking, two main dry needling techniques are used. In addition to deep dry needling, superficial dry needling (SDN) involves inserting a needle into the skin or fascia overlying a TrP, to a depth of 5 to 10 mm. The SDN technique was proposed by Dr. Peter Baldry in the 1980s as a means to allay safety concerns related to deeper needling of muscles such as the scaleni, in view of the risk of pneumothorax (Baldry, 2002, 2005). TrP-DN entails the insertion of the needle directly into a TrP to elicit local twitch responses (LTRs), which are associated with improved outcomes (Hong, 1994; Simons et al., 1999). Needling therapies appear to be effective for relieving pain (Cummings & White, 2001; Furlan et al., 2005).

TrP injection therapy, which was primarily developed by Dr. Janet Travell, involves the dynamic injection of local anesthetic into the TrP with the concurrent elicitation of LTRs (Travell, 1968; Simons et al., 1999). Recent research has supported the contention that, generally speaking, the needling effect is related to mechanical needling stimulation and elicitation of LTRs rather than being a direct effect of the anesthetic or fluid injection (Lewit, 1979; Hong, 1994). Exceptions include injections with botulinum toxin or serotonin antagonists, which do have injectate-specific mechanisms (Kuan et al., 2002; Müller & Stratz, 2004; Reilich et al., 2004; Qerama et al., 2006).

The neurophysiological mechanisms of TrP-DN are not fully understood, but credible explanations for them have been proposed (Dommerholt & Gerwin, 2010b). TrP-DN has been shown to reduce nociceptive chemical concentrations in the vicinity of active TrPs when LTRs are elicited (Shah et al., 2005, 2008). Reducing peripheral nociception in TrPs may eliminate central sensitization and, therefore, be clinically useful for the treatment of pain and motor dysfunction (Fernández-de-las-Peñas et al., 2007). In a rabbit model, TrP-DN proved effective at diminishing motor endplate noise when LTRs were elicited (Chen et al., 2001). Evidence gained from animal studies suggests that other modes of action may include effects on the descending pain inhibition system and circulation (Takeshige et al., 1992a, 1992b; Takeshige & Sato, 1996).

Accurate localization of TrPs forms the basis for safe and effective TrP-DN. This consideration is of paramount importance to allow for direct needling of the TrP zone and to avoid needling in areas such as neurovascular bundles or organs such as the lung. Clinicians should have good anatomic knowledge and be cognizant of muscle attachments, fiber direction, and muscle layers, among other aspects of the anatomy. The effectiveness of TrP-DN is related to the clinician's ability to insert the needle in the TrP zone, as this area is the most responsive part of the muscle and provides for maximum LTRs. The TrP zone is usually the area of greatest stiffness and tenderness. There is no gold standard test for the identification of TrPs in clinical practice; instead, clinicians need to rely on palpation techniques—that is, skilled flat or pincer grip palpation (Simons et al., 1999; Simons, 2004; Dommerholt & McEvoy, in press). Given that the reliability of TrP palpation in accessible muscles depends on the practitioner's expertise and skill, clinical training is of high importance in this area of practice (McEvoy & Huijbregts, 2011). Chapter 15 provides further information on identification of myofascial trigger points.

The effectiveness of TrP needling therapies for the treatment of pain was supported by a meta-analysis, but questions about their efficacy beyond the level produced by placebo remain unanswered owing to the challenges associated with placebo needling design (Cummings & White, 2001). TrP-DN has been found to offer pain relief and improvement in quality of life measures in older patients with osteoarthritic hip and knee pain (Bajaj et al., 2001; Itoh et al., 2008), neck pain (Itoh et al., 2007), and low back pain (Itoh et al., 2004). In a study on hemiparetic shoulder pain syndrome, TrP-DN, as part of a rehabilitation program, provided superior results compared to standard rehabilitation alone (Dilorenzo et al., 2004). In patients with bilateral shoulder pain, unilateral TrP-DN of active TrPs in the infraspinatus muscle increased the active and passive range of shoulder internal rotation, increased the pressure-pain threshold of TrPs, and reduced pain, compared to the control group (Hsieh et al., 2007). In addition, this study demonstrated that TrP-DN of a primary active TrP in the infraspinatus muscle inhibited activity in satellite TrPs situated in the referral zone of the primary TrP in the anterior deltoid and extensor carpi radialis longus muscles on the same side (Hsieh et al., 2007). TrP-DN of the extensor carpi radialis longus muscle decreased the pain intensity and increased the pressure-pain threshold in the ipsilateral trapezius muscle, with a subsequent increase in cervical spine range of motion being noted in patients with active TrPs in the upper trapezius (Tsai et al., 2010).

Referred pain from TrPs in the posterior cervical, head, and shoulder muscles can mimic pain areas observed in patients with head and neck pain (Travell, 1967; Fernández-de-las-Peñas et al., 2007a, 2007b, 2010). Furthermore, TrPs contribute to migraine symptoms, illustrating that peripheral nociceptive input from TrPs might potentially enhance the sensitization level of central sensory neurons (Giamberardino et al., 2007).

In patients with myofascial pain and headaches, TrP-DN has yielded results similar to those seen with lidocaine injection, with and without corticoids, in terms of levels of pain intensity, frequency and duration, obtainment time, and duration of relief (Venancio Rde et al., 2008). TrP anesthetic infiltration in migraineurs, when compared to control migraineurs and normal subjects, was found to improve migraine symptoms and increase threshold sensitivity in TrP-referred areas (Garcia-Leiva et al., 2007). In a comparison of TrP-DN and metoprolol medication, TrP-DN produced a similar reduction in frequency and duration of migraine attacks (Hesse et al., 1994). TrP-DN was superior to metoprolol in terms of side effects (Hesse et al., 1994). TrP-DN techniques for addressing muscles relevant to headache have been previously described (Dommerholt & Gerwin, 2010a).

Interest in TrP-DN in physical therapy practice increased dramatically in the last decade. TrP-DN is now included in the scope of physical therapy practice in an increasing number of countries around the world, including Canada, Chile, Ireland, the Netherlands, South Africa, Spain, Switzerland, and the United Kingdom, and in a growing number of jurisdictions in the United States (Dommerholt et al., 2006).

The American Physical Therapy Association (APTA) and the American Academy of Orthopaedic Manual Physical Therapists (AAOMPT) have both identified TrP-DN as being within the scope of physical therapy practice. Nevertheless, this therapy should be carried out only by clinicians who are trained and competent and in jurisdictions where TrP-DN is considered under the scope of practice. Clinicians should also carry suitable insurance.

The growth of TrP-DN has brought with it a new urgency focused on ensuring patient safety. There are no studies directly assessing TrP-DN safety and adverse reactions. The British Medical Acupuncture Society (BMAS), which represents health-care professionals including medical doctors and physiotherapists, has published an entire edition of the journal *Acupuncture in Medicine* addressing safety and adverse reactions in acupuncture (Filshie & Cummings, 2001). Notwithstanding the technical, theoretical, philosophical, and historical differences between TrP-DN and acupuncture, acupuncture safety research acts as a useful framework for needling therapies. Potential risks associated with TrP-DN include, but are not limited to, pneumothorax, infection, nerve and blood vessel injury, organ injury, aggravation of pain, and clinician needlestick injury. Traumatic complications can be avoided by having an outstanding understanding and awareness of anatomy and by carefully identifying the landmarks relevant to the muscle that is to be needled (Peuker & Gronemeyer, 2001). Clinicians should ensure patients give informed consent prior to performing needling, and local guidelines should be followed. Procedural issues such as forgetting needles, reusing needles, or losing needles can be avoided by adhering to treatment protocols. As an example, clinicians should account for all needles used and employ sterile one-use disposable needles only.

Large epidemiologic studies of acupuncture have shown that the risk of serious adverse events (SAE) with this therapy is very rare. The cumulative worldwide risk of SAE has been estimated to be 0.02 per 10,000 treatments (White & Cummings, 2008). A prospective study of 32,000 acupuncture treatments, delivered by 78 physiotherapists and medical doctors, reported one potential SAE of cellulitis in a previously edematous leg (White et al., 2001). In another prospective study that examined 34,000 treatments given by 574 professional acupuncturists, no serious adverse reactions were reported (MacPherson et al., 2001).

A large prospective observational study, in which 229,230 patients received 2.2 million treatments by 13,579 physicians, was carried out in Germany (Witt et al., 2009). Nerve injury or local infection was rare—0.14 event per 10,000 treatments, or 0.014% of patients. Pneumothorax was also rare—0.01 event per 10,000 treatments, or 0.001% of patients. Essentially, the pneumothorax risk was one in 1.1 million from acupuncture treatment given by German physicians (Witt et al., 2009). No visceral injury was reported in this study.

Another German study of 97,733 patients, who collectively received 760,000 treatments from physician acupuncturists, reported 6 potential SAEs, with a rate of 0.078 per 10,000 treatments (Melchart et al., 2004). Two cases of pneumothorax occurred, representing a rate of 0.026 per 10,000 treatments, or essentially one event per 380,000 treatments.

Significant minor events in acupuncture, such as severe nausea, fainting, and prolonged aggravation of symptoms, have been reported to occur at a rate of 13 to 14 per 10,000 treatments (MacPherson et al., 2001; White et al., 2001). Minor events, such as bleeding, are seen in approximately 7% of treatments or patients (Melchart et al., 2004; White et al., 2008). In one study of 229,230 individuals, 8.6% of patients reported at least one adverse event, with 2.2% of patients requiring medical treatment for such complications (Witt et al., 2009). Clinicians should be familiar with the potential minor and severe adverse reactions associated with TrP-DN and discuss them with patients as part of the informed consent process where appropriate (Witt et al., 2009).

Needling muscle requires a keen awareness of the structures in the vicinity of the TrP. It also requires a well-developed kinesthetic awareness. At all times, the clinician must be able to visualize the pathway the needle takes within the body (Dommerholt et al., 2006).

Post-needling care can prevent or minimize local bleeding, help restore and maintain range of motion, and facilitate a return to normal function. Hemostasis must be accomplished. In general, the use of Coumadin (warfarin) is a relative contraindication to needling, except for the very experienced clinician. The use of platelet inhibitors is generally not a contraindication to needling, but requires care to achieve hemostasis.

APPROACH TO NEEDLING TRIGGER POINTS IN ALL MUSCLES

The following general steps apply to the TrP-DN technique for TrPs:

1. Palpate the muscle(s) to identify the TrP(s) responsible for a referred pain pattern.
2. Palpate along the TrP taut band to identify the region of greatest hardness (greatest resistance) and tenderness.

3. Identify the landmarks associated with the muscle to be treated (e.g., the borders of the muscle or of underlying bone, such as the infraspinatus muscle and the borders of the scapulae).

4. Prepare to use the needle for dry needling.

5. Recheck the landmarks, making certain to identify or note the structures that are to be avoided when placing the needle.

6. Disinfect the skin at the needle site with an alcohol wipe or spray, if so desired. Note that an alcohol wipe does not really disinfect the skin. Guidelines on such care vary in different countries.

7. The angle of initial needle entry is always perpendicular to the skin surface. For TrP-DN, a solid filament needle is employed. The length of needle is determined based on the depth of the TrP. The diameter of the needle is determined by the muscle and its location. In the hand and facial muscles, shorter needles with a smaller diameter are used. It is recommended to maintain approximately 1 cm of the needle outside the skin. With this practice, in the very unlikely event of a needle breakage at the hub, the broken needle could still be retrieved with tweezers.

8. The needle is moved in and out (or up and down) into the targeted TrP by drawing the needle back to the subcutaneous tissue and the skin and reinserting it into the muscle until no more twitch responses occur at that location. If the needle remains within the muscle, it will follow the same original path through even if the direction of the needle above the skin is changed. In that case, the needle will curve as it is inserted back into the muscle.

9. Post-needling muscle stretching is always done in a direction opposite to the action of the muscle. Stretching is intended to restore normal muscle length. Overstretching is not necessary. Stretching may not be indicated in patients who are hypermobile.

10. The patient should always be lying down when being needled, because of the possibility of vasodepressive syncope. Lying down also facilitates better relaxation.

11. If the clinician is not absolutely certain where the needle is going, needling should not be done. When in doubt, stay out!

NECK MUSCLES

Splenius Capitis Muscle

- Anatomy: The splenius capitis muscle arises from the occipital ligamentum nuchae of the mastoid process, and inserts on the posterior spinous processes of C7 to T3–T4.
- Function: Extension, lateral bending, and rotation of the neck.
- Innervation: Cervical spinal nerves.
- Needling technique: The patient is in a lateral decubitus or prone position, and the clinician stands or sits at the patient's head. TrPs are identified manually. One finger is placed on the distal part of the taut band. The needle is inserted into the taut band in a rostral (superior) to caudal (inferior) direction (**Figure 21.1**).
- Precautions: Avoid needling in a rostral direction to be absolutely certain that the needle will not pass through the foramen magnum.

Semispinalis Capitis Muscle

- Anatomy: The semispinalis capitis muscle arises from the occipital ligamentum nuchae and inserts on the articular processes of C4 to C6 and the transverse processes of T1 to T6.
- Function: Extension, lateral bending, and rotation of the neck.
- Innervation: Cervical spinal nerves.

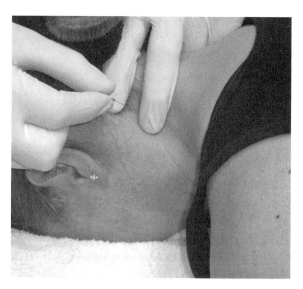

Figure 21.1 Dry Needling of the Splenius Capitis Muscle

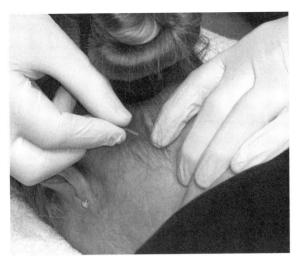

Figure 21.2 Dry Needling of the Semispinalis Capitis Muscle

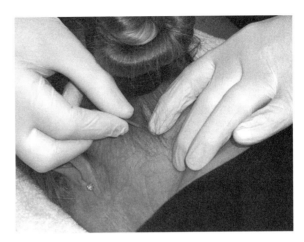

Figure 21.3 Dry Needling of the Splenius Cervicis Muscle

- Needling technique: The patient is in a lateral decubitus or prone position, and the therapist sits or stands at the patient's head. If the patient is in the lateral decubitus position, the clinician is positioned behind the patient. The needle is directed downward from the most rostral part of the TrP in upper-neck TrPs. In more caudal TrPs, the needle can be directed more perpendicularly into the muscle (**Figure 21.2**).
- Precautions: The downward or caudal direction of the needle ensures that the vertebral artery will not be penetrated and that the needle will not penetrate the cervical spine. The caudal direction of the needle also ensures that the foramen magnum will not be penetrated.

Splenius Cervicis Muscle

- Anatomy: The superior attachment of the splenius cervicis muscle is to the anterior aspect of the transverse processes of C1 to C3. The inferior or caudal attachment is to the posterior spinous processes of T2 to T6.
- Function: Extension of the neck and rotation of the head.
- Innervation: Cervical spinal nerves.
- Needling technique: The patient is in a prone or lateral decubitus position, and the therapist stands or sits at the patient's head. If the patient is in the lateral decubitus position, the clinician is positioned behind the patient. The TrP is fixed between two fingers. The needle is inserted

perpendicularly to the skin over the muscle into the taut band at the area of maximum tenderness. It may be directed medially because the muscle is situated laterally away from the cervical spine foramina. The insertion may be through the upper fibers of the trapezius muscle (**Figure 21.3**).
- Precautions: None.

Semispinalis Cervicis Muscle

- Anatomy: The rostral (superior) attachment is to the posterior spinous processes of C2 to C5. The inferior attachment is to the transverse processes of T1 to T5–T6.
- Function: Neck extension and contralateral cervical rotation.
- Innervation: Cervical nerves.
- Needling technique: The patient is in a prone or lateral decubitus position, and the therapist stands or sits at the patient's head. If the patient is in the lateral decubitus position, the clinician is positioned behind the patient. The taut band of the TrP is fixed by the index and long fingers of the non-needling hand. The needle is inserted perpendicularly to the skin at the most tender part of the taut band. It may be directed parallel to the posterior processes or slightly laterally (**Figure 21.4**).
- Precautions: The vertical or slightly lateral direction of the needle minimizes the danger of inserting the needle through the spine into the epidural space, the subarachnoid space, or the spinal cord.

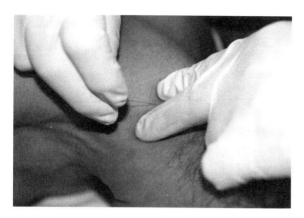

Figure 21.4 Dry Needling of the Semispinalis Cervicis Muscle

Multifidi Muscles

- Anatomy: The rostral (superior) attachment is the posterior processes of C2 to C5. The caudal (inferior) attachment is the articular processes of C2 to C7. The muscle crosses two to four vertebral levels.
- Function: Stabilization of the cervical spine. These muscles may assist in extension and rotation of the spine.
- Innervation: Cervical nerves.
- Needling technique: The patient is in a prone or lateral decubitus position, and the clinician sits or stands by the head of the patient. If the patient is in the lateral decubitus position, the clinician is behind the patient. TrPs are not palpable directly. The level to be treated is identified by determining the level of neurotrophic changes in the skin (changes in skin moisture, edema, or segmental sensitivity to noxious stimuli, such as a pinpoint drag across the skin). The level can also be determined by identifying the innervation of neck and shoulder muscles affected by muscle TrPs. For example, the multifidi at C5 are treated if the C5-innervated infraspinatus muscle has active TrPs. Once the level is identified, the needle is inserted perpendicular to the skin and parallel to the posterior spinous processes, approximately 1 cm lateral to the spinous process. The level above and the level below can be reached from a single needle insertion (**Figure 21.5**).
- Precautions: Avoid directing the needle medially to minimize the risk of penetrating the structures within the spinal canal (epidural or subarachnoid space, spinal cord).

Sub-Occipital Muscles

- Anatomy: The rectus capitis posterior major muscle and oblique capitis inferior muscle attach medially to the posterior spinous process of the axis (C2). The rectus capitis posterior minor muscle attaches medially to the posterior spinous process of the atlas (C1). The oblique capitis superior muscle attaches inferiorly and laterally to the transverse process of the atlas. The rectus capitis posterior major and minor muscles and the oblique capitis superior muscle all attach to the occiput. The oblique capitis inferior muscle is the only one that does not attach to the skull; it attaches to the transverse process of the atlas (C1).
- Function: The rectus capitis posterior major and minor muscles and the oblique capitis superior muscle extend the neck. The oblique capitis superior muscle assists in ipsilateral side bending. These three muscles are more postural control muscles than primary movers of the head. The oblique capitis inferior muscle is a powerful ipsilateral rotator of the head.
- Innervation: C1 nerve.
- Needling technique: Only the oblique capitis inferior muscle is easily and safely needled because of the proximity of the vertebral artery above the arch of the atlas. The patient is in a prone or lateral decubitus position, and the clinician sits or stands at the patient's head. The clinician is behind the patient when the patient lies in the lateral decubitus position. The muscle is located by placing one finger on the transverse process of C1 and the other finger on the posterior

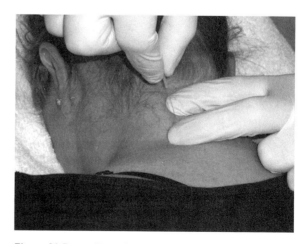

Figure 21.5 Needling of the Multifidi Muscles

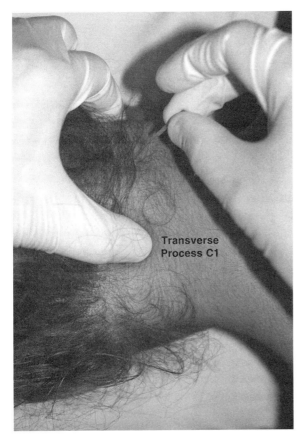

Figure 21.6 Dry Needling of the Sub-Occipital Muscles

process of C2. The point to be needled is located midway between these two markers. The needle is inserted perpendicular to the skin directly into the muscle. A small radius of muscle can be needled from one skin penetration (**Figure 21.6**).

- Precautions: Avoid directing the needle upward or needling too laterally to prevent inadvertent penetration of the vertebral artery.

Sternocleidomastoid Muscle

- Anatomy: The two heads of the sternocleido-mastoid muscle attach superiorly to the mastoid process by a single tendon. The sternal or medial head attaches inferiorly to the manubrium. The clavicular or lateral head attaches inferiorly to the medial third of the clavicle.
- Function: Acting together, the two sternocleido-mastoid muscles flex the neck against resistance or against gravity. Acting unilaterally, the muscle side-bends the head to the same side, and

rotates the head to the opposite side. It also tilts the chin upward and to the opposite side.

- Innervation: The muscle is innervated by the accessory nerve (XI pars) and by the C2 and C3 spinal nerves.
- Needling technique: The patient is in a supine or lateral decubitus position, and the therapist sits or stands at the head of the patient. When the patient is in the lateral decubitus position, the muscle is easily reached by coming over the top of the patient's head. The muscle is grasped by pincer palpation after identifying the carotid artery. The two heads, clavicular and sternal, must both be grasped within the fingers. The needle is inserted either perpendicular to the skin in a posterior direction or in a posterior-lateral direction. The needle should penetrate both heads of the muscle. Two insertions of the needle may be needed to clear the TrPs (**Figure 21.7**).
- Precautions: The carotid artery lies medial to the sternocleidomastoid muscle, next to the trachea. Lift the sternocleidomastoid muscle away from the carotid artery and only needle between the fingers holding the muscle in a pincer grasp, directing the needle as described previously, to avoid needling the carotid artery.

Levator Scapulae Muscle: Superior Portion

- Anatomy: The cervical portion of the levator scapulae muscle is palpated on its lateral border, which is identified as the first muscle belly ventral to the upper part of the trapezius muscle. It is generally felt

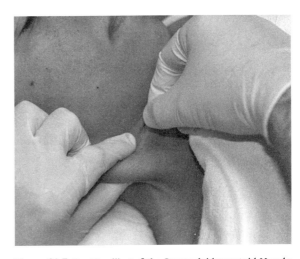

Figure 21.7 Dry Needling of the Sternocleidomastoid Muscle

as a ropy muscle of approximately 5 mm diameter in lateral extent, between the anterior (ventral) border of the upper trapezius and the transverse process of C1. The inferior attachment is to the lateral border of the scapula between the scapular spine and the superior medial border of the scapula.

- Function: The levator scapulae muscle extends and side-bends the neck. When the head is turned to the opposite side and forward flexed, the levator scapulae rotates the head toward the midline. The muscle rotates the scapula glenoid fossa downward when the neck is fixed. Acting with the trapezius, the two muscles elevate the shoulder.
- Innervation: Cervical spinal nerves C3 and C4, and C5 through the dorsal scapular nerve.
- Needling technique: The patient is in a lateral decubitus position, and the clinician sits or stands behind the patient. The muscle is identified and fixed along its length between the index and long fingers. The needle is inserted perpendicular to the skin at the most tender point (**Figure 21.8**).
- Precautions: Do not needle the lowest 2 cm of the muscle above the anterior border of the upper trapezius because of the danger of penetrating a high-positioned apex of the lung.

Scalene Muscles

- Anatomy: The anterior scalene muscle lies deeply beneath the sternocleidomastoid muscle, originating on the anterior aspect of the transverse processes of C3 to C6. It inserts on the

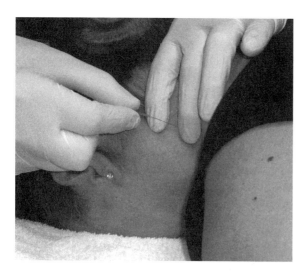

Figure 21.8 Dry Needling of the Levator Scapulae Muscle (Superior Portion)

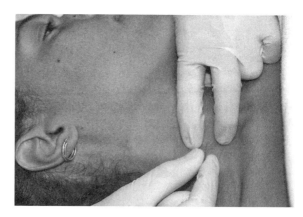

Figure 21.9 Dry Needling of the Scalene Muscles

first rib anterior to the neurovascular bundle. The medium scalene arises from the transverse processes of C3 to C7. It attaches inferiorly to the first rib posterior to the neurovascular bundle.

- Function: Side-bending to the same side. The anterior scalene also assists in rotating the head to the opposite side. Both anterior and medial scalene muscles are accessory respiratory muscles through elevation of the first rib.
- Innervation: The anterior scalene muscle is innervated by spinal nerves C4 to C6. The medium scalene muscle is innervated by C3 to C8.
- Needling technique: The patient is in a supine or lateral decubitus position, and the therapist sits or stands behind the patient. The muscles can be identified by having the patient sniff sharply (activation of the respiratory component of the muscle function). The anterior scalene is reached in the triangle formed by the jugular vein laterally, the lateral edge of the clavicular head of the sternocleidomastoid muscle, and the clavicle as the base (**Figure 21.9**).
- Precautions: The medial head of the scalene muscle must not be needled at the base of the neck. Needle it only one fingerbreadth or more above the base of the neck to avoid a high-positioned apex of the lung.

HEAD MUSCLES

Corrugator Muscle

- Anatomy: The corrugator muscle is located in the medial aspect of the eyebrow, lying deep to the orbicularis oris and the frontalis muscles. At the medial insertion, it may arch downward over the eyebrow.

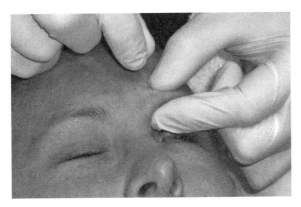

Figure 21.10 Dry Needling of the Corrugator Muscle

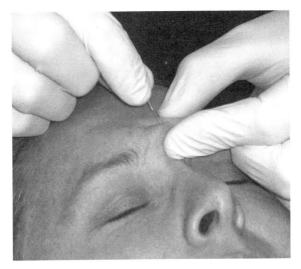

Figure 21.11 Dry Needling of the Procerus Muscle

- Function: The corrugator muscle draws the eyebrow medially, furrowing the forehead.
- Innervation: Facial nerve (temporal branches).
- Needling technique: The patient is in a supine position, and the clinician sits at the head of the table. The muscle is palpated with the free hand. The approach is from either the medial or the lateral aspect of the muscle, directed toward its midportion. The needle is inserted through the skin at a shallow angle, and advanced into the muscle. The entire muscle may be approached with one penetration (**Figure 21.10**).
- Precautions: None.

Procerus Muscle

- Anatomy: The procerus muscle covers the bridge of the nose, with fibers arising from the nasal fascia.
- Function: Wrinkles the skin of the bridge of the nose.
- Innervation: Facial nerve (buccal branches).
- Needling technique: The patient is in a supine position, and the therapist sits at the head of the table. The needle is directed from superior to inferior, coming from the forehead toward the nose. The needle is inserted through the skin at a shallow angle. The needle is directed to various parts of the muscle, keeping a shallow angle (**Figure 21.11**).
- Precautions: None.

Masseter Muscle

- Anatomy: The three layers of the masseter muscle arise from the zygomatic process. The superficial layer inserts into the angle and lateral surface of the mandible. The middle layer inserts

into the midportion of the mandibular ramus. The deep layer inserts into the upper mandibular ramus and the coronoid process.
- Function: Closes the mouth by elevating the mandible.
- Innervation: Mandibular branch of trigeminal nerve.
- Needling technique: The patient is in a supine or lateral decubitus position, and the clinician sits at the head of the table. The needle is inserted perpendicularly to the skin, directly into the TrP taut band identified by palpation (**Figure 21.12**).
- Precautions: None.

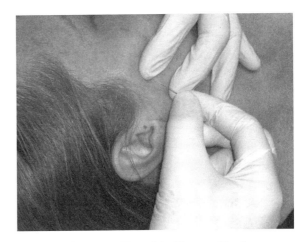

Figure 21.12 Dry Needling of the Masseter Muscle

Temporalis Muscle

- Anatomy: The temporalis muscle arises in the temporal fossa; its insertion is the mandibular coronoid process and the posterior mandibular ramus.
- Function: Closes the mouth by elevating the mandible.
- Innervation: Trigeminal nerve, mandibular branch.
- Needling technique: The patient is in a supine or lateral decubitus position, and the therapist sits at the head of the table or at the side. TrP taut bands are identified by palpation and fixed in place by the index and long fingers of the non-needling hand. The needle is inserted perpendicularly to the skin directly into the taut band (**Figure 21.13**).
- Precautions: Identify the superficial temporal artery to avoid penetrating it with the needle.

Zygomatic Muscle

- Anatomy: The zygomatic major and minor muscles arise from the zygomatic bone and insert into the muscles of the mouth (the orbicularis oris, levator, and depressor anguli oris).
- Function: Elevates the angle of the mouth, as in smiling.
- Innervation: Facial nerve.
- Needling technique: The patient is in a supine position, and the clinician stands or sits at the patient's head. The muscle is identified by pincer

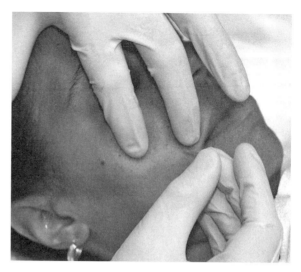

Figure 21.14 Dry Needling of the Zygomatic Muscle

or flat palpation. With the pincer palpation, one palpating digit is inside the cheek against the buccal mucosa and one digit is on the external surface of the skin. With the flat palpation, the taut band is held in between the fingers. The zygomatic muscle may be thin and difficult to feel. The needle is inserted at the most tender spot and angled toward the zygomatic bone. The needle is moved in and out of the muscle, keeping the palpating fingers in place while needling the TrP (**Figure 21.14**).

- Precautions: None.

SHOULDER MUSCLES

Trapezius Muscle: Upper Portion

- Anatomy: The superior attachment of the upper trapezius muscle is to the medial third of the occipital nuchal ridge. The mid-fibers attach to C7 posterior spinous processes. The horizontal fibers attach to the lateral third of the clavicle, to the acromion process, and to the scapular spine.
- Function: Unilaterally ipsilateral side-bending of the head, contralateral rotation of the head, and elevation of the shoulder; bilateral extension of the neck.
- Innervation: Accessory nerve (C-XI) and cervical spinal nerves C3 and C4.
- Needling technique: The patient is in a lateral decubitus position, and the clinician sits or stands

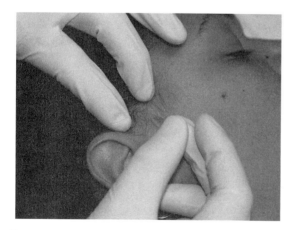

Figure 21.13 Dry Needling of the Temporalis Muscle

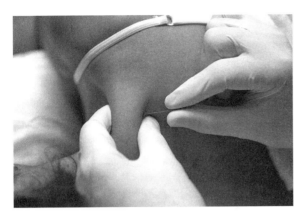

Figure 21.15 Dry Needling of the Trapezius Muscle (Upper Portion)

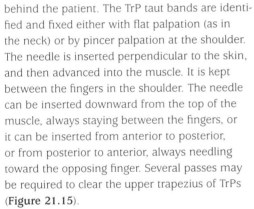

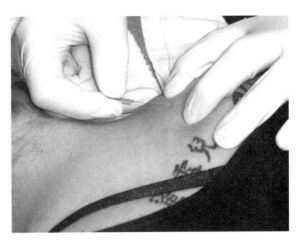

Figure 21.16 Dry Needling of the Levator Scapulae (Inferior Portion)

behind the patient. The TrP taut bands are identified and fixed either with flat palpation (as in the neck) or by pincer palpation at the shoulder. The needle is inserted perpendicular to the skin, and then advanced into the muscle. It is kept between the fingers in the shoulder. The needle can be inserted downward from the top of the muscle, always staying between the fingers, or it can be inserted from anterior to posterior, or from posterior to anterior, always needling toward the opposing finger. Several passes may be required to clear the upper trapezius of TrPs (**Figure 21.15**).

- Precautions: The most common serious adverse event arising from needling the upper trapezius is penetration of the lung that produces a pneumothorax. The danger of this SAE occurring can be minimized by needling strictly between the fingers holding the muscle in a pincer grasp, or needling to the opposing finger.

Levator Scapulae: Inferior Portion

See the section "Levator Scapulae: Superior Portion" for anatomy, function, and innervation of the inferior levator scapulae.

- Needling technique: The patient is in a lateral decubitus position, and the therapist sits or stands behind the patient. The insertion of the muscle on the scapula is located at the medial border of the scapula between the scapular spine and the upper medial border of the scapula. The needle is inserted through the skin at a shallow angle, and directed toward the upper, medial border of the scapula. Movement of the needle is directed toward the scapula (**Figure 21.16**).
- Precautions: The danger with needling the levator scapula in the thorax is penetration of the lung with consequent pneumothorax. This danger is minimized by keeping the angle of the needle shallow and directing the needle toward the medial border of the scapula.

REFERENCES

Bajaj P, Bajaj P, Graven-Nielsen T, et al. Trigger points in patients with lower limb osteoarthritis. *J Musculoskeletal Pain* 2001;9:17–33.

Baldry P. Superficial versus deep dry needling. *Acupunct Med* 2002;20:78–81.

Baldry P. *Acupuncture, Trigger Points and Musculoskeletal Pain.* Edinburgh: Churchill Livingstone; 2005.

Chen JT, Chung KC, Hou CR, et al. Inhibitory effect of dry needling on the spontaneous electrical activity recorded from myofascial trigger spots of rabbit skeletal muscle. *Am J Phys Med Rehabil* 2001;80:729–735.

Cummings TM, White AR. Needling therapies in the management of myofascial trigger point pain: a systematic review. *Arch Phys Med Rehabil* 2001;82:986–992.

Dilorenzo L, Traballesi M, Morelli D, et al. Hemiparetic shoulder pain syndrome treated with deep dry needling during early rehabilitation: a prospective, open-label, randomized investigation. *J Musculoskeletal Pain* 2004;12:25–34.

Dommerholt J, Gerwin RD. Needling of head, neck, and shoulder muscle trigger points relevant to headache. In: Fernández-de-las-Peñas C, Arendt-Nielsen L, Gerwin RD, eds. *Tension-Type and Cervicogenic Headache: Pathophysiology, Diagnosis, and Management.* Sudbury, MA: Jones and Bartlett; 2010a:421.

Dommerholt J, Gerwin RD. Neurophysiological effects of trigger point needling therapies. In: Fernández-de-las-Peñas C, Arendt-Nielsen L, Gerwin RD, eds. *Tension-Type and Cervicogenic Headache: Pathophysiology, Diagnosis, and Management.* Sudbury, MA: Jones and Bartlett; 2010b:247–259.

Dommerholt J, McEvoy J. The myofascial trigger point release approach. In: Davis WCA, ed. *Orthopedic Manual Physical Therapy: From Art to Evidence.* In press.

Dommerholt J, Mayoral O, Grobli C. Trigger point dry needling. *J Manual Manipulative Ther* 2006;14:E70–E87.

Fernández-de-las-Peñas C, Cuadrado ML, Arendt-Nielsen L, et al. Myofascial trigger points and sensitization: an updated pain model for tension-type headache. *Cephalalgia* 2007a;27:383–393.

Fernández-de-las-Peñas C, Simons D, Cuadrado ML, Pareja JA. The role of myofascial trigger points in musculoskeletal pain syndromes of the head and neck. *Curr Pain Headache Rep* 2007b;11:365–372.

Fernández-de-las-Peñas C, Ge HY, Alnso-Blanco C, et al. Referred pain areas of active myofascial trigger points in head, neck, and shoulder muscles, in chronic tension type headache. *J Bodyw Mov Ther* 2010;14:391–396.

Filshie J, Cummings M. *Acupunct Med* 2001;XIX(2):83–139.

Furlan A, Tulder M, Cherkin D, et al. Acupuncture and dry-needling for low back pain: an updated systematic review within the framework of the Cochrane collaboration. *Spine* 2005;30:944–963.

Garcia-Leiva JM, Hidalgo J, Rico-Villademoros F, et al. Effectiveness of ropivacaine trigger points inactivation in the prophylactic management of patients with severe migraine. *Pain Med* 2007;8:65–70.

Giamberardino MA, Tafuri E, Savini A, et al. Contribution of myofascial trigger points to migraine symptoms. *J Pain* 2007;8:869–878.

Hesse J, Mogelvang B, Simonsen H. Acupuncture versus metoprolol in migraine prophylaxis: a randomized trial of trigger point inactivation. *J Intern Med* 1994;235:451–456.

Hong CZ. Lidocaine injection versus dry needling to myofascial trigger point: the importance of the local twitch response. *Am J Phys Med Rehabil* 1994;73:256–263.

Hsieh YL, Kao MJ, Kuan TS, et al. Dry needling to a key myofascial trigger point may reduce the irritability of satellite MTrPs. *Am J Phys Med Rehabil* 2007;86:397–403.

Itoh K, Katsumi Y, Kitakoji H. Trigger point acupuncture treatment of chronic low back pain in elderly patients: a blinded RCT. *Acupunct Med* 2004;22:170–177.

Itoh K, Katsumi Y, Hirota S, Kitakoji H. Randomised trial of trigger point acupuncture compared with other acupuncture for treatment of chronic neck pain. *Complement Ther Med* 2007;15:172–179.

Itoh K, Hirota S, Katsumi Y, et al. Trigger point acupuncture for treatment of knee osteoarthritis: a preliminary RCT for a pragmatic trial. *Acupunct Med* 2008;26:17–26.

Kuan TS, Chen JT, Chen SM, et al. Effect of botulinum toxin on endplate noise in myofascial trigger spots of rabbit skeletal muscle. *Am J Phys Med Rehabil* 2002;81:512–520; quiz 521–523.

Lewit K. The needle effect in the relief of myofascial pain. *Pain* 1979;6:83–90.

MacPherson H, Thomas K, Walters S, Fitter M. A prospective survey of adverse events and treatment reactions following 34,000 consultations with professional acupuncturists. *Acupunct Med* 2001;19:93–102.

McEvoy J, Huijbregts P. Reliability of myofascial trigger point palpation: a systematic review. In: Dommerholt J, Huijbregts P, eds. *Myofascial Trigger Points: Pathophysiology and Evidenced-Informed Diagnosis and Management.* Sudbury, MA: Jones & Bartlett Learning; 2011; 65–88.

Melchart D, Weidenhammer W, Streng A, et al. Prospective investigation of adverse effects of acupuncture in 97 733 patients. *Arch Intern Med* 2004;164:104–105.

Müller W, Stratz T. Local treatment of tendinopathies and myofascial pain syndromes with the 5-HT3 receptor antagonist tropisetron. *Scand J Rheumatol Suppl* 2004; 119:44–48.

Peuker E, Gronemeyer D. Rare but serious complications of acupuncture: traumatic lesions. *Acupunct Med* 2001;19:103–108.

Qerama E, Fuglsang-Frederiksen A, Kasch H, et al. A double-blind, controlled study of botulinum toxin A in chronic myofascial pain. *Neurology* 2006;67:241–245.

Reilich P, Fheodoroff K, Kern U, et al. Consensus statement: botulinum toxin in myofascial pain. *J Neurol* 2004;251: 136–138.

Shah JP, Phillips TM, Danoff JV, Gerber LH. An in vivo microanalytical technique for measuring the local biochemical milieu of human skeletal muscle. *J Appl Physiol* 2005;99:1977–1984.

Shah JP, Danoff JV, Desai MJ, et al. Biochemicals associated with pain and inflammation are elevated in sites near to and remote from active myofascial trigger points. *Arch Phys Med Rehabil* 2008;89:16–23.

Simons DG. Review of enigmatic MTrPs as a common cause of enigmatic musculoskeletal pain and dysfunction. *J Electromyogr Kinesiol* 2004;14:95–107.

Simons DG, Travell JG, Simons L. *Travell and Simons' Myofascial Pain and Dysfunction: The Trigger Point Manual.* Baltimore: Williams & Wilkins; 1999.

Takeshige C, Sato M. Comparisons of pain relief mechanisms between needling to the muscle, static magnetic field, external qigong and needling to the acupuncture point. *Acupunct Electrother Res* 1996;21:119–131.

Takeshige C, Kobori M, Hishida F, et al. Analgesia inhibitory system involvement in nonacupuncture point-stimulation-produced analgesia. *Brain Res Bull* 1992a;28:379–391.

Takeshige C, Sato T, Mera T, et al. Descending pain inhibitory system involved in acupuncture analgesia. *Brain Res Bull* 1992b;29:617–634.

Travell J. Mechanical headache. *Headache* 1967;7:23–29.

Travell J. *Office Hours: Day and Night. The Autobiography of Janet Travell, M.D.* New York: World Publishing; 1968.

Tsai CT, Hsieh LF, Kuan KS, et al. Remote effects of dry needling on the irritability of the myofascial trigger point in the upper trapezius muscle. *Am J Phys Med Rehabil* 2010;89:133–140.

Venâncio Rde A, Alencar FG, Zamperini C. Different substances and dry-needling injections in patients with myofascial pain and headaches. *Cranio* 2008;26:96–103.

White A, Cummings M. *An Introduction to Western Medical Acupuncture.* Edinburgh: Churchill Livingstone/Elsevier; 2008.

White A, Hayhoe S, Hart A, et al. Survey of adverse events following acupuncture (SAFA): a prospective study of 32,000 consultations. *Acupunct Med* 2001;19:84–92.

Witt CM, Pach D, Brinkhaus B, et al. Safety of acupuncture: results of a prospective observational study with 229,230 patients and introduction of a medical information and consent form. *Forsch Komplementmed* 2009;16:91–97.

Vestibular Rehabilitation for Vestibular Migraine and Motion Sensitivity

Nicole Elizabeth Acerra, PT, PhD

INTRODUCTION

Migraineurs frequently report vestibular symptoms such as vertigo, dizziness, and motion sickness. Diagnosis and treatment are challenging, as this heterogeneous patient population consists of people with vestibular migraine, motion sensitivity, or vestibular dysfunction. Almost half of all long-term migraineurs develop motion sensitivity or motion sickness (Kayan & Hood, 1984; Drummond, 2005). In addition to motion sensitivity, 9% of migraineurs experience specific vestibular symptoms such as vertigo and meet the inclusion criteria for vestibular migraine (VM) (Neuhauser et al., 2001). In brief, VM describes episodic vertigo in association with migraine (**Table 22.1**). Some VM patients report persistent vertigo, dizziness, and motion sensitivity before or after their migraine, and many of these individuals have vestibular dysfunction on neuro-otologic testing (von Brevern et al., 2005). Migraineurs are more likely than

Table 22.1 Diagnostic Criteria for Definite and Probable Vestibular Migraine

Definite Vestibular Migraine

A. Episodic vestibular symptoms of at least moderate severity.
B. Current or previous history of migraine according to the 2004 criteria of the IHS.
C. One of the following migrainous symptoms during two or more attacks of vertigo: migrainous headache, photophobia, phonophobia, visual aura, or other aura.
D. Other causes ruled out by appropriate investigations.
Comment: Vestibular symptoms include rotational vertigo or another illusory self- or object motion. They may be spontaneous or positional. Vestibular symptoms are "moderate" if they interfere with but do not prohibit daily activities; they are "severe" if patients cannot continue daily activities.

Probable Vestibular Migraine

A. Episodic vestibular symptoms of at least moderate severity.
B. One of the following: (1) current or previous history of migraine according to the 2004 criteria of the IHS; (2) migrainous symptoms during vestibular symptoms; (3) migraine precipitants of vertigo in more than 50% of attacks: food triggers, sleep irregularities, or hormonal change; or (4) response to migraine medications in more than 50% of attacks.
C. Other causes ruled out by appropriate investigations.

Source: Modified from Neuhauser H, Lempert T. Vestibular migraine. *Neurol Clin* 2009;27:379–391.

the general population to have a coexisting vestibular condition, such as Ménière's disease or benign paroxysmal positional vertigo (BPPV). Fortunately, vestibular dysfunction and motion sensitivity can be managed with a customized vestibular rehabilitation program.

This chapter reviews vestibular migraine, motion sensitivity, and vestibular rehabilitation. It examines these conditions' assessment, prevention measures, and management of vestibular dysfunction, imbalance, and motion sensitivity.

VESTIBULAR MIGRAINE

Incidence

An association between episodic vertigo and migraine was described by Aretaeus of Cappadocia in AD 131 and later by Liveing in 1873 (Sachs, 1970). Today, episodic vertigo is reported in 27% to 33% of migraineurs (Selby & Lance, 1960; Kayan & Hood, 1984). Vestibular symptoms related to migraine have been referred to as benign recurrent vertigo, migrainous vertigo, migraine-associated dizziness (MAD), migraine-related vestibulopathy, and, most commonly, vestibular migraine (Neuhauser & Lempert, 2009).

Approximately 13% to 16% of the general population suffers from migraines, with women affected two to three times more frequently than men (Breslau et al., 1991; Rasmussen et al., 1991; Edmeads et al., 1993; Lipton et al., 2001). Similarly, dizziness and vertigo are common in the general population, with a lifetime prevalence of 7.9% (Neuhauser et al., 2005). However, 10% to

59% of migraineurs experience vertigo and 50% experience motion sickness (Kayan & Hood, 1984; Neuhauser et al., 2001). VM affects 1% of the general population and 10% of patients who present at dizziness clinics (Lempert & Neuhauser, 2009).

Diagnosis

Unfortunately, the International Headache Society (IHS, 2004) has not yet included VM in its classification scheme. Neuhauser and colleagues (Neuhauser et al., 2001, 2004; Neuhauser & Lempert, 2009) proposed diagnostic criteria for *definite* and *probable* VM (Table 22.1) that are widely accepted by clinicians and researchers (Shepard, 2006; Cha, 2010). Clinically, VM presents with attacks of spontaneous or positional vertigo lasting seconds, minutes, hours, or days that may or may not occur with migraine. Migraine accompaniments such as headache, photophobia or phonophobia, and auras are common but are not mandatory for diagnosis. Hearing loss and tinnitus (often high-pitched) may also occur (Lempert & Neuhauser, 2009). Many patients have a long-standing history of migraine prior to developing vestibular symptoms or VM.

The lack of clear VM diagnostic criteria leads to inconsistencies in diagnoses. Diagnosis is further complicated by the high incidence of coexisting vestibular disorders and migraine-related motion sensitivity in migraineurs. The relationship between migraine and vestibular disorders such as Ménière's disease, BPPV, motion sensitivity, cerebellar dysfunction, and nonvestibular disorders is unclear (as discussed later in this chapter). Thus clinicians must carefully differentiate whether vestibular symptoms are due to VM, migraines in general, a coexisting vestibular condition, or some combination (Shepard, 2006; Lempert & Neuhauser, 2009).

Neuro-Otologic Findings and Pathophysiology

It is not clear whether VM is a central or peripheral vestibular disorder. During an acute VM attack, vestibular symptoms commonly include vertigo (30%), positional vertigo (30%), and head-motion intolerance (30%), and oculographic recordings indicate pathological nystagmus in 70% of patients, central vestibular dysfunction in 50%, peripheral vestibular dysfunction in 15%, and an indeterminate site of lesion in 35% (von Brevern et al., 2005). The lack of consistency across patients is staggering; for example, pathological spontaneous nystagmus can range from 3° to 33° per second and present as horizontal, vertical, or torsional nystagmus (von Brevern et al., 2005). In one study, during the symptom-free period, 8.6% of VM patients experienced central vestibular dysfunction (saccadic hypometria), 20% demonstrated unilateral peripheral vestibular loss on caloric testing, and all had reduced balance reactions (Çelebisoy et al., 2008). This wide range in clinical and neuro-otologic findings underscores the need for a thorough examination and a multimodal approach to treatment.

The presence of neuro-otologic findings in the symptom-free period suggests that permanent neurologic damage can occur as a result of migraine. However, the pathophysiology underlying VM remains unclear. Hypothesized explanations include trigeminovascular activation causing plasma extravasation, spreading depression in the brainstem, and cortical spreading depression in the vestibular or oculomotor areas, such as the parieto-temporal cortex (Koo & Balaban, 2006; Richter et al., 2008). Another mechanism may be related to the generalized increase in sensitivity to sensory stimulation such as light or noise (Straube & Rauch, 2010). This hypothesis suggests a redefinition of migraine, with migraine being perceived as a global disturbance of sensory signal processing in which headache is a common manifestation as opposed to a headache disorder with adjunctive symptoms such as photophobia and auras (Straube & Rauch, 2010). This view of migraine may explain the high incidence of motion sensitivity. Thus both peripheral and central vestibular dysfunction can occur with VM. In addition, coexisting vestibular conditions may occur.

Management

VM management is usually multimodal and based on the patient's symptoms, functional level, and treatment goals (**Table 22.2**). In brief, management typically involves

Table 22.2 Overview of Migraine Management

Stress Reduction and Deconditioning

- Consider ways to reduce stress, such as yoga, tai chi, meditation, biofeedback, or relaxation techniques.
- Patients should maintain adequate restorative sleep daily. They should try to not oversleep or change sleep times.
- Patients should gradually increase physical activity until they can sustain 60% to 80% of their maximum heart rate for at least 30 minutes, three to five times per week.
- Stress may temporarily worsen symptoms.

Diet and Dietary Habits

- Patients may be prescribed a migraine diet.
- Patients should eat meals at regular times daily, on both weekends and weekdays.
- Patients should avoid low blood sugar (hypoglycemia) by eating something every 6 to 8 hours.

Nicotine

- When possible, individuals should not smoke or chew products that contain nicotine.

Estrogens

- Many women notice a change in their migraine pattern with menstruation.
- When appropriate, patients should avoid use of exogenous estrogens such as oral contraceptives or estrogen replacement therapy.

Medications

- The physician may prescribe medications to prevent migraines or treat new migraines.

Rehabilitation

- The physiotherapist may provide specific exercises for motion sickness, vertigo, dizziness, blurred vision, or imbalance.

Diary of Symptoms and Triggers

- Patients should note the time and date of headaches/migraines and possible triggers in the 24 hours prior to their onset.
- Patients should also note environmental triggers, such as strong smells, changes in air temperature, and cleaning products.

Source: Modified from Tusa RJ. Migraines, Ménière's disease, and motion sensitivity. In: Herdman S, ed. *Vestibular Rehabilitation*. Philadelphia: F. A. Davis Company; 2007;188–201.

migraine prevention, pharmacological agents (prophylactic or abortive medical therapy), behavioral modifications, and a customized vestibular rehabilitation program to address any vestibular symptoms, dysfunction, and motion sensitivity; these measures are discussed later in this chapter.

SENSITIVITY TO MOVEMENT AND VISUAL STIMULI

Motion Sickness and Motion Sensitivity

Descriptions of motion sickness date back to 400 BC when Hippocrates wrote, "Sailing on the sea shows that motion disorders the body" (Adams, 1849). Motion sickness, or travel sickness, describes the uncomfortable feelings associated with repetitive angular and linear acceleration and deceleration. Motion sickness is not merely a primitive vestibular reflex, but rather the consequence of disruption in spatial orientation (Reason & Brand, 1975). Its symptoms commonly increase with exposure to the stimulus (such as cars, trains, airplanes, ships, or fairground rides) and include nausea, vomiting, pallor, cold sweats, hypersalivation, hyperventilation, headaches, and general malaise (Reason & Brand, 1975; Spinks et al., 2007).

Another form of motion sickness can occur when an individual is sitting still. This condition may be a separate phenomenon in which the person experiences motion-sickness symptoms due to visual stimuli. Thus motion sensitivity can be caused by either real or apparent motion. Examples include watching an action-oriented movie on a large screen or standing in a busy environment such as a crowd or supermarket. This sensitivity to visual stimuli has been called visual vertigo (VV), visual–vestibular mismatch, space and motion discomfort, and motorists' disorientation syndrome (Pavlou, 2010).

 . Patients can present with symptoms caused by movement (e.g., car travel or with repetitive body motions such as head shaking) or visual-conflicting stimuli (e.g., large-screen movies). It is important to distinguish between these two forms of motion sensitivity. Failure to do so may reduce the effectiveness of rehabilitation, as each condition requires separate assessment and management (Pavlou et al., 2006).

Some people are more susceptible to motion sickness than others, and there is no way to reliably predict who will develop this condition (Baloh & Halmagyi, 1996; Quarck et al., 2000). Approximately one-third of adults experience motion sickness (8% to 24% of the general public and 30% of ocean-liner passengers), whereas

26% to 60% of migraineurs experience severe motion sickness (Childs & Sweetnam, 1961; Kuritzky et al., 1981; Kayan & Hood, 1984; Lawther & Griffin, 1988). Researchers have attempted to define the most provocative stimuli, in particular to reduce motion sickness for astronauts and people using transportation such as tilting trains (Bos & Bles, 1998; Golding et al., 2001; Donohew & Griffin, 2004; Golding & Gresty, 2005; Persson, 2008). In reality, motion sickness may be more complicated than simply measuring exposure to stimuli; instead, it may reflect the individual's sensitivity to conflicting information provided by the three balance centers (visual, vestibular, and proprioceptive) during the activity.

Pathophysiology

The underlying cause of motion sensitivity is unknown, as is its relationship to migraine. In addition, the pathophysiology may differ between subjects. Proposed etiologies include abnormal vestibular responses, cerebrospinal fluid dynamics, sensory weighting, excitability of brainstem circuits, neurophysiological wiring in the area postrema or cerebellum, central sensitization causing heightened susceptibility to visual or movement stimuli, and vestibular dysfunction secondary to vasomotor disturbances due to migraine attacks (Crampton, 1993; Drummond, 2005). Much of our current knowledge comes from space research: as many as 70% of astronauts experience motion sickness on their first space missions (Lackner & Dizio, 2006). Research indicates that astronauts vary in how they naturally deal with weightlessness and the lack of a horizon, with space sickness perhaps being related to excessive suppression of vestibular responses under these abnormal conditions (Watt & Lefebvre, 2003). Impaired vestibular–ocular reflexes (VOR) and perception of tilt have been reported in some people prone to motion sickness (Golding & Gresty, 2005). Migraineurs may have central sensitization to stimuli (Burstein, 2001; Straube & Rauch, 2010), although sensory stimuli are not believed to cause migraine or motion sensitivity (Drummond, 2005). An alternative proposal suggests that motion-sick people may have vestibular system dysfunction. One study reported that 17 of 20 people with VV had a peripheral vestibular disorder (Guerraz et al., 2001). However, not all people with vestibular dysfunction experience motion sickness or VV.

The most widely accepted explanation for motion sensitivity is based on the notion of sensory conflict (Money, 1970; Reason, 1970; Reason & Brand, 1975; Yardley, 1992). This hypothesis postulates that each person has an internal representation of body movement that is continually updated by visual, vestibular, and proprioceptive (muscles, tendon, and joint mechanoreceptor) inputs. Repeated and sustained mismatches from these sensory systems may cause conflict in the expected internal model. An example of movement-induced conflict is when your visual system tells you that you are sitting still in the hull of a boat, while your vestibular system simultaneously tells you that the boat is bobbing up and down. An example of visual-stimuli conflict is when you are sitting still at the movie theater but the movie screen visually indicates that you are flying in a plane. The visual stimuli may cause nystagmus (Bronstein, 2005) or the conflict in sensory inputs may cause motion-sickness symptoms. The precise pathophysiology is unclear but may involve inappropriate central integration of vestibular–visual–proprioceptive inputs in the cerebellum or the brainstem's velocity storage system (Linàs et al., 1975; Hoffer et al., 2003).

An extension of this hypothesis is that symptoms result from abnormal weighting of sensory inputs (vestibular–visual–proprioceptive) related to spatial orientation. Some healthy adults rely more on vision (visual-field dependence), whereas others depend more heavily on vestibulo-proprioceptive cues. Posturography data suggest that patients with VV are overly visually dependent when maintaining balance, although not all patients with imbalance have VV (Guerraz et al., 2001; Pavlou et al., 2006). This understanding may be important for rehabilitation because a person's preferred sensory weighting can be trained in such a way as to reduce symptoms. Thus patients can learn to be less visually dependent, which can in turn reduce their VV symptoms (Acerra, unpublished data).

Mal de débarquement (MdD) syndrome may occur as the result of similar mechanisms. MdD is characterized by the perception of motion, such as swaying, when the individual is motionless, with this sensation occurring at least 3 days after prolonged exposure to motion such as via open-ocean travel (Cha, 2009). It has been thought that MdD patients have reduced reliance on vestibular–visual inputs and an increased dependence on somatosensory input to maintain balance (Nachum et al., 2004). Thus rehabilitation that changes this sensory weighting can improve balance and reduce the internal feeling of postural sway.

It is not clear why children are more sensitive to sensory conflict than adults, or why some adults are more sensitive to motion/visual stimuli than others. It is also unclear why migraineurs more frequently develop motion sensitivity than non-migraineurs. This difference may reflect migraine-related changes in the noradrenergic system causing increased sensitivity to sensory stimuli (Vingen et al., 1988; Main et al., 1997; Tusa, 2007). Thus patients with motion sensitivity may represent a heterogeneous population in terms of their disorder. A better understanding of the pathophysiology underlying sensitivity to motion and visual stimuli is imperative, as it could provide important insight into prevention and management of motion sensitivity.

Management

Treatment of motion sensitivity is often multimodal and may include pharmacological, rehabilitation, or behavioral interventions (**Table 22.3**). The optimal management plan is customized based on a thorough clinical examination (as discussed in the next section).

Table 22.3 Overview of Motion Sensitivity Management

Walking Program

- When able, patients should walk 20 minutes or more daily outside or on uneven surfaces.
- Be aware that treadmills may worsen symptoms because the patient *feels* as if he or she is running forward but his or her vision *sees* that the individual is running in place. This causes a "conflict" within the balance centers.

Medications

- The physician may provide medications to prevent or treat motion sickness.

Rehabilitation

- The physiotherapist may provide specific exercises for motion sickness, visual blurring, vertigo, or dizziness.
- The patient may be provided with balance exercises and eye (vision) exercises.

Stress Reduction

- Consider ways to reduce stress and ensure that the patient gets adequate sleep daily. Patients should try to not oversleep.
- Be aware that stress may temporarily worsen symptoms.
- The physiotherapist may provide stress-reduction exercises or specific tasks to perform when a patient has symptoms.

Managing Triggers

- The clinician and patient should discuss specific strategies to manage the situations that trigger symptoms. Avoidance is not always the best answer; patients may be able to tolerate their triggers with practice and new strategies.

VESTIBULAR ASSESSMENT AND REHABILITATION

Vestibular rehabilitation (VR) describes the constellation of interventions available to rehabilitation specialists to assist in the prevention, treatment, and management of vestibular disorders. An overview of interventions is provided here, though it should be noted that these options are not prescriptive to any individual. Clinicians with advanced training and expertise can provide a customized program for any vestibular dysfunction or motion sensitivity related to VM.

Each component of the assessment (history, physical examination, and medical investigations) is important for diagnosis and treatment. The importance of the history cannot be overstated. Vestibular function tests are indirect, as there are no gold-standard tests for diagnosis. Even if definitive tests were available, a history would still be necessary, as symptoms, symptom intensity, and functional goals vary and are incorporated into the rehabilitation program. A complete review of assessment and management is beyond the scope of this chapter but can be found in other sources (Davies, 2004; Hansson, 2007; Herdman, 2007).

Taking a Vestibular History

A time-consuming and challenging aspect of VR is taking a complete and accurate history. This effort is worth the investment, however, as the average vestibular patient sees 4.5 health-care professionals prior to the definitive diagnosis being made and 69% of clinicians report that diagnosis requires important information from the history (Polensek et al., 2008). Patients can be vague in reporting symptoms and do not conveniently report that they have a "VOR deficit"; instead, they complain of dizziness and blurred vision with specific activities. Moreover, each person has his or her own definition of "dizziness." Careful probing can elucidate the specific symptom and necessary details to inform a diagnosis and management plan.

Vestibular dysfunction can cause a wide range of symptoms, and many patients will have had symptoms for years. Furthermore, many patients have different symptoms during an acute event, such as a migraine, than in day-to-day life. For each symptom, the clinician should determine its onset, intensity, tempo, and aggravating and easing factors, as well as any changes in the symptom from its onset to the present day. Note the impact that stress has on symptoms. Consider all relevant orthopaedic, neurologic, and cardiovascular issues, especially after trauma. Also, consider past medical history, comorbidities, family supports, work responsibilities, pastimes, and driving ability.

Notably, vertigo (illusion of spinning or tilt), dizziness (giddiness), light-headedness (faintness), and disorientation are widely reported symptoms. The most common visual symptom is oscillopsia, often described as blurred vision with head movement, reading, or walking. Autonomic symptoms can include nausea, vomiting, sweating, and panic. Fluctuations or changes in hearing and tinnitus can occur in the high- or low-pitch range. Note headaches, migraines (with/without aura), and temporomandibular (TMJ), neck, and back symptoms. Balance impairments may include dysequilibrium, near-falls, and falls with specific activities. Note the impact of being in the dark, changes in body or head position such as rolling in bed, and walking on uneven surfaces or stairs. Other questions may focus on somatosensory changes, facial symptoms, fainting, ear fullness, or ear pain.

Prior to attempting neck mobilization or manipulation, clinicians should ask questions designed to ferret out possible vestibular–basilar artery insufficiency, including diplopia, dysarthria, dysphagia, and drop attacks (Terrett, 2001). Also note the impact of anxiety, panic, and depression. Motion sensitivity assessment is discussed later in this chapter.

Especially challenging is determining which pieces of the history are important and which are not relevant to the current diagnosis. For example, many patients have a history of middle ear infections as a child, which is infrequently related to the current diagnosis.

Questionnaires for Vestibular Symptoms

Symptoms, impairments, and disabilities can be quantified with outcome measures such as a visual or numeric rating scale (VAS or NRS) for a specific symptom (Katz & Melzack, 1999), the Dizziness Handicap Inventory (DHI; Jacobson & Newman, 1990), or the Activities Specific Balance Scale (ABC; Powell & Myers, 1995). Functional recovery can be assessed with the Vestibular Rehabilitation Benefit Questionnaire (VRBQ; Morris et al., 2009). Motion sensitivity assessment instruments are discussed later in this chapter.

Vestibular Clinical Examination

Clinical tests of vestibular function include tests of peripheral vestibular nerve function, otoconia in the semicircular canals (for BPPV), central vestibular function, motion sensitivity, and balance/gait impairments (**Table 22.4** and **Table 22.5**). The testing order may vary based on the

Table 22.4 Clinical Tests of Vestibular Function

Test	Peripheral Test	Central Test
Spontaneous nystagmus	√ (acute)*	√
Ocular alignment (phoria, trophia, skew)	√ (acute)*	√
Extraocular movements		√
Vergence and convergence		√
Conjoint eye movement		√
Smooth pursuit		√
Gaze-evoked nystagmus	√ (acute)*	√
Saccadic eye movements		√
VOR to slow head movements		√
VOR-cancellation		√
Ocular tilt reaction (OTR) and skew deviation	√ (acute)*	√
Optokinetic nystagmus		√
Positional nystagmus	√ (under Frenzel)	√
Head-shaking test (20-plus times, speed > 2 Hz)	√ (under Frenzel)	√
Head-thrust test (HTT)	√	
Dynamic visual acuity (DVA) test	√	
Dix-Hallpike and supine roll tests	√ (for BPPV only)	

VOR, vestibular-ocular reflex.
*Can be seen in the acute phase, but is uncommon in the chronic phase.

patient's specific presentation or irritability with movement. Tests may include vertebrobasilar artery screening and assessment for cervicogenic dizziness. Tests are described with treatment of each dysfunction later in this section.

Vestibular Function Tests and Medical Investigations

A review of vestibular function test interpretation is beyond the scope of this chapter, but discussions of this topic can be found elsewhere (Baloh & Halmagyi, 1996; Herdman, 2007). **Table 22.6** highlights commonly performed tests that may provide some insight into vestibular dysfunction. Importantly, no single test confirms or rules out any particular vestibular diagnosis, and these tests cannot provide a diagnosis in isolation. No standardized tests are available for higher-order sensory integration, motion intolerance, or autonomic response to vestibular or visual stimuli. Medical imaging, such as MRI, is usually negative. Thus clinicians must consider the overall picture, including the history and clinical findings, to determine a diagnosis (**Figure 22.1**).

Differential Diagnosis

The differential diagnosis of vestibular migraine is challenging, as it requires integrating a great deal of information, some of which may not be relevant to the current diagnosis (Figure 22.1). The history is the most powerful tool to determine a differential diagnosis; the combination of specific symptoms often suggests the most likely diagnosis.

Table 22.5 Commonly Used Balance and Gait Tests

Balance Reactions	Gait Tests
Static, eyes open/closed	Walk in straight line, eyes open/closed
Response to perturbations	Tandem walk, eyes open/closed
Response to retropulsion	Walk with head movement (horizontal/vertical)
	Timed up and go (TUG), self-paced
Static and Dynamic Balance	TUG, as fast as you can
	TUG, with physical or cognitive task
Romberg, eyes open/closed	Speed up/slow down while walking
Sharpened Romberg, eyes open/closed	Walk while talk test
Single-leg stance, eyes open/closed	Walk on toes/heels
Modified clinical test of sensory organization and balance (CTSIB)	Walk backward, eyes open/closed
Limit of stability (anterior–posterior; medial–lateral)	Side-stepping; braided walking
Ankle–knee–hip strategy	Ability to negotiate obstacles, steps or stairs
Functional reach	Endurance (6-minute walk test)
Fukuda step test	

Table 22.6 Vestibular Function Tests and Medical Investigations

Test Name	Brief Description	What It Tests
Caloric testing	Warm and cold water irrigation (various protocols may be used).	HC and PVN (superior division). May indicate side of lesion.
Electronystagmogram (ENG)	Tests can vary, including smooth pursuit, saccades, and nystagmus. Can also test for positional nystagmus.	Central vestibular function. Nystagmus with position changes (e.g., side-lying and Dix-Hallpike maneuver).
Rotary chair	Seated in a fixed chair in the dark, the patient is rotated and nystagmus is measured.	HC and PVN (superior division). Does not indicate side of lesion.
Computerized dynamic visual acuity (cDVA)	Quantifies clinical DVA findings.	HC and PVN (superior division).
Subjective visual vertical (SVV)	Tests the patient's ability to orient a vertical line in the dark.	Utricular function or PVN (inferior division).
Vestibular evoked myogenic potential (VEMP)	Tests sternocleidomastoid (SCM) response to a loud click (60 to 94 dB).	Saccular function or PVN (superior division).
Electrocochleaography (ECOG)	Electrode in eardrum or ear canal may indicate inner ear pressure.	May suggest presence of hydrops or Ménière's disease.
Pure tone audiograms	High- and low-frequency hearing test.	Indicates any pure tone hearing loss in right and left ears.
Computerized dynamic posturography (CDP)	Tests standing balance reactions to changes in visual, somatosensory, and vestibular inputs.	Indirect insight into vestibular spinal reflex (VSR) function and contributions of various systems.
Medical imaging	Numerous tests and protocols exist for use with CT and MRI (e.g., gadolinium-enhanced MRI).	Provides structural information on brain regions; type depends on test and protocol used.

HC, horizontal canal; PVN, peripheral vestibular nerve; DVA, dynamic visual acuity; CT, computerized tomography; MRI, magnetic resonance imaging.

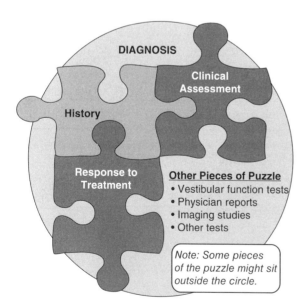

Figure 22.1 Vestibular Differential Diagnosis is Determined Based on the History, Clinical Examination, Vestibular Function Tests, and Response to Treatment. Some information may not be relevant to the current diagnosis and some patients have coexisting conditions, such as motion sensitivity.

In addition, some coexisting vestibular disorders such as Ménière's disease (MD), multiple sclerosis, and BPPV are more common in migraineurs (Kayan & Hood, 1984; von Brevern et al., 2007). Neuhauser and Lempert (2009) reviewed in detail the high frequency and potential links between VM and other vestibular disorders, including Ménière's disease, BPPV, motion sickness, cerebellar dysfunction, and nonvestibular dizziness such as panic/anxiety. Differentiating early MD, migraine, and BPPV can be challenging because of the similarity in symptoms (**Table 22.7**) (Shepard, 2006; Tusa, 2007). Thus migraineurs may present in the clinic with VM, vestibular dysfunction, motion sensitivity, or any combination of these conditions.

Vestibular Disorders Assessment and Management

Vertigo and dysequilibrium caused by migraines respond similarly to other vestibular disorders (Tusa, 2007). Medical management of VM is similar to migraine and can be divided into prophylactic and abortive medical

Table 22.7 Symptom Comparison

Test	Migraine	Ménière's Disease	BPPV
Spontaneous nystagmus	Rare; can occur in an acute event (lasting seconds to hours)	Common with acute events (usually lasts hours)	Rare
Vertigo and positional nystagmus	Can occur with acute events or in the symptom-free period	Can occur with acute events or due to UVL damage	Yes, in specific positions
Tinnitus	High-pitched	Low-pitched, roar	Uncommon
Ear fullness	Can occur	Common	Uncommon
Phonophobia and photophobia	Common	Uncommon	Uncommon
Visual auras	Common	Uncommon	Uncommon
Short naps	Usually help symptoms	Do not usually help	Do not help
Motion sickness	Common	Uncommon	Uncommon

BPPV, benign paroxysmal positional vertigo; UVL, unilateral vestibular loss.

therapy as reviewed in previous chapters (for a review, see Neuhauser & Lempert, 2009). In addition to preventive measures, VR can be segmented into interventions to treat peripheral vestibular dysfunction, central vestibular dysfunction, and motion sensitivity (see the overview of VR in **Table 22.8**).

Migraine Prevention

Prevention of migraines may improve migraine incidence or associated symptoms such as motion sensitivity, vertigo, and dizziness (Table 22.2). The focus for the patient and clinician is to identify triggers and determine

Table 22.8 Overview of Vestibular Rehabilitation for Vestibular Migraine and Motion Sensitivity

Vestibular Disorder	Clinical Tests	Potential Treatments
Benign paroxysmal positional vertigo (BPPV)	Dix-Hallpike test Supine roll test	Canalith-repositioning technique, such as the Epley maneuver.
Peripheral dysfunction (unilateral vestibular loss)	Head thrust test Dynamic visual acuity test Balance/gait assessment	Adaptation exercises; may also include habituation, substitution, balance/gait, and motion exercises.
Peripheral dysfunction (bilateral vestibular loss)	Head thrust test Dynamic visual acuity test Balance/gait assessment	Adaptation, habituation, and substitution, exercises. Balance and gait retraining. May need motion exercises.
Central vestibular dysfunction	Central vestibular tests Balance/gait assessment	Adaptation, habituation, substitution, balance/gait, and motion sensitivity exercises.
Motion sensitivity to body movement and visual stimuli	All peripheral and central tests Balance/gait assessment Tests for motion sensitivity (MST) and visual stimuli	Rehabilitation for motions and visual stimuli that cause symptoms. Treatment of any peripheral or central vestibular dysfunction. May need balance/gait retraining.
Vestibular migraine (VM)	All peripheral, central, and motion sensitivity tests	Treat based on assessment findings (may include peripheral, central, and/or motion sensitivity). Trigger prevention. Walking/exercise program.
Balance/gait impairments	Notice impact on balance with peripheral, central, and motion sensitivity tests	Balance and gait retraining program based on assessment findings.

MST, motion sensitivity test.

strategies to reduce exposure to these stimuli. Subjects respond differently to triggers, of course, and it can take months or years to determine the optimal plan for an individual patient. Maintaining a careful diary of potential triggers that occurred in the 24 hours prior to the migraine can facilitate this process (Tusa, 2007; Salhofer et al., 2010). Common triggers discussed here include stress, aerobic activity, dietary habits, and exposure to nicotine and estrogen. In addition, some evidence suggests that certain environmental factors, such as strong smells, changes in air temperature, gasoline, and cleaning products, can trigger migraines (Fukui et al., 2008).

Stress and Deconditioning   Patients frequently notice their symptoms are more intense when they are under "stress." Examples include increased dizziness when stressed at work or increased motion sickness with tiring long-distance travel. "Stress" can take many forms, including fatigue, emotional stress, and immunological stress such as a common cold. Fukui et al. (2008) reported that 64% of migraineurs' attacks were triggered by emotional stress. Patients often feel more in control of their symptoms when they understand the potential effects of stress and the difference between increased perception of symptoms due to stress versus the development of a "new event" such as an acute migraine. This understanding can reduce overall stress and symptoms. Thus a stress-management plan is essential for migraineurs.

Stress reduction can take many forms, including yoga, tai chi, meditation, biofeedback, and relaxation programs (Holroyd & Penzien, 1990; Sándor & Afra, 2005). Some patients may benefit from a settling or structured-rest exercise (**Table 22.9**). In fact, adequate restorative sleep is strongly recommended (Tusa, 2007). Oversleep

and changes in sleeping time can also trigger migraines, however (Fukui et al., 2008).

Aerobic exercise is an excellent vehicle to reduce stress, improve immune function, and improve deconditioning. Aerobic exercises can alleviate depression and may play a role in migraine prevention (Koseoglu et al., 2003). This intervention may be especially important in migraineurs who avoid movement due to motion sensitivity. Aerobic exercise can provide a fun way to integrate vestibular exercises into daily life. Patients gradually increase physical activity until they can sustain 60% to 80% of the maximum heart rate for at least 30 minutes, three to five times per week (Canada Pulmonary Hypertension Association, 2010). Consideration is given to selecting appropriate activities based on the patient's symptoms and goals. Most patients start with a walking program with an emphasis on walking or hiking on uneven surfaces. Running, swimming, tennis, skiing, and cycling are much more challenging activities, as they require repetitive movements and quick head turns. Treadmill running is often challenging for people with motion sensitivity, likely due to the sensory conflict that results from running in place. Activities can be modified as necessary with changes in cardiovascular fitness and vestibular symptoms.

Diet and Dietary Habits   Patients are encouraged to eat meals at regular times daily and to avoid hypoglycemia by eating something at least every 6 to 8 hours (Tusa, 2007; Fukui et al., 2008). Many foods have been posited to cause migraine, such as cheese, chocolate, sausage, salami, monosodium glutamate (MSG), milk, alcohol, red and white wine, coffee, soft drinks, citrus fruits, ice cream, and nuts (Tusa, 2007). Patients are recommended to follow a migraine diet that calls for eliminating or minimizing tyramine and other substrates known to exacerbate migraine (Shulman et al., 1989). Some foods may immediately trigger a migraine (e.g., red wine, MSG), whereas others may instigate a migraine on the following day after their consumption (e.g., chocolate, nuts, cheeses) (Tusa, 2007). Some food additives such as sucralose (Splenda) or aspartame have also been shown to provoke migraine (van Den Eeden et al., 1994; Patel et al., 2006). Recently, Alpay et al. (2010) reported a randomized trial in which a customized diet that restricted IgG antibodies foods reduced migraine frequency. For each person, 266 dietary items were tested; items producing high levels of IgG antibodies were then eliminated from the patient's diet (Alpay et al., 2010). A low-fat diet may also reduce headache frequency (Bic et al., 1999). Readers are referred to

Table 22.9 Structured Rest/Settling Exercise

This exercise is intended to reduce or settle symptoms. Patients are given the following instructions:
- Lie comfortably on your back (or sit in a firm, comfortable chair with your arms and legs supported and your head resting against the wall). It is important that you are comfortable and not distracted. Close your eyes and attend to your surroundings, noticing the surface you are lying/sitting on. Slowly count backward from 50 to 0. Afterward, continue to rest or gradually return to your previous activities.
- Repeat this exercise if your dizziness or nausea reaches an intensity that interferes with your daily activities.
- Discuss with your physiotherapist any triggers that you believe caused you to need this exercise and describe how you use this exercise to settle your symptoms.

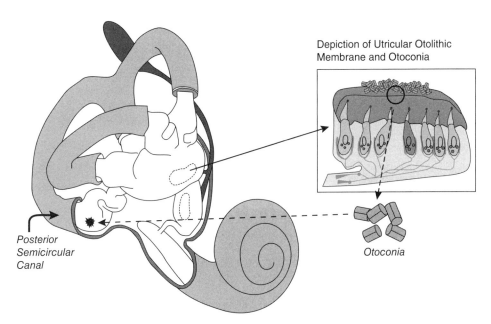

Figure 22.2 Normally, Head Movement Moves the Endolymph Within the Semicircular Canals that in Turn Deflects the Cupula. Displacement of the cupula stimulates the vestibular-ocular reflex (VOR) that controls eye movement. Normally otoconia (calcium-carbonate crystals) reside on the gravity-sensitive gelatinous membrane in the maculae (utricle and saccule). If the otoconia migrates into a semicircular canal they can cause an excitation of that canal with specific head movements, such as looking up/ down or rolling in bed. This excitation causes vertigo and associated nystagmus (direction depends on the affected canal and type of BPPV). This picture depicts otoconia resting in the posterior semicircular canal within the vestibular labyrinth.

Chapters 29 and 30 of the current textbook for more information on nutritional aspects of migraine care.

Nicotine and Estrogen Like all individuals, patients with migraine are encouraged to quit smoking or chewing tobacco (Tusa, 2007; Fukui et al., 2008). The effect of nicotine patches or gums on migraine is not well understood.

Migraine incidence varies with menstruation in more than 50% of women, with most women reporting migraines in the premenstrual period (Fukui et al., 2008). When appropriate, patients are encouraged to avoid or reduce use of exogenous estrogens, such as oral contraceptives and estrogen replacement therapy (Tusa, 2007).

Benign Paroxysmal Positional Vertigo

BPPV is the most common peripheral vestibular dysfunction, with a lifetime incidence of 2.4% (von Brevern et al., 2007). It is unknown why BPPV occurs more commonly in migraineurs (Ishiyama et al., 2000).

Figure 22.2 provides an overview of BPPV pathophysiology. In brief, the calcium particles (otoconia) that normally weigh down the otolithic membrane become dislodged, with the sediment collecting in one or more of the three semicircular canals, thereby changing the fluid dynamics inside the canals. When the otoconia is free-floating, the condition is known as canalithiasis; if the particles become bound to the cupula, it is called cupulolithiasis. In both forms of BPPV, the otoconia disrupts the normal fluid dynamics within the canal, causing characteristic symptoms such as brief (less than 2 minutes) bouts of vertigo often associated with mild nausea, dysequilibrium, and light-headedness.

The Dix-Hallpike (DH) test can identify BPPV in both the anterior (AC) and posterior (PC) semicircular canals (**Figure 22.3**) (Dix & Hallpike, 1952). Prior to testing, clinicians should test the vertebrobasilar artery (Magarey et al., 2004) and ensure that patients do not have any contraindications (Humphriss et al., 2003). For the DH maneuver, the patient is placed in a long-sitting position; the examiner then turns the patient's head 30–45° to one side and lays the person down so that the head is 20–30° below the horizon, either by using pillows or by placing the patient's head over the edge of the bed. A latent response of torsional nystagmus associated with vertigo lasting less than 2 minutes is considered a positive response. The direction of nystagmus indicates the canal. Nevertheless, test interpretation is not always straightforward and some patients cannot tolerate the

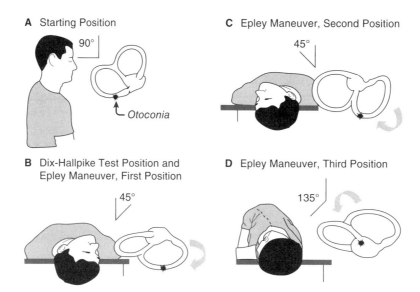

Figure 22.3 The Dix-Hallpike (Dh) Test Assesses for Posterior Canal BPPV (A–B). If detected, BPPV is commonly treated with a series of head movements that slowly moves the crystals back into the utricle, often referred to as canalith-repositioning techniques (CRT). The Epley maneuver is a common CRT (depicted in A–D). Positions B–D are maintained for 1–2 minutes to allow the otoconia adequate time to move within the canal. Modifications to the Epley and other maneuvers are available to treat various forms of BPPV.

testing process (Humphriss et al., 2003). Most commonly, otoconia consists of free-floating particles (80% of time) that settle in the PC (85% to 95% of cases) (Parnes et al., 2003).

The supine roll test identifies horizontal canal (HC) BPPV (Nuti et al., 1998). In this test, with the patient supine and the neck flexed 20–30°, the examiner quickly rotates the patient's head 90°, notes the direction of nystagmus, and compares the right and left responses to determine the affected side. Further information on this test and its alternatives, such as the side-lying test, is available elsewhere (Herdman, 2007; Bhattacharyya et al., 2008; Fife et al., 2008).

Treatment of BPPV most commonly involves a series of head movements that slowly moves the crystals back into the utricle, often referred to as canalith-repositioning techniques (CRT). Several CRT maneuvers have been developed; the clinician must distinguish the type of BPPV and the affected canal to determine the appropriate CRT. A recent systematic review reported that the best diagnostic test for PC canalithiasis is the DH test and the best treatment is the modified Epley maneuver, as shown in Figure 22.3, part D (Epley, 1992; Bhattacharyya et al., 2008). Another systematic review reported that the Epley maneuver is a safe and effective treatment for BPPV (Hilton & Pinder, 2002). One study reported reduced symptoms in 89% of patients after a single session and a resolution of symptoms in 95% of people

after three treatments (Del Rio & Arriaga, 2004). The Epley maneuver can also be provided as a home treatment should BPPV reoccur (Bhattacharyya et al., 2008). Clinical practice guidelines, textbooks, and journal articles provide detailed explanations of BPPV assessment and treatment (Herdman, 2007; Bhattacharyya et al., 2008; Fife et al., 2008).

BPPV is more common with migraine, but the precise relationship between the two entities and the pathophysiology underlying BPPV remain unknown (Neuhauser et al., 2001). One study reported that 34% of BPPV patients had migraine (von Brevern et al., 2007). These patients are also at a greater risk for falls and BPPV recurrence (Uneri, 2004). BPPV is more common with peripheral vestibular dysfunction, which has been reported in VM patients but not in non-dizzy migraine patients. Further research is needed to elucidate this relationship.

Peripheral Vestibular Dysfunction

Unilateral vestibular loss (UVL) refers to one-sided peripheral vestibular nerve dysfunction, whereas bilateral vestibular loss (BVL) refers to two-sided loss. Diagnosis of these conditions is based on history, clinical tests, and vestibular function tests such as calorics. Approximately 15% to 20% of VM patients have peripheral vestibular dysfunction, possibly due to their migraines or to a coexisting vestibular disorder such as Ménière's disease.

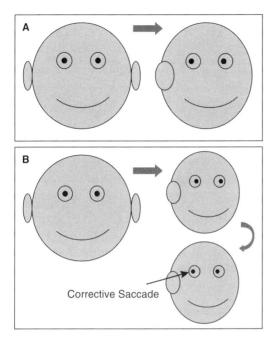

Figure 22.4 Head Thrust Test (HTT). (A) A negative HTT is when the patient flawlessly maintains visual fixation on the examiner's nose. (B) A positive HTT is when the patient looks to the side of the examiner with the head-thrust and needs to make a voluntary rapid eye movement (i.e. corrective saccade) back to the examiners' nose.

UVL and BVL can be identified with two clinical tests: the head thrust test (HTT) or head impulse test (HIT) (Halmagyi & Curthoys, 1988) and the dynamic visual acuity (DVA) test (Demer et al., 1994). The HTT is a direction-specific assessment that can test all six semicircular canals individually (**Figure 22.4**, part A). Neck range of motion is evaluated prior to testing. During the HTT, the examiner sits in front of the patient and asks the patient to keep the neck relaxed and look at the examiner's nose. For the horizontal canal (HC), the examiner orients the canal to the horizon by flexing the patient's neck forward 15–20°, then slowly turns the patient's head right and left at a speed of less than 2 Hz (this portion is a central test). The examiner then imposes a very quick and unpredictable head thrust 20–30° in one direction and observes whether the patient maintained visual fixation on the examiner's nose, which tests that canal's VOR.

In a negative HTT, the patient flawlessly maintains visual fixation. In a positive test, that canal's VOR provides insufficient feedback to the eyes, which in turn results in the eyes moving with the head; therefore the patient looks to the side of the examiner and needs to make a voluntary rapid eye movement (i.e., corrective saccade) back to the examiner's nose. Therefore,

a left UVL involving the HC would have a negative head thrust to the patient's right and a positive head thrust to the patient's left (Figure 22.4, part B). With repetition, patients can "learn" to compensate for their VOR loss, so the HTT must be unpredictable and identified quickly. During testing, the examiner must ensure that the patient does not blink. Experienced clinicians can also test the posterior and anterior canals.

The DVA can quantify oscillopsia with head movement (Demer et al., 1994; Schubert et al., 2002). In this test, the patient is seated and reads a visual-acuity chart such as the Snellen or Eligible-E instrument. The patient then rereads the chart with smooth and consistent head motion at a speed of at least 2 Hz (two rotations per second). A difference of one or two lines is considered normal, but a variation by three or more lines is indicative of impaired visual acuity with head movement. The DVA test is reliable for both horizontal and vertical testing (Schubert et al., 2002).

VR for UVL and BVL includes habituation, adaptation, and substitution exercises (Herdman et al., 2003, 2007). Moderate to strong evidence suggests that VR is safe and effective (Hillier & Hollohan, 2008). The rationale, indications, and examples for various exercises are outlined in **Table 22.10**. Physical activity, motion sensitivity, cervicogenic dizziness, and balance/gait retraining can also be addressed as part of VR (Hansson, 2007; Herdman, 2007). Exercises are progressed in intensity and complexity over 6 to 8 weeks.

For example, gaze-stabilization exercises are designed to improve oscillopsia with head movement. The patient may be provided with a fixed target, such as an "X" on a business card, and taught to maintain visual acuity with head movement. The direction, duration, and progression of the exercise will vary based on the individual, but will likely involve progression to standing, walking, and functional tasks (Hansson, 2007).

VR exercises are safe and effective when delivered as a home-based program and progressed by the physical therapist (Yardley et al., 1998). Some evidence indicates that adaptation (e.g., gaze stabilization) and habituation (e.g., repetitive movements) may be equally beneficial in reducing symptoms (Clendaniel, 2010). Further information on treatment plans for UVL and BVL is available in other sources (Hansson, 2007; Herdman, 2007).

Central Vestibular Dysfunction

Central vestibular loss (CVL) refers to any disruption of vestibular function within the central nervous system. The heterogeneous patient population affected by CVL

Table 22.10 Adaptation, Habituation, and Substitution Exercises

Exercise	Brief Description
Adaptation	Theory: Refers to long-term changes in vestibular response to input (i.e., plasticity). Indications: Predominantly used to change (increase/decrease) VOR gain, which commonly occurs with peripheral vestibular loss (i.e., positive HTT and DVA tests). Example: Gaze stabilization exercises, where the person is seated and moves the head back and forth while trying to maintain focus on a visual target such as an "X" (improves oscillopsia with practice). Can be performed right/left, up/down, or on a diagonal. Can be progressed to include standing, walking, and functional tasks. Other progressions include changing target size or adding target movement or a background.
Habituation	Theory: Repeated exposure to a provocative stimulus reduces pathological symptoms. Indications: Motion sensitivity, peripheral vestibular loss, central vestibular loss. Example: When using the MST, choose up to four movements that cause mild-to-moderate symptoms. Practice the movement 2 to 10 times, twice per day. It is important to let symptoms settle between repetitions; all symptoms should cease within 30 minutes of each practice session. Treatment normally takes 2 to 4 months, but symptoms should improve within approximately 4 weeks. Exercises should be progressed and include functional tasks.
Substitution	Theory: Mechanisms other than adaptation promote recovery or function. Indications: Includes visual/somatosensory cues and central loss. Example: Alterations in somatosensory cues (such as standing on foam) or visual cues (such as eye–head movement strategies or target practice with eyes open and then eyes closed to promote proprioception). Exercise progression varies based on the goals.

VOR, vestibular-ocular reflex; HTT, head thrust test; DVA, dynamic visual acuity test; MST, motion sensitivity test.

includes individuals with strokes, cerebellar degeneration, multiple sclerosis, and migraine (Karatas, 2008). Many clinical tests for central vestibular function have been developed, including those highlighted in Table 22.6. Test interpretation is beyond the scope of this chapter, in particular because some central tests also test peripherally function in the acute phase (Davies, 2004; Herdman, 2007). For example, spontaneous nystagmus may occur with an acute labyrinthitis or any cerebellar or brainstem disorder (Bronstein, 2005). With experience and training, clinicians can use these tests to inform their diagnosis and management plans.

VR for CVL may include habituation, adaptation, substitution exercises, motion sensitivity, and balance/gait exercises, as shown in Table 22.10 (Herdman, 2007). Rehabilitation can be effective for CVL (Brown et al., 2006), and some data suggest that migraineurs specifically improve with VR. One study reported improved symptoms and outcome measures for VM and migraine patients who did a home-based VR program over 4 months, with a mean of 4.9 physical therapy visits required to progress exercises (Whitney et al., 2000). Another study reported similar results in migraineurs with vestibular symptoms over a mean of 3.3 months, with a mean of 4.1 physiotherapy appointments required (Wrisley et al., 2002). Exercise frequency, intensity,

duration, and complexity are progressed over a 3- to 6-month program based on the patient's presentation and goals. In addition, postural instability, falls risk, and eye–head coordination are addressed. Motion sensitivity is common in affected patients; VR to mitigate this condition is described later in this chapter.

Balance, Gait, and Functional Impairments

A complete review of balance and gait impairments is beyond the scope of this chapter. However, balance and gait disturbances are important dysfunctions to be considered, as 95% of patients with an acute VM present with imbalance (von Brevern et al., 2005). Prior to testing balance- and gait-related functional abilities, the clinician should consider the patient's available joint range of motion, muscle tone and strength, postural control, and motor control.

The line between "static" and "dynamic" balance is somewhat blurry, as individuals are usually in motion and people perpetually "lose" and "regain" their balance as they move through space (e.g., in the transition from sitting to standing). However, formal tests can be (somewhat artificially) subdivided into tests for balance reactions, static balance tests, dynamic tests, gait tests, and functional outcomes. Table 22.5 identifies many commonly used tests, including composite measures such as the Dynamic Gait Index, which is particularly helpful for dizzy patients (Teggi et al., 2008).

When evaluating the impact of vestibular loss on balance/gait, emphasis is placed on tests that incorporate head movement, body movement, and eyes closed. The influence of vision and visual intrusion on balance and motion sensitivity should be considered as well. Rehabilitation of these impairments varies and is based on assessment findings (Herdman, 2007).

MOTION SENSITIVITY ASSESSMENT

No clear diagnostic criteria or biologic markers are available to define sensitivity to motion or visual stimuli. Instead, motion sensitivity is a clinical diagnosis based on the history and clinical findings.

History

When taking a history, the clinician should determine the specific circumstances that cause symptoms. It is often helpful to provide several examples to determine whether symptoms are related to body movement, visual-field movement, or both. Note sensitivity to motion (e.g., car/boat/ferry/air travel, repetitive movements), body movement (e.g., speeding up/down when walking or in a car, elevators), and visual stimuli (e.g., watching action movies, supermarket aisles, crowds, cars moving at an intersection, virtual-reality environments). Some examples are difficult to interpret; for example, if supermarkets cause symptoms, the clinician should determine whether it is the visual "busyness" of the environment or the frequent head turns performed that causes symptoms.

For each trigger, the examiner should identify whether symptoms are predominantly gastrointestinal (nausea, vomiting), somatic (dizziness, weakness, fatigue), objective (body temperature, skin humidity, heart rate), or emotional (anxiety, fear, anger) in nature. Irritability and sensitivity are important for developing a rehabilitation program and are useful objective outcomes. Note the length of exposure time prior to symptom onset, the intensity of each symptom (on a numeric rating scale or a visual analogue scale), and the duration of symptoms prior to returning to baseline. For numeric scales, 0 means no symptom and 10 means the worst possible intensity of the given symptom (Katz & Melzack, 1999). Also, consider the impact of symptoms on function; for example, light-rail transit may cause fewer symptoms than travel on a bus that stops and starts or changes lanes frequently and unpredictably.

Several questionnaires are available to quantify motion-related symptoms, including the Motion Sickness Questionnaire (MSQ), the Simulator Sickness Questionnaire (SSQ), and the Vertigo Symptom Scale (VSS) (Yardley et al., 1992; Kennedy et al., 1993; Gianaros et al., 2001). Other questionnaires used for dizziness may be appropriate as well.

Clinical Tests

Objective clinical testing of motion sensitivity is challenging. Sensitivity to motion can sometimes be detected on peripheral and central vestibular testing; often, however, such tests are normal but the patient complains of symptoms such as nausea with visually demanding tasks. Studies have reported mild deficits in DVA testing (horizontal and vertical) or with functional tasks such as walking on a floating dock or scuba diving (Rine et al., 1999). Balance and gait should also be assessed. A VR program can be prescribed to remedy vestibular deficits.

A valid and reliable tool to quantify motion-provoked dizziness is the Motion Sensitivity Test (MST) (Akin & Davenport, 2003). The MST is an excellent tool that calculates the intensity and duration of symptoms evoked for 16 body movements and combines the results into a quotient (abbreviated MSQ). Many patients also have symptoms in positions other than those provided on the MST. Anecdotally, other body movements can be tested with the MST approach. Similarly, visual stimuli that cause symptoms can be tested in the clinic and rated on a 0–10 scale or through the questionnaires mentioned earlier. Identification of these triggers (motion and visually induced) is important to developing an appropriate treatment plan.

Managing Motion Sensitivity

Treatment of motion sensitivity is often multimodal (Table 22.3). Unfortunately, high-quality evidence to guide clinicians in customizing a management plan is lacking. Optimal management may include pharmacological, rehabilitation, or behavioral interventions that will vary based on the person's initial presentation, symptoms, and goals.

Pharmacological Agents

New classes of drugs are currently being studied to improve symptomatic relief (Golding & Gresty, 2005; Spinks et al., 2007; Furman et al., 2011). A wide variety of drugs may provide some symptomatic relief, such as antiemetics, antimuscarinics, H$_1$ antihistamines, and antianxiety medications. Some drugs are effective alone, whereas others might work in combination, such as scopolamine plus dexamphetamine (Golding & Gresty, 2005). Unfortunately, many drugs do not relieve motion sensitivity and, anecdotally, others slow rehabilitation, such as the vestibular system suppressants prochlorperazine (Stemetil) and valium (Diazepam). Ginger may reduce gastrointestinal symptoms (Grontved et al., 1988). Drugs that accelerate plasticity, such as stimulants (e.g., amphetamines), have not been reported to improve VR (Clement et al., 2007). In general, VR programs, such as those incorporating habituation exercises, have been more effective than medications for treating motion sickness (Cowings & Toscano, 2000). More targeted pharmaceutical agents will likely be identified as research further elucidates the mechanisms underlying motion sensitivity.

Behavioral Techniques

Behavioral techniques can prevent or reduce symptoms from motion or visual stimuli (Golding & Gresty, 2005). Countermeasures include reducing head movements (number of repetitions, distance traveled, speed, direction), aligning the head and body in the direction of the forces, obtaining a stable horizontal reference such as the horizon, and reducing "conflicting" sensory input such as running outside instead of on a treadmill. Sitting in the front of the car and taking rest breaks from provocative stimuli can reduce symptoms. Controlled breathing can reduce nausea for short-term exposure to noxious stimuli (Yen-Pik-Sang et al., 2003a, 2003b). Anecdotally, some patients appear to be able to reduce their nausea in a given situation by closing their eyes, taking a few deep breaths, and relaxing their neck and abdominal muscles (Acerra, unpublished data). This technique may be similar to various forms of medication, mindfulness, or centering.

Currently there is no evidence to support acupuncture/acupressure wristbands as effective countermeasures (Miller & Muth, 2004). One study supported the contention that diet can modify symptoms, as people on a high-protein diet reported less motion sickness (Levine et al., 2004). Anecdotally, education, awareness of triggers, and emotional support can reduce symptoms; patients have reported reduced symptom onset, intensity, and duration with understanding of their triggers paired with coping strategies to manage provocative situations (Acerra, unpublished data).

Vestibular Rehabilitation

A growing body of evidence indicates that VR can effectively treat vestibular dysfunction and reduce the incidence and severity of motion sensitivity to movement and visual stimuli. Further research into the mechanisms underlying motion sensitivity will undoubtedly provide insight into ways to better promote motion sensitivity rehabilitation management. VR may accelerate adaptation, habituation, and desensitization to noxious stimuli; correct vestibular and balance impairments; or correct abnormal weighting of sensory inputs.

In general, customized exercise programs are based on the individual's presentation and goals and are progressed over a 3- to 12-month period. Programs commonly include gaze stabilization, habituation, exposure to sensory-conflicting stimuli, and balance/gait activities. Patients can learn strategies for prevention and management, including stress and trigger reduction techniques (Table 22.3).

Rehabilitation and Sensory-Conflict Training Visual–vestibular habituation exercises increase tolerance to visual stimulation, decrease somatosensory preference and dependence, and improve postural control. The mechanisms underlying recovery are unclear, but likely involve central mechanisms (Miles & Braitman, 1980; Golding, 2006). Education can help patients manage how much conflict is appropriate during training and day-to-day life.

Few studies to date have directly compared treatments. Instead, much of our knowledge comes from astronaut research, case studies, and experienced clinicians. Astronauts routinely use habituation for space sickness (Lackner & Dizio, 2006). Cowings and Toscano (2000) reported superior reduction in motion sickness with habituation compared to drugs. Rine et al. (1999) described progressively exposing a motion-sick patient to increasingly provocative stimuli over 10 weeks to attain goals such as return to driving, work, and leisure activities. Exercises included gaze stabilization exercises such as dynamic visual acuity tasks with reduced somatosensory information (e.g., marching in place on dense foam or when turning). Whitney et al. (2000) and Wrisley et al. (2002) reported habituation to specific stimuli that cause dizziness or vertigo (e.g., lying in bed) in vestibular migraineurs. To be effective, exercises must be stimulation specific and be practiced for an adequate length of time, often multiple times per day (e.g., 2 to 5 minutes of training, two to five times per day) (Herdman, 2007). Rest between repetitions is also believed to be important.

Some VV patients are overdependent on visual cues. Visual stimuli can also modify—either enhance or suppress—the VOR (Bronstein, 2005). VR can shift visual dependence, retrain the VOR, influence central preprogramming, and desensitize patients to visual-conflicting stimuli (Guerraz et al., 2001; Herdman et al., 2001; Lopez et al., 2006). VV is diminished with exposure to optokinetic stimuli (such as disco ball), when such treatment is progressively intensified over 6 to 10 weeks (Vitte et al., 1994; Tsuzuku et al., 1995; Pavlou et al., 2004). Initially exercises are started with the patient seated, then while standing, then while walking (with or without head movement), and finally with functional tasks that recreate work or leisure situations (Bronstein, 2005). Pavlou (2010) reported exposure to optokinetic stimuli (via visual environment rotator or DVD) during rehabilitation was superior to a program without visual stimuli for treating dizziness, postural instability, and VV. Patients can be exposed to postural stability tasks that manipulate whether sensory inputs are congruent or incongruent with the goal of teaching patients to rely more on proprioceptive and vestibular cues (Shumway-Cook & Horak, 1990). Exercises may also need to be prescribed to address specific peripheral or central vestibular dysfunction and balance/gait retraining, as many motion-sensitive patients have impaired postural responses (Hoffer et al., 2003).

Stress Reduction and Physical Activity Management of motion sensitivity also involves education of patients on the effects of stress and triggers, specific strategies for trigger prevention and coping skills, and a plan to limit the deleterious effects of deconditioning. For example, patients may notice increased symptoms on a treadmill compared to running outside, likely due to the incongruence of running in place. Many patients are provided with a walking program (e.g., at least 20 minutes outside and on uneven surfaces) as it is a sensory-congruent activity that challenges their balance. In addition, many patients are encouraged to participate in regular aerobic exercise (Table 22.3). Stress reduction was described in detail earlier in this chapter.

PROGNOSIS

Overviews of management and VR treatment are provided in Tables 22.2, 22.3, and 22.9. Moderate to strong evidence indicates that VR provides resolution of vestibular symptoms for BPPV, unilateral vestibular loss, and bilateral vestibular loss (Hilton & Pinder, 2004; Fife et al., 2008; Hillier & Hollohan, 2008). In addition, evidence shows that VR can improve symptoms with VM and central vestibular loss. Case studies and small clinical trials indicate that motion sensitivity can be improved with VR and management strategies.

The prognosis can be poorer in patients with comorbidities such as neurologic conditions (e.g., multiple sclerosis or traumatic brain injury). After completion of the program, many patients are placed on a home maintenance exercise plan to maintain function (e.g., one or two exercises practiced one to three times per week). Patients need to be aware that symptoms can return under some circumstances—for example, after prolonged illness, following deconditioning, or due to new acute events such as a migraine. This loss of function is usually termed decompensation. Patients can learn to prevent or manage their decompensation through a maintenance program and specific coping strategies.

CONCLUSIONS

Migraineurs can present with vestibular migraine, motion sensitivity, or coexisting vestibular disorders. Differential diagnosis is a challenge, in particular due to the current lack of inclusion of VM in the IHS classification scheme. The history is the key to determining a diagnosis and optimal treatment plan. Clinical and neuro-otologic tests are available to determine whether symptoms are related to visual- versus motion-induced sensitivity and to central versus peripheral vestibular dysfunction. Experienced rehabilitation specialists can provide a safe and effective customized vestibular rehabilitation program to address migraine prevention and treatment of vestibular dysfunction and motion sensitivity related to migraine.

REFERENCES

Acerra NE. A retrospective chart review of 62 patients sensitive to motion and visual stimuli. Unpublished data.

Adams F. *The Genuine Works of Hippocrates Translated From the Greek.* London: Sydenham Society; 1849.

Akin FW, Davenport MJ. Validity and reliability of the motion sensitivity test. *J Rehabil Res Development* 2003;40: 415–421.

Alpay K, Ertas M, Orhan EK, et al. Diet restriction in migraine, based on IgG against foods: a clinical double-blind, randomised, cross-over trial. *Cephalalgia* 2010;30:829–837.

Baloh RW, Halmagyi GM. *Disorders of the Vestibular System.* Oxford, UK: Oxford University Press; 1996.

Bhattacharyya N, Baugh RF, Orvidas L, et al. Clinical practice guideline: benign paroxysmal positional vertigo. *Otolaryngology-Head Neck Surg* 2008;139: S47–S81.

Bic Z, Blix GG, Hopp HP, et al. The influence of a low-fat diet on incidence and severity of migraine headaches. *J Women's Health Gender-Based Med* 1999;8:623–630.

Bos JE, Bles W. Modelling motion sickness and subjective vertical mismatch detailed for vertical motions. *Brain Research Bull* 1998;47:537–542.

Breslau N, Davis GC, Andreski P. Migraine, psychiatric disorders, and suicide attempts: an epidemiologic study of young adults. *Psychiatry Research* 1991;37:11–23.

Bronstein AM. Visual symptoms and vertigo. *Neur Clinics* 2005;23:705–713.

Brown KE, Whitney SL, Marchetti GF, et al. Physical therapy for central vestibular dysfunction. *Arch Phys Med Rehabil* 2006;87:76–81.

Burstein R. Deconstructing migraine into peripheral and central sensitization. *Pain* 2001;89:107–110.

Canada Pulmonary Hypertension Association. *Canada's Physical Activity Guide.* Active Living; 2010.

Çelebisoy NFG, Gökcay F, Sirin H, Bicak N. Migrainous vertigo: clinical, oculographic and posturographic findings. *Cephalalgia* 2008;28:72–77.

Cha YH. Mal de débarquement. *Sem Neurol* 2009;29:520–527.

Cha YH. Migraine-associated vertigo: diagnosis and treatment. *Sem Neurol* 2010;30:167–174.

Childs AJ, Sweetnam MT. A study of 104 cases of migraine. *Br J Industrial Med* 1961;18:234–236.

Clement G, Deguine O, Bourga M, et al. Effects of vestibular training on motion sickness, nystagmus, and subjective vertical. *J Vestibular Res* 2007;17:227–237.

Clendaniel RA. The effects of habituation and gaze stability exercises in the treatment of unilateral vestibular hypofunction: preliminary results. *J Neurol Phys Ther* 2010;34:111–116.

Cowings PS, Toscano WB. Autogenic-feedback training exercise is superior to promethazine for control of motion sickness symptoms. *J Clin Pharmacol* 2000;40:1154–1165.

Crampton GH. Research strategies for motion and space sickness. *J Oto-Rhino-Laryngology Related Specialties* 1993;55:175–179.

Davies R. Bedside neuro-otological examination and interpretation of commonly used investigations. *J Neurol Neurosurg Psychiatry* 2004;5:32–44.

Del Rio M, Arriaga MA. Benign positional vertigo: prognostic factors. *Otolaryngology-Head Neck Surg* 2004;130:426–429.

Demer JL, Honrubia V, Baloh RW. Dynamic visual acuity: a test for oscillopsia and vestibulo-ocular reflex function. *Am J Otolaryngology* 1994;15:340–347.

Dix R, Hallpike CS. The pathology, symptomatology and diagnosis of certain common disorders of the vestibular system. *Ann Otology Rhinology Laryngology* 1952;6:987.

Donohew BE, Griffin MJ. Motion sickness: effect of the frequency of lateral oscillation. *Aviation, Space, and Environmental Medicine* 2004;75:649–656.

Drummond PD. Triggers of motion sickness in migraine sufferers. *Headache* 2005;45:653–656.

Edmeads J, Findlay H, Tugwell P. Impact of migraine and tension-type headache on life style, consulting behaviour, and medication use: a Canadian population survey. *Can J Neurol Sci* 1993;20:131–137.

Epley JM. The canalith repositioning procedure: for treatment of benign paroxysmal positional vertigo. *Otolaryngology-Head Neck Surg* 1992;107:399–404.

Fife TD, Iverson DJ, Lempert T, et al. Practice parameter: therapies for benign paroxysmal positional vertigo (an evidence-based review). Report of the Quality Standards Subcommittee of the American Academy of Neurology. *Neurology* 2008;70:2067–2074.

Fukui PT, Gonçalves TR, Strabelli CG, et al. Trigger factors in migraine patients. *Arquivos De Neuro-Psiquiatria* 2008;66:494–499.

Furman JM, Marcus DA, Balaban CD. Rizatriptan reduces vestibular-induced motion sickness in migraineurs. *J Headache Pain* 2011;12:81–88.

Gianaros P, Muth E, Mordkoff T, et al. A questionnaire for the assessment of the multiple dimensions of motion sickness. *Aviation Space Environmental Med* 2001;72:115–119.

Golding JF. Motion sickness susceptibility. *Aut Neuroscience* 2006;129:67–76.

Golding JF, Gresty MA. Motion sickness. *Curr Opinion Neurobiol* 2005;18:29–34.

Golding F, Mueller AG, Gresty MA. A motion sickness maximum around the 0.2 Hz frequency range of horizontal translational acceleration. *Aviation Space Environmental Med* 2001;72:188–192.

Grontved A, Brask T, Kambskard J, et al. Ginger root against seasickness: a controlled trial on the open sea. *Acta Oto-Laryngologica* 1988;105:45–49.

Guerraz M, Yardley L, Bertholon P, et al. Visual vertigo: symptom assessment, spatial orientation and postural control. *Brain* 2001;124:1646–1656.

Halmagyi GM, Curthoys IS. A clinical sign of canal paresis. *Arch Neurol* 1988;45:737–739.

Hansson EE. Vestibular rehabilitation: for whom and how? A systematic review. *Adv Physiother* 2007;9:106–116.

Herdman SJ, ed. *Vestibular Rehabilitation.* Philadelphia: F. A. Davis Company; 2007.

Herdman SJ, Schubert MC, Tusa RJ. Role of central preprogramming in dynamic visual acuity with vestibular loss. *Arch Otolaryngology-Head Neck Surg* 2001;127:1205–1210.

Herdman SJ, Schubert MC, Das VE, et al. Recovery of dynamic visual acuity in unilateral vestibular hypofunction. *Arch Otolaryngology-Head Neck Surg* 2003;129:819–824.

Herdman SJ, Hall CD, Schubert MC, et al. Recovery of dynamic visual acuity in bilateral vestibular hypofunction. *Arch Otolaryngology-Head Neck Surg* 2007;133:383–389.

Hillier SL, Hollohan V. *Vestibular Rehabilitation for Unilateral Peripheral Vestibular Dysfunction* [Review]. John Wiley & Sons; 2008.

Hilton M, Pinder D. The Epley manoeuvre for benign paroxysmal positional vertigo: a systematic review. *Clin Otolaryngology* 2002;27:440–445.

Hilton M, Pinder D. The Epley (canalith repositioning) manoeuvre for benign paroxysmal positional vertigo. *Cochrane Database Systematic Reviews* 2004;2:CD003162.

Hoffer ME, Gottshall K, Kopke RD, et al. Vestibular testing abnormalities in individuals with motion sickness. *Otology Neurotology* 2003;24:633–636.

Holroyd KA, Penzien DB. Pharmacological versus non-pharmacological prophylaxis of recurrent migraine headache: a meta-analytic review of clinical trials. *Pain* 1990;42:1–13.

Humphriss RL, Baguley DM, Sparkes V, et al. Contraindications to the Dix-Hallpike manoeuvre: a multidisciplinary review. *Int J Audiology* 2003;42:166–173.

International Headache Society (IHS). ICHD-II. International Classification of Headache Disorders. 2nd edition. *Cephalalgia* 2004;24:1–160.

Ishiyama A, Jacobson KM, Baloh RW. Migraine and benign positional vertigo. *Ann Otology Rhinology Laryngology* 2000;109:377–380.

Jacobson GP, Newman CW. The development of the Dizziness Handicap Inventory. *Arch Otolaryngology-Head Neck Surg* 1990;116:424–427.

Karatas M. Central vertigo and dizziness: epidemiology, differential diagnosis, and common causes. *Neurologist* 2008;14:355–364.

Katz J, Melzack R. Measurement of pain. *Surg Clin North Am* 1999;79:231–252.

Kayan A, Hood JD. Neuro-otological manifestations of migraine. *Brain* 1984;107:1123–1142.

Kennedy R, Lane N, Berbaum K, et al. Simulator sickness questionnaire: an enhanced method for quantifying simulator sickness. *J Aviation Psychol* 1993;3:203–220.

Koo JW, Balaban CD. Serotonin-induced plasma extravasation in the murine inner ear: possible mechanism of migraine-associated inner ear dysfunction. *Cephalalgia* 2006;26:1310–1319.

Koseoglu E, Akboyraz A, Soyuer A, et al. Aerobic exercise and plasma beta endorphin levels in patients with migrainous headache without aura. *Cephalalgia* 2003;23:972–976.

Kuritzky A, Ziegler DK, Hassanein R. Vertigo, motion sickness and migraine. *Headache* 1981;21:227–231.

Lackner JR, Dizio P. Space motion sickness. *Exp Brain Res* 2006;175:377–399.

Lawther A, Griffin MJ. A survey of the occurrence of motion sickness amongst passengers at sea. *Aviation Space Environmental Med* 1988;59:399–406.

Lempert T, Neuhauser H. Epidemiology of vertigo, migraine and vestibular migraine. *J Neurol* 2009;256:333–338.

Levine ME, Muth ER, Williamson MJ, et al. Protein-predominant meals inhibit the development of gastric tachyarrhythmia, nausea and the symptoms of motion sickness. *Alimentary Pharmacol Ther* 2004;19:583–590.

Linàs R, Walton L, Killman DE, et al. Inferior olive: its role in motor learning. *Science* 1975;190:1230–1231.

Lipton RB, Stewart WF, Diamond S, et al. Prevalence and burden of migraine in the United States: data from the American Migraine Study II. *Headache* 2001;41:646–657.

Lopez C, Lacour M, Magnan J, et al. Visual field dependence-independence before and after unilateral vestibular loss. *Neuroreport* 2006;17:797–803.

Magarey ME, Rebbeck T, Coughlan B, et al. Pre-manipulative testing of the cervical spine review, revision and new clinical guidelines. *Man Ther* 2004;9:95–108.

Main A, Dowson A, Gross M. Photophobia and phonophobia in migraineurs between attacks. *Headache* 1997;37:492–495.

Miles FA, Braitman DJ. Long-term adaptive changes in primate vestibuloocular reflex II: electrophysiological observations on semicircular canal primary afferents. *J Neurophysiol* 1980;43:1426–1436.

Miller KE, Muth ER. Efficacy of acupressure and acustimulation bands for the prevention of motion sickness. *Aviation Space Environmental Med* 2004;75:227–234.

Money KE. Motion sickness. *Physiol Rev* 1970;50:1–39.

Morris AE, Lutman ME, Yardley L. Measuring outcome from vestibular rehabilitation, part II: refinement and validation of a new self-report measure. *Int J Audiology* 2009;48:24–37.

Nachum Z, Shupak A, Letichevsky V, et al. Mal de debarquement and posture: reduced reliance on vestibular and visual cues. *Laryngoscope* 2004;114:581–586.

Neuhauser H, Lempert T. Vestibular migraine. *Neurol Clin* 2009;27:379–391.

Neuhauser H, Leopold M, von Brevern M, et al. The inter-relations of migraine, vertigo, and migrainous vertigo. *Neurology* 2001;56:436–441.

Neuhauser HK, von Brevern M, Radtke A, et al. Epidemiology of vestibular vertigo: a neurotologic survey of the general population. *Neurology* 2005;65:898–904.

Nuti D, Agus G, Barbieri MT, et al. The management of horizontal canal paroxysmal positional vertigo. *Acta Oto-Laryngologica* 1998;118:455–460.

Parnes LS, Agrawal SK, Atlas J. Diagnosis and management of benign paroxysmal positional vertigo (BPPV). *Can Med Assoc J* 2003;169:681–693.

Patel RM, Sarma R, Grimsley E. Popular sweetner sucralose as a migraine trigger. *Headache* 2006;46:1303–1304.

Pavlou M. The use of optokinetic stimulation in vestibular rehabilitation. *J Neurol Phys Ther* 2010;34:105–110.

Pavlou M, Lingeswaran A, Davies RA, et al. Simulator based rehabilitation in refractory dizziness. *J Neurol* 2004;251:983–995.

Pavlou M, Davies RA, Bronstein AM. The assessment of increased sensitivity to visual stimuli in patients with chronic dizziness. *J Vestibular Res* 2006;16:223–231.

Persson R. *Motion Sickness in Tilting Trains: Description and Analysis of the Present Knowledge.* Stockholm: Royal Institute of Technology; 2008.

Polensek S, Sterk C, Tusa R. Screening for vestibular disorders: a study of clinicians' compliance with recommended practices. *Med Screen Monitor* 2008;14:CR238–CR242.

Powell LE, Myers AM. The Activities–Specific Balance Confidence (ABC) scale. *J Gerontology* 1995;50A:M28–M34.

Quarck G, Etard O, Oreel M, et al. Motion sickness occurrence does not correlate with nystagmus characteristics. *Neurosci Lett* 2000;287:49–52.

Rasmussen BK, Jensen R, Schroll M, et al. Epidemiology of headache in a general population: a prevalence study. *J Clin Epidemiol* 1991;44:1147–1157.

Reason JT. Motion sickness: a special case of sensory rearrangement. *Adv Science* 1970;26:386–393.

Reason JT, Brand JJ. *Motion Sickness.* London: Academic Press; 1975.

Richter F, Bauer R, Lehmenkuhler A, et al. Spreading depression in the brainstem of the adult rat: electrophysiological parameters and influences on regional brainstem blood flow. *J Cerebral Blood Flow Metabol* 2008;28:984–994.

Rine RM, Schubert MC, Balkany TJ. Visual–vestibular habituation and balance training for motion sickness. *Phys Ther* 1999;79:949–957.

Sachs OW. *Migraine: The Evolution of a Common Disorder.* London: Faber and Faber; 1970.

Salhofer S, Lieba-Samal D, Freydl E, et al. Migraine and vertigo: a prospective diary study. *Cephalalgia* 2010;30:821–828.

Sándor PS, Afra J. Nonpharmacologic treatment of migraine. *Curr Pain Headache Rep* 2005;9:202–205.

Schubert MC, Herdman SJ, Tusa RJ. Vertical dynamic visual acuity in normal subjects and patients with vestibular hypofunction. *Otology Neurotology* 2002;23:372–377.

Selby G, Lance JW. Observations on 500 cases of migraine and allied vascular headache. *J Neurol Neurosurg Psychiatry* 1960;23:23–32.

Shepard NT. Differentiation of Ménière's disease and migraine-associated dizziness: a review. *J Am Acad Audiology* 2006;17:69–80.

Shulman KI. Dietary restrictions, tyramine, and the use of monoamine oxidase inhibitors. *J Clin Psychopharmacol* 1989;9:397–402.

Shumway-Cook A, Horak FB. Rehabilitation strategies for patients with vestibular deficits. *Neurol Clin* 1990;8:441–457.

Spinks AB, Wasiak J, Villanueva EV, et al. Scopolamine (hyoscine) for preventing and treating motion sickness. *Cochrane Database Systematic Reviews* 2007;3:CD002851.

Straube A, Rauch SD. Vertigo and migraine: a more than twofold connection. *Cephalalgia* 2010;30:774–776.

Teggi R, Caldirola D, Fabiano B, et al. Rehabilitation after acute vestibular disorders. *J Laryngology Otology* 2008;13:1–6.

Terrett AGJ. *Current Concepts in Vertebrobasilar Complications Following Spinal Manipulation.* Norwalk: Foundation for Chiropractic Education and Research; 2001.

Tsuzuku T, Vitte E, Semont A, et al. Modification of parameters in vertical optokinetic nystagmus after repeated vertical optokinetic stimulation in patients with vestibular lesions. *Acta Otolaryngol Suppl* 1995;520:419–422.

Tusa RJ. Migraines, Ménière's disease, and motion sensitivity. In: Herdman S, ed. *Vestibular Rehabilitation.* Philadelphia: F. A. Davis Company; 2007;188–201.

Uneri A. Migraine and benign paroxysmal positional vertigo: an outcome study of 476 patients. *Ear Nose Throat J* 2004;83:814–815.

Van Den Eeden SK, Koepsell TD, Longstreth WT, et al. Aspartame ingestion and headaches: a randomized crossover trial. *Neurology* 1994;44:1787–1793.

Vingen JV, Pareja JA, Støren O, et al. Phonophobia in migraine. *Cephalalgia* 1988;18:243–249.

Vitte E, Semont A, Berthoz A. Repeated optokinetic stimulation conditions of active standing facilitates recovery from vestibular deficits. *Exp Brain Res* 1994;102:141–148.

Von Brevern M, Zeise D, Neuhauser H, et al. Acute migrainous vertigo: clinical and oculographic findings. *Brain* 2005;128:365–374.

Von Brevern M, Radtke A, Lezius F, et al. Epidemiology of benign paroxysmal positional vertigo: a population based study. *J Neurol Neurosurg Psychiatry* 2007;78:710–715.

Watt D, Lefebvre L. Vestibular suppression during space flight. *J Vestibular Res* 2003;13:363–376.

Whitney SL, Wrisley DM, Brown KE, et al. Physical therapy for migraine-related vestibulopathy and vestibular dysfunction with history of migraine. *Laryngoscope* 2000;110:1528–1534.

Wrisley DM, Whitney SL, Furman JM. Vestibular rehabilitation outcomes in patients with a history of migraine. *Otology Neurotology* 2002;23:483–487.

Yardley L. Motion sickness and perception: a reappraisal of the sensory conflict approach. *Br J Psychol* 1992;83:449–471.

Yardley L, Masson E, Verschuur C, et al. Symptoms anxiety and handicap in dizzy patients: development of the vertigo symptom scale. *J Psychomotor Res* 1992;36:731–741.

Yardley L, Burgneay J, Andersson G, et al. Feasibility and effectiveness of providing vestibular rehabilitation for dizzy patients in the community. *Clin Otolaryngology* 1998;23:442–448.

Yen-Pik-Sang F, Billar JP, Golding JF, et al. Behavioral methods of alleviating motion sickness: effectiveness of controlled breathing and music audiotape. *J Travel Med* 2003a;10:108–112.

Yen-Pik-Sang F, Golding JF, Gresty MA. Suppression of sickness by controlled breathing during mild nauseogenic motion. *Aviation Space Environmental Med* 2003b;74:998–1002.

OTHER THERAPIES FOR MIGRAINE

The Placebo Response in Migraine Treatment

David Peters, MB, ChB, DRCOG, DMSMed, MFHom, FLCOM

INTRODUCTION

The term "placebo effect" (PE) is widely used in medicine and medical science, yet the nature of placebos and their effects are far from clear. Other terms that have been used to describe these effects relate to explanatory mechanisms: expectancy effects (Crow et al., 1999), context effects (Di Blasi et al., 2001), and meaning response (Moerman, 2002). The placebo effect is neither a trick nor simply an effect that is "all in the mind." In fact, our growing understanding of the placebo effect is blurring the boundary between so-called subjective and objective worlds. Moreover, because contextual effects occur whenever a treatment takes place, the placebo effect raises fundamental questions about the nature of treatment and treatment outcomes as a whole. Given that these effects influence the course of a disease and the response to a therapy at a physiological level, they are making medicine rethink what it means to ask "what works"—even to rethink what "working" means.

This chapter considers the scope, size, and mechanisms of the placebo effect, its influence in the treatment of migraine, and some implications for research and practice.

UNDERSTANDING THE PLACEBO EFFECT

The Size and Variability of the Placebo Effect

Evaluating drug treatments for acute migraine and its prevention clearly calls for placebo-controlled randomized trials. Nonetheless, the results of these trials reveal extraordinarily high and variable rates of placebo response. To improve future studies, the factors influencing placebo responses must be better understood. The more straightforward factors related to clinical trials include expectations, blinding and unblinding, the route and site of administration, the age and gender of the patient, and the geographic distribution of the trials.

Harrington (1997), in his fascinating book about the placebo effect, explains that, historically speaking, science's relationship to the placebo effect has followed the three stages of an artifact. Initially, an artifact is ignored; subsequently, its presumed contaminating effects are controlled for; and finally, it is recognized and investigated as a phenomenon in its own right. Although the world of medical science may have once dismissed the placebo effect as simply noise in the experimental system or identified it with self-delusion and trickery, that time is over. What started out as a nuisance variable to be explained away is proving to be of great importance. In fact, it might be argued that Henry Beecher's (1955) paper "The Powerful Placebo" served as the impetus for this third stage. Beecher, after considering 26 studies, estimated their average placebo response rate at 32.5%. The erroneous but often repeated medical folklore that a fixed one-third of the population are "placebo-responders," or that a fixed one-third of a treatment outcome is due to placebo effects, probably arose out of a misunderstanding of Beecher's work. What Beecher actually discovered was that in a favorable context, the response rate can be far higher. Roberts et al. (1993) later established that when both the practitioner and the patient believe a treatment to be effective, the power of nonspecific effects can account for as much as two-thirds of successful treatment outcomes.

For their study, Roberts et al. (1993) selected five medical and surgical treatments that were once considered efficacious, but that had subsequently been abandoned when controlled trials ruled out their efficacy. Before their abandonment, for these five treatments combined, outcomes had been reported as 40% excellent, 30% good, and 30% poor. Roberts et al. concluded that "under conditions of heightened expectation the power of nonspecific effects far exceeds that commonly reported in the literature." Thus placebo rates can be very high—but they can also vary enormously.

A 1997 study collected data on postoperative pain relief from five high-quality placebo-controlled single-dose parallel-group randomized controlled trials (RCTs) in which 132 of the 525 patients received placebo. The proportion who obtained more than 50% of the maximum possible pain relief with placebo varied from 7% to 37% across the trials; for the active drugs, the corresponding

variation ranged from 5% to 63% (McQuay et al., 1996). This is generally the case in double-blind placebo-controlled RCTs: outcomes in different trials for similar drugs vary greatly, and it is assumed that the variability of the placebo response contributes considerably to this variation. For example, a systematic review of 117 peptic ulcer studies of cimetidine or ranitidine found that the response rates in the placebo arms varied from 0 to 100%, which was a much greater variation than the response rates in the active arms of the same studies (Moerman, 2002).

What Is the True Placebo Effect in Practice?

These migraine studies remind us that many unknown factors are at work in the clinical encounter. Placebo effects are inherent in all clinical work, so their evaluation is complex, and it is difficult for clinicians to attribute outcomes to inputs. Given this uncertainty, it would be unwise for them to rely solely on their impressions: although they might want to know whether a treatment "works," for a number of reasons this determination is not so easy to make.

Consider, for example, a doctor who prescribes some tablets to a patient who gets migraine. In addition to any specific effects the tablets might elicit, three other factors will contribute to the outcome. The first is natural history: migraines may get better without treatment. Also, given that patients tend to take medicines or consult clinicians when their symptoms are at their worst, improvement due to a regression toward the mean would be expected, too. Second, symptoms tend to improve when they are being observed (the Hawthorne effect), and patients often want to make their practitioner (or researchers) happy by reporting improvements. Collectively, these "natural history effects" and "reporting effects" are likely to amplify estimates of effectiveness. However, neither is truly a placebo effect, a term that applies correctly only to the third of these nonspecific factors: the impact on symptoms—and physiology—of the encounter with an inert treatment may have in the clinical (or research) context (Ernst, 1995). (See **Figure 23.1**.)

In reality, a great deal is going on when that inert tablet is prescribed and taken. Medical encounters take place in a particular setting, and against a cultural backdrop, where two mind-sets—the patient's and the clinician's—interact. Both mind-sets will have been influenced by impressions and pressures from beyond the consulting room. Thus the natural tendency toward recovery intertwines with expectancy and conditioning, and

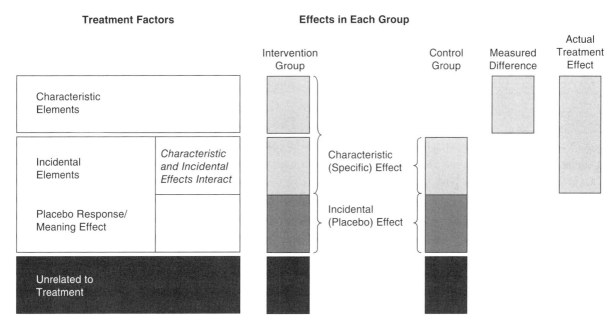

Figure 23.1 The effects of any treatment can be divided into "characteristic effects" (the specific effects of the intervention on the target disorders), and incidental effects (also called non-characteristic effects, context effects, the meaning response or placebo effects), which are a complex combination of all the other factors affecting the outcome (box on left of diagram). In many complex interventions, such as physical therapy, there is an interaction between characteristic elements (e.g., muscle strengthening) and incidental elements (e.g., motivation by the therapist). This can lead to under-estimation of the effect of an intervention if a classical RCT is used to test, as such trial design only measures the difference between characteristic elements and non-characteristic elements.

perhaps with goal-driven and meaning effects as well. These factors may potentially augment the efficacy of any active treatment, especially if the clinician and the patient believe the therapy works. Truly, the existence of placebo effects demonstrates that nothing goes into the mouth without simultaneously going through the imagination as well.

If placebo-like effects are at work in any therapeutic setting, and expectancy and conditioning influence outcomes even when no specific intervention has been given, the resulting scenario is confusing for everyone. For instance, a treatment might have added little or nothing to the powerful triad of natural history, reporting bias, and true placebo effects—yet if the patient improves after taking the medicine, this outcome would convince both the practitioner and the patient that the treatment "worked."

What are clinicians to make of this seeming contradiction? It would make little sense for them to ignore the possibility that how they communicate will either enhance or undermine a patient's capacity for natural recovery. Does this suggest they should harness placebo effects to the full, thereby maximizing the overall effectiveness of the clinical encounter (i.e., the treatment plus the context)? Keith Thomas (1987), a U.K. general

practitioner tested this proposition in his 1987 study of 200 patients who came to him with symptoms but in whom no definite diagnosis could be made. He randomly selected patients for one of four consultations: a "positive consultation" with and without treatment or a "negative consultation" with and without treatment. His article reporting on this study was entitled "General Practice Consultations: Is There Any Point in Being Positive?"— and indeed it seems there is some benefit from positive consultation, for patient satisfaction was significantly greater in the positive groups in Thomas's study. Even more interesting, however, was the lack of difference in satisfaction between the treated and untreated groups. Even more surprising, 2 weeks after consultation, 64% of those patients who received a positive consultation had gotten better, compared with 39% of those who received a negative consultation. By comparison, only 53% of those treated had gotten better compared with 50% of those not treated.

The Importance of Placebo Effects in Research

A clinical intervention will always be a mixture of human and technical elements, and Thomas, like any clinician, might want to boost the overall effectiveness of a treatment. The researcher, however, might view his or her job as being to establish a treatment's specific efficacy: the impact of its purely technical/pharmacological aspects. Yet the fact that it is so difficult to disentangle what is given to a patient from the persons involved, and from the circumstances in which the intervention takes place, makes it extremely difficult to judge what it is that is actually "working." Consequently, medicine's track record abounds with treatments once commonly practiced but now known to be ineffective or actually harmful. Only 50 years ago, insulin coma therapy was a mainline treatment for schizophrenia; less than a decade ago, the finding that hormone replacement therapy actually did not prevent cardiovascular disease shocked the medical world (Rossouw et al., 2002). As Roberts showed, doctors' convictions about the value of treatments subsequently found to be ineffective not only perpetuated their use, but also for a time made treatments that had no inherent efficacy actually effective—treatments such as gastric freezing for peptic ulcers, or internal mammary artery ligation for angina. More recently, knee arthroscopic debridement was once widely practiced (and produced useful pain relief); nevertheless, in one controlled trial (Moseley et al., 2002), it was found to be no more effective than placebo surgery. It seems practitioners and patients are biased and rather poor at judging what works. Therefore they need more robust ways of discriminating the good that medicine can do from its potential to harm.

Over the last 50 years, the chosen yardstick has come to be the RCT and, increasingly, the systematic collection and synthesis of RCTs into data sets that can be meta-analyzed. Because the variables are so large and unpredictable, evaluating a treatment outcome means accounting for and cancelling out these factors through judicious randomization, and by removing patients' and clinicians' observation bias and reporting bias through blinding and the inclusion of control groups. Only then—and providing that the sample size is commensurate with the expected effect-size of the treatment—can small differences in outcomes between treatment and control groups be attributed to the specific treatment. It has taken more than half a century of quality improvement to iron out the RCT's many potential design faults. Even so, many trials remain badly designed, small and under-powered, and inadequately controlled (Lilford, 2002).

The necessary work of improving RCT quality continues, and the great variability of placebo effects across trials presents ongoing, considerable challenges to RCT

design. Only the inclusion of a third (nontreated) arm in RCTs would allow the full range of nonspecific factors to be comprehended. RCT design may have to change as placebo responses are better understood (Enck et al., 2008).

The Neurobiology of Placebo Effects

Placebo effects are not simply a matter of subjective feelings, but rather trigger a cascade of physiological events in the brain and body. These events can be explored using brain imaging techniques, agonist–antagonist studies, and studies in which drugs are administered openly or without the subject's knowledge. Most of our emerging understanding of placebos' neurobiological effects comes from studies of pain and analgesia and from research into placebo effects on depression, the immune system, and Parkinson disease. Placebo effects depend on different psychological processes operating through different brain circuits and based on expectation, anxiety, reward, and a variety of learning phenomena, such as Pavlovian conditioning, cognitive, and social learning. Various neurotransmitter systems operate in different brain regions—in particular, in the anterior cingulate cortex, dorso-lateral prefrontal cortex, and basal ganglia (Oken, 2008). As would be expected given that placebo effects depend on brain chemistry, some experimental evidence supports the existence of genetic variants in placebo responsiveness (Oken, 2008).

Placebo analgesia is initiated and maintained mainly by expectations of symptom change and changes in motivation and emotions (Price et al., 2008). The neural networks involved are modulated by the release of opioids, cholecystokinin, and dopamine. Endogenous opioids activated by placebo administration can even inhibit respiratory centers and perhaps slow the heart by opposing beta-adrenergic sympathetic pathways. Placebos also affect 5-HT secretion from the pituitary and adrenal glands, potentially mimicking the action of the 5-HT inhibitor anti-migraine triptan drugs (Colloca & Benedetti, 2005).

When effectiveness is reduced in someone who is given an active drug but who believes it to be ineffective, this nocebo effect, according to Benedetti et al. (2005), involves cholecystokinin pathways. Conditioning is important in pain relief as well, as previous experiences with effective analgesia tend to improve the outcome with subsequent pain treatments. Goal-directed processes such as the desire or motivation for improvement—mediated by dopamine pathways—are another aspect of the placebo effect.

Pain is something conscious and placebo analgesia is mediated by expectancy, whereas placebo effects act on unconscious physiological functions, such as hormonal secretion, immune functions, and respiratory functions, which depend on processes of classical conditioning mediated through cholecystokinin (CCK) pathways. Placebo effects on the motor disturbances associated with Parkinson disease specifically involve dopamine release in the basal ganglia circuitry (Price et al., 2008).

Benedetti et al.'s (2005) review of the neurobiological mechanisms of the placebo effect highlighted findings from 15 brain studies of placebo, regulation of emotions, and activation by opiate drugs. The researchers discovered a significant degree of co-location in the frontal cortex of areas consistently activated by these diverse processes, which suggested to Benedetti and colleagues that a general system for self-regulation applies to both emotions and pain. Moreover, the areas engaged by placebo may be part of a general circuit that underpins the voluntary regulation of emotion-related responses.

The finding that placebo effects reduce amygdala activation suggests that they decrease the threat value of pain-predicting cues. Perhaps such an increase in the sense of safety might permit shifts in executive attention and produce more effective self-distraction. However, as Benedetti points out, this hypothesis does not explain the widespread activation in frontal systems reported across studies. In fact, when prefrontal functioning is impaired (for instance, in Alzheimer's-type dementia), expectancy responses are reduced or totally lacking (Benedetti et al., 2006). This finding supports the idea that this general circuit may also be subservient to the process of meaning-generation, such that effective placebo treatment might prompt active reevaluation of pain's significance. This process would, in turn, engage frontal and prefrontal systems in moderating pain perception and emotional processing.

As far as Benedetti is concerned, although a complete psychological explanation of placebo effects remains to be elucidated, the placebo effect is strongly linked with human self-regulatory faculties that have evolutionary survival value because they contribute to humankind's social, emotional, and physical health. Benedetti's research on the neurobiology of expectancy effects suggests that they genuinely make analgesic drugs more effective. This leads him to recommend that clinicians should communicate about their treatments in ways that increase positive expectations so as to activate the brain chemistry that mediates placebo responses. Conversely, because negative expectations may make some symptoms worse and even interfere with recovery from a disease, he counsels clinicians to communicate in ways that avoid nocebo

effects. Benedetti predicts that because nocebo hyperalgesia is mediated by CCK, new CCK-antagonists could be developed for the treatment of anxiety-related pain (Benedetti, 2007).

THE PLACEBO EFFECT IN MIGRAINE AND MIGRAINE RESEARCH

The Placebo Effect in Studies of Acute Migraine Episodes

Response rates for placebo treatment of acute headache episodes are higher than corresponding rates in headache prophylaxis. In addition, invasive procedures such as injections have a higher placebo response compared with oral drugs (Diener et al., 2008a).

Triptan Trials

Clinical trials have provided convincing evidence that migraine responds well to placebo treatment. Loder et al. (2005) published a systematic review that included data from 31 studies (1991 to 2002) of oral triptan medication. The main endpoints in studies of acute migraine are typically percentage of headache relief at 2 hours, percentage of subjects pain free at 2 hours, and tolerability. The levels of placebo response and their variability might seem surprising: For 2-hour pain relief, the response rate ranged from 17% to 50% (mean: 28.5% $\pm$ 8.7%). Pain-free rates ranged from 5% to 17% (mean: 6.1% $\pm$ 4.4%), and nocebo effects (i.e., side effects in the placebo arm) varied dramatically between 4.9% and 74% (mean: 23.4% $\pm$ 14%). Triptan studies suggest that the placebo effect is greater when pain is mild (as is the effect of active medication), and that the nocebo effect is reduced when effervescent placebos are used.

Speciali, Peres, and Bigal (2010) published a very useful summary of the field exploring the significance of placebos and the placebo effect in migraine treatment and prevention, and their importance for future research. These authors highlighted the difficulties of measuring the placebo effect in acute migraine, noting that the placebo effect (which is greater in tension headaches than in migraine in general) will be influenced by several basic elements in the trial. Chief among them are whether a study is of a single attack or a series of attacks, the age and gender of the subjects, their prior experience in clinical trials, and previous exposure to the drug being tested. The method and route of administration also strongly influences the placebo response rate (Diener et al., 2008b).

The placebo effect is greater in mild attacks, in attacks without aura, in children, and with nasal administration (rather than oral administration). Surprisingly, a smaller effect is observed for triptans than for non-triptans, although this difference may reflect the fact that triptan trials tend to involve more severe forms of migraine.

In addition, it is well established that the color and shape of a tablet will influence how its effects and effectiveness are perceived: red tablets work better as placebo stimulants, whereas blue tablets are more sedating; tablets in general have a smaller placebo effect than capsules (De Craen et al., 1996). Some studies suggest that the placebo effect may increase if additional placebo tablets are taken, and if they are attractively packaged and more expensive (Colloca & Benedetti, 2006). The placebo effects of an injection or acupuncture are larger than those of tablets (Kaptchuk et al., 2006). Proper adherence to placebos has even been found to have an association with decreased mortality (Simpson et al., 2006).

The nocebo effect (number of patients reporting adverse events from placebos) in migraine trials is lowest for soluble tablets and highest for injectables. According to this review, the placebo effects were high in a trial of suppositories for migraine, in which placebos produced pain relief in 39% of the control group (Speciali et al., 2010).

The Placebo Effect in Studies of Migraine Prevention Drugs

As Speciali et al. (2010) point out, prevention trials often take place over several months, so there is more opportunity for research subjects to guess whether they are taking active medication or placebo. This unblinding tends to increase the nonspecific effects of the active arm of a trial: the greater the expectation of being given an active drug, the higher the potential placebo (and nocebo) effect. Consequently, the more treatment arms a study has (and, therefore, the greater the chance of receiving placebo), the lower the total placebo effect in the trial.

In reviews of prevention trials, the placebo effect also varied greatly according to the drug used in the study: 31% for propranolol, 22% for bisoprolol, 14% to 21% for valproate, and 16% for magnesium. A recent meta-analysis of 32 studies of migraine prophylaxis drugs gave a pooled estimate of patients who improved due to placebo response as 21% (Macedo et al., 2008).

The study design makes a difference, too. A parallel-design clinical trial compares the results of a treatment on two separate groups of patients. A cross-over study compares the results of two treatments on the same group of patients. Placebo response rates are significantly higher in studies with a parallel design than in cross-over studies (Macedo et al., 2008).

Placebo response rates have been significantly higher in European investigations than in North American studies, although, interestingly, nocebo events—which occurred in 30% of the placebo groups overall—were significantly more frequent in North American studies (Macedo et al., 2008). What might we read into this finding: greater expectancy because of trust in Europe's doctors, or more cynicism among U.S. patients, perhaps?

Speciali et al. (2010) commented that, in migraine prophylaxis studies, the size of the placebo effect varies more than in studies of treatment in acute attacks. This is to be expected, given that responses are tracked over many months in migraine prevention studies and, therefore, will inevitably vary far more than those measured over a few hours. Similarly, in long-term prophylaxis trials, nocebo effects are more widespread. Predictably, because consent procedures forewarn subjects of the potential side effects of the active drug being tested, these are the nocebo symptoms that most commonly occur (Amanzio et al., 2009).

The Placebo Effect in Studies of Nonpharmaceutical Prevention

The control group in a drug trial can be given a physiologically inactive substance. When "active" interventions entail physical interventions, however, it is far more difficult to develop reliable placebos that cannot be unblended. This problem arises in all trials of nonpharmacological intervention for migraine, including behavioral, biofeedback, and psychological treatments, as well as manipulation, acupuncture, injections, or massage. In addition, if a control treatment generates a high rate of placebo response, the "double-positive effect" and "efficacy paradox" rear their heads whenever the placebo effect is disproportionately large for a nonblinded therapy (Walach, 2001). For example, a hands-on therapy (acupuncture or manipulation) may have greater efficacy when compared with a drug. When it is compared with an appropriate sham treatment, however, the study is likely to find little treatment effect. Thus the combination of the nonspecific and specific effects may be high even though the specific effect is small. In surgical procedures, for instance, nonspecific beneficial effects may be very significant, but a sham surgery control group is rarely provided. In fact, it may prove impossible to provide a perfect control group when evaluating psychological and behavioral interventions.

Botulinum Toxin (Botox)

Some years ago, after people began having botulinum toxin (Botox) injections for facial wrinkles, reports of headache improvement with this treatment began to surface, including from some migraine sufferers. Several studies followed, but their results were disappointing. The placebo response rate for injections is, of course, impressive; indeed, in Botox studies it may have been so large that it obscured their efficacy. Nevertheless, the available randomized clinical trials provided little evidence that botulinum injections helped with either migraine or tension headache. Controversy about their efficacy persisted (Roach, 2008), and though a recent trial has found it superior to placebo (Diener, 2010), the example of Botox remains an instructive one.

Injections into the head will generate strong contextual, meaning, and expectancy effects; the possibility of positive cosmetic side effects and reputedly benign adverse-effect profile would merely add to Botox's appeal. The active arm in a trial of Botox cannot be blinded, however, because patients in the placebo arm would not experience the expected local muscle paralysis; therefore, they would know they were in the active arm, which would in turn boost their expectancy response. Thus the placebo effect must contribute greatly to the response in Botox trials. The typical primary endpoint in headache trials is a better than 50% reduction in headache frequency; as Speciali et al. (2010) point out in their review, more than 40% of subjects in the placebo arm of a Botox trial (Diener et al., 2010) achieved this goal. These effects were increased after each placebo injection and persisted for 9 months. Migraine can, of course, remit spontaneously, but not at this level, and not among a group of patients who, in some cases, had been getting migraines for more than 20 years. It seems reasonable to conclude that nonspecific self-regulatory responses contributed to the therapeutic outcomes in the active arm as well as the placebo arm of the Botox trial.

Complementary Therapies

Evaluating drug treatments for acute migraine and its prevention calls for placebo-controlled randomized clinical trials. Nonetheless, the results of these trials reveal extraordinarily high and variable rates of placebo response. As previously noted, placebo response rates in the treatment of acute headache episodes are higher than in prophylaxis, and invasive procedures (injections, for example) provoke a higher placebo response than oral drugs. A review of nonpharmaceutical treatments

for migraine was surprisingly positive in its findings (Schiapparelli, 2010). The reviewers found evidence for the prophylactic use of riboflavin and coenzyme Q10, and the prophylactic use of magnesium, particularly for children and menstrually related migraine. The herbal medicine butterbur has been found to significantly decrease attack frequency as well. The efficacy of feverfew was not confirmed in a Cochrane review, however, probably because of the great variations in concentration dosage of its active principal ingredient.

Acupuncture for Migraine: Further Problems with Placebos?

Placebos for RCTs of orally administered herbal remedies and nutritional supplements are relatively easy to design. In contrast, the problems for those wishing to devise RCTs for body-oriented treatments such as acupuncture are twofold: (1) designing effective placebos and (2) distinguishing nonspecific effects that may be intrinsic to the treatment from extrinsic contextual placebo effects. The effects of interventions such as massage, acupuncture, chiropractic, and osteopathy depend on the deliberate and skillful application of touch. Different practitioners will apply such therapy in significantly different ways. No doubt a practitioner's style and quality of touch embodies various unknown nonspecific elements that may potentially influence outcomes either positively or negatively. But would it be correct to describe them as nonspecific contributors to outcome when they are so much part and parcel of the treatment? Would they be better referred to as specific nonspecific effects? If they are placebo-generators, then how are researchers to design controls for such effects, given that such complex and participative interventions rely on a high degree of interaction and communication between the patient and the practitioner (Paterson & Dieppe, 2005)? Practitioners, who cannot be blinded to whether they are giving true or sham treatment, are likely to behave differently depending on which arm of an RCT they are proving "treatment" for, which will presumably alter the contextual effects.

In a qualitative study, Paterson et al. (2008) sought to determine how the RCT context affected participants in an acupuncture study, including whether it distorted their behavior and the outcomes. The 10 participants, 6 of whom were female, and who collectively ranged in age from 23 to 70 years, had severe migraine, for which conventional treatment had been of limited benefit. They were satisfied with the organization of the trial and no acupuncture was perceived as obviously "sham."

The study concluded that because most participants and the practitioner involved played active parts in the trial, their "roles" were different from their usual ones of "patient" and "doctor." This shift altered their expectations and behavior, which in turn influenced how the intervention was delivered and experienced. For instance, there was a reduction in talking, explanations, and participation, and treatment focused on the migraine problem to the exclusion of other conditions, even where participants considered those other conditions to be a cause or a trigger of the migraine. Consequently, the authors concluded that treatment in the trial differed from that described in studies of "real life" traditional acupuncture; furthermore, these differences affected not only the needling—the characteristic or specific intervention—but also contextual factors. The researchers concluded that this limitation of trial design seems inevitable when using a sham-control group to study an intervention based on holistic and participative treatment strategies. Therefore, the design and interpretation of RCTs of complex interventions such as acupuncture have to take these factors into account.

RCTs of acupuncture for migraine ought to help clinicians and patients make informed decisions about treatment. Yet, their results are confusing: some trials find acupuncture to be superior to sham (placebo) acupuncture, while others suggest it is superior to usual care but not to sham acupuncture, and still others conclude that usual care is superior. Subsequent meta-analyses have typically reached indeterminate conclusions about acupuncture as a therapy for migraine, because most acupuncture research (until recently) has involved small trials of poor quality that yielded conflicting results. Such studies are unsuitable grist for the meta-analyst's mill.

Fortunately, this situation is changing. The increasing number of larger, well-designed studies has now allowed a formerly inconclusive Cochrane review to be updated through the inclusion of 12 more RCTs. This review (Linde et al., 2009) of 22 RCTs of acupuncture for migraine prophylaxis—which included data on 4,419 participants—suggests that acupuncture is at least as effective as, or possibly more effective than, prophylactic drug treatment, and has fewer adverse effects. Six trials (including two large trials with 401 and 1,715 patients) comparing acupuncture to no prophylactic treatment or routine care only found that after 3 to 4 months, patients receiving acupuncture had higher response rates and fewer headaches. Fourteen trials compared a "true" acupuncture intervention with a variety of sham interventions. Because pooled analyses did not show any statistically significant superiority for true acupuncture,

the authors stated there is no evidence for an effect of "true" acupuncture over sham interventions. They highlighted, however, that this "true/sham" distinction is a problematic one, as exact point location could be of limited importance. Further, as Moerman and Jonas (2002) state in their excellent article, saying that treatments such as acupuncture are not better than placebo clearly does not mean that they do nothing.

But the problem is that placebo acupuncture does not "do nothing" either. Placebo acupuncture entails inserting needles superficially (so-called minimal acupuncture) or into non-acupoints, or using retractable sham needles with blunt tips. Sometimes, in conditions such as low back pain and knee osteoarthritis, true acupuncture has been shown to be more potent than either minimal acupuncture or conventional non-acupuncture treatment. However, in clinical studies of migraine, both acupuncture and minimal acupuncture have been found to significantly alleviate migraine. For example, sham acupuncture was statistically and clinically superior to guideline-based conventional care for chronic back pain in a recent large ($n = 1,162$) RCT (Haake et al., 2007). This finding has led some authors to conclude that neither "sham" acupuncture nor minimal acupuncture is a valid placebo control in RCTs of acupuncture (Lund et al., 2009). This unsuitability is partly a matter of unblinding: "true" acupuncture treatment often involves stimulating acupoints until the deqi sensation of tingling, numbness, warmth, or heaviness is obtained. Although deqi could also be achieved by needling a "sham" point, the authors point out that even with minimal acupuncture (where no deqi is provoked, or where sham needles are glued to the skin), the procedure could nevertheless evoke activity in cutaneous afferent nerves. Given that this effect may result in what the authors term a "limbic touch response," the so-called sham would not, in fact, be clinically inert. Lund et al. (2009) also question whether the responses to "true" acupuncture and minimal acupuncture would differ depending on the etiology of the pain, and suggest that patients and healthy individuals might respond differently.

Clearly, placebo control acupuncture remains problematic, because even nonpenetrating needles may be potent modulators of target-directed expectation (Benedetti et al., 1999; Pariente et al., 2005) and may condition responses even more than placebo pills (Kaptchuk et al., 2006). Both placebo analgesia and acupuncture elicit the production of endogenous opiates: placebo analgesia elicited with an injection of saline solution can be reversed with the opiate antagonist naloxone (Pomeranz & Chiu, 1976), and enhanced with the opiate agonist proglumide (Benedetti & Amanzio, 1997).

The GERAC study (Haake et al., 2007)—one of the largest acupuncture trials undertaken—tested real acupuncture against minimal acupuncture as a control, comparing it with drug prophylaxis in migraine patients. The researchers concluded there was no difference between the responses of the three groups. In this study, conventional pharmacological prevention performed no better than the acupuncture or control, however, and on some secondary outcome measures it performed significantly worse than the allegedly ineffective acupuncture (Diener et al., 2008a). Therefore, if all three arms were better than no treatment, but no better than "sham acupuncture," ought we to assume that both real acupuncture and drug prophylaxis are ineffective?

Homeopathy, Migraine, and the Placebo Problem

Homeopathic texts tell us that headaches respond well to homeopathy. Skeptics attribute such responses purely to the placebo effect. In fact, homeopathy, like acupuncture, presents some difficult questions about the nature of placebos, and challenges the validity of RCTs as research tools, arguably placing the placebo effect as a central element in all therapeutics. Thus it is useful to examine these issues through the lens of homeopathy.

In the 1990s, when research demonstrating homeopathy's efficacy began to emerge in leading medical journals, the challenge was pithily summed up in a rather polemical *Lancet* editorial (1994) suggesting that either homeopathy works or the RCT does not. Although homeopathy has been inherently controversial throughout its 200-year existence, the debate has continued to heat up, to the point where in 2009 some doctors and politicians proposed that the U.K. National Health Service should cease funding it (*Guardian,* 2010a, 2010b). Perhaps for those who are already convinced that it works, no evidence is required, whereas for those who believe homeopathy could possibly work, no amount of evidence will suffice to disprove its utility. Homeopathy's detractors decry its nonscientific principles, whereas its supporters insist that even though we do not understand how it could work, it is undoubtedly helpful clinically. While its promoters point to research that supports efficacy (Spence et al., 2005), critics cite studies showing no superiority over placebo.

The world of therapeutics is no stranger to such contradictions, which is why systematic reviews and meta-analyses have been put forward as a solution. Systematic reviews combine diverse data from many trials; meta-analyses synthesize the numerical data to provide a single estimate of effect. Together, these methodologies constitute the main tools of evidence-based medicine. Nevertheless, systematic reviews have been criticized because sources of bias are not controlled for by the method, and a surprising degree of subjective interpretation often appears to be used in summarizing evidence and making recommendations. A good meta-analysis of badly designed studies will still result in bad statistics (www.cochrane-net), and the clinical relevance of the resulting conclusions is also open to question. Such studies' rigid structure, detachment from clinical practice, and failure to address the values that should come into play in deciding between alternatives mean their results do not easily translate into individual clinical decisions, and indeed the amassed data are open to many different interpretations (National Center for the Dissemination of Disability Research [NCDDR], 2008).

Thus the solutions to conflicting findings have themselves proved contentious, especially where complementary therapies are concerned, and perhaps most heatedly around homeopathy. Consider, for example, the accomplished meta-analysis by Linde et al. (1997). Based on 32 trials (28 placebo-controlled trials, 2 trials comparing homeopathy and another treatment, and 2 trials comparing homeopathy and both placebo and another treatment) involving a total of 1,778 patients, it concluded that the effects of homeopathic medicines are greater than those of placebos. The authors, however, commented that methodological shortcomings and inconsistencies made the evidence unconvincing. Subsequently, at least six reanalyses of this meta-analysis have been undertaken (Ernst, 2002) and they have shown that as homeopathy RCT design has improved, the effect sizes found have grown smaller, to the extent that the overall benefits of homeopathy become insignificant. However, as Ernst (2002) points out, the validity of conducting systematic reviews of systematic reviews is uncertain, they create no new information, and reviewer bias is difficult to account for.

The take-home message in almost all systematic reviews of complementary therapy studies seems to be that better-designed and far-larger trials are needed to distinguish relatively small specific effect sizes (e.g., homeopathy) from these therapies' large nonspecific effects. Until such large high-quality clinical studies have been conducted, combining data from small, poorly designed trials tends to be a fruitless exercise. A typical early systematic review of trials for homeopathic prophylaxis of headaches and migraine (Ernst, 1999) was based on only four available double-blind RCT studies—all of them small, totaling only 284 participants in the active arm and control groups. Predictably, the conclusion was that homeopathy is not effective in the prophylaxis of migraine or headache beyond its placebo effect. A more recent review stated that because the studies reviewed possessed several flaws in design, there is still insufficient evidence to support or refute the use of homeopathy for managing tension-type, cervicogenic, or migraine headache (Owen & Green, 2004).

ARE RANDOMIZED CONTROLLED TRIALS A RELIABLE RESEARCH METHOD?

In a summary of evidence for homeopathy, David Reilly (2006), a leading homeopathy trialist (Reilly & Taylor, 1985; Reilly et al., 1986, 1994; Taylor et al., 2000), explains that his group's initial position was that the placebo effect explained homoeopathy's effectiveness. However, all four of their trials refuted this position, instead producing patterns of results clearly favoring homoeopathy over placebo. The researchers had to conclude either that homoeopathy works or that basic flaws in the RCT method produce predictable and reproducible false-positive results often enough to undermine its use as a scientific way of evaluating treatments.

Indeed, homoeopathy highlights issues related to trial design and interpretation. In particular, it brings up questions about the number of participants required to detect a change greater than would be attributable to chance or placebo in situations where "placebo/context-enhanced nonspecific healing impact" (Reilly, 2006) applies because the placebo group shows significant improvements.

To bolster his argument, Reilly (2006) cites an example of what he calls a "double positive trial": the Lewith et al. (2002) study of homeopathy for asthma, which was reported as negative. In this study, both groups showed a significant and clinically useful improvement. In view of the small size of any difference between specific effects and nonspecific effects (i.e., in studying any treatment that generates a substantial rate of placebo response), a very large study will be needed to tease out the specific action. Reilly (2006) warns that rejecting "double positive trials" risks "throwing out treatments that have clinically important efficacy because they also show high effectiveness just because these studies lack the statistical power." Walach (2001) also proposes that homeopathy's contextual effects are much larger than in conventional medicine, and its specific effects smaller, and, therefore, that many homeopathic RCTs have failed to prove efficacy because they were been statistically underpowered. To illustrate the

statistical relationship between specific effect size and sample size, consider the following scenario: if 50% of people respond to placebo and 80% respond to an active treatment, the researcher would need 40 people per group to be sure of detecting the effect; if the rates were 50% and 70%, respectively, then 100 people per group would be necessary; but if the rates were 50% and 60%, respectively, 400 people per group would be required. Very few trials of nonpharmaceutical treatments aspire to such large numbers.

IS HOMEOPATHY A "SUPER-PLACEBO"?

Placebo effects can be large and their size varies considerably between trials, leading some critics to suggest that homeopath's lengthy case-taking and practitioner empathy produce enhanced placebo effects. Furthermore, it has been proposed that because homeopathy's nonspecific effects are substantially higher than those associated with conventional medicine, they tend to mask any specific effect of the remedies themselves.

Is there evidence to support these ideas? Two recent studies contradict each other on this point. Nuhn et al. (2010) identified 25 RCTs of classical homeopathy, each of which the researchers were able to compare with at least three matching conventional trials. In 13 of the matched sets, the placebo effect in the homeopathic trials was larger than the average placebo effect in the conventional trials. In 12 of the matched sets, it was lower ($P = 0.39$). Clinicians might be anxious to learn just what determined why this effect was higher or lower, but subgroup analysis yielded no significant differences. Consequently, these authors simply concluded that the overall placebo effect in homeopathy RCTs is no larger than that observed in conventional medicine trials. Nuhn et al. (2010) admit the limitations of their study (limitations typical of systematic reviews in this area: small size of primary trials, small size of included sample, low statistical power, poor matching of studies, and heterogeneity because of substantial differences in study design, intensity of treatment, duration and severity of diseases, and other factors). Consequently, the extracted placebo effects could not be interpreted across, but only within, the matched sets. Recognizing this constraint, the authors suggested that further research should employ trial designs that allow for differentiating treatment effects into specific and nonspecific (context) effects.

Just such a study has recently been published. In this study—an RCT involving patients who had active but relatively stable rheumatoid arthritis—Brien et al. (2011) made the opposing case: that the homeopathic setting creates a super-placebo. Their study's aim was to find whether any benefits from adjunctive homeopathic intervention were due to the homeopathic consultation, to the homeopathic remedies, or to both. The authors concluded that patients did realize clinically relevant benefits but stated that these improvements were associated with the homeopathic consultation rather than the remedies themselves—that is, by "the ritual of the collaborative and highly individualized consultation necessary to identify a homeopathic remedy and the associated symbolic meaning response for that patient."

Ernst (2010) commented in his Pulse blog that Brien et al. (2011) had established no evidence for that assumption, and questioned "whether ineffective therapies can be vindicated through the non-specific effects they generate. A useless surgical operation for instance would not become useful and recommendable because it generates a host of non-specific effects which are typical of that setting." It would be unwise to disagree: surgery carries high risks, but homeopathy and acupuncture carry virtually none. Thus Ernst has cut to the heart of the dilemma created by Reilly's "double positive studies": if the active and the placebo group both produce significant and prolonged symptom relief, which is better than "usual care," then why would the active therapy not be "useful and recommendable" despite its outcomes depending on "a host of non-specific effects"? Ernst insists, however:

> If homeopathic remedies are ineffective and empathetic therapeutic encounters are helpful, as responsible healthcare professionals, we should discard the ineffective and adopt the helpful. If we do this, we must tell our patients that homeopathic remedies are placebos. We should be equally clear that the therapeutic relationship is important. I think (some) GPs could learn a lesson here.

Yet, one question has not been settled by this or any research so far: would the homeopathic consultation be as effective if no remedy (albeit a sugar pill) were prescribed, or if the prescriber did not believe that the whole package of consultation plus remedy was effective? Thus the dilemma may be less straightforward than Ernst suggests. Although placebo responses are triggered by the psychosocial context, words, and the rituals of the therapeutic act, brain studies nonetheless show that they change chemistry and activate particular areas in the patient's brain. Neurochemical and neuroimaging evidence shows specific neural pathways for placebo effects exist in different conditions. Moreover, the mechanisms activated by placebos are no different from those activated by drugs: the endogenous anti-nociceptive system during placebo analgesia,

and dopamine release in the nigro-striatal system during placebo reduction of motor impairment in patients with Parkinson disease (Pollo & Benedetti, 2009).

IMPLICATIONS FOR PRACTICE (AND OPTIMIZING THE "HUMAN RESPONSE")

In favorable circumstances, most control groups tend to improve. Thus the whole notion of nonspecific factors focuses our mind on the nature of individual resilience, natural remission, and the effects of a good practitioner–client relationship. Good health care is a skilled human activity, wherein the art of communication has a prominent role. Through research into placebo effects, we are learning how context and language can change physiological processes in the body and the brain.

The placebo response is of particular interest to those whose clinical work involves skilled use of hands, heart, or language: complementary therapies, psychotherapies, and much of family medicine have proved difficult to fit into the RCT framework. In these complex interventions, nonspecific factors are of great significance. Practitioners who have the requisite skills to harness such factors might feel they can take heart from the "efficacy paradox." Indeed, those clinicians who require little technology to do their work, and who perhaps think they need no hard-science basis for what they do, may nonetheless feel reassured that the expectancy and meaning their work engenders can (as Benedetti and others have shown) have such powerful effects on brain and body. Yet if their "inactive" interventions can produce outcomes larger than some "active" interventions, and their skills produce real neurobiological modulators, how are clinicians to explain this strange paradox to patients? Ought they to tell patients "the treatment I will use is likely to be of benefit, providing we both expect it to be"?

At the time when George Engel (1977) set out his framework for a biopsychosocial model, psychophysiology was relatively undeveloped. Nowadays neurobiology has better maps and we can cite examples of beneficial psychobiological effects, with the placebo response being one of them. This evolution in understanding reminds us that mind and body are, indeed, a single open system contiguous with the world they inhabit. It is no longer allowable to blithely dismiss the placebo response as a nuisance variable or pious fraud, nor to equate it with nontechnical aspects of care that medicine can afford to marginalize. Paradoxically, twenty-first-century knowledge of placebos' power and pathways makes it unscientific for practitioners to place them on the sidelines of the art of medicine.

CONCLUSIONS

Benedetti et al. (2005) suggest that in the public mind, the realization that placebo effects have a physiological reality is a message about enhanced self-regulation, perhaps fortifying aspirations to harness the human capacity for endogenous self-healing. Neuroscience is identifying physiological correlates for hitherto intangible subjective phenomena, and this line of research is leading medicine to take more seriously how context, values and beliefs, perception, and emotion affect homeostatic processes and health. At a time when health-care costs are becoming unsustainable, and medical technology has met with limited success in treating epidemic chronic degenerative diseases, the question of how to catalyze resilience has come to the fore.

The ground-breaking pain management work carried out by Connie Peck and Grahame Coleman convinced them of the wholeness of the mind–body. In their seminal 1991 article about placebos and pain (Peck & Coleman, 1991), they referred to the holistic perspective of Jerome Garb, Professor of Medicine and Chemistry at the University of Leiden, who wrote in 1747:

In his thoughts, to be sure, the physician can abstract body from mind and consider it separately in order to be less confused in the marshalling of ideas. But in the actual practice of his art, where he has to do with man as he is, should the physician devote all of his efforts to the body alone and take no account of the mind, his curative endeavors will pretty often be less than happy and his purpose either wholly missed or part of what pertains to it neglected. (Quoted in Rather, 1965)

I can do no better in ending this chapter than to reiterate, more than 20 years after Peck and Coleman's article, their conclusion: today, it is not merely a holistic notion of the patient that is needed, but a holistic notion of the medical context itself.

REFERENCES

Amanzio M, Corazzini LL, Vase L, Benedetti F. A systematic review of adverse events in placebo groups of anti-migraine clinical trials. *Pain* 2009;146:261–269.

Beecher HK. The powerful placebo. *JAMA* 1955;159:1602–1606.

Benedetti F. The placebo and nocebo effect: how the therapist's words act on the patient's brain. *Karger Gazette* 2007;7–9.

Benedetti F, Amanzio M. The neurobiology of placebo analgesia: from endogenous opioids to cholecystokinin. *Prog Neurobiol* 1997;52:109–125.

Benedetti F, Arduino C, Amanzio M. Somatotopic activation of opioid systems by target-directed expectations of analgesia. *J Neurosci* 1999;19:3639–3648.

Benedetti F, Mayberg HS, Wager TD, et al. Neurobiological mechanisms of the placebo effect. *J Neurosci* 2005;25:10390–10402.

Benedetti F, Arduino C, Costa S, et al. Loss of expectation-related mechanisms in Alzheimer's disease makes analgesic therapies less effective. *Pain* 2006;121:133–144.

Brien S, Lachance L, Prescott P, et al. Homeopathy has clinical benefits in rheumatoid arthritis patients that are attributable to the consultation process but not the homeopathic remedy: a randomized controlled clinical trial. *Rheumatology* 2011;50:1070–1082.

Cochrane. Systematic reviews. 2002. Available at: www.cochranenet.org/openlearning/html/mod3-2.htm.

Colloca L, Benedetti F. Placebos and painkillers: is mind as real as matter? *Nat Rev Neurosci* 2005;6:545–552.

Colloca L, Benedetti F. How prior experience shapes placebo analgesia. *Pain* 2006;124:126–133.

Crow R, Gage H, Hampson S, et al. The role of expectancies in the placebo effect and their use in the delivery of health care: a systematic review. *Health Technol Assess* 1999;3:1–96.

De Craen AJ, Roos PJ, Leonard de Vries A, Kleijnen J. Effect of colour of drugs: systematic review of perceived effect of drugs and of their effectiveness. *BMJ* 1996;313:1624–1626.

Di Blasi Z, Harkness E, Ernst E, et al. Influence of context effects on health outcomes: a systematic review. *Lancet* 2001;357:757–762.

Diener HC, Kronfeld K, Boewing G, et al. Efficacy of acupuncture for the prophylaxis of migraine: a multicentre randomised controlled clinical trial. *Lancet Neurol* 2008a;7:475.

Diener HC, Schorn CF, Bingel U, Dodick DW. The importance of placebo in headache research. *Cephalalgia* 2008b;28:1003–1011.

Diener HC, Dodick DW, Aurora SK, et al. Onabotulinumtoxin A for treatment of chronic migraine: results from the double-blind, randomized, placebo-controlled phase of the PREEMPT 2 trial. *Cephalalgia* 2010;30:804–814.

Editorial: Reilly's challenge. *Lancet* 1994;344:1585.

Enck P, Benedetti F, Schedlowski M. New insights into the placebo and nocebo responses. *Neuron* 2008;59:195–206.

Engel GL. The need for a new medical model: a challenge for biomedicine. *Science* 1977;196:129–136.

Ernst E. Homeopathic prophylaxis of headaches and migraine: a systematic review. *J Pain Sympt Manage* 1999;18:353–357.

Ernst E. A systematic review of systematic reviews of homeopathy. *Br J Clin Pharmacol* 2002;54:577–582.

Ernst E. Patients must be told homeopathic remedies are placebos. 2010. Available at: www.pulsetoday.co.uk/story.

Ernst E, Resch KL. Concept of true and perceived placebo effects. *BMJ* 1995;311:551–553.

Guardian. Stop homeopathy funding says Commons committee. 2010a. Available at: www.guardian.co.uk/society/2010/feb/22.

Guardian. Ban homeopathy from NHS, *say* doctors. 2010b, June 29. Available at: www.guardian.co.uk/society.

Haake M, Muller HH, Schade-Brittinger C, et al. German acupuncture trials (GERAC) for chronic low back pain:

randomized, multicenter, blinded, parallel-group trial with 3 groups. *Arch Intern Med* 2007;167:1892–1898.

Harrington A. *The Placebo Effect.* Cambridge, MA: Harvard University Press; 1997.

Kaptchuk TJ, Stason WB, Davis RB, et al. Sham device versus inert pill: randomised controlled trial of two placebo treatments. *BMJ* 2006;332:391–397.

Lewith GT, Watkins AD, Broomfield JA, et al. Use of ultramolecular potencies of allergen to treat asthmatic people allergic to house dust mite: double blind randomized controlled clinical trial. *BMJ* 2002;324:5203.

Lilford RJ. The ethics of underpowered clinical trials. *JAMA* 2002;288:2118–2119.

Linde K, Clausius N, Ramirez G, et al. Are the clinical effects of homoeopathy placebo effects? A meta-analysis of placebo-controlled trials. *Lancet* 1997;350:834–843.

Linde K, Allais G, Brinkhaus B, et al. Acupuncture for migraine prophylaxis. *Cochrane Database of Systematic Reviews* 2009;1:CD007587.

Loder E, Goldstein R, Biondi D. Placebo effects in oral triptan trials: the scientific and ethical rationale for continued use of placebo controls. *Cephalalgia* 2005;25:124–131.

Lund I, Näslund J, Lundeberg T. Minimal acupuncture is not a valid placebo control in randomised controlled trials of acupuncture: a physiologist's perspective. *Chin Med* 2009;4:1.

Macedo A, Baños JE, Farré M. Placebo response in the prophylaxis of migraine: a meta-analysis. *Eur J Pain* 2008;12:68–75.

McQuay H, Carroll D, Moore A. Variation in the placebo effect in randomised controlled trials of analgesics: all is as blind as it seems. *Pain* 1996;64:331–335.

Moerman DE. Explanatory mechanisms for placebo effects: cultural influences and the meaning response. In: Guess HA, Kleinman A, Kusek JW, Engel LW, eds. *The Science of the Placebo.* London: BMJ Books; 2002:77–107.

Moerman DE, Jonas WB. Deconstructing the placebo effect and finding the meaning response. *Ann Internal Med* 2002;136:471–476.

Moseley JB, O'Malley K, Petersen NJ, et al. A controlled trial of arthroscopic surgery for osteoarthritis of the knee. *N Engl J Med* 2002;347:81–88.

National Center for the Dissemination of Disability Research (NCDDR) 2008 Webcast Task Force on Systematic Review and Guidelines. September 3, 2008. Available at: www.ncddr.org/webcasts/11/index.html.

Nuhn T, Lüdtke R, Geraedts M. Placebo effect sizes in homeopathic compared to conventional drugs: a systematic review of randomised controlled trials. *Homeopathy* 2010;99:76–82.

Oken BS. Placebo effects: clinical aspects and neurobiology. *Brain* 2008;131:2812–2823.

Owen JM, Green BN. Homeopathic treatment of headaches: a systematic review of the literature. *J Chiropr Med* 2004;3:45–52.

Pariente J, White P, Frackowiak RS, Lewith G. Expectancy and belief modulate the neuronal substrates of pain treated by acupuncture. *Neuroimage* 2005;25:1161–1167.

Paterson C, Dieppe P. Characteristic and incidental (placebo) effects in complex interventions such as acupuncture. *BMJ* 2005;330:1202–1205.

Paterson C, Zheng Z, Xue C, Wang Y. Playing their parts: the experiences of participants in a randomized sham-controlled acupuncture trial. *J Altern Compl Med* 2008;14:199–208.

Peck C, Coleman G. Implications of placebo theory for clinical research and practice in pain management. *Theoret Med Bioethics* 1991;12:247–270.

Pollo A, Benedetti F. The placebo response: neurobiological and clinical issues of neurological relevance. *Prog Brain Res* 2009;175:283–294.

Pomeranz B, Chiu D. Naloxone blockade of acupuncture analgesia: endorphin implicated. *Life Sci* 1976;19:1757–1762.

Price DD, Finniss DG, Benedetti F. A comprehensive review of the placebo effect: recent advances and current thought. *Annu Rev Psychol* 2008;59:565–590.

Rather JL. *Mind and Body in Eighteenth Century Medicine: A Study Based Upon Jerome Garb's De Regimine Mentis.* Berkeley: University of California Press; 1965.

Reilly D. The evidence for homoeopathy, D. September 2006. Available at: www.adhom.com, V8.3.

Reilly DT, Taylor MA. Potent placebo or potency? A proposed study model with initial findings using homoeopathically prepared pollens in hay fever. *Br Homoeopathic J* 1985;74:6575.

Reilly DT, Taylor MA, McSharry C, Aitchison T. Is homoeopathy a placebo response? Controlled trial of homoeopathic potency, with pollen in hay fever as model. *Lancet* 1986;2:1272.

Reilly DT, Taylor MA, Campbell J, et al. Is evidence for homoeopathy reproducible? *Lancet* 1994;344:1601–1606.

Roach ES. Questioning botulinum toxin for headache: reality or illusion. *Arch Neurol* 2008;65:151–152.

Roberts AH, Kewman DG, Mercier L, Hovell M. The power of nonspecific effects in healing: implications for psychosocial and biological treatments. *Clin Psychol Review* 1993;13:375–391.

Rossouw JE, Anderson GL, Prentice RL, et al. Risks and benefits of estrogen plus progestin in healthy postmenopausal women: principal results from the Women's Health Initiative randomized controlled trial. *JAMA* 2002;288:321–333.

Schiapparelli P, Allais G, Castagnoli Gabellari I, et al. Non-pharmacological approach to migraine prophylaxis: part II. *Neurol Sci* 2010;31:137–139.

Simpson SH, Eurich DT, Majumdar SR, et al. A meta-analysis of the association between adherence to drug therapy and mortality. *BMJ* 2006;333:15.

Speciali JG, Peres M, Bigal ME. Migraine treatment and placebo effect. *Expert Rev Neurother* 2010;10:413–449.

Spence DS, Thompson EA, Barron SJ. Homeopathic treatment for chronic disease: a 6-year, university-hospital outpatient observational study. *J Altern Complement Med* 2005;11:793–798.

Taylor MA, Reilly D, Llewellyn Jones RH, et al. Randomised controlled trial of homoeopathy versus placebo in perennial allergic rhinitis with overview of four trial series. *BMJ* 2000;321:4716.

Thomas KB. General practice consultations: is there any point in being positive? *BMJ* 1987;294:1200–1202.

Walach H. Das wirksamkeitsparadox in der komplementärmedizin [The effectiveness paradox in complementary medicine]. *Forsch Komplementarmed Klass Naturheilkd* 2001;8:193–195.

Biobehavioral and Psychological Management of Migraine

Frank Andrasik, PhD, and Dawn C. Buse, PhD

INTRODUCTION

Biobehavioral approaches have long been applied for treatment of migraine, beginning with the early biofeedback investigations in the late 1960s and early 1970s. These early biofeedback treatments were guided more by clinical acumen than by theory, along with a dose of serendipity. When recording psycho-physiological responses from a patient with migraine, researchers at the Menninger Clinic in Topeka, Kansas (Sargent et al., 1972, 1973) noticed that the patient's hand temperature spiked approximately 12 °F midway through the session. In talking to the patient afterward, they learned she began the session with a debilitating migraine, which abated around the time her peripheral temperature increased. The researchers then began to pilot-test ways to teach patients to increase their hand temperature as a method for combating migraine. They added certain features of autogenic therapy (Schultz & Luthe, 1969) and referred to this combination of thermal biofeedback and autogenic therapy as "autogenic biofeedback." Although the precise mechanisms underlying this approach are still not fully known, decades of research support it as a viable treatment for migraine.

Thermal biofeedback uses a highly sensitive thermistor (thermometer) to monitor finger temperature. During or preceding a headache, a person's body may enter the "fight or flight" state, with the sympathetic nervous system becoming activated. As sympathetic activity increases, circulation to the extremities decreases, causing a corresponding decrease in surface temperature. When sympathetic arousal is dampened, circulation and extremity temperature increase. Thus finger temperature is now viewed as providing an indirect measure of autonomic arousal. Patients are taught that higher finger temperature corresponds to a more relaxed state; their goal is to raise their finger temperature. In essence, hand-warming biofeedback serves as a general-purpose way to promote a state of relaxation—suggesting that it can be of value for a host of disorders characterized by excessive arousal.

It was not long before investigators tried more direct means of promoting relaxation, including progressive muscle relaxation (systematic tensing and contracting of major muscles), diaphragmatic breathing, meditation, and the like. The next wave of treatment focused more on stress and environmental factors that served to precipitate, exacerbate, and maintain headache; these strategies were variously termed stress coping training, stress management, and, more recently, cognitive-behavioral therapy, which in practice often combines elements of all of the preceding approaches. The next sections describe these three major approaches in somewhat greater detail. Before exploring them, however, it is important to note the crucial role of patient education—the foundation for all such self-management treatments.

PATIENT EDUCATION, MOTIVATION, AND ADHERENCE

Patient Education

Common to all of these biobehavioral and psychological approaches to migraine is active engagement by the patient. Education and patient "buy-in" are essential, as patients subsequently make the majority of therapeutic decisions about which technique(s) to apply and when to do so. Education alone can lead to significant improvements in pain frequency, intensity, and duration; better functional status and quality of life; and decreased symptoms of depression and service utilization (Lemstra et al., 2002; Blumenfeld & Tischio, 2003; Harpole et al., 2003; Rothrock et al., 2006). Indeed, brief patient education has been shown to improve adherence and efficacy for medication alone (e.g., abortive medications) (Holroyd et al., 1989).

No single discipline has a corner on the education market—physicians, nurses (Cady et al., 2007), psychologists, and other team members can all be effective educators—and the material may take on varied formats—individual consultation, formal group classes, or patient self-guided learning. The American Council for Headache Evaluation (ACHE), an online forum sponsored by the American Headache Society, contains helpful information designed specifically for headache patients (http://www .achenet.org/). Patients are taught the relationship between their behaviors and lifestyle choices, which can enhance self-efficacy, promote a more internal locus of control, and solidify the patient–provider collaborative relationship.

Some of the most important areas to include in patient education are summarized in this chapter. Patients need to be provided with a basic understanding of migraine pathology, apprised of the typical course of this chronic disease (characterized by episodic manifestations), reassured of the benign nature of migraine (once other causes have been eliminated), and instructed about the proper application of medication, if indicated. Research has shown that patients who grasp the therapeutic mechanism of their prescription and the way in which it meshes with their treatment plan are twice as likely to fill the prescription (Cameron, 1996). This interaction also provides an occasion to discuss the potential for medication-overuse headache, adverse effects of medications, and possible deleterious drug interactions, as well as the effects and interactions of any over-the-counter agents and herbal treatments patients may be taking. More specifically, by keeping detailed diary records, patients can determine the relationship between their thoughts, behaviors, emotions, and lifestyle choices, which is facilitated by monitoring prodromal symptoms and triggers.

The level of patient understanding and the agreement need to be evaluated by requesting feedback and employing certain communication strategies. For example, the "ask–tell–ask" strategy was used with great effectiveness in the American Migraine Communication Study—2 (Hahn et al., 2008). This strategy is based on the theory that effective education requires assessing what the patient already knows and believes, then building on (or correcting when necessary) that understanding. The "ask–tell–ask" strategy can be used for any medical communication, but in this study, it was used primarily to ensure optimal communication about migraine frequency in headache days. This strategy is based on three simple steps (**Table 24.1**). Strategies such as use of open-ended questions, the "ask–tell–ask" technique, active listening, and "being fully present" with the patient can significantly improve the quality of the medical relationship, resulting in positive and more satisfying outcomes for both patient and health-care provider.

Rains et al. (2006b) believe the following topics are critical to an effective education:

1. Limit instructions to three to four major points during each discussion.
2. Use simple, everyday language, especially when explaining diagnoses and treatment instructions (model or demonstrate, when possible).

Table 24.1 The "Ask–Tell–Ask" Strategy

Step 1	**Ask** the patient to explain or restate the issue, problem, or treatment in his or her own words. This step, which allows the health-care provider to assess the patient's personal beliefs, emotional responses, and understanding of the situation, helps guide the clinician in furthering effective communication.
Step 2	**Tell** the patient the relevant facts, diagnosis, and/or treatment plan, using language at a level that he or she will understand. This provides opportunities to correct any misunderstanding or incorrect information communicated by the patient in response to the first question and to reinforce and validate the correct information that the patient shared.
Step 3	**Ask** the patient to rephrase the information given in step 2 ("tell") in his or her own words. This will allow the health-care provider to reassess the patient's level of understanding and give the patient an opportunity to ask questions and express concerns.

Source: Hahn SR. Communication in the care of the headache patient. In: Silberstein SD, Lipton RL, Dodick DW, eds. *Wolff's Headache and Other Head Pain.* New York: Oxford University Press; 2008:805–824.

3. Supplement oral instructions with written materials.
4. Involve the patient's family members or significant others.
5. Ask patients to restate recommendations back to you ("I want to make sure I am being clear and you are understanding what I am saying, so please tell me in your own words what we just covered").
6. In conclusion, repeat and reinforce the concepts that were discussed.

Point 4 emphasizes the importance of capitalizing on social support, which may be obtained during informal conversation in the physician's waiting room, over the Internet, or via participation in organized support groups (which can be especially valuable to patients) (Klapper et al., 1992; Alemi et al., 1996). Patients appreciate opportunities to converse with someone who "truly understands" how headaches affect their lives. Many countries and states have associations that sponsor support groups and mechanisms for facilitating patients contacting one another.

Adherence and Motivation

Adherence refers to an active and collaborative involvement by the patient in the implementation of a therapeutic regimen. Compliance refers to the degree to which patients follow medical recommendations of their health-care providers (Urquhart, 1996; Rains et al., 2006a). Although these terms are sometimes used interchangeably, we prefer to use the term "adherence" in headache care to emphasize the importance of the patient's participation in effective treatment.

Non-adherence can pose a significant barrier to effective headache management in many ways. Common problems of adherence in headache treatment include misuse of medication (including unfilled, overused, underused, incorrectly used, and non-advised discontinuation of prescribed medications or treatments) (Gallagher & Kunkel, 2003), difficulties in appointment keeping (Edmeads et al., 1993; Spierings & Miree, 1993), failure to perform record keeping (diaries), and unwillingness or inability to follow clinical suggestions. Improper medication use may not only limit relief, but also aggravate the primary headache condition (e.g., lead to medication-overuse or rebound headache) (Rains et al., 2006a).

Adherence declines with more frequent and complex dosing regimens (Claxton et al., 2001), increased side effects (Dunbar-Jacob et al., 2000), and increased costs (Motheral & Henderson, 1999), and is worse in chronic conditions compared to acute conditions (Dunbar-Jacob & Mortimer-Stephens, 2001). The majority of these factors come into play with headache care. Further, rates of adherence with behavioral recommendations—such as dietary modifications, weight loss, exercise, smoking cessation, and treatment for alcohol or substance use, which are some of the primary components of behavioral headache management—are even lower than rates of adherence with prescribed medication regimens (Claxton et al., 2001). In addition, sociodemographic factors play a role in predicting adherence, although the patient's perceived level of self-efficacy is an even more important consideration.

In his social learning theory, Albert Bandura (1986) posited that two components predict and mediate behavior: self-efficacy (i.e., confidence in one's ability to perform an action) and outcome efficacy (i.e., the belief that a behavior or set of behaviors will have a desirable result) (Bandura, 1977). In general, most models that explain health-related behaviors share the hypothesis that health-related behavior change and motivation are based on three components:

- The patient's readiness for change
- Self-efficacy
- Outcome efficacy (Elder et al., 1999; Jensen, 2002; Miller & Rollnick, 2002)

Following this line of reasoning, skills or knowledge alone are not sufficient to ensure behavior change. Rather, the patient must want to change, believe that he or she can change, and believe that the necessary actions will accomplish the desired goal(s).

In an attempt to operationalize these concepts, Miller et al. (2002) drew upon a theoretical framework (the transtheoretical model) (Prochaska et al., 1997) and applied it clinically (motivational interviewing [MI]) (Miller, 1996) to assess and enhance patients' motivation for change. The transtheoretical model proposes that patients' readiness and motivation for change can be categorized into one of five stages:

1. Precontemplation: The patient is not thinking about changing behavior and does not recognize the need or a problem.
2. Contemplation: The patient recognizes a need or problem and begins to think about changing behavior and may be developing a plan, but has not taken any action.
3. Preparation: The patient has done research, developed a plan, and may begin making minor changes or actions.
4. Action: The patient is actively engaged in the behavior change or new actions.
5. Maintenance: The patient is continuing behaviors necessary to maintain changes.

In the case of headache management, health-care providers should consider a patient's stage of readiness for change and tailor their interventions, clinical advice, and education accordingly. MI focuses on the patient's stage of readiness and explores his or her beliefs, concerns, perspective, and ambivalence about behavior change. The objective is for health-care providers to help patients realize the importance of change while maintaining an empathic, supportive, and nonjudgmental approach. Motivation for change is increased when patients examine the pros and cons of change and participate and engage in making decisions jointly with their health-care providers rather than being passive recipients of instructions. Rains et al. (2006a) provide several behavioral strategies to enhance patient adherence and maximize headache management that are worth considering.

EMPIRICALLY SUPPORTED BIOBEHAVIORAL THERAPIES FOR MIGRAINE

Nonpharmacological treatments for migraine can be broadly divided into the categories of behavioral treatments (cognitive-behavioral therapy and biobehavioral training, such as biofeedback, relaxation training, and stress management), physical therapies, and education including lifestyle modification. This chapter reviews empirically supported and efficacious biobehavioral approaches to the treatment and management of migraine. These techniques include strategies for both patients and health-care providers and are essential components of a comprehensive headache management plan. Once learned, patients can benefit from these strategies throughout their entire lives.

The concept of empirically supported or "evidence-based" medicine is defined as "The conscientious, explicit and judicious use of current best evidence in making clinical decisions about the care of patients . . . thereby integrating individual clinical care with the best available clinical evidence" (Eddy, 2001). Biobehavioral treatments with demonstrated empirical efficacy for headache management have become standard components of specialty headache centers and multidisciplinary pain management programs. Several empirical biobehavioral approaches to headache management are endorsed by the American Medical Association, the World Health Organization, and the National Institutes of Health, as well as by other professional organizations.

The U.S. Headache Consortium has developed evidence-based guidelines for the treatment and management of migraine based on an extensive review of the medical literature and compilation of expert consensus. Published guidelines include data and recommendations on the utility of nonpharmacological (i.e., behavioral and physical) treatments, among other issues related to migraine diagnosis and management (Campbell et al., 2000). In addition, the U.S. Headache Consortium has reported on the efficacy of behavioral interventions in the prevention of attacks, although some of these behavioral interventions may also provide relief once an attack has begun. The following goals have been established for behavioral interventions as preventive treatment for headache:

1. Reduced frequency and severity of headache
2. Reduced headache-related disability
3. Reduced reliance on poorly tolerated or unwanted pharmacotherapies
4. Enhanced personal control of migraine
5. Reduced headache-related distress and psychological symptoms

Biofeedback: Then and Now

Biofeedback involves monitoring physiological processes of which the patient may not be consciously aware or over which the patient does not believe he or she has voluntary control. The goal of biofeedback is to increase patient awareness of and bring under voluntary control specific physiological functions associated with or presumed to underlie headache (Penzien & Holroyd, 1994; Schwartz & Andrasik, 2003). Biological or physiological information is sensed, converted into a signal that is understandable to the patient, and then "fed back" via some type of display to facilitate voluntary control. Specific modalities are used for certain conditions, but multiple modalities are typically combined to create the biofeedback program.

Biofeedback takes one of two general approaches. The first approach seeks to facilitate overall relaxation, such as discussed for autogenic feedback. Feedback of muscle tension and sweat gland activity can be helpful in this regard as well. When used in this manner, training in various relaxation skills is often added, such as diaphragmatic breathing or visualization to induce the "relaxation response" (Benson, 1975); this response is designed to reduce sympathetic nervous system activity and activate the parasympathetic nervous system—approaches discussed more fully in the next section. The second approach targets specific response systems pivotal to migraine genesis and maintenance; thus it is more conceptually linked to the underlying physiology of migraine. These techniques include blood volume pulse (BVP) and electroencephalography (EEG) biofeedback. Recent literature on the neurophysiology of migraine and fMRI studies of pain networks suggests that behavioral interventions may be another way to target neuromodulation (Andrasik & Rime, 2007).

BVP biofeedback involves monitoring blood flow in the temporal artery and providing feedback to teach patients how to decrease or constrict blood flow. This approach, as first envisioned (Friar & Beatty, 1976), can be thought of as the nonpharmacologic counterpart to an abortive agent. The accumulated body of research is sufficient to establish it as an evidence-based approach (see the later section for further detail).

Techniques focusing on EEG activity take one of two approaches. The first derives from research examining the links between certain EEG frequency bands and the experience of pain (Jensen et al., 2008). This research suggests that the experience of pain is associated with lower amplitudes of slow brain wave activity (delta,

theta, and alpha) and higher amplitudes of faster brain wave activity (beta). Several reports involving uncontrolled series have appeared in the literature, but more well-controlled investigations are needed before making specific claims.

The second-line approach takes a different tack, focusing on the contingent negative variation response (CNV). The CNV is a slow cortical event-related potential that examines EEG activity occurring between presentations of a warning stimulus followed by an imperative stimulus—that is, a stimulus requiring a response by the individual. This potential reflects resource mobilization (e.g., expectation, attention, and motivation) (Elbert, 1993), with its amplitude arising from activation in the striato-thalamo-cortical loop (Elbert & Rockstroh, 1987). Studies with children and adults reveal that migraineurs have a heightened response (i.e., increased amplitude) to novel stimuli and that they do not habituate as readily over repeated trials as do non-migrainous controls (Kropp et al., 2002). The CNV response is regarded as reflecting anticipation of a migraine attack because its amplitude and habituation patterns change during the headache-free interval. Abnormalities gradually increase in the days before a migraine attack, with the most pronounced changes occurring just prior to the attack (Siniatchkin et al., 2006).

One study (the only one published on this topic to date) explored whether child migraineurs could learn, via biofeedback, to alter their CNV activity and whether this technique would favorably alter the subsequent course of the participants' migraine attacks (Siniatchkin et al., 2000). Ten child migraineurs, without aura, were provided with CNV biofeedback where they were taught how to both decrease and increase EEG negativity (bidirectional control of a physiological response is assumed to reflect a greater level of self-regulation). Following 10 sessions of treatment, children were able to regulate their CNV activity, but only when feedback was provided. The number of biofeedback sessions administered was low, considering that EEG treatment sessions for other conditions typically utilize 20 to 40 sessions. A greater number of sessions might have led to greater response generalization. Of more interest is the finding that baseline or tonic levels of CNV negativity changed over treatment, so much so that the child migraineurs were no longer distinguishable from a matched sample of healthy controls, and suggesting their level of cortical excitability may have diminished. CNV biofeedback led to improvements on most measures of headache activity when compared to a group of child migraineurs who comprised a waiting-list control group. These preliminary findings add to those previously briefly mentioned for other EEG biofeedback approaches, suggesting further investigations of this strategy are warranted.

Relaxation Training

Relaxation techniques focus on minimizing physiological responses to stress and decreasing sympathetic arousal. The classic procedure "Progressive Muscle Relaxation Training" (PMRT), first introduced by Jacobson in a publication in 1938, is based on muscle discrimination training and is implemented by systematically tensing and relaxing various muscle groups while taking note of the contrasting sensations. By exaggerating and then relaxing muscle tension levels, the patient learns how to discriminate various tension states and the associated feelings. Also, when vigorous contractions are stopped, the muscles reflexively return to a lower state of tension (through the process of homeostasis), further enhancing discrimination learning. As patients become increasingly aware of rising tension states, they can then engage in strategies to counteract tension buildup.

Because it is impossible to experience tension and relaxation at the same time, Wolpe (1958) used PMRT as part of the desensitizing procedure for treatment of phobias. Soon afterward, PMRT became an essential tool in the treatment of anxiety, phobias, and other related disorders; it is now used for a variety of conditions characterized by hyperarousal, including migraine pain. Other commonly utilized clinical relaxation techniques include visual or guided imagery, cue-controlled relaxation, diaphragmatic breathing, hypnosis (therapist- or self-applied), meditation, prayer, yoga, listening to pleasant music, and any other method the patient finds effective for quieting the mind and body (Hall, 2011; Rime & Andrasik, 2011; see Chapter 25 of the current textbook).

Relaxation training is usually taught by clinical professionals, such as psychologists, social workers, occupational therapists, and other health-care providers, but it can also be self-taught by patients with print or audio support materials. Regular practice in the patient's day-to-day setting is required to realize the full benefits and implement the strategies when needed.

Cognitive-Behavioral Therapy

Cognitive-behavioral therapy (CBT) has been demonstrated to be an effective intervention for headache management (Campbell et al., 2000). CBT is also effective in treating depression, anxiety, panic attacks, obsessive–compulsive disorder, eating disorders, and sleep disorders, among other conditions. These conditions are frequently noted to be comorbid with migraine.

CBT, as the name implies, consists of both cognitive and behavioral strategies. Cognitive strategies focus on identifying and challenging maladaptive or dysfunctional thoughts, beliefs, and responses to stress (Beck et al., 1979; Holroyd & Andrasik, 1982; McCarran & Andrasik, 1987). Behavioral strategies identify and modify behaviors that may precipitate, increase, or maintain undesirable or unhealthy states; in the case of headache, this includes modifying triggers and promoting healthy lifestyle habits.

Cognitive targets of CBT for headache management include enhancing self-efficacy (Bandura, 1977), reducing "catastrophizing" (a hopeless and overwhelming thinking pattern, which has been shown to predict poor outcome and reduced quality of life; (Holroyd et al., 2007), and helping patients adopt an internal locus of control (i.e., a belief that the mechanism for change lies within oneself) as opposed to an external locus of control (i.e., the belief that only the physician, medication, or medical procedures have the power for change) (French et al., 2000; Heath et al., 2008). Other targets of CBT for headache include assertiveness training, increased coping and problem-solving skills, and stress management.

Behavioral targets of CBT for migraine include a focus on healthy lifestyle habits, avoidance of triggers (which often includes the use of headache daily diaries), and lifestyle modification. To maintain stability in the autonomic nervous system, persons with headache should strive to maintain a regular and healthy lifestyle, including a regular sleep–wake schedule, a regular and healthy diet, regular exercise, avoidance of excessive caffeine or alcohol consumption, refraining from smoking or using nicotine, and regular practice of stress management, relaxation techniques, and self-care, especially during times when they are most vulnerable to an attack (e.g., premenstrually).

Some patients have the benefit of fairly predictable migraine attacks. For these patients, particular triggers, time periods, and prodromal symptoms provide windows of opportunity in which to deploy behavioral tools to stop or slow the process of migraine early, even before headache onset. It is important for patients to keep a diary to note these associations. Of course, some triggers cannot be changed or avoided, such as the menstrual cycle; in such cases, patients should be aware of their vulnerability to headache during this time and protect themselves by following a very healthy lifestyle. By doing so, they may reduce the number of headache attacks, although it is unlikely that they will disappear altogether. Patients may be able to modify or eliminate other triggers as well.

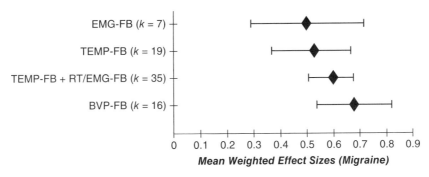

Figure 24.1 Mean Weighted Effect Sizes for the Different Feedback Modalities in the Treatment of Migraine. Outcome is measured in headache pain. Mean effect sizes are displayed with their individual 95% confidence intervals (*k* = number of independent effect sizes). EMG/FB, electromyographic feedback; TEMP-FB, peripheral temperature feedback; RT, relaxation training; BVP-FB, blood-volume pulse feedback.

EMPIRICAL EVIDENCE BASE FOR BIOBEHAVIORAL THERAPIES

Biobehavioral treatments have been the subject of many evidence-based reviews, including both quantitative (meta-analyses) and qualitative (study-by-study reviews conducted by evidentiary panels) reviews. Meta-analyses abound and uniformly support the utility of these approaches (see Andrasik, 2007, for a historical summary and Nestoriuc & Martin, 2007, and Nestoriuc et al., 2008, for recent examples).

The most recent meta-analysis (Nestoriuc et al., 2008) is contained in a comprehensive efficacy ("white paper") review of existing investigations of biofeedback for migraine (as well as for tension-type headache).

Efficacy recommendations were provided as part of this analysis, according to guidelines jointly established by the Association for Applied Psychophysiology and Biofeedback (AAPB) and the International Society for Neurofeedback and Research (ISNR) (LaVaque et al., 2002). Effect sizes were computed for nearly 100 outcome studies that met rigid inclusion criteria, of which we report only those for migraine. Medium-to-large mean effect sizes were found for biofeedback treatment of migraine in adults, with effects being maintained over an average follow-up period of 14 months (both in completer and intention-to-treat analyses; see **Figure 24.1**). Nestoriuc et al. (2008) examined effects for secondary variables as well, something not included in prior analyses. **Figure 24.2** (which also reports findings for various

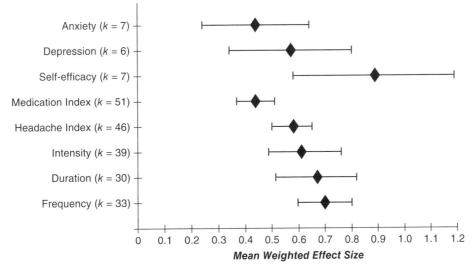

Figure 24.2 Mean Weighted Effect Sizes for the Different Outcome Variables in the Biofeedback Treatment of Migraine. Outcome is measured in headache pain over all biofeedback modalities. Mean effect sizes are displayed with their individual 95% confidence intervals (*k* = number of independent effect sizes).

headache indices) shows that biofeedback led to significant improvements in perceived self-efficacy, symptoms of depression and anxiety, and medication use. The authors concluded that biofeedback can be supported as an efficacious treatment option for migraine with a confidence of Level 4 evidence (efficacious) according to the AAPB/ ISNR criteria, which corresponds to a grade of 1A + according to van Kleef et al. (2009).

A more expanded meta-analysis of nonpharmacological treatments for migraine sponsored by the U.S. Agency for Healthcare Research and Quality (AHRQ) identified 355 studies of behavioral and physical treatments (Goslin et al., 1999). Few of these investigations (70 of 355) were controlled trials of behavioral treatments, and fewer yet (39 of 355) met the criteria for inclusion in the meta-analysis. Nevertheless, these authors found similar support for biobehavioral treatments of migraine.

A number of consensus-based reviews, conducted by expert panels, have also weighed the evidence for CBT treatments, with the most ambitious of these analyses being commissioned by the U.S. Headache Consortium. One large panel of experts included representatives from the American Academy of Family Physicians, American Academy of Neurology, American Headache Society, American College of Emergency Physicians, American College of Physicians, American Society of Internal Medicine, American Osteopathic Association, and National Headache Foundation (Campbell et al., 2000). The U.S. Headache Consortium was charged with developing "scientifically sound, clinically relevant practice guidelines on chronic headache in the primary care setting," and asked to "propose diagnostic and therapeutic recommendations to improve the care and satisfaction of migraine patients" based on a review of the current literature (Goslin et al., 1999). It used the following grading system based on the quality of evidence (Fiore et al., 1996), which closely approximates the scheme of van Kleef et al. (2009):

- Grade A: Multiple well-designed randomized clinical trials, directly relevant to the recommendation, yielded a consistent pattern of findings.
- Grade B: Some evidence from randomized clinical trials supported the recommendation, but the scientific support was not optimal (e.g., either few randomized trials existed, existing trials were somewhat inconsistent, or trials were not directly relevant to the recommendation).

The Consortium awarded grade A to the following treatments: relaxation training, thermal biofeedback combined with relaxation training, electromyographic biofeedback, and cognitive-behavioral therapy (for prevention of migraine). Grade B was assigned to the evidence for behavioral therapy combined with preventive drug therapy to achieve added clinical improvement for migraine.

The U.S. Headache Consortium pointed out conditions where biobehavioral approaches might be particularly well suited:

- Patients who have a preference for nonpharmacological interventions
- Patients who display a poor tolerance for specific pharmacological treatments
- Patients who exhibit medical contraindications for specific pharmacological treatments
- Patients who have insufficient or no response to pharmacological treatment
- Patients who are pregnant, are planning to become pregnant, or are nursing
- Patients who have a history of long-term, frequent, or excessive use of analgesic or acute medications that can aggravate headache problems (or lead to decreased responsiveness to other pharmacotherapies)
- Patients who exhibit significant stress or deficient stress-coping skills

Biobehavioral techniques have also demonstrated efficacy with children and adolescents (Hermann et al., 1995; Holden et al., 1999; Hermann & Blanchard, 2002). Migraine commonly first occurs during adolescence or early adulthood. By encouraging patients to train their physiological responses through biofeedback and relaxation, adopt healthy lifestyle habits, and recognize and mediate the effects of stress in their lives, health-care providers can give these individuals a set of tools that can last a lifetime.

INTEGRATING BIOBEHAVIORAL TREATMENT WITH PHARMACOLOGICAL TREATMENT

The previously mentioned therapies may be offered individually or in conjunction with a pharmacologic regimen, with the latter being the most common approach. Meta-analyses comparing behavioral and pharmacological (prophylactic) treatments have shown similar efficacy between the two approaches (Holroyd & Penzien, 1990; Penzien et al., 1990; Holroyd et al., 1991, 1992). These meta-analytic findings of comparable outcomes for behavioral and medication treatments are consistent with the findings from the few direct comparisons that have been conducted for migraine headache (Mathew, 1981; Holroyd et al., 1988).

The combination of pharmacological and nonpharmacologic approaches has been demonstrated to be more effective than either approach on its own (Holroyd et al., 1995), to help maintain positive outcomes (Grazzi et al., 2002; Andrasik et al., 2009), and to improve treatment adherence (Rains et al., 2006a, 2006b).

MIGRAINE AND PSYCHOLOGICAL COMORBIDITIES, HEALTH-RELATED QUALITY OF LIFE, AND PRODUCTIVITY

Migraine is associated with increased odds for a number of comorbid psychiatric conditions, including depression, anxiety, panic disorder, obsessive–compulsive disorder, bipolar disorder, childhood abuse and neglect, posttraumatic stress disorder (PTSD), and suicide attempts (Breslau & Davis, 1993; Jette et al., 2008). In a cross-sectional analysis, the gender-adjusted odds ratio for migraineurs for these disorders ranged from 2.6 for phobias to 6.6 for panic disorder. Migraine and depression are bidirectional; thus individuals who experience one of these conditions are at a higher risk for developing the other (Breslau & Davis, 1993).

Screening, assessment, referral, and education about common psychiatric comorbidities should be included in routine headache care. Brief screening instruments can be used to assess depression and anxiety (Maizels et al., 2006). The PHQ-4 is a two-item screening instrument that has been empirically shown to detect the presence of depression and anxiety; it contains two screening items for each disorder (Whooley et al., 1997). The PHQ-9 (adapted from Prime MD Today, developed by Spitzer et al., 2006) can be used to conduct a more thorough depression assessment and assign a diagnosis based on DSM-IV criteria (American Psychiatric Association, 2000), while the GAD-7 can be used to assess generalized anxiety (Spitzer et al., 2006). Questionnaires may be used at a screening or initial visit or to track progress or changes over time (Lemstra et al., 2002).

Migraine negatively affects quality of life, with its effects being felt on many aspects of sufferers' lives. Lipton et al. (2003) found that migraineurs scored significantly worse in eight of the nine domains and the two scores of the SF-36. Migraine is also associated with headache-related disability and lost time and productivity during work, family, and leisure time (Dueland et al., 2004). Migraine can place a significant burden on sufferers' lives, both during attacks and interictally (Buse et al., 2007).

Chronic migraine—an ICHD-2 diagnosis given for 15 or more headache days per month over the past 3 months, of which at least 8 headache days per month meet criteria for migraine without aura or respond to migraine-specific treatment (ICHD-II, 2004)—is especially burdensome. Compared with people with episodic migraine, individuals with chronic migraine have greater migraine-related disability, more impairment in quality of life, greater headache-related disability, worse healthcare costs and lost productivity, and more medical and psychiatric comorbidities (Buse et al., 2010). Migraine can be conceptualized as a chronic disorder with episodic manifestations (Haut et al., 2006). Patients with migraine may spontaneously remit for unknown reasons, they may continue to have intermittent attacks for many decades, or they may develop chronic migraine headache (i.e., progression). Biobehavioral techniques can be employed to reduce the risk of progression of migraine from episodic to chronic migraine. Several risk factors for progression have been identified (Bigal & Lipton, 2006), some of which are nonremediable (e.g., gender, age, race), and some of which are especially well targeted by biobehavioral techniques (e.g., frequency of migraine attacks, obesity, acute medication overuse, caffeine overuse, stressful life events, depression, anxiety, and sleep disorders).

CONCLUSIONS

A large and constantly growing body of published evidence has examined the use of behavioral therapies for migraine (and other forms of headache), including meta-analytic studies and evidence-based reviews (Andrasik, 2007; Nestoriuc & Martin, 2007). Evidence-based nonpharmacological (biobehavioral) treatments for migraine management include biofeedback, relaxation training, cognitive-behavioral therapy, education, and lifestyle modification. These behavioral treatments have been found to be superior to various control conditions, and the benefits from these treatments are generally maintained over time. They may be used individually or in conjunction with pharmacological and other interventions, and may augment the effectiveness of other treatments or minimize the need for their use. A combination of pharmacological and nonpharmacological approaches has been demonstrated to be superior to either approach on its own, so as to help maintain positive outcomes and to improve treatment adherence.

Patients can be taught ways to modify thoughts, feelings, and behavior with CBT. CBT interventions aid in headache management by making patients more aware of triggers, including the relationship between stress and headache, and by identifying and challenging counterproductive or self-defeating beliefs and ideas. Patients can be taught to manage the physiological effects of stress with biofeedback and relaxation training. They should be encouraged to adopt an internal locus of control and to consider treatment to be a collaborative process. Patients should be educated about times and situations in which they may be most vulnerable to an attack. During these periods, they need to be especially aware of potential triggers and the importance of avoiding stress, engage in relaxing and nurturing activities, and maintain a very regular and healthy lifestyle.

Stress, depression, anxiety, and other psychological and emotional factors are related to migraine, and many psychological conditions have elevated rates of comorbidity with migraine. Patients should be routinely assessed and appropriately treated or referred for management of these psychological comorbidities. Improvements in psychological comorbidities may translate into improvements in headache status, and vice versa.

The treatments and strategies reviewed in this chapter can help build feelings of self-efficacy and encourage patients to actively participate in the management of their migraines. Some behavioral techniques can be incorporated by health-care providers during an appointment (e.g., communication strategies, education, diaphragmatic breathing, and guided imagery), some can be self-taught and practiced by the patient (e.g., relaxation practice and stress management), and some require a referral to an appropriately trained professional (e.g., biofeedback training, CBT).

Biobehavioral tools should be used prophylactically and practiced on a regular basis so as to maintain homeostasis and manage stress, thereby ensuring that the patient does not allow these factors to trigger a headache attack in the first place. Health-care providers can utilize these strategies with their patients on a daily basis, whether by helping patients gain a more realistic understanding of their illness, helping patients recognize the effort and contribution that they themselves must make in their treatment (i.e., enhancing self-efficacy and encouraging an internal locus of control), or instructing patients to maintain a headache diary to facilitate assessment and treatment planning. By encouraging patients to train their physiology through biofeedback and relaxation, adopt healthy lifestyle habits, and recognize and mediate the effects of stress in their lives through CBT, the health-care provider gives patients a set of tools that can last a lifetime.

REFERENCES

Alemi F, Mosavel M, Stephens RC, et al. Electronic self-help and support groups. *Med Care* 1996;34:OS32–OS44.

American Psychiatric Association. *Diagnostic and Statistical Manual of Mental Disorders.* 4th ed. Washington, DC: American Psychiatric Press; 2000.

Andrasik F. What does the evidence show? Efficacy of behavioral treatment for recurrent headaches in adults. *Neurol Sci* 2007;28:S70–S77.

Andrasik F, Rime C. Can behavioural therapy influence neuromodulation? *Neurol Sci* 2007;28:S124–S129.

Andrasik F, Buse DC, Grazzi L. Behavioral medicine for migraine and medication overuse headache. *Curr Pain Headache Rep* 2009;13:241–248.

Bandura A. Self-efficacy: Toward a unifying theory of behavioral change. *Psychol Rev* 1977;84:191–215.

Bandura A. *Social Foundations of Thought and Action: A Social Cognitive Theory.* Englewood Cliffs, NJ: Prentice Hall; 1986.

Beck AT, Rush AJ, Shaw BF, et al. *Cognitive Therapy of Depression.* New York: Guilford Press; 1979.

Benson H. *The Relaxation Response.* New York: William Morrow; 1975.

Bigal ME, Lipton RB. Modifiable risk factors for migraine progression. *Headache* 2006;46:1334–1343.

Blumenfeld A, Tischio M. Center of excellence for headache care: group model at Kaiser Permanente. *Headache* 2003;43:431–440.

Breslau N, Davis GC. Migraine, physical health and psychiatric disorder: a prospective epidemiologic study in young adults. *J Psychiatr Res* 1993;27:211–221.

Buse DC, Bigal ME, Rupnow MFT, et al. The Migraine Interictal Burden Scale (MIBS): results of a population-based validation study. *Headache* 2007;47:778.

Buse DC, Manack A, Serrano D, et al. Socio-demographic and co-morbidity profiles of chronic migraine and episodic migraine sufferers. *J Neurol Neurosurg Psychiatry* 2010;81:428–432.

Cady R., Farmer K, Beach ME, et al. Nurse-based education: an office-based comparative model for education of migraine patients. *Headache* 2007;48:564–569.

Cameron C. Patient compliance: recognition of factors involved and suggestions for promoting compliance with therapeutic regimens. *J Adv Nurs* 1996;24:244–250.

Campbell JK, Penzien DB, Wall EM. Evidence-based guidelines for migraine headache: behavioral and physical treatments. US Headache Consortium; 2000. Available at: http://www.aan.com. Accessed July 2008.

Claxton AJ, Cramer J, Pierce C. A systematic review of the associations between dose regimens and medication compliance. *Clin Ther* 2001;23:1296–1310.

Dueland AN, Leira R, Burke TA, et al. The impact of migraine on work, family, and leisure among young women: a multinational study. *Curr Med Res Opin* 2004;20:1595–1604.

Dunbar-Jacob J, Mortimer-Stephens MK. Treatment adherence in chronic disease. *J Clin Epidemiol* 2001;54:S57–S60.

Dunbar-Jacob J, Erlen JA, Schlenk EA, et al. Adherence in chronic disease. *Annu Rev Nurs Res* 2000;18:48–90.

Eddy DM. *Evidence-Based Clinical Improvements.* Presentation at Directions for Success: Evidence-Based Health Care

Symposium sponsored by Group Health Cooperative; Tucson, AZ; May 7–9, 2001.

Edmeads J, Findlay H, Tugwell P, et al. Impact of migraine and tension-type headache on life-style, consulting behaviour, and medication use: a Canadian population survey. *Can J Neurol Sci* 1993;20:131–137.

Elbert T. Slow cortical potentials reflect the regulation of cortical excitability. In: McCallum WC, Curry SH, eds. *Slow Potential Changes in the Human Brain*. New York: Plenum; 1993:235–251.

Elbert T, Rockstroh B. Threshold regulation: a key to understanding the combined dynamics of EEG and event-related potentials. *J Psychophysiol* 1987;4:317–333.

Elder JP, Ayala GX, Harris S. Theories and intervention approaches to health-behavior change in primary care. *Am J Prev Med* 1999;17:275–284.

Fiore M, Bailey W, Cohen S, et al. *Smoking Cessation Clinical Practice Guideline No. 18*. Rockville: Agency for Health Care Policy and Research, U.S. Department of Health and Human Services; 1996.

French DJ, Holroyd KA, Pinell C, et al. Perceived self-efficacy and headache-related disability. *Headache* 2000;40:647–656.

Friar LR, Beatty J. Migraine: management by trained control of vasoconstriction. *J Consult Clin Psychol* 1976;44:46–53.

Gallagher RM, Kunkel R. Migraine medication attributes important for patient compliance: concerns about side effects may delay treatment. *Headache* 2003;43:36–43.

Goslin RE, Gray RN, McCrory DC, et al. Behavioral and physical treatments for migraine headache. Technical review 2.2 February 1999. Prepared for the Agency for Health Care Policy and Research under Contract No. 290-94-2025. Available at: http://www.clinpol.mc.due.edu. Accessed July 2008.

Grazzi L, Andrasik F, D'Amico D, et al. Behavioral and pharmacologic treatment of transformed migraine with analgesic overuse: outcome at three years. *Headache* 2002;42:483–490.

Hahn SR. Communication in the care of the headache patient. In: Silberstein SD, Lipton RL, Dodick DW, eds. *Wolff's Headache and Other Head Pain*. New York: Oxford University Press; 2008:805–824.

Hahn SR, Lipton RB, Sheftell FD, et al. Healthcare provider–patient communication and migraine assessment: results of the American Migraine Communication Study (AMCS) Phase II. *Curr Med Res Opin* 2008;24:1711–1718.

Hall, H. Hypnosis. In: Waldman SD, ed. *Pain Management*. Vol. 2, 2nd ed. Philadelphia: Saunders-Elsevier; 2011.

Harpole L, Samsa G, Jurgelski A, et al. Headache management program improves outcome for chronic headache. *Headache* 2003;43:715–724.

Haut SR, Bigal ME, Lipton RB. Chronic disorders with episodic manifestations: focus on epilepsy and migraine. *Lancet Neurol* 2006;5:148–157.

Heath RL, Saliba M, Mahmassani O, et al. Locus of control moderates the relationship between headache pain and depression. *J Headache Pain* 2008;9:301–308.

Hermann C, Blanchard EB. Biofeedback in the treatment of headache and other childhood pain. *Appl Psychophysiol Biofeedback* 2002;27:143–162.

Hermann C, Kim M, Blanchard EB. Behavioral and prophylactic pharmacological intervention studies of pediatric migraine: an exploratory meta-analysis. *Pain* 1995;20:239–256.

Holden EW, Deichmann MM, Levy JD. Empirically supported treatments in pediatric psychology: recurrent pediatric headache. *J Pediatr Psychol* 1999;24:91–109.

Holroyd KA, Andrasik F. A cognitive-behavioral approach to recurrent tension and migraine headache. In: Kendall PC, ed. *Advances in Cognitive-Behavioral Research and Therapy*. Vol. 1. New York: Academic; 1982:275–320.

Holroyd KA, Penzien DB. Pharmacological versus non-pharmacological prophylaxis of recurrent migraine headache: a meta-analytic review of clinical trials. *Pain* 1990;42:1–13.

Holroyd KA, Holm JE, Hursey KG, et al. Recurrent vascular headache: home-based behavioral treatment vs. abortive pharmacological treatment. *J Consult Clin Psychol* 1988;56:218–223.

Holroyd KA, Cordingley GE, Pingel JD, et al. Enhancing the effectiveness of abortive therapy: a controlled evaluation of self-management training. *Headache* 1989;29:148–153.

Holroyd KA, Penzien DB, Cordingley GE. Propranolol in the management of recurrent migraine: a meta-analytic review. *Headache* 1991;3:333–340.

Holroyd KA, Penzien DB, Rokicki LA, et al. Flunarizine vs. propranolol: a meta-analysis of clinical trials. Headache 1992;32:256.

Holroyd KA, France JL, Cordingley GE, et al. Enhancing the effectiveness of relaxation–thermal biofeedback training with propranolol hydrochloride. *J Consult Clin Psychol* 1995;63:327–330.

Holroyd KA, Drew JB, Cottrell CK, et al. Impaired functioning and quality of life in severe migraine: the role of catastrophizing and associated symptoms. *Cephalalgia* 2007;27:1156–1165.

ICHD-II. Headache Classification Subcommittee of the International Headache Society. The International Classification of Headache Disorders, 2nd ed. *Cephalalgia* 2004;24(suppl 1):1–160.

Jacobson E. *Progressive Relaxation*. Chicago: University of Chicago Press; 1938.

Jensen MP. Enhancing motivations to change in pain treatment. In: Turk DC, Gatchel RJ, eds *Psychological Approaches to Pain Management: A Practitioner's Handbook*. 2nd ed. New York: Guilford Press; 2002:71–93.

Jensen MP, Hakimian S, Sherlin LH, Fregni F. New insights into neuromodulatory approaches for the treatment of pain. *J Pain* 2008;9:193–199.

Jette N, Patten S, Williams J, et al S. Co-morbidity of migraine and psychiatric disorders: a national population-based study. *Headache* 2008;48:501–516.

Klapper J, Stanton J, Seawell M. The development of a support group organization for headache sufferers. *Headache* 1992;32:193–196.

Kropp P, Siniatchkin M, Gerber WD. On the patho-physiology of migraine: links for empirically based treatment with neurofeedback. *Appl Psychophysiol Biofeedback* 2002;27:203–213.

LaVaque TJ, Hammond DC, Trudeau D, et al. Template for developing guidelines for the evaluation of the clinical efficacy of psycho-physiological interventions. Efficacy Task Force. *Appl Psychophysiol Biofeedback* 2002;27:273–281.

Lemstra M, Stewart B, Olszynski W. Effectiveness of multi-disciplinary intervention in the treatment of migraine: a randomized clinical trial. *Headache* 2002;42:845–854.

Lipton RB, Liberman JN, Kolodner KB, et al. Migraine headache disability and health-related quality-of-life: a population-based case-control study from England. *Cephalalgia* 2003;23:441–450.

Maizels M, Smitherman TA, Penzien DB. A review of screening tools for psychiatric comorbidity in headache patients. *Headache* 2006;46:S98–S109.

Mathew NT. Prophylaxis of migraine and mixed headache: a randomized controlled study. *Headache* 1981;21:105–109.

McCarran MS, Andrasik F. Migraine and tension headaches. In: Michelson L, Ascher M, eds. *Anxiety and Stress Disorders: Cognitive-Behavioral Assessment and Treatment.* New York: Guilford Press; 1987:465–483.

Miller WR. Motivational interviewing: research, practice, and puzzles. *Addictive Behaviors* 1996;21:835–842.

Miller WR, Rollnick S. *Motivational Interviewing: Preparing People for Change.* 2nd ed. New York: Guilford Press; 2002.

Motheral BR, Henderson R. The effect of copay increase on pharmaceutical utilization, expenditures, and treatment continuation. *Am J Manag Care* 1999;5:1383–1394.

Nestoriuc Y, Martin A. Efficacy of biofeedback for migraine: a meta-analysis. *Pain* 2007;128:111–127.

Nestoriuc Y, Martin A, Rief W, Andrasik F. Biofeedback treatment for headache disorders: a comprehensive efficacy review. *Appl Psychophysiol Biofeedback* 2008;33:125–140.

Penzien DB, Holroyd KA. Psychosocial interventions in the management of recurrent headache disorders II: description of treatment techniques. *Behav Med* 1994;20:64–73.

Penzien DB, Johnson CA, Carpenter DE, et al. Drug vs. behavioral treatment of migraine: long-acting propranolol vs. home-based self-management training. *Headache* 1990;30:300.

Prochaska JO, Redding A, Evers KE. The transtheoretical model and stages of change. In: Glanz K, Lewis FM, Rimer BK, eds. *Health Behavior and Health Education.* San Francisco: Jossey-Bass; 1997:60–84.

Rains JC, Lipchik GL, Penzien DB. Behavioral facilitation of medical treatment for headache. Part I: review of headache treatment compliance. *Headache* 2006a;46:1387–1394.

Rains JC, Penzien DB, Lipchik GL. Behavioral facilitation of medical treatment for headache. Part II: theoretical models and behavioral strategies for improving adherence. *Headache* 2006b;46:1395–1403.

Rime C, Andrasik F. Relaxation techniques and guided imagery. In: Waldman SD, ed. *Pain Management.* Vol. 2, 2nd ed. Philadelphia: Saunders/Elsevier; 2011.

Rothrock JF, Parada VA, Sims C, et al. The impact of intensive patient education on clinical outcome in a clinic-based migraine population. *Headache* 2006;46:726–731.

Sargent JD, Green EE, Walters ED. The use of autogenic training in a pilot study of migraine and tension headaches. *Headache* 1972;12:120–124.

Sargent JD, Green EE, Walters ED. Preliminary report on the use of autogenic feedback training in the treatment of migraine and tension headaches. *Psychosom Med* 1973;35:129–135.

Schultz JH, Luthe W. *Autogenic Therapy.* Vol. 1. New York: Grune & Stratton; 1969.

Schwartz MS, Andrasik F. Headache. In: *Biofeedback: A Practitioner's Guide.* 3rd ed. New York: Guilford Press; 2003:275–348.

Siniatchkin M, Hierundar A, Kropp P, et al. Self-regulation of slow cortical potentials in children with migraine: an exploratory study. *Appl Psychophysiol Biofeedback* 2000;25:13–32.

Siniatchkin M, Averkina N, Andrasik F, et al. Neurophysiological reactivity before a migraine attack. *Neurosci Lett* 2006;400:121–124.

Spierings EL, Miree LF. Non-compliance with follow-up and improvement after treatment at a headache center. *Headache* 1993;33:205–209.

Spitzer RL, Kroenke K, Williams JB, et al. A brief measure for assessing generalized anxiety disorder: the GAD-7. *Arch Intern Med* 2006;166:1092–1097.

Urquhart J. Patient non-compliance with drug regimens: measurement, clinical correlates, economic impact. *Eur Heart J* 1996;17(suppl A):8–15.

van Kleef M, Mekhail N, van Zundert J. Evidence-based guidelines for interventional pain medicine according to clinical diagnoses. *Pain Practice* 2009;9:247–251.

Whooley MA, Avins AL, Miranda J, et al. Case-finding instruments for depression: two questions are as good as many. *J Gen Intern Med* 1997;12:439–445.

Wolpe J. *Psychotherapy by Reciprocal Inhibition.* Stanford: Stanford University Press; 1958.

Hypnosis for Pain Management

Nicole Malaise, MA, Irène Salamun, MA, Valérie Palmaricciotti, MA, and
Marie-Elisabeth Faymonville, MD, PhD

INTRODUCTION

Chronic and persistent pain syndromes are as much physical and medical problems as behavioral and psychological problems. Chronic headache or migraine is not detectable or measurable on the basis of the traditional, physical, tissue-oriented medical disease model. Pain evaluation requires acknowledging and understanding a multifaceted biopsychosocial model that transcends the usual, more limited disease model.

The segments of the pain patient population termed "medically treatable up to a point" represent the majority of pain sufferers, and many of these patients can benefit from hypnosis.

A mounting body of evidence indicates that focused psychological intervention can improve pain management outcomes by helping pain patients learn self-management techniques and build coping skills.

Although hypnosis has probably been known since antiquity, its contemporary use for pain management was first documented in the nineteenth century, as Elliotson (1843) reported using "mesmeric sleep" as an effective anesthetic during surgery. Since then, hypnosis has enjoyed a long-standing history of relieving pain (Barber, 1996; Patterson & Ptacek, 1997).

In the twentieth century, hypnosis was greatly developed both from a clinical perspective and a conceptual point of view by psychologists and psychiatrists (Erickson et al., 1976). Recent research has described it as an empirically supported clinical intervention, often being incorporated as part of a treatment program, for a number of psychological and medical conditions (Lynn et al., 2000).

More particularly, hypnosis is considered as an interesting option for the relief of many forms of pain and is widely taught and used for this purpose in clinics, hospitals, burn care centers, and dental offices. Applications include the treatment of acute or chronic pain, as well as hypnosedation in surgery, an anesthetic technique combining hypnosis, local anesthesia, and light intravenous sedation, that allows the patient to remain conscious and feel comfortable during interventional radiology and different and various surgical procedures (Defechereux et al., 2000; Lang et al., 2000; Faymonville et al., 2006).

The purposes of this chapter are fourfold: (1) to provide a brief definition of hypnosis, hypnotic process, and self-hypnosis; (2) to describe briefly the neurophysiological correlates of hypnosis and hypnotic analgesia; (3) to provide a short review of recent literature concerning the effectiveness of clinical hypnosis in chronic pain, emphasizing more specifically research on the effectiveness of hypnosis with migraine; and (4) to address questions about this modality's clinical use.

SOME DEFINITIONS

It remains quite difficult to define hypnosis, although many authors have proposed their own definitions, reflecting their particular clinical perception and theoretical approaches (Green et al., 2005). "Hypnosis" as a word has been overused; indeed, the tendency to describe many different experiences as "hypnosis" yields ample opportunities for misconceptions to arise.

Hypnosis is defined as a set of techniques designed to enhance concentration, minimize one's usual distractions, and heighten responsiveness to suggestions to alter one's thoughts, feeling, behavior, or physiological state. The American Psychological Association's website includes a definition and description of hypnosis targeted toward informing clinicians, researchers, and the lay public alike. Nevertheless, there remains no commonly accepted definition and no single unifying theory to account for all the various facets of hypnosis.

Clinical hypnosis can be introduced as a system of skilled and influential communication that teaches how words can heal. Arranging the concepts and techniques of hypnosis into a useful definition is a difficult task (Edmonston, 1991):

- Hypnosis is a natural, altered state of consciousness. A person enters in a hypnotic state through a natural process.
- An individual in a hypnotic state is usually physically relaxed, while being mentally alert and focused.

- Hypnosis is a hypersuggestible state. The person enters a very relaxed state of mind and body and subsequently is more responsive to suggestion.
- The patient in a hypnotic state experiences suggested sensations, perceptions, and cognitions associated with his or her targeted therapeutic goals. Responses to these suggestions may seem as if they occur on their own.

The induction of hypnosis usually involves some sort of ritual for inducing an alteration in consciousness from whatever is an individual's typical state of mind and mood to a different relaxed, imagination-dominated state. The person "shifts" into this particular state. Hypnosis is a highly subjective experience, however. Some psychological characteristics, such as selective attention, dissociation, and increased responsiveness to suggestion, as well as physical characteristics, such as muscular relaxation, changes in breathing rate and pulse rate, and eye closure with fluttering eyelids, are observed. Each of these characteristics may be used as a general indicator of hypnosis, but no single sign by itself suffices to explain what the patient or volunteer is actually experiencing internally. Anything that focuses the patient's attention and facilitates feelings of comfort and well-being can be used to deepen the hypnotic process. Disengagement is the final stage of hypnotic interaction. When and how to disengage are a matter of individual clinical judgment, based on the overall treatment plan. Experimented hypnotists can easily proceed less formally and make use of conversational techniques.

Self-hypnosis consists of inducing the experience of hypnosis by oneself. This practice requires previous training with a hypnotist, most often in a classical way, and is furthered by practicing regularly alone, with or without the support of recorded tapes. Exercises are proposed based on the goals defined with the patient, including pain relief, and patients may also be encouraged to make use of their creativity to find by themselves interesting imaginative or memory supports. Other exercises aiming at modifying perception of oneself or one's behaviors in daily life may also be proposed, most often through a brief therapy or cognitive-behavioral perspective.

NEUROPHYSIOLOGICAL CORRELATES OF HYPNOSIS AND ITS PAIN MODULATION

Modern neuroimaging technologies have facilitated efforts for an improved understanding of the brain mechanisms involved in the pain experience, hypnosis, and pain modulation by hypnosis. Functional imaging techniques such as position emission tomography (PET) scanning and functional magnetic resonance imaging (fMRI) provide a means of evaluating modified brain function before, during, and after pain stimulation or hypnotic interventions that are independent of subjective reports.

Brain imaging with PET has identified some of the main cerebral structures in the central network activated by pain. The basic pain network is composed of approximately four functional groupings (Jones et al., 1991; Peyron et al., 1999; Büchel et al., 2002; Petrovic et al., 2002):

- The *sensory-perceptual component* includes the primary and secondary somatosensory cortices (S1 and S2) as well as portions of the thalamus and of the insular cortex.
- The *motor integratory group* includes the supplementary motor cortex, putamen, globus pallidus, several regions in the cerebellum, and mesencephalic regions.
- The *attentional component* is composed of the anterior cingulate cortex (ACC) and other prefrontal cortex regions and the posterior parietal cortex.
- The fourth system is related to *descending control*. Activation of the mesencephalic periaqueductal group is consistent with the idea that descending control processes can be activated during the administration of experimental pain stimuli. A stimulus response function in the perigenual ACC and the amygdala is also in accordance with the putative role of these areas in the emotional processing of aversive events.

Psychological states are able to modulate the perception of experimentally induced pain. Concerning hypnosis, theoretical debates on the mechanisms by which hypnosis produces its effects have stimulated theory-driven research, mainly related to two major theoretical lines of thought. According to proponents of a state theory, hypnosis is a special state of consciousness, characterized by heightened responsiveness to suggestions, and dependent on individual hypnotizability (the ability to enter a deep hypnotic state) (Hilgard & Hilgard, 1983). Proponents of a social-cognitive theory, in contrast, argue that the hypnotic phenomena and the appearance of a "hypnotic-like" state are the results of an active participation and social compliance of the subject, so as to respond to desirable suggestions (Spanos, 1991; Bowers, 1992).

Understanding the neural substrates of hypnosis has been possible with the advent of functional imaging. This technology provides a means of evaluating altered brain function during hypnotic interventions that is independent of subjective reports.

One hypnotic technique based on reliving pleasant autobiographical experiences and pleasant imagery of past events activates area 32 in the ACC—this area is known to become activated during happiness (George et al., 2005) and positive emotions (Vogt, 2005). Mental relaxation and absorbtion in hypnosis correlate with ACC activity (Rainville et al., 2002). It appears that some cognitive functions supported by the dorsolateral prefrontal cortex (DLPF), such as willed action, independent thinking, critical reflection, and initiative, are affected by hypnosis. During hypnosis, suggestions become the predominant content in the working memory buffers, albeit without the higher cognitive control exerted by the DLPF circuits. In addition, a regional decrease in structures such as the right inferior parietal precuneus and posterior cingular cortex occurs (Maquet et al., 1999); these structures are essential for the regulation of consciousness. The decreases in ventromedial prefrontal cortex (VMPFC) activity (Maquet et al., 1999; Rainville et al., 1999) could also reflect the observation of decreased initiative of movements.

Hypnosis researchers have long sought psychophysiological indicators of hypnotic analgesia. Some evidence indicates that hypnotic analgesia is associated with changes in the RIII component of the nociceptive reflexes (Kiernan et al., 1995; Langlade et al., 2002). Electroencephalographic (EEG) and evoked potential (EP) studies have shown some physiological correlates reflecting hypnotic analgesia: they observed reductions in late somatosensory potentials evoked by nociceptive stimuli during hypnosis; the changes were linked to perceived pain intensity changes, which seem not to be under conscious control (Crawford et al., 1998; De Pascalis et al., 1999).

Neuroimaging techniques have demonstrated hypnosis-induced changes in pain perception and its underlying brain mechanisms (Rainville et al., 1997; Faymonville et al., 2000). Such changes were associated with changes in activity in the mid-cingulate cortices (MCC). This functionally heterogeneous region, which is innervated by a multitude of neuromodulatory pathways (Paus, 2001), is thought to modulate interaction.

The anterior MCC appears pivotal to understanding cognitive modulation of pain by hypnosis (Craig et al., 1996; Peyron et al., 1999; Petrovic et al., 2002). This region is involved in assessing the motivational content of both internal and external stimuli as well as in regulating context-dependent behaviors (Devinsky et al., 1995). The hypnotic context, which relies on suggestions for relaxation and instructions to think about pleasant life experiences, lowers both unpleasantness and perceived intensity of the noxious stimuli (Faymonville et al., 2000). Hypnosis decreases both components of pain perception, with this modulatory effect being mediated by the anterior MCC (Rainville et al., 1997; Faymonville et al., 2000). Access of the ACC to the descending noxious inhibitory system (DNIC) may be pivotal to the mechanisms of hypnosis-induced analgesia. The induction of positive emotions during hypnosis activates area 32 and its projections to the periaqueductal gray (PAG) to engage the DNIS (Faymonville et al., 2009). Projections from the PAG inhibit the flow of nociceptive information out of the spinal cord and truncate nociceptive processing through the thalamus (Reynolds, 1969). Studies of functional cerebral connectivity have shown that the hypnosis-induced reduction of pain processing mediated by the MCC (Rainville et al., 1997, 1999; Faymonville et al., 2000) relates to an increased functional modulation between this MCC and a large neural network of cortical and subcortical structures known to be involved in different aspects of pain processing, encompassing the insular cortex, pregenual cortex, thalamus, striatum, prefrontal and pre-supplementar motor cortex, and brainstem (Faymonville et al., 2003). These findings point to a critical role for the ACC and MCC in hypnosis-related alteration of sensory, affective, cognitive, and behavioral aspects of nociception.

HYPNOSIS IN THE TREATMENT OF CHRONIC PAIN

As shown in the literature, hypnosis is useful in the management of chronic pain states (Montgomery et al., 2000; Patterson & Jensen, 2003; Jensen & Patterson, 2006). In their review, Elkins et al. (2007) emphasized that the number of controlled studies using hypnotic techniques is actually adequate to draw meaningful conclusions about the efficacy of hypnosis for chronic pain management. These researchers examined 13 controlled prospective trials of hypnosis for the treatment of chronic pain, excluding headache, and compared outcomes from hypnosis to either baseline data or control conditions, such as physical therapy, biofeedback, no treatment, or standard care conditions. Hypnotic interventions were found to produce a significant decrease in pain associated with a variety of chronic pain problems—namely, cancer pain, low back pain, arthritis, sickle cell disease, temporomandibular joint chronic pain, fibromyalgia, and physical disability of mixed etiologies.

Recently, Jensen (2009) examined four additional clinical trials, all of which supported the efficacy of self-hypnosis training for chronic pain management: idiopathic orofacial pain (Abrahamsen et al., 2008), chronic widespread pain (Grandahl & Rosvold, 2008), multiple sclerosis with chronic pain (Jensen et al., 2009a), and spinal cord injury and chronic pain (Jensen et al., 2009b).

Stoelb et al. (2009) also drew some conclusions about the efficacy of hypnotic analgesia in adults, based on previous reviews and recent randomized, controlled trials of hypnotic analgesia for the treatment of chronic and acute pain in adults. They summarized their conclusions as follows:

- Hypnotic analgesia consistently results in greater pain alleviation as compared to no treatment or standard care.
- Hypnosis frequently outperforms nonhypnotic interventions (e.g., education, supportive therapy) in terms of reductions in pain-related outcomes.
- Hypnosis performs similarly to treatments that contain hypnotic elements (such as progressive muscle relaxation), but is not surpassed in efficacy by these treatments.

Concerning children, Rogovik and Goldman (2007) emphasize in their review of the literature that hypnotic techniques have been systematically applied to children since the 1980s for a number of clinical conditions. In particular, such therapy has been directed toward alleviating pain during bone marrow aspiration, lumbar punctures, anxiety during angulated forearm reduction, postoperative pain and anxiety, and chronic pain states.

CLINICAL HYPNOSIS FOR CHRONIC HEADACHES

Hammond (2007) provides a review of clinical trials addressing the efficacy of hypnosis in the treatment of chronic tension headache and migraine. Among these, several concerned chronic headache. Melis et al. (1991) evaluated the effectiveness of hypnosis sessions (one session per week for 4 weeks, coupled with self-hypnosis training supported by recorded tapes made during each session) on 11 subjects, in comparison with a wait-list control group of 15 subjects. Significant reductions in the number of headache days, the number of headache hours, the intensity of headache pain, and anxiety scores were found at 4-week follow-up for the hypnotic-treatment group compared to the wait-list group. Van Dyck et al. (1991) studied the efficacy of autogenic training versus hypnosis imagery. In this investigation, 55 subjects were randomly assigned into two groups (28 to autogenic training and 27 to hypnosis). Both procedures were found equally effective in reducing headache pain, medication use, depression, and state anxiety.

Zitman et al. (1992) compared 89 patients split into three groups who received, over an 8-week period, an abbreviated form of autogenic training, a hypnotic treatment based on future-oriented pain-free imagery, and the same treatment without presenting it as hypnosis, respectively. All treatments were found equally effective in reducing headache after 1 month, but the hypnosis treatment presented as such was found superior to autogenic training in a 6-month follow-up.

Spanos et al. (1993) studied 136 students with chronic headache. They were randomized into three groups (imagery-based hypnotic treatment, placebo treatment called "subliminal reconditioning," and no-treatment control group). The researchers found, among other results, that the hypnotic treatment was more effective in decreasing medication overuse and headache.

Ter Kuile et al. (1994) evaluated autogenic training, cognitive self-hypnosis training, and a wait-list control condition. At the conclusion of a 6-month treatment regimen, both treatment groups showed a significant reduction in their Headache Index Scores compared with the wait-list control group.

Finally, Mannix et al. (1999) evaluated the effect of guided imagery on 129 patients with chronic tension-type headache, who were asked to listen daily during 1 month to a 20-minute guided imagery audiotape. After 1 month, both the patients in the imagery group and the patients in a control group receiving individual headache therapy (n = 131) were found to have improved in terms of headache frequency, severity global assessment, quality of life, and disability caused by headache. Nevertheless, significantly more patients in the guided imagery group reported that their headaches were much better and had significantly more improvement in pain, vitality, and mental health, as measured with the SF-36 test of quality of life.

EFFICACY OF CLINICAL HYPNOSIS WITH MIGRAINE

Anderson et al. (1975) studied the effectiveness of hypnosis by comparing two groups of subjects—one group receiving hypnotherapy, and the other group receiving standard care with prochlorperazine and ergotamine. The hypnotic treatment included induction, deepening, suggestive therapy, and ego-strengthening; subjects were also instructed in self-hypnosis to prevent migraine attacks and asked to practice self-hypnosis daily. Results showed that the monthly number of migraine headaches was significantly decreased in the hypnotic-treatment group. Alladin (1988), in his review of literature on hypnosis, identified several hypnotic techniques used in the treatment of chronic migraine. Hypnotic training emphasizing relaxation and hand warming, as well as hypnotic suggestions of symptom removal, were shown to be effective in reducing the duration, intensity, and frequency of migraine attacks.

Hammond (2007) reviewed the literature on the effectiveness of hypnosis for treating tension-type and migraine headaches, and discussed three studies, including Anderson's investigation (1975), addressing specifically migraine. Three treatment conditions were compared by Andreychuck and Skriver (1975): self-hypnosis training, biofeedback training with bipolar EEG montage connection in the left and right occipital areas (designed to enhance alpha brain waves), and biofeedback training for hand warming associated with listening to autogenic training tapes. In this study, 32 patients were randomly assigned to one of three groups and received one 45-minutes session per week for 10 weeks, as well as encouragement to practice twice a day between sessions. All groups experienced a significant reduction in migraine levels from pre- to post-treatment.

Olness et al. (1987) conducted a prospective, randomized, double-bind, placebo-controlled study with classic juvenile migraine. Children (aged 6 to 12) were randomly assigned to three groups: placebo/placebo/self-hypnosis, propanolol/placebo/self-hypnosis, or placebo/propanolol/self-hypnosis. At the end of one year, the mean number of migraines per child was significantly lower in the hypnosis group.

Emmerson and Trexler (1999) studied the efficacy of a 12-week hypnosis treatment on a single group of 32 patients, comparing pretreatment trends and post-treatment effects, within a time-series design. Treatment included group hypnosis sessions and use of prerecorded self-hypnosis tapes. Duration of migraine, migraine severity, post-treatment duration of migraine treatment, and medication use were significantly reduced with this regimen.

CONSENSUS ON HYPNOSIS AS AN EFFECTIVE TREATMENT FOR MIGRAINE

According to the report published by the Quality Standards Subcommittee of the American Academy of Neurology entitled "Practice Parameters: Evidence-Based Guidelines for Migraine Headache" (Silberstein, 2000):

1. Relaxation training, thermal biofeedback combined with relaxation training, electromyographic biofeedback, and cognitive therapy may be

considered as treatment options for prevention of migraine (evidence grade A).

2. Behavioral therapy may be combined with preventive drugs to achieve additional clinical improvement for migraine relief (evidence grade B).

3. Evidence-based treatment recommendations regarding the use of hypnosis, acupuncture, transcutaneous electrical nerve stimulation, chiropractic or osteopathic cervical manipulation, occlusal adjustment, and hyperbaric oxygen as preventive or acute therapy for migraine are not yet possible.

However, Hammond (2007), in his more recent review, concludes that the use of hypnosis with headache and migraine represents a well-established evidence-based practice for the treatment of chronic headaches and migraine, which is both efficacious and specific, according to the criteria needed to obtain the status of "well-established psychological treatment" (Chambless et al., 1998; Chambless & Hollon, 1998). Moreover, according to Hammond (2007), hypnosis is a treatment that is relatively brief and cost-effective, is virtually free of side effects or risks of adverse reactions, and reduces the ongoing expense associated with the widely used medication treatments.

PRACTICAL ISSUES

Although hypnotherapy is considered a relevant approach for the treatment of chronic pain, including migraine, several issues concerning its practical use are discussed in this section.

Are Hypnotherapeutic Treatments Suitable for Anyone?

Criteria for hypnotherapy may vary according to different authors, as reviewed by Salem (2004). It is usually assumed that caution must be used in selecting patients for hypnoanalgesic treatment: patients suffering from psychosis, organic psychiatric conditions, or antisocial/borderline personality disorders should not be treated by hypnosis. Due to psychiatric disturbance or psychological instability, there is a risk that the hypnotist may have difficulty in controlling or ending a hypnotic state that has been induced in the patient, or in controlling emotional reactions, which may further destabilize the patient. Patients with severe cognitive or neurologic problems (dementia, deafness) may be unable to cope with hypnotic suggestions as well (Zelinka et al., 2009).

Does Hypnotic Suggestibility Matter?

Jensen and Patterson (2006) indicate that, concerning hypnotic analgesia, hypnotic suggestibility and the ability to experience vivid images are often—but not always—associated with treatment outcomes in hypnosis and treatments including hypnotic elements (progressive muscle relaxation, autogenic training). Several studies have underlined the possibility that even patients with low suggestibility might benefit from hypnosis treatment (Andreychuck & Skriver, 1975; Friedman & Taub, 1984; Holroyd, 1996).

Andreychuck and Skriver (1975), in their study comparing the effectiveness of self-hypnosis and two forms of biofeedback training on migraine, showed, by cutting across the three groups, that highly hypnotizable subjects, as measured with the Hypnotic Induction Profile (Spiegel & Spiegel, 1978), demonstrate significant reduction in migraine as compared to low hypnotizable subjects.

Does Regular Hypnotic Practice Influence Outcomes?

Hypnosis, and especially self-hypnosis, requires the patient to learn and practice on a regular basis. Achieving these goals, in turn, requires motivation and self-discipline. This may be a difficult feat for patients who have often faced several therapeutic failures before attempting hypnosis. Patients may also have wrong impressions of hypnosis, including a requirement of passivity toward the therapist, and be in search of a magical solution that will suppress their symptoms. Although hypnosis may be a natural ability, its development may be related to inter-individual variations, depending on the creativity and resources of the patient. Finally, hypnosis often recruits the attentional resources of the patients and may weaken their capacities of memorization and concentration, lengthening the process of learning self-hypnosis.

Does Hypnosis Require the Collaboration of the Patient?

Hypnosis in the treatment of chronic pain implies an active participation of the patient. It may be limited by a passive or refractory attitude, a previous negative experience, an unrealistic expectation, and a non-adherence to the therapeutic project. In selecting this type of treatment, one must take into account the possibility of resistance to change as well as the primary and secondary benefits associated with relief of the symptoms via hypnosis. It is important to define a realistic and acceptable therapeutic goal before starting the treatment.

Which Type of Hypnotic Treatment Design Is the Best for Migraine?

As the literature review earlier in this chapter indicated, many different hypnotherapeutic treatment designs are used for migraine. The number of sessions, frequency and duration of self-hypnosis practice, and length of treatment are also different. Further research is necessary to elucidate the best way to identify and develop most efficient methods.

Interest in Self-Hypnosis

Hypnosis and especially the practice of self-hypnosis appear to be key elements in the treatment of chronic pain. Given that the duration of the analgesic effect of hypnosis is not well known, a regular practice of self-hypnosis may help the patient to renew the experience of pain improvement. Self-hypnosis increases the ability to cope with pain and limit medication use and related adverse effects. Gaining autonomy may limit medical and pharmacological shopping, with ensuing benefits for both the patient's health and his or her finances. Interestingly, as shown in two follow-up studies of patients suffering spinal cord injury and multiple sclerosis, self-hypnosis may mainly be a skill with which to obtain a temporary decrease in pain, as most of the patients in these studies continued to practice self-hypnosis even when not reporting clinically meaningful improvements in daily pain intensity after one year (Jensen et al., 2008, 2009a, 2009b).

Ethical Guidelines

Hypnosis will acquaint the specialized professional with a dynamic, diverse, and constantly evolving field, and one offering superb therapeutic tools that are widely applicable in many contexts. As the practice of hypnosis is broadened from "doing formal hypnosis" to a model of deliberate and effective communication, increasing numbers of professionals can be expected to integrate hypnotic techniques into their work. As a helping professional, you are assumed to be prepared to use the understandings of human nature and the capacity for interpersonal influence you have in a constructive ethical way.

The first priority is to help, not hurt. It is important to never go beyond your range of expertise. Using hypnotic techniques without adequate knowledge and training is potentially dangerous and damaging. Accredited training programs on hypnosis are available in many qualified centers. Acquiring hypnotic skills is one way to enhance your clinical abilities to obtain lasting results in the therapy work with your patients.

CONCLUSION

Chronic migraine and chronic headache in general are complex phenomena, which have multiple implications for the quality of life of the patient. These entities require a global and multidisciplinary approach, and most often a multifaceted program of treatment. Despite a persistent need for further research to explain the neurophysiological mechanisms that underlie chronic headache and migraine, the use of hypnosis and self-hypnosis can help patients to better cope with it. Hypnosis is not a "magical" solution, but rather an interesting additional or alternative technique in the treatment of migraine. It lacks adverse side effects, yet can contribute to reducing the frequency, severity, and duration of migraine as well as medication use. It is a cost-effective treatment for the patient and the community. The use of hypnosis can be a powerful way to promote self-efficiency and independence in patients, helping them to be more self-assured and self-valuing.

REFERENCES

Abrahamsen R, Baad-Hansen L, Svensson P. Hypnosis in the management of persistent idiopathic orofacial pain: clinical and psychosocial findings. *Pain* 2008;136:44–52.

Alladin A. Hypnosis in the treatment of severe chronic migraine. In: Heap M, ed. *Hypnosis: Current Clinical, Experimental and Forensic Practices.* London: Croom Helm; 1988:159–166.

Anderson JA, Basker MA, Dalton R. Migraine and hypnotherapy. *Int J Clin Exp Hypnosis* 1975;23:48–58.

Andreychuck T, Skriver C. Hypnosis and biofeedback in the treatment of migraine headache. *Int J Clin Exp Hypnosis* 1975;23:172–183.

Barber J. *Hypnosis and Suggestion in the Treatment of Pain.* New York: Norton; 1996.

Bowers KS. Imagination and dissociation in hypnotic responding. *Int J Clin Exp Hypnosis* 1992;40:253–275.

Büchel C, Bornhovd K, Quante M, et al. Dissociable neural responses related to pain intensity, stimulus intensity, and stimulus awareness within the anterior cingulate cortex: a parametric single trial laser functional magnetic resonance imaging study. *J Neurosci* 2002;22:970–976.

Chambless DL, Hollon SD. Update on empirically supported therapies. *J Consulting Clin Psychol* 1998;66:7–18.

Chambless DL, Baker MJ, Baucaom DH, et al. Update on empirically validated therapies II. *Clin Psychologist* 1998;51:3–16.

Craig AD, Reiman EM, Evans A, Bushnell MC. Functional imaging of an illusion of pain. *Nature* 1996;384:258–260.

Crawford HJ, Knebel T, Kaplan L, et al. Hypnotic analgesia: 1. Somatosensory event-related potential changes to noxious stimuli and 2. Transfer learning to reduce chronic low back pain. *Int J Clin Exp Hypnosis* 1998;46:92–132.

Defechereux T, Degauque C, Fumal I, et al. L'hypnosédation, un nouveau mode d'anesthésie pour la chirurgie endocrinienne cervicale. Etude prospective randomisée. *Ann Chir* 2000;125:539–546.

De Pascalis V, Magurano MR, Bellusci A. Pain perception, somatosensory event-related potentials and skin conductance responses to painful stimuli in high, mid and low hypnotizable subjects; effects of differential pain reduction strategies. *Pain* 1999;83:499–508.

Devinsky O, Morell MJ, Vogt BA. Contribution of anterior cingulate cortex to behaviour. *Brain* 1995;118:279–306.

Edmonston W. Anesis. In : Lynn S, Rhue J, eds. *Theories of Hypnosis: Current Models and Perspectives.* New York: Guilford; 1991:197–237.

Elkins G, Jensen MP, Patterson DR. Hypnotherapy for the management of chronic pain. *Int J Clin Hypnosis* 2007;55:275–287.

Elliotson J. *Numerous Cases of Surgical Operations Without Pain in the Mesmeric State.* Lea and Blanchard: Philadelphia, 1843.

Emmerson GH, Trexler G. An hypnotic intervention for migraine control. *Aust J Clin Exp Hypnosis* 1999;27:54–61.

Erickson MH, Rossi EL, Rossi, SI. *Hypnotic Realities: The Induction of Clinical Hypnosis and Forms of Indirect Suggestions.* New York: Irvington; 1976.

Faymonville ME, Laureys S, Degueldre C, et al. Neural mechanisms of antinociceptive effects of hypnosis. *Anesthesiology* 2000;92:1257–1267.

Faymonville ME, Roediger L, Delfiore G, et al. Increased cerebral functional connectivity underlying the antinociceptive effects of hypnosis. *Cog Brain Res* 2003;17:255–262.

Faymonville ME, Boly M, Layreys S. Functional neuroanatomy of the hypnotic state. *J Physiology Paris* 2006;99:463–469.

Faymonville ME, Vogt B, Maquet P, Laureys S. Hypnosis and cingulate-mediated mechanisms of analgesia. In: Vogt B, ed. *Cingulate Neurobiology and Disease.* Oxford, UK: Oxford University Press; 2009:381–400.

Friedman H, Taub HA. Brief psychological procedures in migraine treatment. *Am J Clin Hypnosis* 1984;26:187–200.

George MS, Ketter TA, Parekh PI, et al. Brain activity during transient sadness and happiness in healthy women. *Am J Psych* 1995;152:341–351.

Grandahl JR, Rosvold EO. Hypnosis as a treatment of chronic widespread pain in general practice: a randomized control pilot trial. *BMC Musculoskelet Disord* 2008;9:124.

Green JP, Barabasz AF, Barrett D, Montgomery GH. Forging ahead: the APA division 30 definitions of hypnosis. *Int J Clin Exp Hypnosis* 2005;53:259–264.

Hammond DC. Review of the efficacy of clinical hypnosis with headaches and migraines. *Int J Clin Exp Hypnosis* 2007;55:207–219.

Hilgard ER, Hilgard JR. *Hypnosis in the Relief of Pain.* California: William Kaufmann; 1983.

Holroyd J. Hypnosis treatment of clinical pain: understanding why hypnosis is useful. *Int J Clin Hypnosis* 1996;44:33–51.

Jensen MP. Hypnosis for chronic pain management: a new hope. *Pain* 2009;146:235–237.

Jensen MP, Patterson DR. Hypnotic treatment of chronic pain. *J Behavioral Med* 2006;29:95–124.

Jensen MP, Barber J, Hanley MA, et al. Long-term outcome of hypnotic-analgesia treatment for chronic pain in persons with disabilities. *Int J Clin Exp Hypnosis* 2008;56:156–169.

Jensen MP, Barber J, Romano JM, et al. A comparison of self-hypnosis versus progressive muscle relaxation in patients with multiple sclerosis and chronic pain. *Int J Clin Exp Hypnosis* 2009a;57:198–221.

Jensen MP, Barber J, Romano JM, et al. Effects of self-hypnosis training and EMG biofeedback relaxation training on chronic pain in persons with spinal cord injury. *Int J Clin Exp Hypnosis* 2009b;57:239–268.

Jones AKP, Brown WD, Friston KJ, et al. Cortical and subcortical localization of response to pain in man using positron emission tomography. *Proc R Soc Lond B Biol Sci* 1991;244:39–44.

Kiernan BD, Dane, JR, Phillips LH, Price DD. Hypnotic analgesia reduces R-III nociceptive reflex: further evidence concerning the multifactorial nature of hypnotic analgesia. *Pain* 1995;60:39–47.

Lang EV, Benotsch EG, Fick LJ, et al. Adjunctive non-pharmacological analgesia for invasive medical procedures: a randomized trial. *Lancet* 2000;355:1486–1490.

Langlade A, Jussiau C, Lamonerie L, et al. Hypnosis increases heat detection and heat pain thresholds in healthy volunteers. *Reg Anesth Pain Med* 2002;27:43–46.

Lynn S, Kirsch I, Barabasz A, et al. Hypnosis as an empirically supported clinical intervention: the state of the evidence and a look to the future. *Int J Clin Exp Hypnosis* 2000;48:235–255.

Mannix LK, Chandurkar RS, Rybicki LA, et al. Effect of guided imagery on quality of life for patients with chronic tension-type headache. *Headache* 1999;29:326–334.

Maquet P, Faymonville ME, Degueldre C, et al. Functional neuroanatomy of hypnotic state. *Biol Psychiatry* 1999;45:327.

Melis PM, Rooimans W, Spierings EL, Hoogduin CA. Treatment of chronic tension-type headache with hypnotherapy: a single-blind controlled study. *Headache* 1991;31:686–689.

Montgomery GH, DuHamel KN, Redd WH. A meta-analysis of hypnotically induced analgesia: how effective is hypnosis. *Int J Clin Hypnosis* 2000;48:138–153.

Olness K, MacDonald JT, Uden DL. Comparison of self-hypnosis and propanolol in the treatment of juvenile classic migraine. *Pediatrics* 1987;79:593–597.

Patterson DR, Jensen MP. Hypnosis and clinical pain. *Psychol Bull* 2003;29:495–521.

Patterson DR, Ptacek JT. Baseline pain as a moderator of hypnotic analgesia for burn injury treatment. *J Consulting Clin Psychol* 1997;65:60–67.

Paus T. Primate anterior cingular cortex: where motor control, drive and cognition interface. *Nat Rev Neurosci* 2001;2:417–424.

Petrovic P, Kalso E, Peterson KM, Ingvar M. Placebo and opioid analgesia: imaging a shared neuronal network. *Science* 2002;295:1737–1740.

Peyron R, Garcia-Larrea L, Gregoire MC, et al. Haemodynamic brain responses to acute pain in humans: sensory and attentional networks. *Brain* 1999;122:1765–1780.

Rainville P, Duncan GH, Price DD, et al. Pain affect encoded in human anterior cingulate but not in somatosensory cortex. *Science* 1997;277:968–971.

Rainville P, Hofbauer RK, Paus T, et al. Cerebral mechanisms of hypnotic induction and suggestion. *J Cogn Neurosci* 1999;11:110–125.

Rainville P, Hofbauer RK, Bushnell MC, et al. Hypnosis modulates activity in brain structures involved in the regulation of consciousness. *J Cogn Neurosci* 2002;11:110–125.

Reynolds DV. Surgery in the rat during electrical analgesia. *Science* 1969;164:444–445.

Rogovik AL, Goldman RD. Hypnosis for treatment of pain in children. *Can Family Physician* 2007;53:823–825.

Salem G. Indications, contre-indication, objections. In: Salem G, Bonvin E, eds. *Soigner par l'Hypnose*. Masson: Paris; 2004:64–69.

Silberstein SD. Practice parameter: evidence-based guidelines for migraine headache (an evidence-based review): report of the Quality Standards Subcommittee of the American Academy of Neurology. *Neurology* 2000;55:754–762.

Spanos NP. A sociocognitive approach to hypnosis. In: Lynn S, Rhue J, eds. *Theory of Hypnosis: Current Models and Perspectives*. New York: Guilford; 1991:324–361.

Spanos NP, Liddy SJ, Scott H, et al. Hypnotic suggestion and placebo for the treatment of chronic headache in a university volunteer sample. *Cognitive Ther Res* 1993;17:191–205.

Spiegel H, Spiegel D. *Trance and Treatment: Clinical Uses of Hypnosis*. New York: Basic Books; 1978.

Stoelb BL, Molton IR, Jensen MP, Patterson DR. The efficacy of hypnotic analgesia in adults: a review of the literature. *Contemporary Hypnosis* 2009;26:24–39.

Ter Kuile MM, Spinhoven P, Linssen ACG, et al. Autogenic training and self-hypnosis for the treatment of recurrent headaches in three different subject groups. *Pain* 1994;58:331–340.

Van Dyck R, Zitman FG, Linssen A, et al. Autogenic training and future oriented hypnotic imagery in the treatment of tension headache: outcome and process. *Int J Clin Exp Hypnosis* 1991;39:6–23.

Vogt BA. Pain and emotion interactions in subregions of the cingulate gyrus. *Nature Rev Neurosci* 2005;6:533–544.

Zelinka V, Faymonville ME, Pitchot W, Ansseau M. L'hypnose dans la prise en charge des douleurs chroniques. *Acta Psychiatrica Belgica* 2009;109:21–28.

Zitman FG, Van Dyck R, Spinhoven P, et al. Hypnosis and autogenic training in the treatment of tension headache: a two-phase constructive design with follow-up. *J Psychosom Res* 1992;36:219–228.

Neurostimulation and Neuromodulation in Migraine

Thorsten Bartsch, MD, Koen Paemeleire, MD, PhD,
and Peter J. Goadsby, MD, PhD

INTRODUCTION

The acute and preventive medical treatment of patients with primary headaches such as chronic migraine is challenging, and side effects frequently complicate the course of medical treatment. Recently, there has been considerable progress in neurostimulation techniques in medically intractable chronic headaches. It is very well known that a nonpainful stimulation of peripheral nerves can elicit analgesic effects (Wall, 1978; Woolf & Thompson, 1994). This phenomenon has been used in certain pain syndromes using noninvasive high- or low-frequency transcutaneous electrical nerve stimulation (TENS), percutaneous electrical nerve stimulation (PENS; acupuncture-like TENS [AL-TENS]), and spinal cord stimulation (SCS). The analgesic effect is critically dependent on the intensity of the electrical stimulation. In recent years, minimally invasive neurostimulation techniques and neuromodulatory techniques, such as transcranial magnetic stimulation, have also been applied to patients with migraine. This chapter summarizes the current concepts and outcome data related to invasive and noninvasive device-based neurostimulation and neuromodulatory approaches in migraine.

NEUROSTIMULATION AND NEUROMODULATION: CURRENT CONCEPTS

Gate Control Theory of Pain

Traditionally, the effect of peripheral neurostimulation (PNS) has been attributed to the activation of non-noxious afferent nerve fibers (Aβ fibers), which is thought to modulate Aδ- and C-fiber–mediated nociceptive transmission in the spinal cord, compatible with the gate control theory of pain. The understanding of pain–modulatory mechanisms in the spinal cord as well as in the supraspinal structures has been greatly advanced by the gate control theory advanced by Ronald Melzack and Patrick D. Wall (1965). Although considerably extended and modified since then, their framework, in essence, proposed that the transmission of pain in the spinal cord is modulated by excitatory and inhibitory influences (Dickenson, 2002). These influences may arise from intrinsic factors within the spinal cord, from supraspinal projections onto the spinal cord, or from both. This short- and long-lasting relay function of the spinal cord may play an important role in pathophysiological pain states such as in persistent pain, central sensitization, hyperalgesia, and allodynia (Sandkuhler, 2009). The concept of modulation also implies a changeable, plastic transmission.

Besides the concept of modulation—mediated via decreasing excitation or increasing inhibition—a prerequisite of this arrangement is the convergence of different types of afferent activity. Another prerequisite of an adequate effect of PNS is an intact descending modulatory network.

In accordance with the gate control theory, a similar interplay of multiple mechanisms of segmental spinal inhibiting effects and descending pain inhibitory pathways may mediate the analgesic effects of PNS.

Central Mechanisms of Pain Processing: Central Sensitization, Synaptic Plasticity, and Descending Inhibition

Nociceptive spinal cord neurons can be sensitized due to a strong afferent stimulation by small-fiber afferents. The resulting hyperexcitability is reflected in a reduction of the activation threshold, an increased responsiveness to afferent stimulation, an enlargement of receptive fields, or the emergence of new receptive fields and the recruitment of "silent" nociceptive afferents (see Chapters 5 and 6 for more information on the relationship of sensitization to migraine). The clinical correlates of this central hypersensitivity in migraine patients include the development of spontaneous pain, hyperalgesia, and allodynia (Burstein et al., 2000; Sandkuhler, 2009). The hypersensitivity of the afferent synaptic input in the spinal cord is thought to be due to the stimulation-induced release of various neuropeptides, such as calcitonin gene-related peptide (CGRP), or to augmented glutamate release and action at the N-methyl-D-aspartate (NMDA) receptor, but may also be due to decrease of local segmental spinal inhibition in response to the afferent stimulation (Woolf & Salter, 2000; Sandkuhler, 2009).

It is now well established that the nociceptive inflow to second-order neurons in the spinal cord and the trigeminocervical complex is subject to a modulation by descending inhibitory projections from brainstem structures such as the periaqueductal gray (PAG), nucleus raphe magnus (NRM), and rostral ventromedial medulla (RVM) (Fields & Heinricher, 1985; Sandkuhler et al., 1987; Behbehani, 1995; Ren & Dubner, 2008), as stimulation of these regions produces profound anti-nociception (Fields, 2004; Heinricher & Ingram, 2008) (see Chapter 5). In particular, recent findings suggest that the ventrolateral division of the PAG (vlPAG) has a pivotal role in trigeminal nociception, as stimulation of the vlPAG modulates dural nociception and selectively receives input from trigeminovascular afferents (Keay & Bandler, 1998; Hoskin et al., 2001; Knight & Goadsby, 2001; Knight et al., 2002; Bartsch et al., 2004) (**Figure 26.1**).

In recent years, researchers have shown that the pain-modulating circuits in the brainstem are involved not only in anti-nociception, but also, under certain conditions, in the facilitation of central sensitization and secondary hyperalgesia (Urban & Gebhart, 1999; Ren & Dubner, 2002). These findings suggest that the level of excitability of dura-sensitive neurons in the trigeminocervical complex might potentially be increased by (possibly dysfunctional) brainstem pain-modulatory structures.

Spinal Mechanisms of PNS

In accordance with the gate control theory of pain, a similar interplay of multiple mechanisms on the spinal cord may contribute to the analgesic effects of PNS. Earlier studies in animals showed decreased activity in dorsal horn cells in both spontaneous activity and nociceptive-evoked responses during TENS (Garrison & Foreman, 1994, 1996). Despite similar effects as well as values of stimulation parameters in TENS and PNS, however, it remains unclear whether both methods share the same neuromodulatory mechanisms. As in SCS, PNS may also decrease long-term potentiation of nociceptive wide dynamic range neurons in the spinal dorsal

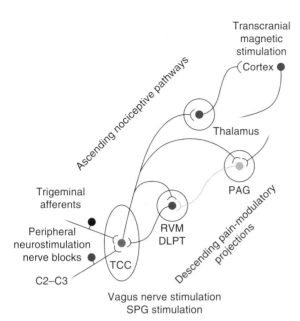

Figure 26.1 Functional Anatomy of Pain-Modulatory Pathways in the Spinal Cord and Supraspinal Structures. Nociceptive and non-nociceptive information is relayed in the spinal dorsal horn, where it is subject to segmental modulatory mechanisms, either intrinsic or extrinsic, from descending projections. The nociceptive input is transmitted to supraspinal relay sites (e.g., the thalamus and cortex) and is subject to inhibitory anti-nociceptive as well as pro-nociceptive projections by pain-modulatory circuits in the brainstem. Pain processing at different levels may be modulated by neurostimulation of peripheral nerves. (RVM, rostral ventromedial medulla; DLPT, dorsolateral pontomesencephalic tegmentum; PAG, periaqueductal gray; TCC, trigeminalcervical complex; SPG, sphenopalatine ganglion.)

Courtesy of Dr. Thorsten Bartsch.

horn (Yakhnitsa et al., 1999; Wallin et al., 2003). With regard to the pathophysiological mechanisms involved in acute and persistent pain states, TENS may depotentiate central sensitization mechanisms in the dorsal horn, including secondary hyperalgesia (Sluka et al., 1998; Ma & Sluka, 2001).

In recent years, several neurotransmitter systems have been identified as being involved in segmental spinal cord effects of TENS. Low-frequency TENS activates serotoninergic ($5-HT_2$ and $5-HT_3$) synaptic transmission, probably reflecting the activation of descending serotoninergic pathways (Radhakrishnan et al., 2003; Sluka et al., 2006; Song et al., 2009). Inhibitory projections in the spinal cord releasing gamma-aminobutyric acid (GABA) are also activated, as TENS increases extracellular GABA concentrations and the effect of PNS is prevented by the blockade of spinal $GABA_A$ receptors (Radhakrishnan et al., 2003; Maeda et al., 2007). Using spinal microdialysis in arthritic rats, the role of the opioidergic-dependent

glutamate and aspartate release in the spinal cord was studied. TENS led to a δ-opioidergic–mediated blockade of the excitatory transmitters glutamate and aspartate (Radhakrishnan & Sluka, 2003; Sluka et al., 2005). Similarly, TENS and SCS activate spinal muscarinic M_1 and M_3 receptors, but not spinal nicotinic receptors (Radhakrishnan & Sluka, 2003; Schechtmann et al., 2008; Song et al., 2008).

The involvement of α_2-noradrenergic receptors in the neuromodulatory effects of TENS was implied by the finding that the application of clonidine augments the analgesic effects of TENS (Sluka & Chandran, 2002). Spinal blockade of α_2-noradrenergic receptors similarly decreases the analgesic effects of TENS (Resende et al., 2004; King et al., 2005). Using immunohistochemistry and reverse transcription polymerase chain reaction (RT-PCR) technology, it was shown that PENS elicited an increased expression of somatostatin in the dorsal root ganglion and spinal dorsal horn in rats (Dong et al., 2005). Interestingly, pharmacological therapy combined with electrical neuromodulation may produce an increased efficacy or delay in analgesic tolerance (Sluka & Chandran, 2002; Wallin et al., 2002).

Supraspinal Mechanisms of PNS

Recent experimental evidence indicates that supraspinal structures, such as PAG, are also involved in mediating the anti-nociceptive effects of neurostimulation (Lindblom et al., 1977; Garrison & Foreman, 1994). A positron emission tomography (PET) study investigating the effect of SCS in pain-free patients with angina pectoris demonstrated increased blood flow in the vlPAG during neurostimulation (Hautvast et al., 1997). Further effects were also observed at the thalamic level (Gildenberg & Murthy, 1980; Olausson et al., 1994).

A microdialysis study on transmitter release in the PAG of rats receiving SCS demonstrated that neurostimulation caused a decrease of GABA levels but not of serotonin or substance P (Lindblom et al., 1977; Garrison & Foreman, 1994). Given that GABA-neurons in the PAG exert a tonic inhibitory effect on the activity in descending pain inhibitory pathways, including trigeminovascular inputs (Knight et al., 2003), it has been suggested that a decreased GABA level in this region following repeated SCS might lead to activation of descending anti-nociceptive projections, with subsequent pain reduction (Duggan & Foong, 1985; Stiller et al., 1995, 1996).

In an experimental arthritis animal model, researchers noted that in animals with joint inflammation, after inducing a central sensitization, application of TENS significantly increased withdrawal thresholds of the paw and knee joint in the group. Reversible functional inactivation of vlPAG prevented the effects of TENS in terms of increased withdrawal thresholds. However, blockade of neuronal pathways in the vlPAG after induction of an inflammation also transiently reversed the behavioral changes indicative of a mechanical hyperalgesia, thus suggesting a role for the vlPAG in the facilitated transmission of pain from deep somatic tissue (DeSantana et al., 2009). Furthermore, blockade of μ- and δ-opioid receptors in RVM prevents the analgesic effects of TENS (Kalra et al., 2001; Ainsworth et al., 2006). In the NRM, PNS modulates synthesis of Orphanin FQ (OFQ), an endogenous ligand for the opioid receptor-like-1 (ORL1) receptor and OFQ peptide level (Dong et al., 2005).

Pharmacology

Since the early studies on PNS, opioidergic mechanisms have been suggested to be involved in the effects of PNS and, at least partly, to contribute to the analgesic effect of PNS. In humans, experimental data show an increased concentration of β-endorphins and methionine-enkephalin in the cerebrospinal fluid after application of high-frequency TENS (Salar et al., 1981; Han et al., 1991). As discussed earlier, the involvement of pain-modulating structures in the midbrain, such as the PAG and RVM, also suggests an involvement of its opioidergic projections (Sabino et al., 2008). Indeed, TENS elicits its analgesic effects by activation of μ- and δ-opioid receptors in the RVM and the spinal cord (Sluka et al., 1999; Kalra et al., 2001; DeSantana et al., 2009). With regard to TENS, low-frequency TENS elicits an anti-hyperalgesic effect through μ-opioid receptor activation, whereas high-frequency TENS leads to anti-hyperalgesia through δ-opioid receptors in the spinal cord. As noted earlier, blockade of μ- and δ-opioid receptors in the spinal cord and RVM prevents the analgesic effect produced by TENS in arthritic rats (Sluka et al., 1999).

NEUROSTIMULATION OF THE OCCIPITAL NERVES IN MIGRAINE

Occipital nerve stimulation (ONS) as a medical option for medically intractable headache was introduced by Weiner and Reed (1999). Recently, there has been a great interest in this new procedure in the treatment of primary headache disorders—an interest reflected in the large number of case reports, case series, and prospective studies on this indication. ONS has been also applied to secondary headaches, including post-traumatic headache and cervicogenic headache, and to cranial neuralgias, including occipital neuralgia.

Several variants on the original Weiner and Reed implantation technique (Weiner & Reed, 1999) have been described. In principle, the procedure can be performed under local or general anesthesia, with a subcutaneous lead (either a cylindrical or paddle style electrode) inserted to cross the greater, lesser, and least occipital nerves via an incision on the midline or a lateral incision close to the mastoid process (Trentman & Zimmerman, 2008; **Figure 26.2**). Alternatively, a recently introduced miniaturized Bion device can be implanted in the suboccipital region (Lipton, 2009). The stimulation parameters, including frequency, pulse width, and voltage, are classically adjusted to make patients experience mild paraesthesia in the stimulated area.

Recent results with the use of ONS to treat intractable chronic migraine, frequently complicated by medication overuse, have been encouraging, with 43 of 51 patients (84%) experiencing at least a 50% improvement

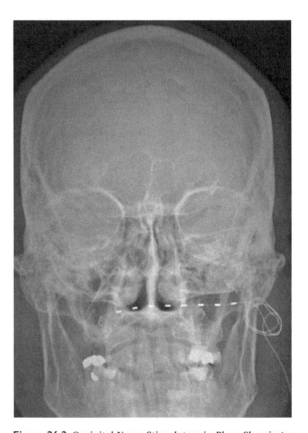

Figure 26.2 Occipital Nerve Stimulators in Place Showing a Lateral Approach with an Eight-Electrode Paddle

Courtesy of Prof. Olav Jansen, Institute of Neuroradiology, University Hospital Schleswig Holstein, Kiel, Germany.

(Matharu et al., 2004; Oh, 2004; Schwedt et al., 2007a). A genuine effect of ONS in intractable chronic migraine is suggested by data from a multicenter, prospective, randomized, single-blind, controlled study (ONSTIM trial; Saper, 2011). Interestingly, most of the patients in this study had experienced chronic migraine for approximately a decade before implantation of the ONS device, suggesting that even chronic headache syndromes might be responsive to neurostimulation. A positive response was defined as a 50% drop in headache days per month or a 3 or more point drop (on a 0–10 scale) in overall pain intensity from baseline at 3-month follow-up. As such, the responder rate was 39% in intractable chronic migraine patients treated with ONS, compared to 8% in a control stimulation group and 0% in the medical management group after 3 months. No unanticipated adverse device events occurred. Lead migration occurred in 12 of 51 (24%) subjects. **Table 26.1** provides a synopsis of published cases on the effects of ONS in migraine.

A retrospective survey aimed at identifying the headache phenotype in 26 patients with medically refractory head pain treated with ONS (Paemeleire et al., 2010). After phenotyping, two main groups emerged: eight patients had "migraine without aura" and eight patients had "constant pain caused by compression, irritation, or distortion of cranial nerves or upper cervical roots by structural lesions." Moreover, overuse of symptomatic acute headache treatments was associated with less favorable long-term outcomes in migraine patients. The authors concluded that clinical phenotyping may help in defining those subgroups of patients with medically refractory headache who are more likely to respond to ONS.

In principle, technical and safety data of ONS are within the normal range of similar procedures, although surgical revisions are frequently required. To date, not a single persistent iatrogenic neurological deficit has been reported. The postoperative infection risk is low if the procedure is performed by experienced hands. Frequently, both traumatic and spontaneous electrode migration are reported within the first year post surgery, reflecting the fact that patients tend to be younger and mobile. Battery replacement and electrode fracture or malfunction may lead to repeated surgery. Few patients experience painful sensations at the site of the generator. To avoid paraesthesia and to save battery power, some patients turn their stimulator off at night. Local discomfort, such as myoclonus, muscle twitching, and allodynia at the electrode site, may occur, as well as slight neck stiffness persisting for some months after surgery. Like all stimulators, the ONS devices may be accidentally switched off by strong magnetic fields.

Current Concepts of Occipital Nerve Stimulation

Most likely, multiple mechanisms involving pain processing circuits in the central nervous system are participating in the analgesic effects of peripheral neurostimulation

Table 26.1 Effects of Occipital Nerve Stimulation in Migraine: Synopsis of Published Cases

Study	Headache Syndrome	Diagnostic Criteria	Type of Study	Number of Patients	Mean Disease Duration (Years) Before Implantation	Number of Improved Patients (> 50% relief) / (%)	Follow-Up (Years)
Popeney & Alo (2003)	Transformed migraine	IHS and Silberstein et al., 1996	P	25	10	22 (88)	1.5
Oh et al. (2004)	Transformed migraine	IHS and Silberstein et al., 1996	P	10	12 +	10 (100)	0.5
Matharu et al. (2004)	Chronic migraine	IHS	O	8	5.8	8 (100)	1.5
Schwedt et al. (2007a)	Chronic migraine	IHS	R	8	N.S.	3 (38)	1.5
Saper et al. (2010) (ONSTIM)	Chronic migraine	IHS	P	76	22/CM: 10	29 (39)	0.25
Lipton et al. (2009) (PRISM)	Migraine/chronic migraine	IHS	P	132		17 (27)	1.0

IHS, International Headache Society; N.S., not stated; CM, chronic migraine; R, retrospective; O, observational; P, prospective.

(Goadsby, 2007; Goadsby et al., 2008). First, direct effects of electrical stimulation on peripheral nerve excitability, such as transient slowing in conduction velocity, increase in electrical threshold, and decrease in response probability, have been suggested (Ignelzi & Nyquist, 1979). Interestingly, ONS did not significantly alter pain thresholds in patients with cluster headache (Magis et al., 2007).

Second, given that projection fibers represent only a minority of fibers within the spinal ascending tracts, whereas propriospinal neurons and interneurons of the spinal dorsal horn outnumber these projection neurons, it has been suggested that the segmental neural network might represent the site of the neuromodulatory effect (Chung et al., 1984; Doubell, 1999; Meyerson & Linderoth, 2006). Indeed, the somatosensory peripheral neurostimulation of afferent Aβ fibers might potentially modulate the nociceptive transmission on a segmental level, thus revisiting the gate control theory proposed by Melzack and Wall (Kolmodin & Skoglund, 1960; Woolf, 1979; Chung et al., 1984; Garrison & Foreman, 1996). Further, experimental data indicate that supraspinal structures, such as the PAG, are at least partly involved in mediating the anti-nociceptive effects of neurostimulation (Lindblom et al., 1977; Garrison & Foreman, 1994). Using a neuropharmacological approach, the pharmacological mechanisms of opioidergic and GABAergic receptor systems involved in ONS have just begun to be studied (Burns, 2010).

Complementary neuroimaging studies investigating the role of supraspinal structures in mediating an anti-nociceptive effect in ONS suggest similar central mechanisms are at work (Matharu et al, 2004). In one study, eight patients with chronic migraine, who responded to a nonpainful high-frequency stimulation (50–120 Hz) of afferents in the greater occipital nerve (GON) using bilaterally implanted neurostimulators, were given PET scans while they were in different states: during stimulation when the patient was pain-free, during nonstimulation with pain and typical clinical features, and during partial activation of the stimulator with different levels of paraesthesia (Matharu et al., 2004). Cerebral blood flow changes during the pain state were observed in the dorsal rostral pons, anterior cingulate cortex (ACC), and cuneus—sites that are known to be active in migraine (Weiller et al., 1995; Bahra et al., 2001). The activation in the dorsal rostral pons strongly suggests that this structure plays a role in the pathophysiology of chronic migraine. In the paraesthesia state during neurostimulation, ACC and left pulvinar activation were observed, indicating that ONS can modulate activity in the thalamus. Indeed, the pulvinar has been suggested to be involved

in pain modulation, as neurosurgical pulvinotomy has been performed to relieve intractable pain (Mayanagi & Bouchard, 1976; Choi & Umbach, 1977).

In conclusion, ONS is a promising treatment for disabling refractory primary headache syndromes. However, several issues need to be critically addressed and evaluated before broad clinical application of this technique comes into sight. Careful clinical phenotyping, which may include an indomethacin test, is mandatory in the preoperative evaluation. Indeed, most patients in an original case series of occipital neuralgia (Weiner & Reed, 1999) were reclassified as migraine patients after clinical review as part of a functional imaging study (Matharu et al., 2004). Identification of clinical predictors of ONS is mandatory. Interestingly, the response to an occipital nerve block seems not to be a predictor of outcomes with ONS (Schwedt et al., 2007b; Goadsby et al., 2009; Paemeleire et al., 2010). There are strong indications that ongoing medication overuse negatively affects the outcome in chronic migraine patients. Patients should be withdrawn from such medications prior to placement of the ONS device, as withdrawal itself may account for improvement by itself (Paemeleire et al., 2010). Technically, specific electrodes need to be developed for ONS, for two reasons: (1) current material for SCS is generally being used and (2) lead migration and revision within 3 years of follow-up are frequent occurrences (Schwedt et al., 2007a). It has been suggested that paddle electrodes, rather than a cylindrical electrode, may be associated with fewer migrations and revisions (Oh, 2004). Rechargeable and miniaturized technology, such as the Bion device, needs to be further explored (Burns et al., 2009). Finally, optimal stimulation parameters need to be determined.

TRANSCRANIAL MAGNETIC STIMULATION

Transcranial magnetic stimulation (TMS) is a noninvasive tool to study excitability changes in cortical neurons by means of a depolarization in the neurons of the brain. TMS delivers a rapidly changing magnetic field from the scalp surface to induce current in adjacent cortical tissue. The therapy is delivered as either a single pulse (sTMS) or repetitive pulses (rTMS). High-frequency rTMS increases neural excitability, whereas low-frequency rTMS decrease neural excitability. TMS was originally developed as an experimental tool to study excitability changes of cortical neurons, but has since been used as a diagnostic tool to study the integrity of descending motor pathways. The observed effects obviously depend on various parameters such as the stimulation protocol, the cortex area stimulated, and the condition of the patient. TMS has been widely used as a tool to study pathophysiological changes of cortical neuronal excitability in migraine (Coppola et al., 2007). Using laser-evoked potentials as a surrogate marker in migraine patients in migraine, high-frequency rTMS of the left primary motor cortex (M1) were able to modulate pain-related evoked laser-evoked cortical potentials (de Tommaso et al., 2010). From a clinical standpoint, TMS recently has been evaluated in the treatment of various neuropsychiatric disorders including migraine and neuropathic pain disorders (Lipton & Pearlman, 2010).

Acute Treatment

On an observational cohort level, application of two brief pulses resulted in an analgesic effect and a modulation of autonomic responses—in particular, in patients with a migraine aura (Clarke et al., 2006). In a subsequent study with 42 patients with migraine aura, however, no effect could be seen (Mohamad, 2006). Using a TMS handheld device, a pilot study conducted over 3 months on 12 patients with migraine with aura demonstrated an analgesic effect within 2 hours after two single-pulse TMS applications were delivered after the onset of migraine aura (Mohammad, 2006).

In a Phase 3, randomized, double-blind, parallel-group, two-phase, sham-controlled multicenter trial studying patients with migraine with aura, the effects of sTMS were further evaluated. Patients used a handheld device that applies two pulses of TMS to treat migraine in the aura phase. They were instructed to treat up to three attacks over 3 months while experiencing migraine aura. The primary outcome was a pain-free response 2 hours after the first attack. In the study, 164 patients treated at least one attack with sTMS ($n = 82$) or sham stimulation ($n = 82$). Pain-free response rates after 2 hours were significantly higher with sTMS (39%) than with sham stimulation (22%). Absence of pain was sustained 24 hours and 48 hours after treatment. This trial demonstrated that early treatment of migraine with aura by sTMS results in increased freedom from pain at 2 hours post application compared with sham stimulation (Lipton et al., 2010).

Preventive Treatment

A recent placebo-controlled, blinded study evaluated the therapeutic effects of low-frequency rTMS in 27 migraine patients. The primary endpoint was a reduction of migraine attacks compared with placebo; secondary outcomes included reductions in the total number of headache days, pain intensity, and use of analgesic medication

(Teepker et al., 2009). Although a significant decrease in the number of migraine attacks was described in the treatment group, no significant difference from placebo was observed in terms of the primary and secondary outcome measures. High-frequency rTMS over the left dorsolateral prefrontal cortex (DLPFC) were shown to have a beneficial effect on chronic migraine that lasted up to 1 month after the stimulation session (Brighina et al., 2004).

Mechanisms of Action

The mechanisms of the analgesic effect of TMS are still not clear, but have been attributed to perturbations of cortical nociceptive processing, modulation of thalamo-cortical circuits, changes in long-term potentiation (LTP) in cortical neurones, and activation of descending pain-inhibiting projections (Siebner & Rothwell, 2003). Interestingly, in an animal model, sTMS was shown to inhibit cortical spreading depression in comparison to sham application (Holland, 2009). Further, it has been suggested that high-frequency rTMS may restore cortical excitability in migraine patients (Brighina et al., 2004).

SPHENOPALATINE GANGLION ELECTRICAL STIMULATION

The sphenopalatine ganglion (SPG) is involved in the autonomic innervation of dural vessels. Animal experiments suggest that the parasympathetic outflow is involved in the pathophysiology of migraine, as stimulation of the ganglion induces vasodilatation of cerebral and meningeal vessels (Delepine & Aubineau, 1997; Brennan & Charles, 2010). Interestingly, nasal lidocaine-induced SPG block in migraineurs has a pain-relieving effect (Yarnitsky et al., 2003). Unilateral neurostimulation (1.2 V, 67 Hz, 462 msec) of the SPG in migraineurs did show an acute pain-relieving effect in 5 of 11 patients (Tepper et al., 2009). Similarly, neurostimulation of the SPG seems to have an acute effect in cluster headache (Ansarinia et al., 2010).

VAGUS NERVE STIMULATION

Vagus nerve stimulation (VNS) has been introduced in the neuromodulatory therapy of drug-refractory epilepsies. Experimental evidence suggests that this technology may also have a pain-modulating effect (Multon & Schoenen, 2005; Lenaerts et al., 2008). Anecdotal observations of a pain-modulating effect relative to migraine in patients treated for epilepsy led to a pilot study in patients with chronic cluster and migraine headaches (Sadler et al., 2002; Hord et al., 2003). Two patients with chronic migraines did show some relief with stimulation (Mauskop, 2005). Another pilot study in four patients with drug-refractory chronic migraine associated with depression suggested a beneficial effect of VNS on depression and, in two patients, on migraine as well (Cecchini et al., 2009).

SUPRA-ORBITAL NERVE STIMULATION

Considering the conceptual background of neuromodulation and peripheral nerve stimulation, Reed and colleagues hypothesized that patients with hemicranial-holocephalic primary migraine could benefit from a "dual" neuromodulatory approach of trigeminal and occipital (upper cervical) afferent input (Burns, 2010). Subsequently, bilateral occipital nerve and supra-orbital nerve stimulation was combined in eight patients with chronic drug-resistant migraine (Reed et al., 2010). Although this was a nonrandomized, open-label study with retrospective assessment of outcomes, dual stimulation did result in a greater pain relief than ONS alone for some patients over the follow-up period of 15 months. These observations suggest that a neuromodulation of convergent input of trigeminal and cervical afferents in the trigeminocervical complex may have a stronger effect (Bartsch & Goadsby, 2003).

NERVE BLOCKS

From a practical point of view, it has long been known that nerve blocks can have a beneficial effect in the treatment of migraine, as the analgesic effect may overcome the pharmacokinetically expected duration of the local anesthetic. Typically, local anesthetics such as bupivacaine, lidocaine, mepivacaine, and prilocaine, either in combination (e.g., lidocaine with bupivacaine) or with corticosteroids, are used (Levin, 2010). From a conceptual perspective, nerve blocks are thought to modulate convergent afferent input, as they can modulate pain outside the dermatome injected. However, an additional systemic effect cannot be ruled out.

Most commonly, a greater occipital nerve (GON) block is used for this purpose. In 19 patients with acute migraine and allodynia, a GON block decreased headache in 17 of the patients, but reduced allodynia in all patients (Ashkenazi & Young, 2005). In another study involving patients with acute migraine, 60% of patients experienced rapid pain relief within 5 minutes after injection (Cook, 2006). Moreover, a long-lasting effect of a unilateral GON block with lidocaine and methylprednisolone was seen in 26 of 54 migraine patients studied. Adding the long-acting synthetic corticosteroid

triamcinolone to the local anesthetics used for GON and trigger point injections for chronic migraine did result in headache improvement in both groups (Saracco et al., 2010), although outcomes did not differ significantly between groups.

Further studies are needed, as most studies of nerve blocks for migraine have methodological limitations in terms of sample size, control status, techniques, types, and doses of local anesthetics (Ashkenazi et al., 2010). Interestingly, the positive response to GON block is not predictive of the therapeutic effect from ONS in patients with medically refractory chronic headaches (Schwedt et al., 2007b).

TRANSCRANIAL DIRECT CURRENT STIMULATION

Transcranial direct current stimulation (tDCS) is a noninvasive application of weak electrical currents to the scalp (1–2 mA) intended to modulate the excitability of nerve cells in the CNS by means of a DC brain polarization. tDCS is usually well tolerated. This method is currently being used to study pathophysiological changes in the excitability of cortical neurons in migraine patients (Chadaide et al., 2007; Antal et al., 2008). From a therapeutic point of view, several studies have addressed the treatment effects of tDCS in migraine. Interestingly, with regard to experimental models and future applications, tDCS seems to have a modulating effect on experimentally induced cortical spreading depression (CSD) in animals (Liebetanz et al., 2006; Fregni et al., 2007).

CONCLUSIONS

This chapter summarized clinical and experimental data suggesting that neurostimulation approaches such as ONS and TMS may offer new therapeutic opportunities in patients with migraine. These therapies remain experimental, however, and further data are needed from larger randomized, controlled studies before they come into widespread use. The indications for these procedures and patient management strategies should be decided in specialized and experienced headache treatment centers. Finally, the underlying pathophysiological mechanisms, the predictors for a positive response, and the long-term outcomes when ONS is applied to a broader patient population remain to be determined.

ACKNOWLEDGMENTS

This work was supported by the Sandler Family Trust.

REFERENCES

Ainsworth L, Budelier K, Clinesmith M, et al. Trans-cutaneous electrical nerve stimulation (TENS) reduces chronic hyperalgesia induced by muscle inflammation. *Pain* 2006;120:182–187.

Ansarinia M, Rezai A, Tepper SJ, et al. Electrical stimulation of sphenopalatine ganglion for acute treatment of cluster headaches. *Headache* 2010;50:1164–1174.

Antal A, Lang N, Boros K, et al. Homeostatic metaplasticity of the motor cortex is altered during headache-free intervals in migraine with aura. *Cereb Cortex* 2008;18:2701–2705.

Ashkenazi A, Young WB. The effects of greater occipital nerve block and trigger point injection on brush allodynia and pain in migraine. *Headache* 2005;45:350–354.

Ashkenazi A, Blumenfeld A, Napchan U, et al. Peripheral nerve blocks and trigger point injections in headache management: a systematic review and suggestions for future research. *Headache* 2010;50:943–952.

Bahra A, Matharu MS, Buchel C, et al. Brainstem activation specific to migraine headache. *Lancet* 2001;357:1016–1017.

Bartsch T, Goadsby PJ. The trigeminocervical complex and migraine: current concepts and synthesis. *Curr Pain Headache Rep* 2003;7:371–376.

Bartsch T, Knight YE, Goadsby PJ. Activation of 5-HT1B/1D receptors in the periaqueductal grey inhibits meningeal nociception. *Ann Neurol* 2004;56:371–381.

Behbehani MM. Functional characteristics of the midbrain periaqueductal gray. *Prog Neurobiol* 1995;46:575–605.

Brennan KC, Charles A. An update on the blood vessel in migraine. *Curr Opin Neurol* 2010;23:266–274.

Brighina F, Piazza A, Vitello G, et al. rTMS of the prefrontal cortex in the treatment of chronic migraine: a pilot study. *J Neurol Sci* 2004;227:67–71.

Burns B. "Dual" occipital and supra-orbital nerve stimulation for primary headache. *Cephalalgia* 2010;30:257–259.

Burns B, Marin J, Goadsby PJ. Mechanisms of occipital nerve stimulation (ONS): a double blind, placebo controlled, crossover study using naloxone and flumazenil. *Neurology* 2009;72(suppl 3):A177.

Burstein R, Cutrer MF, Yarnitsky D. The development of cutaneous allodynia during a migraine attack: clinical evidence for the sequential recruitment of spinal and supraspinal nociceptive neurons in migraine. *Brain* 2000;123:1703–1709.

Cecchini AP, Mea E, Tullo V, et al. Vagus nerve stimulation in drug-resistant daily chronic migraine with depression: preliminary data. *Neurol Sci* 2009;30:S101–S104.

Chadaide Z, Arlt S, Antal A, et al. Transcranial direct current stimulation reveals inhibitory deficiency in migraine. *Cephalalgia* 2007;27:833–839.

Choi CR, Umbach W. Combined stereotaxic surgery for relief of intractable pain. *Neurochirurgia (Stuttg)* 1977;20:84–87.

Chung JM, Lee KH, Hori Y, et al. Factors influencing peripheral nerve stimulation produced inhibition of primate spinothalamic tract cells. *Pain* 1984;19:277–293.

Clarke BM, Upton AR, Kamath MV, et al. Trans-cranial magnetic stimulation for migraine: clinical effects. *J Headache Pain* 2006;7:341–346.

Cook B, Malik SN, Shaw JW, et al. Greater occipital nerve (GON) block successfully treats migraine within five minutes. *Neurology* 2006;66:A42.

Coppola G, Pierelli F, Schoenen J. Is the cerebral cortex hyperexcitable or hyperresponsive in migraine? *Cephalalgia* 2007;27:1427–1439.

Delepine L, Aubineau P. Plasma protein extra-vasation induced in the rat dura mater by stimulation of the parasympathetic sphenopalatine ganglion. *Exp Neurol* 1997;147:389–400.

DeSantana JM, Da Silva LF, De Resende MA, Sluka KA. Transcutaneous electrical nerve stimulation at both high and low frequencies activates ventrolateral periaqueductal grey to decrease mechanical hyperalgesia in arthritic rats. *Neuroscience* 2009;163:1233–1241.

de Tommaso M, Brighina F, Fierro B, et al. Effects of high-frequency repetitive transcranial magnetic stimulation of primary motor cortex on laser-evoked potentials in migraine. *J Headache Pain* 2010;11:505–512.

Dickenson AH. Gate control theory of pain stands the test of time. *Br J Anaesth* 2002;88:755–757.

Dong ZQ, Xie H, Ma F, et al. Effects of electroacupuncture on expression of somatostatin and preprosomatostatin mRNA in dorsal root ganglions and spinal dorsal horn in neuropathic pain rats. *Neurosci Lett* 2005;385:189–194.

Doubell T, Mannion RJ, Woolf CJ. The dorsal horn: state dependent sensory processing, plasticity and the generation of pain. In: Melzack PDWR, ed. *Textbook of Pain,* Vol. 59 (4th ed.). Edinburgh: Churchill Livingstone; 1999:165–180.

Duggan AW, Foong FW. Bicuculline and spinal inhibition produced by dorsal column stimulation in the cat. *Pain* 1985;22:249–259.

Fields H. State-dependent opioid control of pain. *Nat Rev Neurosci* 2004;5:565–575.

Fields HL, Heinricher MM. Anatomy and physiology of a nociceptive modulatory system. *Philos Trans R Soc Lond B Biol Sci* 1985;308:361–374.

Fregni F, Liebetanz D, Monte-Silva KK, et al. Effects of transcranial direct current stimulation coupled with repetitive electrical stimulation on cortical spreading depression. *Exp Neurol* 2007;204:462–466.

Garrison D, Foreman R. Decreased activity of spontaneous and noxiously evoked dorsal horn cells during trans-cutaneous electrical nerve stimulation (TENS). *Pain* 1994;58:309–315.

Garrison DW, Foreman RD. Effects of trans-cutaneous electrical nerve stimulation (TENS) on spontaneous and noxiously evoked dorsal horn cell activity in cats with transected spinal cords. *Neurosci Lett* 1996;216:125–128.

Gildenberg PL, Murthy KS. Influence of dorsal column stimulation upon human thalamic somatosensory-evoked potentials. *Appl Neurophysiol* 1980;43:8–17.

Goadsby PJ. Neuro-stimulation in primary headache syndromes *Expert Rev Neurother* 2007;7:1785–1789.

Goadsby PJ, Bartsch T, Dodick DW. Occipital nerve stimulation for headache: mechanisms and efficacy. *Headache* 2008;48:313–318.

Goadsby PJ, Dodick DW, Saper JR, Silberstein SD. Occipital nerve stimulation (ONS) for the treatment of intractable chronic migraine (ONSTIM). *Cephalalgia* 2009;29:133.

Han JS, Chen XH, Sun SL, et al. Effect of low- and high-frequency TENS on Met-enkephalin-Arg-Phe and dynorphin A immuno-reactivity in human lumbar CSF. *Pain* 1991;47:295–298.

Hautvast RW, Ter Horst GJ, DeJong BM, et al. Relative changes in regional cerebral blood flow during spinal cord stimulation in patients with refractory angina pectoris. *Eur J Neurosci* 1997;9:1178–1183.

Heinricher MM, Ingram SL. The brainstem and nociceptive modulation. In: Basbaum A, Bushnell A, eds. *Science of Pain*. Oxford: Academic Press; 2008: 593–626.

Holland P, Schembri CT, Fredrick JP, Goadsby PJ. Trans-cranial magnetic stimulation for the treatment of migraine aura. *Cephalalgia* 2009;72:A250.

Hord ED, Evans MS, Mueed S, et al. The effect of vagus nerve stimulation on migraines. *J Pain* 2003;4:530–534.

Hoskin KL, Bulmer DC, Lasalandra M, et al. Fos expression in the midbrain periaqueductal grey after trigeminovascular stimulation. *J Anat* 2001;198:29–35.

Ignelzi RJ, Nyquist JK. Excitability changes in peripheral nerve fibers after repetitive electrical stimulation: implications in pain modulation. *J Neurosurg* 1979;51:824–833.

Kalra A, Urban MO, Sluka KA. Blockade of opioid receptors in rostral ventral medulla prevents antihyperalgesia produced by transcutaneous electrical nerve stimulation (TENS). *J Pharmacol Exp Ther* 2001;298:257–263.

Keay KA, Bandler R. Vascular head pain selectively activates ventrolateral periaqueductal grey in the cat. *Neurosci Lett* 1998;245:58–60.

King EW, Audette K, Athman GA, et al. Trans-cutaneous electrical nerve stimulation activates peripherally located alpha-2A adrenergic receptors. *Pain* 2005;115:364–373.

Knight YE, Goadsby PJ. The periaqueductal grey matter modulates trigeminovascular input: a role in migraine? *Neuroscience* 2001;106:793–800.

Knight YE, Bartsch T, Kaube H, Goadsby PJ. P/Q-type calcium-channel blockade in the periaqueductal gray facilitates trigeminal nociception: a functional genetic link for migraine? *J Neurosci* 2002;22:1–6.

Knight YE, Bartsch T, Goadsby PJ. Trigeminal antinociception induced by bicuculline in the periaqueductal gray (PAG) is not affected by PAG P/Q-type calcium channel blockade in rat. *Neurosci Lett* 2003;336:113–116.

Kolmodin GM, Skoglund CR. Analysis of spinal inter-neurons activated by tactile and nociceptive stimulation. *Acta Physiol Scand* 1960;50:337–355.

Lenaerts ME, Oommen KJ, Couch JR, Skaggs V. Can vagus nerve stimulation help migraine? *Cephalalgia* 2008;28:392–395.

Levin M. Nerve blocks in the treatment of headache. *Neurotherapeutics* 2010;7:197–203.

Liebetanz D, Fregni F, Monte-Silva KK, et al. After-effects of transcranial direct current stimulation (tDCS) on cortical spreading depression. *Neurosci Lett* 2006;398:85–90.

Lindblom U, Tapper DN, Wiesenfeld Z. The effect of dorsal column stimulation on the nociceptive response of dorsal horn cells and its relevance for pain suppression. *Pain* 1977;4:133–144.

Lipton RB, Pearlman SH. Trans-cranial magnetic simulation in the treatment of migraine. *Neurotherapeutics* 2010;7:204–212.

Lipton R, Goadsby PJ, Cady RK, et al. PRISM study: occipital nerve stimulation for treatment-refractory migraine. *Cephalalgia* 2009;29(suppl 1):30.

Lipton RB, Dodick DW, Silberstein SD, et al. Single-pulse transcranial magnetic stimulation for acute treatment of migraine with aura: a randomised, double-blind, parallel-group, sham-controlled trial. *Lancet Neurol* 2010;9:373–380.

Ma YT, Sluka KA. Reduction in inflammation-induced sensitization of dorsal horn neurons by trans-cutaneous electrical nerve stimulation in anesthetized rats. *Exp Brain Res* 2001;137:94–102.

Maeda Y, Lisi TL, Vance CG, Sluka KA. Release of GABA and activation of GABA(A) in the spinal cord mediates the effects of TENS in rats. *Brain Res* 2007;1136:43–50.

Magis D, Allena M, Bolla M, et al. Occipital nerve stimulation for drug-resistant chronic cluster headache: a prospective pilot study. *Lancet Neurol* 2007;6:314–321.

Matharu M, Bartsch T, Ward N, et al. Central neuromodulation in chronic migraine patients with suboccipital stimulators: a PET study. *Brain* 2004;127:220–230.

Mauskop A. Vagus nerve stimulation relieves chronic refractory migraine and cluster headaches. *Cephalalgia* 2005;25:82–86.

Mayanagi Y, Bouchard G. Evaluation of stereotactic thalamotomies for pain relief with reference to pulvinar intervention. *Appl Neurophysiol* 1976;39:154–157.

Melzack R, Wall PD. Pain mechanisms: a new theory. *Science* 1965;150:971–979.

Meyerson BA, Linderoth B. Mode of action of spinal cord stimulation in neuropathic pain. *J Pain Symptom Manage* 2006;31:S6–S12.

Mohamad YM, Kothari R, Hughes G, et al. Trans-cranial magnetic stimulation (TMS) relieves migraine headache. *Headache* 2006;46:839.

Mohammad TM, Hughes G, Nkrumah M, et al. Self-administered transcranial magnetic stimulation (TMS) during the aura phase improved and aborts headache. *Headache* 2006;46:857.

Multon S, Schoenen J. Pain control by vagus nerve stimulation: from animal to man . . . and back. *Acta Neurol Belg* 2005;105:62–67.

Oh M, Ortega, J, Bellotte BJ, et al. Peripheral nerve stimulation for the treatment of occipital neuralgia and transformed migraine using a C1-2-3 subcutaneous paddle style electrode: a technical report. *Neuromodulation: Technology at the Neural Interface* 2004;7:103–112.

Olausson B, Xu ZQ, Shyu BC. Dorsal column inhibition of nociceptive thalamic cells mediated by gamma-amin-obutyric acid mechanisms in the cat. *Acta Physiol Scand* 1994;152:239–247.

Paemeleire K, Van Buyten JP, Van Buynder M, et al. Phenotype of patients responsive to occipital nerve stimulation for refractory head pain. *Cephalalgia* 2010;30:662–673.

Popeney CA, Aló KM. Peripheral neurostimulation for the treatment of chronic, disabling transformed migraine. *Headache* 2003;43:369–375.

Radhakrishnan R, Sluka KA. Spinal muscarinic receptors are activated during low or high frequency TENS-induced anti-hyperalgesia in rats. *Neuropharmacology* 2003;45:1111–1119.

Radhakrishnan R, King EW, Dickman JK, et al. Spinal 5-HT(2) and 5-HT(3) receptors mediate low, but not high, frequency TENS-induced antihyperalgesia in rats. *Pain* 2003;105:205–213.

Reed KL, Black SB, Banta CJ 2nd, Will KR. Combined occipital and supra-orbital neuro-stimulation for the treatment of chronic migraine headaches: initial experience. *Cephalalgia* 2010;30:260–271.

Ren K, Dubner R. Descending modulation in persistent pain: an update. *Pain* 2002;100:1–6.

Ren K, Dubner R. Descending control mechanisms. In: Basbaum A, Bushnell A, eds. *Science of Pain.* Oxford: Academic Press; 2008: 723–762.

Resende MA, Sabino GG, Candido CR, et al. Local trans-cutaneous electrical stimulation (TENS) effects in experimental inflammatory edema and pain. *Eur J Pharmacol* 2004;504:217–222.

Sabino GS, Santos CM, Francischi JN, de Resende MA. Release of endogenous opioids following trans-cutaneous electric nerve stimulation in an experimental model of acute inflammatory pain. *J Pain* 2008;9:157–163.

Sadler RM, Purdy RA, Rahey S. Vagal nerve stimulation aborts migraine in patient with intractable epilepsy. *Cephalalgia* 2002;22:482–484.

Salar G, Job I, Mingrino S, et al. Effect of transcutaneous electrotherapy on CSF beta-endorphin content in patients without pain problems. *Pain* 1981;10:169–172.

Sandkuhler J. Models and mechanisms of hyperalgesia and allodynia. *Physiol Rev* 2009;89:707–758.

Sandkuhler J, Fu QG, Zimmermann M. Spinal pathways mediating tonic or stimulation-produced descending inhibition from the periaqueductal gray or nucleus raphe magnus are separate in the cat. *J Neurophysiol* 1987;58:327–341.

Saper J, Dodick DW, Silberstein SD, et al. Occipital nerve stimulation for the treatment of intractable chronic migraine headache: ONSTIM feasibility study. *Cephalalgia,* 2011;31:271–285.

Saracco MG, Valfre W, Cavallini M, Aguggia M. Greater occipital nerve block in chronic migraine. *Neurol Sci* 2010;31(suppl 1):S179–S180.

Schechtmann G, Song Z, Ultenius C, et al. Cholinergic mechanisms involved in the pain relieving effect of spinal cord stimulation in a model of neuropathy. *Pain* 2008;139:136–145.

Schwedt TJ, Dodick DW, Hentz J, et al. Occipital nerve stimulation for chronic headache: long-term safety and efficacy. *Cephalalgia* 2007a;27:153–157.

Schwedt TJ, Dodick DW, Trentman TL, Zimmerman RS. Response to occipital nerve block is not useful in predicting efficacy of occipital nerve stimulation. *Cephalalgia* 2007b;27:271–274.

Siebner HR, Rothwell J. Trans-cranial magnetic stimulation: new insights into representational cortical plasticity. *Exp Brain Res* 2003;148:1–16.

Silberstein SD, Lipton RB, Sliwinski M. Classification of daily and near-daily headaches: a field study of revised IHS criteria. *Neurology* 1996;47:871–887.

Sluka KA, Chandran P. Enhanced reduction in hyperalgesia by combined administration of clonidine and TENS. *Pain* 2002;100:183–190.

Sluka KA, Bailey K, Bogush J, et al. Treatment with either high or low frequency TENS reduces the secondary hyperalgesia observed after injection of kaolin and carrageenan into the knee joint. *Pain* 1998;77:97–102.

Sluka KA, Deacon M, Stibal A, et al. Spinal blockade of opioid receptors prevents the analgesia produced by TENS in arthritic rats. *J Pharmacol Exp Ther* 1999;289:840–846.

Sluka KA, Vance CG, Lisi TL. High-frequency, but not low-frequency, transcutaneous electrical nerve stimulation reduces aspartate and glutamate release in the spinal cord dorsal horn. *J Neurochem* 2005;95:1794–1801.

Sluka KA, Lisi TL, Westlund KN. Increased release of serotonin in the spinal cord during low, but not high, frequency transcutaneous electric nerve stimulation in rats with joint inflammation. *Arch Phys Med Rehabil* 2006;87:1137–1140.

Song Z, Meyerson BA, Linderoth B. Muscarinic receptor activation potentiates the effect of spinal cord stimulation on pain-related behavior in rats with mononeuropathy. *Neurosci Lett* 2008;436:7–12.

Song Z, Ultenius C, Mcyerson BA, Linderoth B. Pain relief by spinal cord stimulation involves serotonergic mechanisms: an experimental study in a rat model of mononeuropathy. *Pain* 2009;147:241–248.

Stiller CO, Linderoth B, O'Connor WT, et al. Repeated spinal cord stimulation decreases the extracellular level of gamma-aminobutyric acid in the periaqueductal gray matter of freely moving rats. *Brain Res* 1995;699:231–241.

Stiller CO, Cui JG, O'Connor WT, et al. Release of gamma-aminobutyric acid in the dorsal horn and suppression of tactile allodynia by spinal cord stimulation in mononeuropathic rats. *Neurosurgery* 1996;39:367–374; discussion 374–375.

Teepker M, Hotzel J, Timmesfeld N, et al. Low-frequency rTMS of the vertex in the prophylactic treatment of migraine. *Cephalalgia* 2009;8:8.

Tepper SJ, Rezai A, Narouze S, et al. Acute treatment of intractable migraine with sphenopalatine ganglion electrical stimulation. *Headache* 2009;49:983–989.

Trentman TL, Zimmerman RS. Occipital nerve stimulation: technical and surgical aspects of implantation. *Headache* 2008;48:319–327.

Urban MO, Gebhart GF. Supraspinal contributions to hyperalgesia. *Proc Natl Acad Sci USA* 1999;96:7687–7692.

Wall PD. The gate control theory of pain mechanisms: a re-examination and re-statement. *Brain* 1978;101:1–18.

Wallin J, Cui JG, Yakhnitsa V, et al. Gabapentin and pregabalin suppress tactile allodynia and potentiate spinal cord stimulation in a model of neuropathy. *Eur J Pain* 2002;6:261–272.

Wallin J, Fiska A, Tjolsen A, et al. Spinal cord stimulation inhibits long-term potentiation of spinal wide dynamic range neurons. *Brain Res* 2003;973:39–43.

Weiller C, May A, Limmroth V, et al. Brain stem activation in spontaneous human migraine attacks. *Nat Med* 1995;1:658–660.

Weiner R, Reed K. Peripheral neuro-stimulation for control of intractable occipital neuralgia. *Neuromodulation* 1999;2:217–221.

Woolf CJ. Trans-cutaneous electrical nerve stimulation and the reaction to experimental pain in human subjects. *Pain* 1979;7:115–127.

Woolf CJ, Salter MW. Neuronal plasticity: increasing the gain in pain. *Science* 2000;288:1765–1769.

Woolf C, Thompson J. Stimulation-induced analgesia: transcutaneous electrical nerve stimulation (TENS) and vibration. In: Wall P, Melzack R, eds. *Textbook of Pain.* New York: Churchill Livingstone; 1994:1191–2008.

Yakhnitsa V, Linderoth B, Meyerson BA. Spinal cord stimulation attenuates dorsal horn neuronal hyperexcitability in a rat model of mononeuropathy. *Pain* 1999;79:223–233.

Yarnitsky D, Goor-Aryeh I, Bajwa ZH, et al. Possible parasympathetic contributions to peripheral and central sensitization during migraine. *Headache* 2003;43:704–714.

Botulinum Toxin

Stephen Silberstein, MD

INTRODUCTION

Headache affects more than 45 million individuals in the United States, which makes it one of the most common nervous system disorders in existence (National Institute of Neurological Disorders and Stroke, 2002). In the last decade, the International Headache Society (IHS) diagnostic criteria for headache disorders have been revised to address changing perceptions of these conditions (International Classification of Headache Disorders 2 [ICHD-II], 2004). Headache disorders can be broadly classified as episodic (fewer than 15 headache days per month) or chronic (15 or more headache days per month for more than 3 months) (ICHD-II, 2004).

Migraine is a primary headache disorder characterized by various combinations of neurologic, gastrointestinal, and autonomic changes. The ICHD-II criteria specify a total of seven subtypes of migraine.

Chronic daily headache (CDH) is a heterogeneous group of headache disorders that can include chronic migraine (CM), chronic tension-type headache (CTTH), and other headache types that occur on 15 or more days per month in the absence of structural or systemic disease (Silberstein et al., 2005). CDH affects 4% to 5% of the general population worldwide (Scher et al., 1998; Castillo et al., 1999; Wang et al., 2000). Patients with CDH often overuse acute headache medications (Silberstein et al., 2005) and have greater disability and lower quality of life compared to patients with episodic headache (Wang et al., 2000; Meletiche et al., 2001; Bigal et al., 2003).

HEADACHE TREATMENT

Acute (abortive) migraine treatments, which patients take at the time of headache occurrence in an attempt to relieve pain and disability and prevent progression, include both migraine-specific medications, such as ergots and triptans, and nonspecific agents, such as analgesics and opioids (Silberstein, 2004). In contrast, preventive treatments are designed to reduce the frequency, severity, or duration of migraine attacks. These therapies are indicated when acute medications are ineffective or overused, or when headaches are very frequent or disabling (Silberstein, 2004). Preventive agents include beta-adrenergic blockers, antidepressants, calcium-channel and serotonin antagonists, anticonvulsants, and nonsteroidal anti-inflammatory drugs (Silberstein, 2004).

Although daily oral prophylactic treatments have proved effective, issues such as lack of compliance with daily dosing regimens and adverse effects have limited their usefulness (Blumenfeld et al., 2003; Silberstein, 2004). In turn, health-care providers have looked at other modalities and agents, including botulinum toxins (botulinum neurotoxins; BoNTs), as potential preventive treatments.

BOTULINUM TOXIN IN HEADACHE DISORDERS
Botulinum Toxin Formulations

The seven BoNT serotypes (A, B, C1, D, E, F, and G) produced by *Clostridium botulinum* are synthesized as single-chain polypeptides. All serotypes inhibit acetylcholine release, although their intracellular target proteins, physiochemical characteristics, and potencies differ (Aoki & Guyer, 2001; Mauskop, 2004). Botulinum toxin type A (BoNTA) has been the most widely studied serotype for therapeutic purposes (Aoki & Guyer, 2001).

Currently, BoNT is available for clinical use in the United States as onabotulinumtoxinA (botulinum toxin type A), sold under the brand name Botox (Allergan, Inc., Irvine, California); abobotulinumtoxinA (another botulinum toxin type A), brand name Dysport (Ipsen Ltd., Slough, United Kingdom); incobotulinumtoxinA (another botulinum toxin type A), brand name Xeomin (Merz Pharmaceuticals, Greensboro, North Carolina); and the BoNTB product rimabotulinumtoxinB, brand name Myobloc/Neurobloc (Solstice Neurosciences, Inc., South San Francisco, California, and Solstice Neurosciences Ltd., Dublin, Ireland). Lyophilized Botox is available in vials containing 100 units (U) of BoNTA and is diluted with 2 or 4 mL of preservative-free 0.9% saline to yield a concentration of 5.0 or 2.5 U per 0.1 mL, respectively (BOTOX® package insert, 2004). Reconstituted solutions of Botox can be refrigerated but must be used within 4 hours (BOTOX® package insert, 2004). Myobloc is available in 0.5-, 1-, and 2-mL vials containing 5,000 U per mL (Mauskop, 2004).

Mechanism of Action of Botulinum Toxin in Headache

BoNT inhibits the release of acetylcholine at the neuromuscular junction by binding to motor or sympathetic nerve terminals, then entering the nerve terminals and inhibiting release of acetylcholine, thereby blocking neuromuscular transmission. This inhibition occurs as the BoNT cleaves one of several proteins integral to the successful docking and release of acetylcholine from vesicles situated within nerve endings. Following intramuscular (IM) injection, BoNT produces partial chemical denervation of the muscle, resulting in a localized reduction in muscle activity (Aoki & Guyer, 2001; Mauskop, 2004).

The association between BoNTA use and the alleviation of migraine headache symptoms was discovered during the initial clinical trials of BoNTA treatment for hyperfunctional lines of the face (Binder et al., 2000). BoNTA therapy has been used for a variety of disorders associated with painful muscle spasms. Because migraine attacks are frequently associated with muscle tenderness (Jensen et al., 1998), it was generally believed that intramuscular BoNTA might prevent abnormal sensory signals in the affected muscle from arriving in the central nervous system. If abnormal muscle physiology can trigger migraine, then BoNTA treatment might be expected to work prophylactically only in patients whose migraine attacks develop on the heels of episodic or chronic muscle tenderness.

Jakubowski et al. (2006) have explored neurologic markers that might distinguish migraine patients who could benefit from BoNTA treatment from those who do not. In their study, the prevalence of neck tenderness, aura, photophobia, phonophobia, osmophobia, nausea, and throbbing was similar between responders and nonresponders. The two groups offered different accounts of their pain, however. Among nonresponders, 92% described a buildup of pressure inside their head (exploding headache). Among responders, 74% perceived their head to be crushed, or clamped, or stubbed by external forces (imploding headache); and 13% attested to an eye-popping pain (ocular headache). The finding that exploding headache is not as responsive to extracranial BoNT injections is consistent with the view that migraine pain is mediated by intracranial innervation. The amenability of imploding and ocular headaches to BoNTA treatment suggests that these types of migraine pain involve extracranial innervation as well (Jakubowski et al., 2006).

The precise mechanisms by which BoNTA alleviates headache pain remain unclear. This compound is known to inhibit the release of glutamate and two neuropeptides, substance P and calcitonin gene-related peptide (CGRP), from nociceptive neurons, suggesting that antinociceptive properties are distinct from its neuromuscular activity (Dodick et al., 2005).

BoNTA may inhibit central sensitization of trigeminovascular neurons, which is believed to be key to migraine's development and maintenance (Aoki, 2003; Cui et al., 2004; Oshinsky, 2004; Dodick et al., 2005). In their work, Oshinsky et al. (2004) relied on a preclinical model of sensitizing dorsal horn neurons in the trigeminal nucleus caudalis (TNC) following chemical stimulation of the dura for testing the effects of BoNTA on central sensitization. These researchers used the single-neuron electrophysiology of second sensory neurons in the TNC with cutaneous receptive fields and microdialysis of the TNC to evaluate the effects of pretreatment of the peri-orbital region of the rat with BoNTA. In saline-treated animals, extracellular glutamate increased steadily after 100 minutes following the application of inflammatory soup to the dura. The increase of glutamate reached approximately three times the basal level at 3 hours after the inflammatory soup. Electrophysiologic recordings of neurons in the TNC before and after sensitization confirmed these data. Following the inflammatory soup, the magnitude of the response to sensory stimuli increased, as did the cutaneous receptive field of the second sensory neurons in the TNC.

Afferent–efferent communication occurs in the nerve through axon–axon glutamate secretion, and at the level of the ganglion through nonsynaptic release of glutamate and peptides (CGRP and substance P). Oshinsky (2004) proposed the following explanation for this phenomenon: after chemical stimulation of the dura during a migraine attack and in their rat model, the dural afferents may communicate with other trigeminal afferents on the ophthalmic division of the trigeminal nerve and recruit them to secrete glutamate and neuropeptides. This process would lead to the recruitment of even more afferents, thereby spreading activation and sensitization. The number of afferents activated on the dura is small compared with the total number of afferents in the whole trigeminal system, so activation of the dural afferents alone may not be sufficient to produce the large changes in the central nervous system that lead to central sensitization.

Oshinsky et al. (2004) measured the extracellular level of glutamate following a 5-minute chemical stimulation of the dura and found that there is a two- to threefold increase in its concentration more than 1.5 hours following the stimulation. This increase was blocked by pretreating the face of the rat with BoNTA. Producing large changes in extracellular glutamate levels in the central

nervous system requires a massive sensory activation. The afferents of the dura may recruit the afferents of the face and head, which in turn leads to the sensitization of these areas seen in human and animal studies. BoNT may block the axon-to-axon and interganglionic communication of the afferents, thereby preventing central and peripheral sensitization outside of rat dura. Electrophysiologic studies confirmed that there was no change in the magnitude of the sensory response in the TNC neurons or their receptive field in the BoNTA rats following the inflammatory soup. These data indicate that peripheral application of BoNTA prevents central sensitization elicited by stimulation of the dura with inflammatory mediators (Oshinsky et al., 2004).

BOTULINUM TOXIN TREATMENT TECHNIQUES

Sterile technique should be observed for the entire BoNT injection procedure. Injections do not have to be intramuscular, but we use the muscles as reference sites for injections, which are most commonly administered in the glabellar and frontal regions, the temporalis muscle, the occipitalis muscle, and the cervical paraspinal region.

Three injection protocols are commonly used:

- The fixed-site approach, which uses fixed, symmetrical injection sites and a range of predetermined doses
- The follow-the-pain approach, which adjusts the sites and doses depending on where the patient feels pain and where the examiner can elicit pain and tenderness on palpation of the muscle, and which often employs asymmetrical injections
- A combination approach, using injections at fixed frontal sites, supplemented with follow-the-pain injections (this approach typically uses higher doses of BoNTA) (Blumenfeld et al., 2003)

Table 27.1 lists recommended anatomical sites of injection for headache and the BoNTA (Botox) dose per site used in the PREEMPT trials.

Clinical Comparison of Botulinum Toxin's Efficacy in Headache Disorders

Most studies on BoNT's efficacy and safety in headache treatment have used Botox (Schulte-Mattler & Leinisch, 2008). No large, well-controlled studies using other preparations have been yet published. The clinical trial results discussed in this subsection are summarized in **Table 27.2** (Schulte-Mattler & Leinisch, 2008).

Table 27.1 Botox Dosing for Chronic Migraine by Muscle

	Total Number of Units (U) (Number of IM Injection Sites)	
Head/Neck Area	Minimum Dose	Maximum Dose
Frontalis	20 U (4 sites)	20 U (4 sites)
Corrugator	10 U (2 sites)	10 U (2 sites)
Procerus	5 U (1 site)	5 U (1 site)
Occipitalis	30 U (6 sites)	≤40 U (5 U per site; ≤8 sites)
Temporalis	40 U (8 sites)	≤50 U (5 U per site; ≤10 sites)
Trapezius	30 U (6 sites)	≤50 U (5 U per site; ≤10 sites)
Cervical paraspinal muscle group	20 U (4 sites)	20 U (4 sites)
Total Dose Range	155 U 31 sites	195 U ≤39 sites

Each IM injection site = 0.1 mL = 5 U onabotulinumtoxinA.

Table 27.2 Summary of Randomized, Double-Blind, Controlled Studies of the Efficacy of Botulinum Toxin Type A in the Treatment of Headache

Headache Type	Study Outcome
Migraine	
Silberstein et al., 2000	Decreased migraine frequency and severity and acute medication use with 25 U BoNTA but not with 75 U BoNTA
Brin et al., 2000	Decreased migraine pain compared with placebo with simultaneous frontal and temporal BoNTA injections
Evers et al., 2004	No difference from placebo in decreased frequency of migraine Greater decrease in migraine-associated symptoms with BoNTA 16 U
Saper et al., 2007	Decreased frequency and severity of migraine in BoNTA and placebo groups with no between-group differences
Elkind et al., 2006	Comparable decreases in migraine frequency in both BoNTA and placebo groups with no between-group differences
Chronic Migraine	
Mathew et al., 2005	No difference from placebo on primary efficacy endpoint: change in headache-free days from baseline at day 180 A significantly higher percentage of BoNTA patients had a 50% or greater decrease in headache days/month at day 180 compared with placebo
Dodick et al., 2005	Greater decrease in headache frequency after two and three injections compared with placebo
Silberstein et al., 2005	No difference from placebo on primary efficacy endpoint: change in headache frequency from baseline at day 180 Greater decrease in headache frequency for 225 U BoNTA and 150 U BoNTA than placebo
Aurora et al., 2010; Diener et al., 2010; Dodick et al., 2010	Two large placebo-controlled, double-blinded trials Follow the pain BoNTA is both safe and effective
Chronic Tension-Type Headache	
Silberstein et al., 2006	No difference from placebo on primary efficacy endpoint: mean change from baseline in CTTH headache days Greater percentage of BoNTA patients than placebo recipients with a 50% or greater reduction in headache frequency at 90 and 120 days for several doses of BoNTA

Some studies support BoNTA's efficacy in migraine treatment. A double-blind, vehicle-controlled trial of 123 patients with moderate-to-severe migraine found that subjects treated with a single injection of 25 U BoNTA (but not those treated with 75 U) showed significantly fewer migraine attacks per month, as well as reductions in migraine severity, number of days requiring acute medication, and incidence of migraine-induced vomiting (Silberstein et al., 2000). The lack of a significant effect in the higher-dose group may be related to baseline group differences—for example, fewer migraines or a longer time since migraine onset in the higher-dose group (Silberstein et al., 2000).

Another double-blind, placebo-controlled, region-specific study found a significant reduction in migraine pain among patients who received simultaneous injections of BoNTA in the frontal and temporal regions, as well as an overall trend toward BoNTA superiority to placebo in reducing migraine frequency and duration (Silberstein et al., 2000). A randomized, double-blind, placebo-controlled study compared the efficacy of placebo, 16 U BoNTA, and 100 U BoNTA as migraine prophylaxis injected into the frontal and neck muscles (Evers et al., 2004). There were no statistically significant differences in reduction of migraine frequency among the groups, but the accompanying migraine symptoms were reduced in the group whose members received 16 U BoNTA (Evers et al., 2004).

Later studies, however, have not demonstrated significant improvements for BoNTA over placebo. A recent study (Saper et al., 2007) of patients (N = 232) with moderate to severe episodic migraine (four to eight episodes per month) compared placebo with regional (frontal, temporal, or glabellar) or combined (frontal/temporal/glabellar) treatment with BoNTA. Reductions from baseline in migraine frequency, maximum severity, and duration occurred with BoNTA and placebo, without significant between-group differences being noted (Saper et al., 2007). Elkind et al. (2006) conducted a series of three sequential studies of 418 patients with a history of four to eight moderate-to-severe migraines per month with re-randomization at each stage and BoNTA doses ranging from 7.5 to 50 U. BoNTA and placebo produced comparable decreases from baseline in migraine frequency at each time point examined, with no consistent, statistically significant, between-group differences being observed (Elkind et al., 2006).

Several randomized, double-blind, placebo-controlled studies support the efficacy of BoNT for the treatment of CDH. In a large, placebo-controlled study (N = 355), Mathew et al. (2005) found that while BoNTA did not differ from placebo in the primary efficacy measure

(change from baseline in headache-free days at day 180), significant differences in several secondary endpoints were apparent, including a greater percentage of patients with a 50% or greater decrease in headache frequency and a greater mean change from baseline in headache frequency at day 180. A subgroup analysis of patients not taking concomitant preventive agents (n = 228) revealed that BoNTA patients had a greater decrease in headache frequency compared with patients who received placebo after two and three injections, and at most time points from day 180 to 270 (Dodick et al., 2005). In a similar study (N = 702) by Silberstein et al. (2005) that utilized several doses of BoNTA (75, 150, and 225 U), the primary efficacy endpoint (mean improvement from baseline in headache frequency at day 180) was also not met. However, all groups responded to treatment, and patients taking 150 and 225 U of BoNTA had a greater decrease in headache frequency at day 240 than those who received placebo (Silberstein et al., 2005).

More recently, the PREEMPT clinical program confirmed onabotulinumtoxinA as an effective, safe, and well-tolerated headache prophylaxis treatment for adults with CM. Two Phase 3, multicenter studies (PREEMPT 1 and 2), each of which consisted of a 24-week, double-blind, parallel-group, placebo-controlled phase followed by a 32-week open-label phase, enrolled 1,384 patients with CM. All patients received the minimum IM dose of 155 U of onabotulinumtoxinA administered to 31 injection sites across seven head and neck muscles using a fixed-site, fixed-dose injection paradigm. In addition, as much as 40 U onabotulinumtoxinA, administered IM to 8 injection sites across three head and neck muscles, was allowed using a modified follow-the-pain approach. Thus, the minimum dose was 155 U and the maximum dose was 195 U (Table 27.1). Statistically significant reductions from baseline in terms of frequency of headache days after BoNTA treatment compared to placebo treatment in both PREEMPT 1 and 2 (P = 0.006; P < 0.001) were observed. Statistically significant improvement from baseline after onabotulinumtoxinA treatment compared with placebo was seen for headache episodes in PREEMPT 2 (P = 0.003). Pooled analysis demonstrated that onabotulinumtoxinA treatment significantly reduced the mean frequency of headache days (−8.4 onabotulinumtoxinA, −6.6 placebo; P < 0.001) and episodes (5.2 onabotulinumtoxinA, −4.9 placebo; P = 0.009). Additionally, for several other efficacy variables (i.e., migraine episodes, migraine days, moderate or severe headache days, cumulative hours of headache on headache days, and proportion of patients with severe disability), significant between-group differences favored onabotulinumtoxinA. The PREEMPT results included highly significant improvements in multiple headache symptom measures and demonstrated improvement in patients' functioning, vitality, psychological distress, and overall quality of life. Multiple treatments of 155 U up to 195 U per treatment cycle administered every 12 weeks were shown to be safe and well tolerated (Aurora et al., 2010; Diener et al., 2010; Dodick et al., 2010).

Studies evaluating the efficacy of BoNTA in CTTH have yielded inconsistent results. A double-blind, randomized, placebo-controlled study (Silberstein et al., 2006) of 300 patients found that while all treatment groups, including those who received placebo, improved in mean change from baseline in CTTH-free days per month (primary endpoint) at day 60, patients receiving BoNTA, at any dose or regimen (50 to 150 U), did not demonstrate improvement compared with patients receiving placebo. However, a significantly greater percentage of patients in three BoNTA groups at day 90 and two BoNTA groups at day 120 had a 50% or greater decrease in CTTH days compared to the placebo group (Silberstein et al., 2006). Furthermore, a review evaluating clinical studies of TTH supports the benefit of BoNTA in reducing frequency and severity of headaches, improving quality of life and ratings on disability scales, and reducing the need for acute medication (Mathew & Kaup, 2002). Another review, which also included studies with both Botox and Dysport, concluded that randomized, double-blind, placebo-controlled trials present contradictory results attributable to variable doses, injection sites, and frequency of treatment (Rozen & Sharma, 2006).

Adverse Events Associated with Botulinum Toxin Use

More than two decades of clinical use have established BoNTA as a safe drug (Mauskop, 2004), with no systemic reactions being reported in clinical trials for headache. Rash and flu-like symptoms can rarely occur as a result of an allergic reaction (Mauskop, 2004). However, serious allergic reactions have never been reported. Injection of anterior neck muscles can cause dysphagia (swallowing difficulties) in some patients (Mauskop, 2004). Dysphagia and dry mouth appear to be more common with injections of BoNTB (Myobloc) because of its wider migration pattern (Mauskop, 2004). The most common side effects when treating facial muscles are cosmetic; they include ptosis or asymmetry of the position of the eyebrows (Mauskop, 2004). Another possible, but rare, side effect is difficulty in holding the head erect because of neck muscle weakness (Mauskop, 2004). Headache patients occasionally develop a headache following the injection procedure, although some have immediate relief of an acute attack. The latter is most likely due to trigger point injection effect (Mauskop 2004). Worsening of headaches and neck pain can occur and last for several days or, rarely, weeks after the injections because of the irritating effect of the needling and delay in the muscle relaxing effect of BoNT (Mauskop, 2004).

CONCLUSIONS

Headache disorders, including migraine and CM, are common debilitating conditions that profoundly impact quality of life. Clinical studies suggest that BoNT is a safe treatment and is efficacious for the prevention of some forms of migraine—specifically, chronic migraine and perhaps high-frequency episodic migraine. Further research is needed to elucidate the mechanism of action of BoNT in headache, further establish its safety and efficacy for these indications, and fully develop its therapeutic potential.

REFERENCES

Aoki KR. Evidence for antinociceptive activity of botulinum toxin type A in pain management. *Headache* 2003;43:S109–S115.

Aoki KR, Guyer B. Botulinum toxin type A and other botulinum toxin serotypes: a comparative review of biochemical and pharmacological actions. *Eur J Neurol* 2001;8(suppl 5):21–29.

Aurora SK, Dodick DW, Turkel CC, et al. OnabotulinumtoxinA for treatment of chronic migraine: results from the double-blind, randomized, placebo-controlled phase of the PREEMPT 1 trial. *Cephalalgia* 2010;30:793–803.

Bigal ME, Rapoport AM, Lipton RB, et al. Assessment of migraine disability using the Migraine Disability Assessment (MIDAS) Questionnaire: a comparison of chronic migraine with episodic migraine. *Headache* 2003;43:336–342.

Binder WJ, Brin MF, Blitzer A, et al. Botulinum toxin type A (Botox) for treatment of migraine headaches: an open-label study. *Otolaryngol Head Neck Surg* 2000;123:669–676.

Blumenfeld A, Binder W, Silbrestein SD, Blizter A. Procedures for administering botulinum toxin type A for migraine and tension-type headache. *Headache* 2003;43:884–891.

BOTOX® package insert. Irvine, CA: Allergan, Inc.; 2004.

Brin MF, Swope DM, O'Brien C, et al. Botox for migraine: double-blind, placebo-controlled, region-specific evaluation [Abstract]. *Cephalalgia* 2000;20:421–422.

Castillo J, Munoz P, Guitera V, Pascual J. Epidemiology of chronic daily headache in the general population. *Headache* 1999;39:190–196.

Cui M, Khanijou S, Rubino J, Aoki K. Subcutaneous administration of botulinum toxin A reduces formalin-induced pain. *Pain* 2004;107:125–133.

Diener H-C, Dodick DW, Aurora SK, et al. OnabotulinumtoxinA for treatment of chronic migraine: results from the double-blind, randomized, placebo-controlled phase of the PREEMPT 2 trial. *Cephalalgia* 2010;30:804–814.

Dodick DW, Mauskop A, Elkind AH, et al. Botulinum toxin type A for the prophylaxis of chronic daily headache: subgroup analysis of patients not receiving other prophylactic medications: a randomized double-blind, placebo-controlled study. *Headache* 2005;45:315–324.

Dodick DW, Turkel CC, DeGryse RE, et al. OnabotulinumtoxinA for treatment of chronic migraine: pooled results from the double-blind, randomized, placebo-controlled phases of the PREEMPT clinical program. *Headache* 2010;50: 921–936.

Elkind AH, O'Carroll P, Blumenfeld A, et al. A series of three sequential, randomized, controlled studies of repeated treatments with botulinum toxin type A for migraine prophylaxis. *J Pain* 2006;7:688–696.

Evers S, Vollmer-Haase J, Schwaag S, et al. Botulinum toxin A in the prophylactic treatment of migraine: a randomized, double-blind, placebo-controlled study. *Cephalalgia* 2004;24:838–843.

ICHD-II Headache Classification Committee. The International Classification of Headache Disorders, 2nd edition. *Cephalalgia* 2004;24(suppl 1):1–160.

Jakubowski M, McAllister PJ, Bajwa Z, et al. Exploding vs. imploding headache in migraine prophylaxis with botulinum toxin A. *Pain* 2006;125:286–295.

Jensen R, Bendtsen L, Olesen J. Muscular factors are of importance in tension-type headache. *Headache* 1998;38:10–17.

Mathew NT, Kaup AO. The use of botulinum toxin type A in headache treatment. *Cur Treatment Options Neurol* 2002;4:365–373.

Mathew N, Frishberg B, Gawel M, et al. Botulinum toxin type A (Botox) for the prophylactic treatment of chronic daily headache: a randomized, double-blind, placebo-controlled trial. *Headache* 2005;45:293–307.

Mauskop A. The use of botulinum toxin in the treatment of headaches. *Pain Physician* 2004;7:377–387.

Meletiche DM, Lofland JH, Young WB. Quality of life differences between patients with episodic and transformed migraine. *Headache* 2001;41:573–578.

National Institute of Neurological Disorders and Stroke (NINDS). *Headache: Hope Through Research*. NIH publication -02-158. Bethesda, MD: U.S. Department of Health and Human Services, National Institutes of Health; 2002.

Oshinsky ML. Botulinum toxins and migraine: how does it work. *Practical Neurol* 2004;suppl:10–13.

Oshinsky M, Poso-Rosich P, Luo J, et al. Botulinum toxin A blocks sensitization of neurons in the trigeminal nucleus caudalis [Abstract]. *Cephalalgia* 2004;24:781.

Rozen D, Sharma J. Treatment of tension-type headache with Botox: a review of the literature. *Mt Sinai J Med* 2006;73:493–498.

Saper JR, Mathew NT, Loder EW, et al. A double-blind, randomized, placebo-controlled comparison of botulinum toxin type A injection sites and doses in the prevention of episodic migraine. *Pain Med* 2007;8:478–485.

Scher AI, Stewart WF, Liberman J, Lipton RB. Prevalence of frequent headache in a population sample. *Headache* 1998;38:497–506.

Schulte-Mattler W, Leinisch E. Evidence based medicine on the use of botulinum toxin for headache disorders. *J Neural Transm* 2008;115:647–651.

Silberstein SD. Migraine. *Lancet* 2004;363:381–391.

Silberstein SD, Mathew N, Saper J, Jenkin S. Botulinum toxin type A as a migraine preventive treatment: for the Botox® Migraine Clinical Research Group. *Headache* 2000;40:445–450.

Silberstein SD, Stark SR, Lucas SM, et al. Botulinum toxin type A for the prophylactic treatment of chronic daily headache: a randomized, double-blind, placebo-controlled trial. *Mayo Clin Proc* 2005;80:1126–1137.

Silberstein SD, Gobel H, Jensen R, et al. Botulinum toxin type A in the prophylactic treatment of chronic tension-type headache: a multicentre, double-blind, randomized, placebo-controlled, parallel-group study. *Cephalalgia* 2006;26:790–800.

Wang SJ, Fuh JL, Lu SR, et al. Chronic daily headache in Chinese elderly: prevalence, risk factors and biannual follow-up. *Neurology* 2000;54:314–319.

Chinese and Traditional East Asian Medicine

Stefan Chmelik, MSc, MRCHM, MBAcC, and Mark Bovey, MSc, MBAcC

CHAPTER OUTLINE

BRIEF INTRODUCTION TO TRADITIONAL CHINESE MEDICINE

Ever since European travelers started coming back from East Asia in the seventeenth century, stories about Chinese medicine with its exotic techniques and *Materia Medica* have abounded. The history of medicine in what we today call China goes back some 3,500 years (Unschuld, 1985). *Traditional Chinese medicine* (TCM) is a modern term used to describe a standardized form of traditional medicine as utilized in state hospitals in the People's Republic of China over the last few decades (Unschuld, 1985; Schied, 2002). Although it remains the best-recognized form in the West, Unschuld points out that TCM is only one stream from one school—that of systematic correspondences. The terms *Oriental medicine* (OM) and, increasingly, *traditional East Asian medicine* (TEAM) are being used to encompass the traditional medical practices of the whole vast region in general, including Japan, Tibet, Vietnam, Korea, Taiwan, and Cambodia.

TCM, OM, and TEAM are regarded by their proponents today as total systems of medicine (Maciocia, 1989; Maclean & Lyttleton, 1998, 2010), independent and separate from modern biomedicine, although increasingly partaking of and influenced by the same. These traditional systems incorporate different methods: acupuncture (and its related techniques such as bleeding, cupping, gua sha, plum blossom hammer, and moxibustion), bodywork (such as *tui na* and *shiatsu*), herbal medicine, food and dietary therapy, exercise and movement therapy (such as *Tai Qi* and *Qi Gong*), and meditation or spiritual practice. Acupuncture has attracted the most interest outside of East Asia.

TRADITIONAL EAST ASIAN MEDICINE THERAPIES

TEAM therapies include the following:

- Acupuncture: insertion of solid, fine needles into nonvascular surface anatomy, either at points determined by TEAM assessment or in palpated areas
- Cupping: use of glass or bamboo suction cups over acupuncture channels
- Moxibustion: creating local heat on acupuncture channels through use of smoldering dried *Artemisa vulgaris* (mugwort)
- Gua sha: repetitive rubbing or scrapping of acupuncture channels to create localized heat and inflammation

- Bleeding: pricking of acupuncture points to release small droplets of blood
- Plum blossom hammer: use of a small "hammer" with multiple short needles attached to a flexible handle to tap along acupuncture channels
- Tui na: Chinese physical therapy
- Shiatsu: Japanese physical therapy
- Tai Qi and Qi Gong: forms of movement and exercise designed to strengthen the body and regulate Qi flow

Acupuncture (and its related techniques) and herbal medicine are the two therapies explored in this chapter.

TEAM, although influenced by and interactive with Greco-Roman and Arab medicine and science, essentially developed according to a different worldview, with a corresponding variation in the physiology, and to some extent even the functional anatomy of the human body (Unshuld, 1985). Today, doctors and researchers in China, Japan, and other countries are attempting to correlate traditional TEAM with modern-science medicine and its discoveries, although this is seldom an easy fit. A number of modern explanations have attempted to identify the "mechanism behind" acupuncture, or at least to explain some of its apparent effects. In respect to its analgesic effect (by far the most studied aspect), acupuncture appears to deactivate a complex limbic–paralimbic–neocortical network, mediated by various signal molecules, notably opioid peptides (Zhao, 2008; Hui et al., 2010). Nevertheless, a single unified theory that explains all of the effects claimed for acupuncture by TEAM practitioners has yet to emerge. Perhaps the latest discoveries in soft connective tissue and fascia and its related biophysiological, biochemical, and biosocial effects are coming closer to this point. Discussion of fascia is beyond the scope of this chapter, however.

Practicing TEAM is now a viable profession in most developed countries, with its own regulatory bodies, practitioner organizations, and educational frameworks. In the West, there is considerable discussion about, and variation in, minimum training standards. Indeed, some experts believe that the majority of adverse events associated with acupuncture are caused by physicians who have undertaken only a short training (Walkley, 2010). Less controversially, it has been noted that acupuncture "fatalities are avoidable and a reminder of the need to insist on adequate training for all acupuncturists" (Ernst, 2010).

Use

It is possible that TEAM is the most widely utilized medical intervention worldwide. As Xue et al. (2010)

state, "In its region of origin, TCM is an essential part of the national health care system." Accurate figures are not available for all countries, but TEAM therapies are clearly being used by large and increasing numbers of patients in the United States and the United Kingdom (Bodeker et al., 2005; Barnes et al., 2008; Hunt et al., 2010; Xue et al., 2010). In East Asia, TEAM is ubiquitous, even with the increase in modern biomedicine. As of February 2010, a combined population of more than 1.5 billion people, or 22% of the world's population, lived in these countries—specifically, People's Republic of China (mainland China, Tibet, Hong Kong, Macau), Japan, North Korea, South Korea, and Taiwan. Populations in Vietnam and Cambodia also utilize TEAM. Approximately 70% to 80% of the population of Southeast Asia is believed to use traditional medicines (Xue et al., 2010). A Taiwanese study showed that 62.5% of all beneficiaries of National Health Insurance (which covers 98% of the population) had used TCM/TEAM during the 6-year period examined and that 86% of this group preferred herbal medicine (Chen et al., 2008).

Complementary and Alternative Medicine

The public has increasingly visited complementary and alternative medicine (CAM) practitioners in the West, mostly within the private medical arena, with some private medical insurers now covering the major therapies (such coverage varies significantly by country) and with some provision within the public health services. The public clearly likes CAM therapies. As Gaul et al. (2009) point out, "In the patients' view, scientific data on a CAM therapy of their choice is not the most crucial aspect, as they do not pay attention to evidence-based medicine." Of patients in a recent survey, 65% reported that they would continue their CAM therapies despite negative scientific reports; positive personal experience apparently outweighs scientific data in their minds (Vanderheyden et al., 2005).

Use of TEAM Outside of East Asia

Use and availability of TEAM in hospital or primary medical environments varies widely and has been largely dependent on available funding. **Table 28.1** summarizes estimates of its use in selected non-Asian countries. Patients in Australia and Germany are particularly high users of such therapies, with a prevalence four to five times greater than that in the United Kingdom or United States. A telephone survey in Australia indicated that acupuncture had been used by 9% of respondents during the previous 12 months and that adult Australians made approximately 2.6 million visits to acupuncturists and incurred personal expenditures for such treatments estimated to be $1.58 billion in total (Xue et al., 2006). Twelve-month use of Chinese herbs lagged only slightly behind at 7%, whereas in Germany acupuncture is far more prevalent (Bücker et al., 2008).

Table 28.1 Population Use of Chinese Medicine Modalities

Country/Year	12-Month Prevalence for Each Modality (%) [Lifetime Use in Brackets Where Available]			Author
	Acupuncture	Herbs (TCM/TEAM)	CAM Overall	
Australia, 2005	9.2	7.0	19.3	Xue et al., 2010
Canada, 2001–2005	2.2		12.4	Metcalfe et al., 2010
Germany, 2008	[34.5]	[9.7]	[42.3]	Bücker et al., 2008
Japan, 2001	6.7	>17.2*	76.0	Yamashita et al., 2002
United Kingdom, 1998	1.6 [7.0]		13.6† [32.1]†	Thomas et al., 2001
United Kingdom, 2001	1.6	0.4	10.0†	Thomas & Coleman, 2004
United Kingdom, 2005	3.2	1.6		Hunt et al., 2010
United States, 1999	1.4		28.9	Ni et al., 2002
United States, 2002	1.1 [4.1]			Burke et al., 2006
United States, 2007	1.4		38.3	Barnes et al., 2008
Taiwan, 2001	2.8	24.4		Chen et al., 2007

* Herbs includes over-the-counter (17%) and prescribed (10%) preparations, but not those in health drinks.

† CAM excludes over-the-counter purchases; includes only practitioner visit.

In the United Kingdom, the latest analysis (Hunt et al., 2010) estimates 12-month acupuncture use at 3.2% and TCM at 1.6%. These figures represent a doubling for acupuncture and a fourfold increase in use of herbs since the national survey undertaken 4 years earlier (Thomas & Coleman, 2004). The two data sets are not entirely comparable but probably do highlight a genuine trend. Recent national statistics for the United States (Burke et al., 2006) also indicate an increase in visits to acupuncturists (from 1.1% in 2002 to 1.4% in 2005), which goes against the trend for several other CAM therapies. Relatively greater increases have been seen for the use of herbs (Tindle et al., 2006), and prevalence figures are much higher than for acupuncture (approximately 18% in recent years for 12-month use: Barnes et al., 2008). TEAM herbs probably make up a rather small (and unknown) proportion of this figure, which includes prescribed and over-the-counter use of any non-vitamin, non-mineral natural product. One reason for the rise in TCM/TEAM use in the West may be the increasing body of scientific evidence concerning its safety and effectiveness (Xue et al., 2008).

Use of TEAM Specifically for Migraine and Headache

Table 28.2 summarizes use of acupuncture by headache/migraine patients. A 10-year analysis of patients' visits for migraine treatment in Taiwan found that 30% received combined drug and CAM therapy and that 100% of this group had received herbal medicine (Chang et al., 2009). In a study of tertiary headache outpatient clinics in Germany and Austria, nearly 82% of attendees had used some form of CAM, with the most popular being acupuncture (lifetime use 58.3%) (Gaul et al., 2009).

Acupuncture usage rates from Italian (Rossi et al., 2006) and Swiss (Kozac et al., 2005) surveys were lower than the German and Austrian rate, but still substantial: 27% and 21%, respectively. There is also some indication that migraineurs use acupuncture to a greater degree than patients with tension headache (Rossi et al., 2006).

Research: Biomedical-Oriented Research Paradigms Compared to TEAM and Holistic Approaches

We should perhaps acknowledge the "elephant in the room" when attempting to apply randomized, controlled trial (RCT) or similar research methodology to TEAM, and indeed to many—if not all—CAM therapies. This is an issue also acknowledged by the World Health Organization (WHO) (Xue et al., 2010)—namely, the worldview and very basis on which *holistic* therapies are theorized to work is self-evidently an uncomfortable fit within a reductionist model where the purest results are achieved by *eliminating* or controlling as many parameters as possible. Holism, which was first described by Aristotle, aims to *include* as many parameters as possible in a patient's overall care.

Xue et al. (2010) note:

> The conduct of RCTs on TCM can be more challenging due to a number of intrinsic and external factors. . . . Criticism of the methodological quality of TCM clinical trials remains a challenge, as it is difficult to align traditional medicine philosophies with modern scientific methods. (p. 311)

The same authors also note that RCTs for drug trials are not without potential bias, however.

TEAM utilizes a different model of physiology and biochemistry compared to Western medical science. Any attempt to understand and explain the claims of TEAM

Table 28.2 Use of Acupuncture by Headache/Migraine Patients

Country/Year	Acupuncture		CAM		Author	Sample Characteristics
	12-Month Use (%)	Lifetime Use (%)	12-Month Use (%)	Lifetime Use (%)		
Canada, 2001–2005	2.2		19.0		Metcalf et al., 2010	Migraine—general population
Germany/Austria, 2005–2006		58.3		81.7	Gaul et al., 2009	Primary headache (mainly migraine)— headache clinic
Italy, 2002–2003		27.3	17.1	31.4	Rossi et al., 2005	Migraine—headache clinic
Italy, 2003–2004		17.8	22.7	40.0	Rossi et al., 2006	Tension headache—headache clinic
Switzerland, 1996–1998		20.8		29.8	Kozac et al., 2005	Migraine and tension headache—headache clinic

will, therefore, often have to select a specific aspect of the terminology to study (e.g., "Ascendant Liver Yang" as a cause of "migraine" within TEAM terminology), and then correlate this aspect with a parameter that will make sense to the non-TEAM physician (such as lymphocyte protein expression, to continue the same example). Gabriel (2004) notes, "Complaints, which are apparently not in correlation with the migraine, disappear because of the holistic medical therapy."

Comparing Acupuncture and Herbal Medicine Research

Unlike with acupuncture, where significant controversy and debate exist regarding potential mechanisms of action, few dispute that herbs are simply natural drugs, albeit of a more chemically complex and variable nature. There is no doubt that Chinese herbal medicines are pharmacologically active, as can be attested to by the thousands of research papers identifying active ingredients of Chinese herbs and exploring their pharmacological effects. TEAM physicians may use terminology foreign to Westerners to describe how or why they believe the herbs are working, but the human body just notes the biochemical effects.

Chinese herbal medicines . . . are comprised of a complex multicomponent nature. The activities are aimed at the system level via interactions with a multitude of targets in the body. The formulation principle of multi-herbs intervention strategy is a systems approach for the treatment and prevention of disease. (Wang et al., 2009, p. 40)

A significant issue to acknowledge is the obvious discrepancy between the quantity of research available in English on herbal medicine as opposed to acupuncture. It is immediately apparent upon scoping and searching the literature that significantly less good-quality data are available for herbal medicine. Some noted examples in the West are use of such therapies to treat eczema or dermatitis (Sheehan & Atherton, 1992), endometriosis (Flower et al., 2009), unexplained infertility (Wing & Sedlmeier, 2006), irritable bowel syndrome (Bensoussan et al., 1998), and rheumatoid arthritis (Goldbach-Mansky et al., 2009).

A number of reasons can be postulated to explain this imbalance, and it is worth speculating on these issues briefly to foster a better understanding as well as to direct future researchers and translators to relevant areas.

1. Acupuncture, as a treatment, is more popular than herbal medicine in the West. This preference is interesting because traditionally herbs have always been the main medicine in China, with acupuncture having a much less broad appeal. However, the perceived exotic nature of Asian herbs, the difficulty prescribing them without a TEAM diagnosis (in contrast to medical acupuncture), and the perceived conflict with pharmaceutical drugs seem so far to have limited the expansion of herbs into Western countries, with a presumed effect on research emphasis (Hoizey & Hoizey, 1988).
2. The vast majority of herbal medicine research has not been translated from the original Chinese or Japanese (which makes up the bulk of the literature on this topic). More papers on acupuncture were identified that met the inclusion criteria for this chapter than papers on herbal medicine. However, a quick glance at the TEAM databases in Chinese show thousands of papers on herbs.
3. It may be easier to get a paper on acupuncture published in a Western journal than one on herbal medicine.
4. TEAM doctors tend to start with the premise that herbal medicine works, such that the purpose of their research is simply to put numbers to the success rate. This bias tends to exclude the vast majority of Chinese research (acupuncture and herbs).
5. The possible variables with herbal research are vast, probably even more so than for acupuncture.
6. A significant number of medical professionals now insert solid needles for therapeutic purposes but do so without using a TEAM framework or diagnosis. This provider population includes doctors, physiotherapists, osteopaths, chiropractors, and others. This non-TEAM acupuncture movement has produced a whole new generation of research outside East Asia. The same trend has not occurred with Asian herbal medicine, which is practiced almost entirely by TEAM-trained physicians.

TEAM Theory and Practice: Disease Patterns for Migraine

TEAM herbal remedies are, in the vast majority of cases, prescribed as tailored formulae for a specific individual. Nevertheless, certain patterns emerge with their use that can be identified with modern disease classifications (**Table 28.3**). There are approximately 80 organ-based disease patterns associated with TCM in particular.

The main symptoms of migraine fall into the following patterns (Maclean & Lyttleton, 1998): Liver Qi constraint (also called Liver Qi Stagnation), Liver Fire, Ascendant Liver Yang and Wind (also called Liver Yang Rising), and

Table 28.3 TEAM Pattern Differentiation by Headache Symptom (All Types)

TEAM Pattern	Clinical Features
Wind Cold	Acute, accompanied by chills
Wind Heat	Acute, accompanied by feeling hot
Wind Damp	Heavy sensation, worse in morning and with humidity
Summer-Heat	Acute, accompanied by high fever
Liver Qi Constraint	Recurrent, tight sensation, preceded by related symptoms
Liver Fire	Acute, splitting, related to excesses of behavior
Ascendant Liver Yang and Wind	Recurrent, severe with distention sensation
Cold Affecting Liver and Stomach	Recurrent, accompanied by digestive symptoms and weakness
Phlegm Damp	Dull, distending and tight, provoked by irritant
Wind Phlegm	Acute, pounding with vomiting
Blood Stasis	Recurrent and focal, often related to trauma
Stomach Heat	Frontal and related to food
Stomach and Gallbladder Disharmony	Temporal or frontal with radiation pattern, related to diet and accompanied by vomiting or bile
Qi Deficiency	Background headaches, worse when tired
Blood Deficiency	Background headaches, initiated by menstruation, breastfeeding, or blood loss
Kidney Yin Deficiency	Chronic, empty feeling with mild heat sensation
Kidney Yang Deficiency	Chronic, empty feeling with dull-cold sensation

Source: Adapted from Maclean W, Lyttleton J. *Handbook of Internal Medicine, Vol. 3.* London: Pangolin Press; 2010.

Qi and Blood Stasis. A patient will usually also exhibit an underlying pathology responsible for the migraine mechanism—for example, Qi deficiency, blood deficiency, kidney Yin deficiency, and kidney Yang deficiency.

A full description of TEAM terminology is beyond the scope of this chapter. In addition to specific words that resist translation such as *Qi, Yin,* and *Yang,* words that are commonly translated into English can actually have quite different meanings. Thus *Liver* refers to a host of *functions* in addition to the actual viscus that sits in the right hypochondrium. *Wind* has a complex meaning that includes acute pathology, contagious disease, and spasm or tremor. *Blood* includes, among other things, much of the biochemistry of the body including aspects of the endocrine system. In this chapter, words with specific TEAM meaning have been denoted by the use of capitalization for the first letter of the word.

ACUPUNCTURE FOR MIGRAINE: THE EVIDENCE

Cochrane Review Evidence

The Cochrane systematic review and meta-analysis on migraine prophylaxis (Linde et al., 2009a) is the first starting point in considering the evidence base for acupuncture.

It included randomized trials of acupuncture versus no treatment (except for routine care and for acute attacks) or sham acupuncture or another treatment. Studies of acute migraine, and those with mixed and inseparable headache types, were excluded. Only Western databases were searched, up to 2008. Acupuncture studies were defined as those with needle insertion at specific points: traditionally defined, trigger points or tender spots.

Twenty-two trials were included, with 4,419 participants (median: 42; range: 27–1,715). Prior to 2002, all studies ($n = 11$) were small (range: 30–85). More recent studies have been not only larger but also rated more highly for methodological quality, with most considered to be adequate. All 22 were parallel group designs (cross-over trials are generally problematic for acupuncture due to the high risk of carry-over effects). Controls used in the selected studies included no acupuncture (6 studies), sham acupuncture (14 studies), conventional drugs (4 studies), and other therapies (2 studies). Meta-analysis was carried out within these four types, but it should be recognized that substantial heterogeneity exists as to the nature of the control within each type. Given that debate around sham comparisons forms a central focus of acupuncture evidence evaluation, it is important to understand the nature of sham acupuncture.

Table 28.4 Main Results from Cochrane Meta-Analysis of Acupuncture for Migraine Prophylaxis

Control Group Type	Number of Trials (High Quality)	Number of Trials Favoring Acupuncture (Number Significant)	Responder Proportions (%)		Overall Effect	
			Acupuncture	Control	Risk Ratio	P Value
Normal care	4 (3)	4 (3)	40.7	17.2	2.33	< 0.00001
Sham	11 (5)	8 (2)	43.5	37.7	1.13	0.16
Drugs	2 (2)	2 (0)	46.8	39.1	1.20	0.08
		Alternative Outcome: Headache Frequency				
Drugs	3 (3)	3 (2)			0.26*	0.0008

* Standardized mean difference.

Sham control groups represent an attempt to duplicate the placebo RCT model, which is used as the gold standard for evaluating drug efficacy. This Cochrane review identified five main sham types among the migraine studies:

- Superficial needling of acupuncture points inappropriate for migraine ($n = 2$ studies)
- Superficial needling in locations not identified as classical acupuncture points ($n = 5$)
- Unknown needling procedure in locations that were not acupuncture points but were close to them ($n = 2$)
- Use of specialized "placebo" needles in appropriate acupuncture points—these deliver pricking or pressing sensations but not penetrating the skin, with the action being invisible to the patient ($n = 2$)
- Other nonpenetrating shams, such as mock transcutaneous electrical nerve stimulation (TENS) ($n = 2$)

These techniques differ in their degree of credibility and blinding and in the amount and type of physiological effects they provoke. They are not inert placebos, however (Lundeberg et al., 2011). They answer research questions about whether particular sets of points, or types of needling action, are more effective than others; they do not answer questions about the effectiveness of acupuncture (Birch, 2006).

In addition to the nature of the sham, heterogeneity in most aspects of the acupuncture intervention was apparent—for example, in terms of the number and frequency of treatments, choice of points and degree of standardization in this selection, and needle manipulation techniques. The outcome measures used, the time points, and length of follow-up also varied dramatically. The primary outcome for the meta-analysis was responder proportion, i.e., a 50% or greater reduction in frequency or other headache measure, at 3 to 4 months after randomization.

A summary of the main results is shown in **Table 28.4**. For four trials of acupuncture versus no acupuncture, the overall effect of the intervention was highly significant: risk ratio of 2.33 (95% CI: 2.02–2.69), probability test value $P < 0.001$. The proportions of responders overall were 40.7% in the acupuncture group and 17.2% for routine care. Three of the four trials were rated as high quality; all four individually had positive outcomes in relation to the control group, and three were significantly positive. Only one study included long-term follow-up; in this investigation, acupuncture was still significantly superior 9 months after the end of the trial. *The conclusion was that acupuncture is clearly helpful if added to routine care.*

Of the 14 sham-controlled trials, only 11 could be analyzed together. In 8 of the 11 studies, the acupuncture group had better results than the sham group, but only 2 trials yielded significantly better outcomes with acupuncture. The overall effect was nonsignificant: RR of 1.13 (95% CI: 0.95–1.35; $P = 0.16$). The proportions of responders were 43.5% for acupuncture and 37.7% for sham. A subgroup analysis of the 5 high-quality studies gave similar results. Each of the 3 trials not analyzed with the rest had significantly positive results and may well have swung the overall effect to a significant one if their data could have been included. *The conclusion was that acupuncture was not superior to sham treatment.*

For the comparison with conventional medication, only two trials were available for analysis of responders, but three for headache frequency. All 3 studies were of high quality. Acupuncture outcomes in each trial were superior to drugs, with 0/2 and 2/3 showing statistical significance for responders and frequency, respectively. The overall effect was significantly positive for frequency ($P = 0.0008$) but showed just a positive trend for the response rate ($P = 0.08$). The proportions of responders were 46.8% for acupuncture and 39.1% for drugs. *The conclusion was that acupuncture is at least as good as drugs and is associated with fewer adverse events.*

There were two small trials of acupuncture versus other therapies, but it was not possible to estimate effect sizes from their data.

Although the proportions of responders favored acupuncture in all three trial designs, the lack of statistical significance for the sham comparison means that these results are paradoxical and difficult to interpret. This outcome is not unusual with acupuncture clinical evidence—indeed, it is the norm—but migraine provides a particularly good example. There are now in excess of 20 RCTs focusing on use of acupuncture to treat migraine (many more, if Chinese databases are included), and several are large and of high quality. The results are consistent despite the variable designs and interventions. Their external validity is considered to be reasonable given that the response rates in the RCTs have been found similar to those in observational studies (Linde et al., 2007). On the face of it, acupuncture is no better than sham treatment, but no worse than conventional prophylactic drugs, which themselves have been found superior to sham/placebo in extensive testing. The authors suggested four possible explanations (which will be taken up again later in this chapter):

1. Acupuncture is a potent placebo.
2. Sham acupuncture has direct physiological effects that help migraine.
3. The lack of blinding in non-sham trials introduced bias.
4. The acupuncture quality in trials is not as good as the usual quality found in clinical practice.

They concluded that acupuncture should be considered as a prophylactic treatment option for migraine, especially for those patients refusing drug treatment or suffering unwanted side effects from it (Linde et al., 2009a).

Finally, apart from the effectiveness issue, three other major considerations feed into recommendations related to use of acupuncture in migraine: cost-effectiveness, adverse events, and concerns over conventional drugs.

Adverse Events

As mentioned earlier, acupuncture intervention arms were associated with significantly fewer unwanted effects than medication arms in comparative trials. Nevertheless, acupuncture is an invasive therapy and does carry some risk. In a retrospective literature review for the period 1965–1999, all reported cases of acupuncture adverse

events were assembled and inspected (Lao et al., 2003). It was concluded that acupuncture carried out by trained practitioners, using clean needle techniques, is a generally safe procedure. The risk of serious events from trained practitioners is very low, with estimates per 10,000 treatment sessions ranging from 0.05 to 0.55 over all conditions ("Acupuncture for Tension-Type Headaches and Migraine," 2010) and 0.034 estimated from 3.84 million chronic pain treatment sessions (Weidenhammer et al., 2007).

In a very large prospective observational study in Germany, 8.6% of the (229,230) patients reported at least one adverse event (Witt et al., 2009), while a large U.K. survey estimated this rate to be 10.7% (MacPherson et al., 2004b). No deaths or permanent injuries occurred in either the German or U.K. study. The most commonly reported events in the German study were minor bleeding and bruising at the insertion site (6.17%) and pain (1.7%); in the U.K. study, the counterparts were tiredness and pain.

Practitioner reports of adverse events at much lower frequencies (MacPherson et al., 2001; White et al., 2001) probably indicate a degree of under-reporting, although it is also possible that patients may over-report and assume nonexistent causality (MacPherson et al., 2004a). The vast majority of patients reporting adverse events were content to continue with treatment (MacPherson et al., 2004a). There is no evidence that the adverse event rates and profile of migraine patients deviates significantly from those for patients with chronic pain or the general population (Melchart et al., 2006). Thus acupuncture can be considered comparatively safe (Linde et al., 2009a).

Cost-Effectiveness

Two large pragmatic trials of acupuncture for migraine have been carried out, evaluating the effect of the intervention over and above routine care (Vickers et al., 2004; Jena et al., 2008). In each case, the associated costs were higher with acupuncture, largely due to the cost of providing the treatment, but this factor was outweighed by the value of the benefits related to quality of life (Wonderling et al., 2004; Witt et al., 2008). In both trials, acupuncture was found to be cost-effective according to international standards: $18,403–$15,829 per quality-adjusted life year (QUALY).

Concerns over Conventional Drugs

Verum response rates in migraine drug trials are high—in excess of 50% when response is defined as a 50% or greater reduction in attack frequency. However, dropout rates are also high and long-term follow-up is almost nonexistent, so there are doubts as to their level of helpfulness in routine care (Linde et al., 2009a). In the large German comparison trials of acupuncture and drugs, substantial numbers of dropouts were noted in the drug arms, perhaps because those populations already preferred acupuncture (Diener et al., 2006; Streng et al., 2006; Linde et al., 2007). Acupuncture performs well in real-world settings (Weidenhammer et al., 2007; Jena et al., 2008), for whatever reasons, and may provide valuable long-term benefits (Vickers et al., 2004; Thomas et al., 2005).

Comparison with Other Systematic Reviews of Acupuncture for Migraine

Scott and Deare (2006) employed quite similar inclusion criteria to those used in the Cochrane Review for publications up to 2006. They selected 25 studies, of which 16 overlapped with the Cochrane review. The Cochrane authors excluded 8 of the studies included in Scott and Deare's review, largely based on its questionable validity. Despite the differences, and a responder cut-off of 33% rather than 50%, the meta-analysis results were similar and the headline stories were identical: acupuncture was found to be significantly better than no acupuncture, similar to sham treatment, and as good as or better than medication. *Scott and Deare concluded that acupuncture with or without conventional treatment would be likely to reduce migraine frequency, with minimal side effects.*

Sun and Gan (2008) covered Western database literature up to November 2007, but included tension headache as well as migraine. Of the 17 migraine papers, 13 overlapped with the Cochrane review. All of the 4 different trials were drug comparisons, but unfortunately the review did not present separate migraine and tension headache results. For the comparisons against no acupuncture and against sham treatment, the migraine results matched those found in the other meta-analyses. Notably, for tension headache, acupuncture enjoyed a significant advantage over sham treatment (a result also seen in another Cochrane review [Linde et al., 2009b]).

Pickett and Blackwell (2010) reviewed the evidence for the U.S. Family Physician's Network, and concluded that acupuncture was effective in reducing the frequency of migraines. The strength of their recommendation was accorded the highest level (A).

Narrative Reviews

Endres et al. (2007) concluded that a 6-week course of acupuncture is at least as good as 6 months of prophylactic drugs and recommended that this therapy should be integrated into existing treatment repertoires. The sham trial results were interpreted as indicating that specific Chinese point selection and needle depth are not as important as previously thought. Bongaard (2008) provided a completely different explanation for this outcome: minimal, shallow needling was equated with Japanese-style acupuncture, in contrast to a more vigorous Chinese style in the verum groups. Effective sham treatment indicates that both styles are viable, whether on or near to acupuncture points, thereby circumventing any placebo implications.

These issues were considered in some depth in a review covering chronic back pain, osteoarthritis, and headache (Sherman & Coeytaux, 2009). Acupuncture may be seen as a placebo therapy, but the lack of an accepted inert sham leaves this interpretation open to debate. The authors adopted a pragmatic stance and recommended that acupuncture be added to existing options, albeit not as the clear therapy of choice. Again, similar findings were reported in the latest review ("Acupuncture for Tension-Type Headaches and Migraine," 2010). When the effectiveness data were considered together with trial quality, cost-effectiveness, and adverse events, acupuncture was recommended as a reasonable adjunctive treatment, especially in patients not well managed by medication or looking for nondrug options.

Published Guidelines

- *U.S. Headache Consortium (2000):* "Evidence-based recommendations are not yet available for acupuncture." Evidence grade: C. This assessment was based on the rather small and largely low-quality trials available at that point, so the conclusion is not surprising.
- *British Association for the Study of Headache (BASH) (2007):* "Acupuncture is of little benefit." This is a controversial opinion, as it is based on two of the largest, best-quality studies conducted to date (Linde et al., 2005; Diener et al., 2006). It has set aside the routine care and drug comparison evidence and adopted the line that only superiority over sham is indicative of a real effect.
- *Scottish Intercollegiate Guidelines Network (SIGN) (2008):* "Acupuncture should be considered for preventive management in patients with migraine." Strength of recommendation: B. This guideline is noticeably different in tone from the BASH guideline despite much the same evidence being available to each organization.

Chinese Trials of Acupuncture for Migraine Prophylaxis

Systematic Reviews

A small number of Chinese journals are indexed in Western databases, but most Chinese medicine output is not easily accessible, especially to non-Chinese speakers. A systematic search of both Western and Chinese databases located nine high-quality Western trials and three low-quality Chinese ones (Zhang et al., 2008). The authors concluded that there were no high-quality migraine trials in China. Australian researchers conducted a systematic review of RCTs for migraine prophylaxis using the two largest Chinese databases, up to 2006 (Wang YY et al., 2008). They converted the imprecise Chinese outcome measures into global response rates, similar to those used elsewhere, but were unable to separate short- and long-term outcomes. Study quality was generally low, with none scoring more than 60%. Most did not describe the method of randomization or allocation concealment.

Seventeen trials were included, with a total of 2,097 participants (median: 91; range: 62–414). All except 2 were published after 2000, and none overlapped with the studies included in the Cochrane review (Linde et al., 2009a). All 17 used (largely appropriate) Western drugs for the control group, with no sham. Acupuncture was applied alone in 10 trials, combined with other interventions in 6 studies, and combined with drugs in 1 trial.

For the comparison of acupuncture (alone) and drugs, all 10 trials favored the acupuncture intervention and 5 of the 10 yielded statistically superior results. The overall effect was significant: RR: 1.55; 95% CI: 1.27–1.88; $P < 0.001$. For acupuncture combined with other TCM modalities, the overall effect was significantly positive for TCM. The authors concluded that acupuncture might be an effective prophylactic treatment, used either alone or together with drugs. Better-quality trials are needed to confirm this finding, and adverse events need to be recorded.

Recent Chinese Trials

Since the publication of the Australian review (Wang YY et al., 2008), a number of new Chinese RCTs for migraine prophylaxis have appeared in Western databases. Four completed trials and two protocols are summarized in **Table 28.5**. Although the emphasis in these investigations remained the comparative effectiveness of acupuncture as measured against drugs, some studies also included sham controls. One of these studies (Zhang et al., 2009a), as well as a larger uncompleted follow-up (Zhang et al., 2009b), used a double-dummy design. The largest trial, unpublished as yet in the West except for its protocol (Li XZ et al., 2008), included three

Table 28.5 Summary of Recent Chinese Trials of Acupuncture for Migraine Prophylaxis

Study	Number of Patients	Acupuncture Intervention	Number of Sessions	Control	Responders (%)	
					End of Treatment	3 Months
Huang et al., 2006	100	"Jingjin" therapy	10	Nimodipene	28 versus 7	32 versus 13
Jia et al., 2009	275	Electro-acupuncture, 1 appropriate point	20	Electro-acupuncture, 1 inappropriate point	100 versus 70*	100 versus 70*
Zhang et al., 2009a	60	3 main points + others + sham drug	12	Flunarizine + sham acupuncture	68 versus 24	68 versus 32
Zhong et al., 2009b	253	4 main points + others	Unknown	Flunarizine	93 versus 86	93 versus 86
Unfinished Trials						
Li XZ et al., 2008	480	Specific points on favored channels	20	3 different shams, all penetrating acupuncture		
Zhang et al., 2009b	140			Otherwise identical to Zhang et al., 2009a		

* Outcome time point not specified; global value used.

control groups who received normal needling, either at non-points or less appropriate points. One sham study compared just one appropriate point against one inappropriate point (Jia et al., 2009). The goal of Chinese trials is often not an evaluation of acupuncture but rather a test of one particular protocol against another.

For the four completed trials, the mean responder rates were 74% for acupuncture and 48.5% for the control (Huang et al., 2006; Jia et al., 2009; Zhang et al., 2009a; Zhong et al., 2009b). In those trials comparing acupuncture with medication (Huang et al., 2006; Zhang et al., 2009a; Zhong et al., 2009b), acupuncture was found to be significantly better in terms of the primary migraine outcomes at all time points, even at one year follow-up (Zhong et al., 2009b).

Comparison of Western and Chinese Trials

Despite their lower quality, the Chinese trials substantially add to the evidence base for acupuncture. The Cochrane review (Linde et al., 2009a) included only 2 to 3 trials in the acupuncture versus drug meta-analyses, whereas there were 10 trials when Chinese data were used 10 (Wang YY et al., 2008). In any review that omits Chinese data, there is also always the suspicion that the treatment provided is not the best or most authentic. A comparison of the overall effect sizes estimated from Chinese and Western two-arm drug trials shows a higher value for the former: 1.55 versus 1.20 (Wang YY et al., 2008; Linde et al., 2009a). The more recent Chinese trials feature much improved methodology and reporting quality. Some of these researchers have published their protocols in Western trials registers, which helps protect against publication bias—a notable problem in the past (Vickers at al., 1998). The recent comparative effectiveness studies (Huang et al., 2006; Zhang et al., 2009a; Zhong et al., 2009b) confirm the significant advantage of acupuncture over drugs.

Mechanisms

Preliminary results from a Spanish RCT with verum, sham, and normal care arms (Ramos-Font et al., 2009) showed that verum, but not sham, acupuncture modifies regional cerebral blood flow (measured by brain perfusion tomography), in line with observed clinical improvements in migraine headache. In most acupuncture imaging studies, researchers have observed that verum and sham needling (differentiated by the degree or depth of stimulation, the points needled, and sensation elicited) are associated with different patterns of brain area activation (Harris et al., 2009; Napadow et al., 2009).

Other studies seeking to demonstrate verum–sham differences in respect to acupuncture mechanisms for migraine have investigated arterial dilation (Boutouyrie et al., 2010) and autonomic regulation (Backer et al., 2008). In addition, acupuncture was observed to affect blood flow in the extracranial arteries in a nonblinded study (Park et al., 2009).

Most physiological studies on acupuncture have taken place in China, although only a tiny proportion have been reported in Western databases. Recent examples for migraine indicate that acupuncture may have the following effects:

- Suppress cortical spreading depression and plasma calcitonin gene-related peptide and substance P levels in rats (Shi et al., 2010)
- Increase plasma 5-hydroxytriptamine (5-HT) levels in verum versus sham controls in humans, and produce superior clinical outcomes (Jia et al., 2009)
- Reduce glucose metabolic activity in particular brain areas of migraineurs (Li XZ et al., 2008)
- Regulate inhibitory and stimulatory G protein levels in the brainstem of rats (Wang S et al., 2008)
- Regulate the expression of 5-HT and inducible nitric oxide synthetase mRNA in rat brains (Zhong & Li, 2007)
- Control cranial blood vessel expansion and contraction, and blood flow velocity, more effectively than drugs (Cai & Wang, 2006; Qin & Gu, 2006)

In a review of acupuncture used as treatment for headaches, Zhao et al. (2005) focused on the inhibitory effects on pain processing in the trigeminal nucleus caudalis and dorsal horn but recognized that many pathways and neurotransmitters may be involved. A variable combination of peripheral, spinal and supraspinal, cortical, psychological, and placebo effects are likely to occur with such therapy (Linde et al., 2009a). The relevance of the various experimental physiological changes to long-term clinical outcomes is not clear, however, especially given the much more positive results from sham-controlled studies in basic science than seen in most clinical trials.

Other Evidence
Observational Studies

Observational studies are not generally included in systematic reviews, yet can present aspects of evidence that are absent, or uncertain, in RCTs—in particular, how whole services operate in the real world. In a notable example, under the same umbrella of research designed to evaluate the suitability of acupuncture for reimbursement by

German state health insurance companies, very large observational studies were conducted alongside the RCTs. For 162,229 acupuncture patients with chronic headache, the physicians assessed 79% as having shown a marked or moderate response (21% minimal or no change) (Weidenhammer et al., 2007). A subset of these studies provided migraine-specific data (n = 732) (Melchart et al., 2006). Patients had, on average, 8.6 acupuncture sessions and showed a significant improvement in all headache outcomes both after treatment and at 6-month follow-up. Response rates were similar to those seen in the companion RCTs (Linde at al., 2007).

Qualitative Studies

Qualitative research is increasingly being embedded in clinical trials, partly to explore the perceptions of patients about the trial processes. Within a sham-controlled migraine RCT, patients and practitioners were found not to behave in the same way as in normal practice, which itself could alter the nature of the intervention and render the design invalid (Paterson et al., 2008).

Qualitative research can also provide a more complete picture of the treatment effects. In narrative interviews with 10 women having acupuncture for migraine, the treatment was found to relieve pain, decrease the use of pharmaceuticals, and increase emotional strength. The women felt safer, able to live a fuller life, and as if they had more control over the migraines (Rutberg & Ohrling, 2009).

Expert Opinion

Migraine is firmly believed by traditional acupuncturists to be one of the conditions most amenable to treatment (Maciocia, 2008). A survey among acupuncturists (largely neurologists) reported that treatment of tension headache and migraine gave the best results for all considered conditions, with improvements of more than 50% in 70% of cases (Bijak, 2008).

Acute Migraine Attacks

Very little information has been published in the West on treating acute migraine attacks with acupuncture, although it has been suggested that traditionally Chinese doctors have focused on treating acute attacks rather than preventing them (Guo, 2010). A German trial compared individualized, TCM-based acupuncture with sumatriptan injection and sham injection (Melchart et al., 2003). Acupuncture was found to be equivalent to sumatriptan, and both acupuncture and sumatriptan were better than the placebo for halting the attack. However, a second

dose of the drug was more effective than acupuncture for migraines that persisted after the initial treatment.

A large Chinese study (Zhou et al., 2007) found acupuncture to be superior to standard drug treatment in terms of reducing headache intensity and extending length of remission. Acupuncture consisted of one treatment on one point only, and the inclusion criteria restricted patients to those with one specific TCM-diagnosed pattern.

A recent three-arm Chinese study compared verum to (1) a sham procedure using "Chinese non-acupuncture points" and (2) the same sham treatment but with "Western non-points" (Li et al., 2009). The verum group responded faster and continued to show superiority over both sham groups. After 24 hours, 41% of acupuncture patients had complete pain relief and 80% had no recurrence or aggravation of symptoms.

Effectiveness of Procedures Allied with Acupuncture

Traditional acupuncture is often accompanied by adjunctive procedures such as moxibustion, cupping, or tui na, and needles may be substituted by anything from finger pressure to laser devices. Electro-acupuncture is prevalent in China but there were few examples provided in the review of Chinese migraine trials (Wang YY et al., 2008).

A laser acupuncture trial for children with headache (tension or migraine) showed superiority over sham (Gottschling et al., 2008). Wet cupping (i.e., cupping with some blood-letting, commonly practiced in the Middle East) was tested in a pre-post observational design in Iran (Ahmadi et al., 2008) with 70 mixed migraine and tension headache patients. Headache days were reduced by 12.6 days per month and severity by 66%. No other RCTs of allied procedures were located. Largely, these therapies have been seen in the West as an added complication that would obscure evaluating acupuncture per se, ignoring the fact that, traditionally, acupuncture exists within a Chinese (or East Asian) framework that incorporates many possible interacting components. What constitutes acupuncture per se is highly debatable (Sherman & Coeytaux, 2009).

Adequacy of the Acupuncture Used in Clinical Trials

In one respect, the acupuncture in Chinese trials, as in Chinese routine practice, is very different from that typical in the West: treatment is much more frequent, often daily (compared with 1 or 2 times per week), with more sessions in total (average 30 for Chinese trials versus 7 to 15 in the West). Best practice in Chinese medicine is generally considered to involve individualized diagnosis and treatment that evolves over time. All of the trials in the Cochrane review were based in the West: 55% apparently used individualized acupuncture, 27% used semi-standardized treatment, and 18% used standardized protocols. By comparison, none of the Chinese trials reviewed by Wang YY et al. (2008) followed an individualized route: 77% were entirely formulaic and 23% were semi-standardized. Chinese researchers appear to be less concerned about external validity in the sense of individualization. However, they do specify that treatment is based firmly on TCM principles, which is not the case for all Western trials (Wang YY et al., 2008; Linde et al., 2009a), and do believe that they provide better-quality treatment than in the West (Tu, 2010).

Individualized acupuncture in a RCT can mean many things, but most closely resembles normal practice in open, pragmatic trials where the diagnostic and treatment options are left to the practitioners' discretion for each patient, at each session. As Sherman and Coeytaux (2009) pointed out, "most trials don't evaluate acupuncture as it is actually practiced." These authors went on to describe the salient features of usual acupuncture as delivered either by traditionally or nontraditionally trained practitioners; outside the United States and the United Kingdom the distinction blurs, however, as many conventional doctors use at least some traditionally based acupuncture. None of the reviewed RCTs is likely to have contained all of Sherman and Coeytaux's traditional acupuncture components, which are numerous and cover the theoretical framework, diagnosis, point selection, point stimulation procedures, needling sensations, lifestyle advice, the therapeutic relationship, and the nature of treatment goals and outcomes.

Thus the acupuncture intervention in RCTs may possibly be inadequate or unrepresentative, which could reduce the reliability of the results (Facco et al., 2008; White et al., 2008). Nevertheless, some researchers have certainly gone to great lengths in trying to guard against this possibility (Molsberger et al., 2006).

Application of Acupuncture Quality Criteria in Systematic Reviews

There is little consensus on the treatment parameters that would make up an ideal acupuncture regime; hence there has been little attempt to apply quality criteria in systematic reviews (White et al., 2008). The most likely candidate is the adequacy of the amount of treatment, with four to six sessions suggested as a minimum requirement. Subgroup analysis has sometimes been run on

this basis (Ernst & White, 1998). In the Cochrane review (Linde et al., 2009a), two acupuncture quality grading systems were applied—namely, the authors' assessments of the appropriateness of the regimen and the similarity to their own choices. Culling the low-scoring ones would not appear to significantly alter the meta-analysis outcomes for acupuncture against sham. The same applies if those with fewest treatments were to be omitted. A more substantial change is seen if only those with individualized acupuncture are selected, as this choice would remove all three trials with negative results, leading to a significant advantage for acupuncture over sham treatment. This is not convincing evidence in itself but rather indicates that the nature and adequacy of the intervention may be an important consideration. A swing from marginally missing 95% statistical significance to marginally achieving it can have a disproportionate effect on systematic review conclusions and the perception of those who read them.

Specifying an Acupuncture Protocol for Treating Migraine

Some styles of acupuncture focus strongly on the patient's underlying constitutional characteristics, with little emphasis on the symptoms (Moss, 1999), in which case the idea of a protocol specifically oriented toward migraine has little meaning. However, most practitioners would be familiar with a core group of Chinese medicine patterns that are associated with migraine, whilst still having considerable latitude for individualization. In this section, we will not discuss the differentiations and guidelines provided for acupuncturists in standard textbooks, but rather seek to summarize the protocols and recommendations arising from research studies.

For Western trials, there has been a recent analysis of protocols (Zheng et al., 2010). The Chinese authors located six trials where acupuncture was either better than sham treatment or as good as standard drug therapy (positive trials), and contrasted them with three studies where this was not the case (negative trials). For each group, they summarized the choice of points, needling characteristics, and amount of treatment. The positive studies were used to inform protocol recommendations:

- The main formula should include these points: GB20, EX-HN5, Du20, Liv3, Ren 12, and Sp6. Another four optional points were identified.
- Manual, bilateral needling is recommended, and eliciting "deqi" is obligatory.
- There should be at least 18 sessions in all, twice weekly, with approximately 20 needled points per session.

Comparison with the negative trials shows that the latter differ only in having slightly fewer sessions and in the choice of some of the points. Altogether this was not a convincing exercise, with several of the recommendations based on flimsy evidence.

In the systematic review of Chinese trials (Wang YY et al., 2008), five points were used more commonly than the rest: GB20, GB8, EX-HN5, LI4, and Liv3. Three of these points overlap with the Western core group of points mentioned previously. No two studies used the same formula. The average number of sessions was 30, usually daily, which constitutes an entirely different regimen than that used in the Western versions. Few data on the acupuncture dose-response relationship exist, but one headache study recorded a greater decrease in pain intensity with increasing numbers of sessions (Lefaki et al., 2009): this would give credence to the supposition that the better results in the Chinese trials come, at least in part, from larger numbers of treatments.

The general approach has been quite consistent from ancient times (Zhao et al., 2009) to modern days (Hu et al., 2009), with the focus on the Gallbladder (GB) channel, and secondarily the San Jiao (SJ) channel, and using combinations of local and distal points. Every author has a different formula, however, with only one point featuring in almost every core protocol—GB20. Western point formulae have tended to be fairly similar to Chinese ones.

Whether built into a fixed formula or presented more flexibly, the most important guiding principle for point selection is that of channel differentiation (Molsberger et al., 2006; Zhang et al., 2008; Zhao et al., 2009; Guo, 2010); that is, the location of the symptoms is used to guide one to the most relevant channel(s). Migraines typically belong to the Shaoyang (GB and SJ) region, although other channels may be implicated.

The next most frequently used approach is based on differentiation by syndrome—a cornerstone of contemporary TCM. It depends strongly on identifying patterns in the patient's presenting symptoms but also typically gathers information from radial pulse palpation and tongue inspection. For example, seven main syndromes were chosen to guide treatment in an Italian RCT, with 4 to 7 points specified for each syndrome, and each patient individually diagnosed on this basis (Facco et al., 2008). The syndromes most commonly found among participants were excess of Liver Yang (39%) and exogenous Wind-Cold attack (23%). The excess Liver Yang and Liver Fire patterns have been found to be the most characteristic TCM diagnoses for differentiating migraine from tension-type headache, according to German trial data (Bowing et al., 2010).

Traditional protocols also often include local tender ("ahshi") points. Some preliminary evidence suggests that palpation for sensitive ear points (Allais et al., 2010) or local trigger points (Calandre et al., 2006) may indicate effective locations for needling when treating migraine.

Acupuncture, Sham Treatment, and Placebo

Now we return to the paradoxical situation described in most of the recent migraine reviews (Scott & Deare, 2006; Linde et al., 2009a; Sherman & Coeytaux, 2009; "Acupuncture for Tension-Type Headaches and Migraine," 2010): acupuncture seems not to be superior to sham treatment but is as good as evidence-based conventional treatment. It has been suggested that acupuncture may provide a particularly potent placebo (Linde et al., 2009a), owing to its close therapeutic relationship, relaxed atmosphere, mysterious ritual, and potential to reframe patients' experiences and illness. Of course, this is in itself an admirable quality. Promoting patients' own self-healing capabilities, by whatever route, is the key to affordable long-term health care for chronic conditions.

A fundamental consideration is the definition of acupuncture and hence what can legitimately be called a sham. For most practitioners, all of the placebo-enhancing factors listed in the preceding paragraph, plus other components as well, are part and parcel of the complex intervention that is acupuncture (Sherman & Coeytaux, 2009). Thus an appropriate control to test its effectiveness would need to "sham" all of these components (Wayne et al., 2009). It is not known what the active part of acupuncture is or what the specific effect is (Sherman & Coeytaux, 2009); most likely, verum and placebo effects interact and confound estimation. The assumption has been that acupuncture could be defined just by its use of specific points on the body, with the needling procedures being used to stimulate those sites. If acupuncture is seen as part of a whole system, however, then investigating just the needling is not useful (Sherman & Coeytaux, 2009).

A sham procedure should mimic acupuncture but not mimic its physiological effects. Of course, this condition is difficult to achieve (unlike with drugs) when the relevant physiological and psychosocial mechanisms are unknown (Wayne et al., 2009). Most sham interventions used in acupuncture trials (Linde et al., 2009a) are not inert. Not only do they approach the clinical outcomes of acupuncture, but they are also as effective as drugs, and considerably more effective than drug placebos. Although some of this potency may be attributed to placebo mechanisms (expectations, conditioning), other parts come through direct physiological routes—for example, the touch effect on C-type fibers (Lundeberg et al., 2011). Neuroimaging studies indicate that different mechanisms may underlie apparently similar verum and sham responses (Wayne et al., 2009) despite the fact that endogenous opioids are implicated in both (VanderPloeg & Yi, 2009). The delayed onset of action after acupuncture and the possibility for long-term effects after cessation of treatment are not characteristic of placebo and would probably rely on different mechanisms (VanderPloeg & Yi, 2009).

Some styles of acupuncture use shallow or even nonpenetrating needling (Birch, 2003), so sham controls employing shallow needling or "placebo" needles that press but do not penetrate the skin can be seen merely as lighter styles of the same therapy—equivalent to comparing Chinese and Japanese styles of acupuncture, for example (Molsberger, 2006; Bongaard, 2008). Other sham treatments use non-acupuncture points or points deemed appropriate for the condition. Such designs merely test whether one group of points works better than another; they do not test whether acupuncture works in general. In addition, classical points have not been exactly defined and cannot be reproducibly located (Tao et al., 2009), nor were they until recently assigned specific functions of the sort used to define "appropriate" and "inappropriate"; also, they all interconnect according to acupuncture meridian theory (Scott & Deare, 2006). Thus concepts of "right" and "wrong" points, or actual and non-points, are vague and may lead to erroneous conclusions being drawn from sham RCTs. Different styles, schools, and individuals provide a plurality of approaches, such that one person's sham may be another's active treatment.

Blinding of practitioners while still allowing them to function normally has not been achieved: generally, sham-controlled acupuncture studies aim to blind the patients and assessors. Some may argue that no blind practitioners delivering verum treatment would be more potent. However, those knowingly providing sham treatments may invest more care and attention in their patients, thereby boosting their outcomes.

In summary, we can make the following statements about sham treatments and placebo:

- Sham controls are not physiologically inactive and equate more to different styles of acupuncture than to placebos.
- They produce physiological effects that may differ from those evoked by verum acupuncture.

- Lack of practitioner blinding might conceivably favor either the verum group or the sham.
- Various contextual factors, as well as the many components of the treatment itself, may have a significant impact.
- Sham controls have been used to test the specificity of point selections and needling methods, but may be confounded even in such studies.
- Sham treatments are not appropriate tools for determining whether acupuncture is effective.
- On balance, theoretical expectations are that sham controls would underestimate the size of the verum effects (Wayne et al., 2009), which would explain the paradoxical evidence.

Application of Evidence Scoring

Following the evidence scoring system of VanKleef et al. (2009), the following conclusions can be drawn about acupuncture and migraine:

- *Benefits: Risks and Burdens.* The benefit of the effectiveness is greater than the risk and burden of complications. Major complications are very rare for properly trained practitioners, most of whom have never experienced a serious adverse event in their professional lifetimes. Comparative trials show acupuncture is associated with significantly fewer adverse events than conventional drugs.
- *Grade of Evidence (Grade A).* There have been more than 20 RCTs of acupuncture in the West and at least as many in China. At least 8 are of high quality.
- *Outcomes (Evaluation: +).* Cochrane meta-analysis results indicate that acupuncture is at least as good as evidence-based medication, while the addition of the therapy to routine care provides a significant extra benefit. Sham studies were not statistically significant, although 11 out of 14 favored acupuncture, as did the overall response rates.

Those wedded to the idea that the only valid test of an intervention is its comparison against placebo would look no further than the sham trial results. Unfortunately, we cannot say that these shams actually are providing sham control (Wayne et al., 2009), leading to endless debate about the interpretation of the study results. With this caveat in mind, many acupuncture researchers have called for a move away from sham-controlled trials and toward pragmatic, comparative effectiveness and cost-effectiveness studies (together with a variety of non-RCT designs). Given that acupuncture appears to be cost-effective, may potentially be better than drugs, and improves outcomes compared to routine care alone, then this leads us to score the evidence as positive: *Overall Score = 1A +*.

We recommend that acupuncture be part of the available repertoire for the prophylactic treatment of migraine. This position is in accord with recent reviews (Scott & Deare, 2006; Endres et al., 2007; Bongaard, 2008; Linde et al., 2009a; Sherman & Coeytaux, 2009; "Acupuncture for Tension-Type Headaches and Migraine," 2010; Pickett & Blackwell, 2010) and at least one national guideline (Scottish Intercollegiate Guidelines Network, 2008). In fact, many established orthodox interventions have no comparable weight of evidence behind them.

Little is known so far about which subgroups of types of patients might respond to acupuncture better than others (Linde et al., 2009a). Understandably, acupuncture is particularly recommended for people whose health does not improve with medication (Linde et al., 2009a; "Acupuncture for Tension-Type Headaches and Migraine," 2010). During the near future, the most pertinent question may be "How can acupuncture (and Chinese medicine and other complementary therapies) be best used together with various conventional approaches to fashion optimal care packages?" (Institute for Integrative Health, 2009). This is what patients are seeking, largely through their own experimentation, and researchers should design trials that are relevant for them.

HERBAL MEDICINE

The Issue of Formulae Versus Active Ingredients in Research

Herbs are ubiquitous. It is common knowledge that these treatments have been used by traditional societies around the world for a long time. East Asia and China in particular have an extremely diverse geography and flora and fauna, which is reflected in the pharmacopeia of the People's Republic of China, which contains nearly 1,000 herbal monographs. In addition, herbs in TEAM are virtually always given as a combination of ingredients, or formula, based on empirical clinical experience where specific combinations have frequently been used for some time (perhaps as long as 3,000 years).

This practice presents real issues for both research and pharmaceutical manufacture. A single herb may contain dozens of "active ingredients." Chen and Chen (2001) list at least 40 such ingredients for Chuan xiong, for instance, although these are simply the main ingredients that have

been studied to varying extents. A formula of, say, 15 herbs will have hundreds, and potentially thousands, of these "active ingredients."

Although it is understandably tempting, at least to the pharmaceutical industry, to try to isolate *the* ingredient that provides an individual herb with its specific action for a particular disease, clearly it is difficult or impossible to do so for single herbs, let alone a formulation. Indeed, it may well be some synergistic action of all the ingredients that gives a formula its effects.

Consider the story of Zemaphyte. A Cochrane review (Zhang et al., 2004) found that Chinese herbal mixtures may be effective in the treatment of atopic eczema, in particular looking at the evidence for Zemaphyte, the only Chinese herbal product to have been licensed for use in the United Kingdom, with all the attendant expense involved. The product is no longer manufactured, as doctors did not take it up. This example illustrates why no private concern is enthusiastic about funding herbal research, as it is extremely unlikely that the investment would be recovered.

East Asian Traditional Herbal Phytopharmacology

The construction of a classical Chinese herbal formula is designed to maximize its therapeutic potential, yet simultaneously minimize its potential adverse effects. Classical formulae (defined as combinations that have been in consistent and continuous use prior to 1911) are structured around the hierarchy of the Emperor's Imperial Court:

- *Emperor:* the principal substance generating the main therapeutic effect of the formula (e.g., Tonify Blood or Release the Exterior).
- *Minister:* used to enhance the therapeutic actions of the Emperor.
- *Assistant:* provides treatment for (1) accompanying symptoms, (2) counteracting harsh or toxic herbs, (3) assisting the Emperor and Ministers, and (4) providing a warming or cooling effect.
- *Messenger/Envoy:* either guides the formula to certain meridians, organs, or body regions, or balances the prescription.

This is not just a fanciful tradition harking back to olden times. We can use this formula as a sort of practical mnemonic to illustrate that therapeutic action is enhanced and adverse reactions reduced through balancing the activity of a formulation, according to the theory of classical TEAM. **Table 28.6** illustrates the Chinese medicine

Table 28.6 Individual Herbs Used in Treating Migraine by TEAM Anatomic Division

Yangming (Frontal)	Shaoyang (Temporal)	Taiyang (Occipital)	Jueyin (Vertex)
Bai zhi	Chuan xiong	Qiang huo	Wu xhu yu
Cang er zi	Chai hu	Gao ben	Gao ben
Man jing zi	Ju hua	Ge gen	Gou teng
Ju hua	Gou teng	Chuan xiong	Tian ma
Sheng ma	Bai ji li		Shi jue ming
Chuan xiong	Shi jue ming		Chuan xiong

Sources: Maciocia, 1994; Maclean W, Lyttleton J. *Handbook of Internal Medicine, Vol. 3.* London: Pangolin Press; 2010.

concept of the Six Divisions, which can also be used as a method of herb selection.

Categories of Herbs

Between 18 and 20 categories of herbs are recognized in the *Materia Medica* (Bensky & Gamble, 1993; Chen & Chen, 2001). Only herbs from the first two categories listed below are discussed in this chapter, but ingredients from several categories could be included in actual migraine formulae in clinical practice:

- Blood-Invigorating and Stasis-Removing Herbs
- Liver-Calming and Wind-Extinguishing Herbs
- Qi-Regulating Herbs
- Tonic Herbs (Qi, Blood, Yin, Yang)
- Exterior-Releasing Herbs

Table 28.7 illustrates another expert opinion on the most common presentation of TEAM disease patterns and their related formulae (Jiang, 2004). A small selection of herbs that feature in the cited migraine-oriented formulae are described in more detail in the next subsection.

Individual Herbs

Although there are insufficient data from the studies that have been included in this chapter to provide anything close to a definitive list, certain herbs do crop up in formulae more often than others, and this is also the case in the classical literature. More than 400 herbs are described in detail in the main *Materia Medica* translated into English (Bensky & Gamble, 1993; Chen & Chen, 2001). Note that this list of herbs is in no way a "formula" and would not be prescribed in this combination in the clinic.

Special note should be made of Chuan xiong, which features in most of the formulae listed. It is regarded variously as mainly a treatment for menstrual headaches (Chen & Chen, 2001) or temporal headaches (Maclean & Lyttleton, 2010), but can be used for almost any severe or stubborn headache in practice, making it especially useful for migraine. The "acrid," "warm," and "dispersing" (in TEAM terms) nature of Chuan xiong means that it is prescribed alongside tonic herbs to moderate its action.

Table 28.7 Differentiation of the Four Main TEAM Migraine Patterns with Suggested Formulae

Exterior Wind-Cold Accumulation	Liver Qi Constraint/Liver Wind Agitating Within	Qi Constraint and Blood Stasis	Liver and Kidney Yin Deficiency with Qi Constraint and Blood Stasis
Formulae			
Jiu wei qiang huo tang	Zheng tian wan	Shu gan wan	Zhi bai di huang wan
Chuan xiong cha tiao san	Yan hu zhi tong jiao nong	Jia wei xiao yao wan	Geng nian an wan
		Xiao yao wan	Yan hu zhi tong jiao nong
		Yan hu tong jiao nang	Xue fu zhu yu wan
		Xue fu zhu yu wan	

Source: Jiang D. Management of migraine using traditional Chinese medicine. *J Chin Med* 2004;76:40–44.

The normal dosage range for Chuan xiong is 3 to 9 g per day. Nevertheless, when it is used for severe headaches, doses as large as 50 g can be used, during the duration of the headache and only when combined with Dang gui ± Bai shao to moderate its strong blood-dispersing action.

Chuan Xiong

Radix ligustici chuanxiong
Category: Blood-Invigorating and Stasis-Removing Herbs
Family: Umbelliferae
First described: *Shen Nong Ben Cao Jing* (*The Divine Farmer's Materia Medica*), from 300 BC
Properties: warm, acrid
Enters the following channels: Liver, Gallbladder, Pericardium
Actions: activates Qi and Blood circulation; disperses Wind and alleviates pain; specific for headaches
Dosage: 3–10 g (and see the preceding paragraph)
Chemical composition: alkaloids (chuanxiongzine, tetramthylpyrazine, L-isoleucine-L-valine anhydride, L-valine-L-valine anhydride, trimethylamine, choline, perlolyrine, cnidiumlactone, chuanxingol, 4-hydroxy-3 butyl-phthalide, lugustilide, neocnidilide); organic acids (ferulic acid, sedanoic acid, folic acid, vanillic, caffeic acid, protocatechuic acid, palmitic acid, linolenic acid, chrysophanol, methyl phenylacetate, sedanoic acid lactone, methyl pentadecanoate); and essential oils (ethyl pentadecanoate, ethyl palmitate, ethyl heptadecanoate, ethyl isoheptadecanoate, ethyl octadecanoate, ethyl isoctadecanoate, methyl palmitate, methyl linolenate)

Tian Ma

Rhizoma gastrodiae elatae
Category: Liver-Calming and Wind-Extinguishing Herbs
Family: Orchidaceae
First described: *Shen Nong Ben Cao Jing* (*The Divine Farmer's Materia Medica*)
Properties: sweet, neutral
Enters the following channels: Liver
Actions: Calms the Liver, extinguishes Wind, controls spasm and tremor; relieves obstruction and alleviates pain (especially headache)
Dosage: 3–10 g/day
Chemical composition: gastrodin, 4-hydroxybenzyl alcohol, daucosterol, succinic acid, vannillyl alcohol, vanillin, β-sitosterol, gastrodioside, vitamin A

Gou Teng

Ramulus cum uncis uncariae
Category: Liver-Calming and Wind-Extinguishing Herbs
Family: Rubiaceae
First described: *Ming Yi Za Zhu* (*Miscellaneous Records of Famous Physicians*) by Tao Hong-Jing in 500 AD
Properties: sweet, cool
Enters the following channels: Heart, Liver
Actions: extinguishes Wind, alleviates spasm; drains Liver heat and pacifies Liver yang
Dosage: 6–15 g/day
Chemical composition: rhynchophylline, isorhynchophylline, corynoxeine, isocorynoxeine, corynantheine, diydrocorynatheine, trifolin, hyperin, nicotinic acid, hirsutine, hirsuteine

Dang Gui

Radacis angelicae sinensis
Category: Blood Tonic
Family: Umbelliferae
First described: *Shen Nong Ben Cao Jing* (*The Divine Farmer's Materia Medica*)
Properties: sweet, acrid, warm
Enters the following channels: Heart, Liver, Spleen
Actions: Tonifies Blood; Invigorates Blood circulation and relives pain
Dosage: 5–15 g/day
Chemical composition: essential oils 0.2% to 0.4% (ligustilide, *n*-butylidene phthalide, *n*-butylphthalide, *n*-valero-phenone-*O*-carboxylic acid); ferulic acid, scopletin; sequiterpenes; carvacrol; dihydrophthalic anhydride; sucrose, vitamin B_{12}, carotene, β-sitosterol

Utilization of Nonplant Ingredients

East Asian medicine has always used animal and mineral ingredients in addition to plants. In fact, in almost every category of herbs, nonplant ingredients are the strongest of all medicinal components listed. Traditionally, such formulae have included a number of animal parts that are now on the international endangered species list (Convention on International Trade in Endangered Species of Wild Fauna and Flora [CITES]), and it should be noted that these are correctly banned and will not be used by any registered professional. CITES also lists a number of plants, such as members of the orchid family, that are threatened and can be imported only under license. The legal status of nonplant ingredients varies throughout Western countries.

The use of nonplant ingredients has a long traditional history of use, and offers a wide-ranging group of therapeutic ingredients with potentially strong actions. Further research is needed to explore the potential and ethical, safe use of this category of medicine. The substances potentially used in the treatment of migraine are listed here:

- Animals: Ling yang jiao, Gui ban, Lu jiao
- Insects: Quan xie, Wu gong, Jiang can, Di long
- Minerals: Shi gao, Shi jue ming, Long gu, Zhen zhu mu, Zhu sha

These ingredients are classified as having the following functions: (1) stop pain and spasm; (2) descend Liver Yang; (3) disperse Blood Stasis; (4) clear Heat; and (5) nourish Yin.

Safety of Herbs

MacPherson and Liu (2005) reported no serious adverse effects and 32 minor adverse events among 169 patients receiving Chinese herbal medicine in the United Kingdom. Analysis of European adverse events associated with herbs shows that they are associated with lack of professional regulation, poor herbal quality assurance, and inadequately trained practitioners (Blackwell, 1996). Wang et al. (2009) maintain that "proper processing and multi-herbs formulation can reduce the level of toxic components."

On a practical level, Blackwell (2009) points out that professional indemnity insurance premium for practitioners in the United Kingdom is a fraction of that for physicians ($207–$3,980). This difference is a significant indicator of herbs' safety, as insurers carefully set their rates according to perceived risk and in line with the number of claims related to a particular occupation.

Efficacy and Effects of Herbs for Treating Migraine

Summary of Studies and Trials

In this analysis of herbal treatment of migraine, Western databases were searched and Chinese studies were included only where a translated abstract was available. Although migraine was the focus, given the paucity of material, some studies of headache in general were also included. Classical TEAM herbal formulae, modern clinical research formulae, and single-herb research were all included. Seventeen papers were located to review. Controls used in the selected studies included a mixture of treatment versus drug, treatment versus herb, and treatment versus or combined with TCM, including

acupuncture. Substantial heterogeneity exists as to the nature of the control within each type.

The Herbs Used and Their Characteristics

Three herbs in particular appear most frequently in the formulae used in the studies: Dang gui, Chuan xiong, and Bai shao. This accords with theoretical and clinical practice, as all three have a particular focus on targeting the Liver, effecting Blood circulation, and alleviating pain. Gan cao and Fu ling also appear frequently because they are used in a large number of formulae generally, rather than for any headache-specific properties. Sheng jiang appears in many formulae, but also has a migraine-specific action. **Table 28.8** summarizes the ingredients of formulae used in migraine studies (organized in alphabetical order).

We have highlighted the use of Chuan xiong in this chapter, as part of a balanced TEAM formula. Peng et al. (2009) suggest that the volatile oils in this plant are ultimately responsible for its headache-relieving effects. This relationship would be consistent with the traditional classification of this herb as "acrid" or "pungent." **Table 28.9** shows the herbs most frequently used in migraine studies.

Yarnell and Abascal (2007) cite more than 15 herbs, most of them used by TEAM practitioners, as having "importance in remedying headaches effectively and safely." One of these ingredients, *Zingiber officinale* (ginger), has also been the subject of research indicating that it appears to thin the blood by interfering with the ability of blood platelets to clump together (Srivastava, 1984; Backon, 1986). It is also interesting to note that ginger is one of the three substances (along with vitamin C and vitamin B_6) that are tested for in the Migraine Profile Platelet Studies (an assessment of an individual's blood for migraine substance reactivity) at Biolab Medical Unit in London, which is used by many doctors for sensitivity testing.

Japanese Herbal Medicine

Japanese herbal medicine is referred to by the term *Kanpo/kampo,* literally meaning "medicine of the Han," or Chinese medicine. Goshuyuto is the Japanese name for Wu zhu tang (*Evodia decoction*), which has been the subject of multiple studies in Japan. Two of its ingredients have been found to inhibit platelet aggregation (Hibino et al., 2008), and autonomic nervous system effects have also been noted (Wakasugi et al., 2008). Clinical efficacy for migraine prophylaxis has been established by Ishida and Sato (2006), when combined with Senkyuchachosan

Table 28.8 Ingredients of Formulae Used in Migraine Studies (Alphabetical)

No. 1 Traditional Chinese Medicine	No. 2 Traditional Chinese Medicine	Chotosan (Diao Teng San)*	Geng Nian An Wan	Goshuyuto (Wu Zhu Yu Tang)
Ling yang jiao	Zhen zhu†	Shi gao	*Shu di huang*	Wu zhu yu
Quan xie	*Ling yang jiao*	Ju hua	He shou wu	*Sheng jiang*
Dang gui	Zhu sha	*Sheng jiang*	Ze xie	Suan zao ren‡
Chuan xiong	Yuan zhi	Chen pi	*Fu ling*	Renshen
Tao ren	Suan zao ren	Ren shen	Wu wei zi	
Hong hua	Shi chang pu	Mai men dong	Zhen zhu mu	
Chi shao	Bai he	Fu ling	Xuan shen	
Bai shao	Hu po	Gou teng	Fu xiao mai	
Ju hua	*Dang gui*	Ban xia	Lu hui	
Man jing zi	*Bai shao*	*Gan cao*	*Dang gui*	
Gan cao	*Hong hua*	*Sheng jiang*		
	Chuan xiong	*Fang feng*		
	Lu rong			
	Renshen			
	Huang qi			
	Fu ling			
	Xi xin			
	Quan xie			
	Gan cao			

Gou Teng San/Yin*	Fu Fang Dan Shen Di	Jiu Wei Qiang Huo Tang	Long Dan Xie Gan	Senkyuchachosan (Chuan Xiong Cha Tiao)
Gou teng	Dan shen	Qiang huo	Long dan cao	*Bo he*
Ren shen	San qi	*Fang feng*	Huang qin	*Chuan xiong*
Ling yang jiao	Bing pian	Cang zhu	Zhi zi	Jing jie
Tian ma		*Xi xin*	Zie xie	Qiang huo
Quan xie		*Chuan xiong*	Mu tong§	*Bai zhi*
Gan cao		*Bai zhi*	Che qian zi	*Gan cao*
		Huang qin	Sheng do huang	*Fang feng*
		Sheng di huang	*Dang gui*	*Xi xin*
		Gan cao	*Chai hu*	(taken with green tea)
		Sheng jiang		

Shu Gan Wan	Tian Ma Gou Teng Yin (Li and Li)*	Tian Ma Gou Teng Yin (Classical)*	Xiao Yao Wan	Jia Wei Xiao Yao
Chuan lian zi	*Tian ma*	*Tian ma*	*Chai hu*	*Chai hu*
Yan hu suo	*Gouteng*	*Gou teng*	*Dang gui*	*Dang gui*
Bai shao	Shi jue ming	Shi jue ming	*Bai shao*	*Bai shao*
Jiang huang	Huang qin	Huang qin	*Bai zhu*	Bai zhu
Mu xiang	Ze lan	Zhi zi	*Fu ling*	*Fu ling*
Chen xiang	Bai jie zi	Yi mu cao	*Gan cao*	*Gan cao*

Table 28.8 Ingredients of Formulae Used in Migraine Studies (Alphabetical)(Continued)

Shu Gan Wan	Tian Ma Gou Teng Yin (Li and Li)*	Tian Ma Gou Teng Yin (Classical)*	Xiao Yao Wan	Jia Wei Xiao Yao
Dou kou ren		Niu xi	*Bo he*	Mu dan pi
Hou po		Du zhong	*Sheng jiang*	Zhi zi
Chen pi		Sang ji sheng		*Bo he*
Zhi ke		Ye jiao teng		*Sheng jiang*
Fu ling		Fu shen		
Sha ren				

Xue Fu Zhu Yu Wan	Yan Hu Zhi Tong Jiao Nong	Yangxueq Qingnao Grain	Zheng Tian Wan	Zhi Bai Di Huang Wan
Tao ren	Yan hu suo	*Dang gui*	*Chuan xiong*	*Shu di huang*
Hong hua	Bai zhi	*Chuan xiong*	*Dang gui*	Shan zhu yu
Dan shen		*Bai shao*	*Hong hua*	Mu dan pi
Chuan xiong		Yan hu suo	*Fang feng*	Shan yao
Dang gui		*Shu di huang*	Du huo	*Fu ling*
Niu xi		Zhen zhu mu	*Bai shao*	Ze xie
Zhi ke		Xia ku cao	*Shu di huang*	Zhi mu
Chi shao		Jue ming zi	*Tao ren*	Huang bai
Jie geng		Ji xue teng	*Xi xin*	
Chai hu		*Gou teng*	Fu zi	
Shu di huang				
Gan cao				

Notes: Herbs in italics are the most frequently cited. Formula names in brackets are the Chinese name for the Kanpo formula.

* Different versions of these formulae appear in the literature; all versions have been included here for completeness.

† Probably refers to Zhen zhu mu (mother of pearl) rather than pearl itself.

‡ Should be Da zao.

§ Tong cao is often substituted today.

(Chinese: Chuan Xiong Cha Tiao) for pain relief, and also by Odaguchi et al. (2006) in comparison with placebo.

Liver Yang Patterns

Several authors have highlighted the fact that the majority of patients presenting with migraine, and the herbs used to treat them, fall within the category of Ascending Liver Yang (Liver Yang Rising) or Liver Fire with Wind (**Table 28.10**).

Expression ubiquitin (a protein found in all eukaryotic cells that plays a role in cell-cycle regulation and repair) may provoke migraines, and some studies have suggested that it is closely linked to the TCM concept known as "Hyperactivity of Liver Yang." In one study, an aconite solution was used to induce Hyperactive Liver

Yang in mice; proteins in the herbal treatment group returned to normal in comparison to the control group (Hu et al., 2008). Details of the herbal formulae were not given in the study paper, however.

Tian ma gou teng yin (TMGTY, or *Gastrodia* and *Uncaria* decoction) is a primary formula for treating migraine due to Ascendant Liver Yang. Li et al. (2006) measured protein expression differences in rat brains induced with Ascendant Liver Yang and migraine, establishing that the distribution pattern in those given TMGTY was markedly different from that observed in the control group. These authors proposed that this effect may be associated with the cure mechanism for migraine.

One recent study examined lymphocyte protein expression (Zhong et al., 2009a). Cure rates were higher in the treatment group compared to the control (87.5%

Table 28.9 Most Frequently Used Herbs in Migraine Studies

Herb	Frequency	Herb Category
Chuan xiong	9	Blood-Invigorating and Stasis-Removing Herbs
Dang gui	9	Blood Tonic
Bai shao	8	Blood Tonic
Sheng jiang	6	Exterior-Releasing Herbs
Gou teng	6	Liver-Calming and Wind-Extinguishing Herbs
Shi di	5	Liver-Calming and Wind-Extinguishing Herbs
Xi xin	4	Exterior-Releasing Herbs
Hong hua	4	Blood-Invigorating and Stasis-Removing Herbs
Fang feng	4	Exterior-Releasing Herbs
Chai hu	4	Exterior-Releasing Herbs
Tian ma	3	Liver-Calming and Wind-Extinguishing Herbs
Tao ren	3	Blood-Invigorating and Stasis-Removing Herbs
Yan hu suo	3	Blood-Invigorating and Stasis-Removing Herbs
Bai zhi	3	Exterior-Releasing Herbs
Bo he	3	Exterior-Releasing Herbs
Ling yang jiao	3	Liver-Calming and Wind-Extinguishing Herbs
Quan xie	3	Liver-Calming and Wind-Extinguishing Herbs
Niu xi	3	Blood-Invigorating and Stasis-Removing Herbs
Gan cao	10	Qi Tonic
Fu ling	7	Drain Dampness

versus 75.0%, respectively), and related symptoms (vertigo, restlessness and tantrum, and facial heat) also improved to a greater extent in the treatment group ($P < 0.05$). The researchers noted an improved TCM score (as devised for this study) and suggested that the effects on migraine patients with Hyperactivity of Liver Yang syndrome may be related to regulating the blood lymphocyte protein expression.

Other Findings

A few other papers are worthy of mention. Guo and Shi (2007) proposed a theoretical basis for developing TCM treatment for migraine based on their findings that herbal formulae (not specified) regulate constriction and dilation of cerebral blood vessels through restraining excessive expression of meningeal NF-κB genes.

Another novel trial (Hu et al., 2006) involved the clinical application of a classical Liver-oriented formula taken as nasal drops (presumably for rapid effect). Xiao yao wan Nose Drops (XYWND, also known as Free and Easy) demonstrated dramatic differences in the clinical total effective rate and headache-alleviating rate compared to the control group, with these rates being 93.3% and 96.7%, respectively, for the treated group and 18.3% and 20.0%, respectively, for the control group.

Two trials specifically compared herbal therapy to conventional treatment. In one study, individualized formulae (as opposed to standardized over-the-counter herbal pills) were found to be effective in migraine patients who had responded poorly to pharmaceutical treatments (Melchart et al., 2004). The other study compared TEAM or stellate ganglion block treatment for people with obstinate headaches (Su et al., 2005). The researchers concluded that chronic relapse rates were lowest in the combined-therapy group, thus posing an

Table 28.10 Main Formulae for Treating Liver Disease Patterns with Migraine Modifications

Liver Qi Constraint Xiao Yao San	Ascendant Liver Yang Tian Ma Gou Teng Yin	Liver Fire Long Dan Xie Gan Wan
Migraine Modification		
Add:	Add:	Add:
Chuan xiong	Chuan xiong	Gou teng
Man jing zi	Bai shao	Bai ji li
	Gou qi zi	Xia ku cao
		Niu xi
		Jue ming zi

Source: Maclean W, Lyttleton J. *Handbook of Internal Medicine, Vol. 1.* Washington DC: Macarthur; 1998.

Table 28.11 Summary of Conclusions for Formulae Where Ingredients Have Not Been Specified or for Single Herbs

Herb	Author	Conclusion
Guixin granule (GXG)	Fu et al., 2003a	Improves migraine symptoms through a decrease of plasma viscosity and increase of serum magnesium
Chuanju zhitong (CJZT)	Wang et al., 2002	Can be used to prevent and treat migraine by decreasing plasma-endothelin level
Shutianning granule (STNG)	Hu et al., 2002	Improves cerebrovascular function, raises plasma beta-endorphins level, lowers plasma neuropeptide-Y level, and alleviates vascular tension in migraine patients
New zhengtian pill (NZTP)	Zhu et al., 2001	The markedly effective rate and total effective rate were higher than for the flunarizine control group ($P < 0.05$ and $P < 0.01$)
New zhengtian pill (NZTP)	Wang et al., 1996	Mechanism on migraine may be due to the herbs' action on platelet absorption, and releasing and regulation of 5-HT
Yangxueqingnaokeli (YXQN)	Luo et al., 2001	The total number and duration of migraine attacks were markedly reduced after treatment in the therapeutic group (3.1 ± 2.5 and 4.2 ± 2.7) compared to the placebo group (31.0 ± 48.0 and 51.2 ± 73.8)
Alkaloid extracts of Dang gui and black cohosh	Burke et al., 2002	Reduced the average frequency of menstrual migraine attacks to 10.3 (± 2.4) in placebo-treated patients and to 4.7 (± 1.8) ($P < 0.01$) in the treatment group
Petasites hybridus	Lipton et al., 2004	Migraine attack frequency was reduced by 48% over 4 months of treatment

interesting argument for integration. Two traditional herbal formulae are described in Table 28.9.

One Chinese study (He et al., 2009) compared herbs combined with acupuncture against herbal treatment alone. Perhaps unsurprisingly, the combined-treatment group fared better in terms of symptom reduction ($P < 0.05$), although both groups experienced reductions in the frequency and duration of their attacks ($P < 0.01$). Other studies have compared herbal formulae to migraine drugs. The herbal formula Yangxue Qingnao Grain was found to be effective for migraine, albeit not superior to the calcium-channel blocker flunarizine (Sibelium) (Zhao et al., 2008). This result may still be worthwhile given that side effects are reasonably common with this drug. The same herbal formula has also been investigated for migraine in relation to its microcirculation effects (Feng et al., 2004).

Proprietary Formulae

Our search revealed a number of papers where the formula name is given, but the ingredients are not specified. For example, Guixin granules are the subject of a large number of papers in Chinese, but the English abstracts do not list their ingredients (Fu et al., 2003a, 2003b). This seems to be part of a trend that has developed over the last few years. Whereas previously open communication and reporting of findings were the norm, more recently the level of secrecy surrounding the ingredients

of new research formulations has been increasing. This trend likely reflects—at least in part—the difficulties in claiming intellectual property rights for natural products. **Table 28.11** covers the group of formulae that are not discussed specifically in the main text, as their individual ingredients are not listed in the research literature.

In Context: A TEAM Hospital in the West

Germany houses one of the few working TCM hospitals outside of East Asia, an 81-bed hospital for traditional Chinese in Kötzting, treating approximately 1,000 patients with chronic disease each year since 1991. An estimated 20% of these patients seek help for chronic headaches, 14% of them for migraine—the single most prevalent condition treated at the hospital. Treatment costs are reimbursed under public health insurance schemes.

In addition to providing medical services, the hospital supports educational and research programs. In one RCT, patients with headache (migraine, tension-type headache, or both) who received 4 weeks of TCM therapy were compared to a waiting list control (Melchart et al., 2004). The treatment group, who had been traditionally diagnosed, received an individually tailored herbal prescription that was changed as they progressed. Acupuncture, Chinese manual therapy (tui na massage), and a specific relaxation technique (Qi Gong) were also available.

A reduction of more than 50% in headache days was observed in 52% of the patients in the experimental group and 16% of the waiting list group. Patients with migraine improved more than those with tension-type headaches. In another study at the same hospital, the number of days with headaches per month decreased from 9 days (median) at baseline to 4 days at discharge; it was 3 days per month at 12 months' follow-up. Other outcomes also improved (Melchart et al., 2006).

Application of Evidence Scoring

VanKleef et al. (2009) have assessed evidence scoring as it relates to acupuncture and drawn the following conclusions:

- *Benefits: Risks and Burdens.* The benefit of the effectiveness with herbal preparations for migraine is greater than the risk and burden of complications. Serious adverse reactions are rare; most reactions consist of minor transient gastrointestinal disturbance. Most events are associated with lack of professional regulation, poor herbal quality assurance, and inadequately trained practitioners, all of which continue to improve.
- *Grade of Evidence (Grade B).* There have been few RCTs in the West, and most reports of Chinese studies have not been translated. Many more observational studies and nonrandomized comparisons exist. The one systematic review available for Western review covers just a single herbal formula out of the hundreds of classical formulae in common use.
- *Outcomes (Evaluation +).* Cochrane meta-analysis is unavailable for TEAM herbal medicine but the studies cited appear to show good results

for observed outcomes and when compared to pharmaceutical drugs. Physiological activity has been demonstrated for many herbs.
- *Overall Score 1B +.*

More research into the potential for use of TEAM herbal treatments for migraine is needed, and translation and publication in Western journals of high-quality research from East Asia should be an objective. TEAM herbal therapy seems to show promise as a stand-alone or adjunct therapy for the treatment of migraine or tension-type headache. Formulae appear to be more effective than single herbal ingredients or extracts of active ingredients.

APPENDIX

Latin Names for the Most Frequently Used Herbs

Pin Yin	Latin
Bai shao	*Radix paeoniae lactiflorae*
Bai zhi	*Radix angelicae dahuricae*
Bo he	*Herba mentha haplocalycis*
Chai hu	*Radix bupleuri*
Chuan xiong	*Radix ligustici chuanxiong*
Dang gui	*Radix angelicae sinensis*
Fang feng	*Radix ledebouriellae divaricatae*
Fu ling	*Sclerotium poria cocos*
Gan cao	*Radix glycyrrhizae uralensis*
Gou teng	*Ramulus cum uncis uncariae*
Hong hua	*Flos carthami tinctorii*
Ling yang jiao	*Cornu antelopis*
Quan xie	*Buthus martensi*
Sheng jiang	*Rhizoma zingiberis officinalis recens*
Shu di	*Radix Rehmanniae glutinosae preperatae*
Tao ren	*Semen persica*
Tian ma	*Rhizoma gastrodiae elatae*
Xi xin	*Herba cum radice asari*
Yan hu suo	*Rhizoma corydalis*

REFERENCES

Acupuncture for tension-type headaches and migraine. *Drug Therap Bull* 2010;48:62–65.

Ahmadi A, Schwebel DC, Rezaei M. The efficacy of wet-cupping in the treatment of tension and migraine headache. *Am J Chin Med* 2008;36:37–44.

Allais G, Romoli M, Rolando S, et al. Ear acupuncture in unilateral migraine pain. *Neurol Sci* 2010;31:S185–S187.

Backer M, Grossman P, Schneider J, et al. Acupuncture in migraine: investigation of autonomic effects. *Clin J Pain* 2008;24:106–115.

Backon J. Ginger: inhibition of thromboxane synthetase and stimulation of prostacyclin: relevance for medicine and psychiatry. *Med Hypotheses* 1986;20:271–278.

Barnes PM, Bloom B, Nahin RL. Complementary and alternative medicine use among adults and children: United States, 2007. *Natl Health Stat Report* 2008;12:1–23.

Bensky D, Gamble A. *Chinese Herbal Medicine Materia Medica*. Vista, CA: Eastland Press; 1993.

Bensoussan A, Talley NJ, Hing M, et al. Treatment of irritable bowel syndrome with Chinese herbal medicine. *JAMA* 1998;280:1585–1589.

Bijak M. What can be achieved by using acupuncture and related techniques in neurology? Expert evidence. *Rev Internacional Acupuntura* 2008;2: 231–237.

Birch S. Grasping the sleeping tiger's tail: perspectives on acupuncture from the edge of the abyss. *N Amer J Orient Med* 2003;11:20–23.

Birch S. A review and analysis of placebo treatments, placebo effects, and placebo controls in trials of medical procedures when sham is not inert. *J Altern Complement Med* 2006;12:303–310.

Blackwell R. Adverse events involving certain Chinese herbal medicines and the response of the profession. *J Chinese Med* 1996;50:12–22.

Blackwell R. *Acupuncture and Chinese Herbal Medicine Evidence.* Research document for the Northern College of Acupuncture; 2009.

Bodeker G, Ong CK, Grundy C, et al. *WHO Global Atlas of Traditional, Complementary and Alternative Medicine.* Kobe: World Health Organization, WHO Centre for Health Development; 2005.

Bongaard B. Using acupuncture for headache treatment: getting the point. *Altern Med Alert* 2008;11:49–60.

Boutouyrie P, Corvisier R, Ong KT, et al. Acute and chronic effects of acupuncture on radial artery: a randomized double blind study in migraine. *Artery Res* 2010;4:7–14.

Bowing G, Zhou J, Endres HG, et al. Differences in Chinese diagnoses for migraine and tension-type headache: an analysis of the German acupuncture trials (GERAC) for headache. *Cephalalgia* 2010;30:224–232.

British Association for the Study of Headaches. BASH management guidelines, 3rd edition. April 2007. Available at: http://216.25.88.43/upload/NS_BASH /BASH_guidelines_2007.pdf

Bücker B, Groenewold M, Schoefer Y, Schäfer T. The use of complementary alternative medicine (CAM) in 1 001 German adults: results of a population-based telephone survey. *Gesundheitswesen* 2008;70:E29–E36.

Burke A, Upchurch DM, Dye C, Chyu L. Acupuncture use in the United States: findings from the National Health Interview Survey. *Altern Ther Health Med* 2006;12: 639–648.

Burke BE, Olson R, Cusack B. Randomized, controlled trial of phytoestrogen in the prophylactic treatment of menstrual migraine. *Biomed Pharmacother* 2002;56:283–288.

Cai YY, Wang S. [Therapeutic effect of point-through-point acupuncture on migraine and its effects on brain blood flow velocity]. *Zhongguo Zhen Jiu.* 2006;26:177–179.

Calandre EP, Hidalgo J, García-Leiva JM, Rico-Villademoros F. Trigger point evaluation in migraine patients: an indication of peripheral sensitization linked to migraine predisposition? *Eur J Neurol* 2006;13:244–249.

Chang SC, Hou MC, Hu NZ, et al. The joint usage of conventional medicine and alternative medicine for migraine in Taiwan. *Journal of the Neurological Sciences.* Conference: 19th World Congress of Neurology, Bangkok, Thailand. Conference Publication; 2009;285:S315.

Chen FP, Chen TJ, Kung YY, et al. Use frequency of traditional Chinese medicine in Taiwan. *BMC Health Serv Res* 2007;7:26.

Chen J, Chen T. *Chinese Medical Herbology and Pharmacology.* City of Industry, CA: Art of Medicine Press; 2001.

Chen YC, Chen FP, Chen TJ, Chou LF, Hwang SJ. Patterns of traditional Chinese medicine use in patients with inflammatory bowel disease: a population study in Taiwan. *Hepatogastroenterology* 2008;55:467–470.

Diener HC, Kronfeld K, Boewing G, et al. Efficacy of acupuncture for the prophylaxis of migraine: a multicentre randomised controlled clinical trial. *Lancet Neurol* 2006;5:310–316.

Endres HG, Diener HC, Molsberger A. Role of acupuncture in the treatment of migraine. *Expert Rev Neurother* 2007;7:1121–1134.

Ernst E. Deaths after acupuncture: a systematic review. *Intern J Risk Safety Med* 2010;22:131–136.

Ernst E, White AR. Acupuncture for back pain: a meta-analysis of randomized controlled trials. *Arch Intern Med* 1998;158:2235–2241.

Facco E, Liguori A, Petti F, et al. Traditional acupuncture in migraine: a controlled, randomized study. *Headache* 2008;48:398–407.

Feng JL, Zeng AY, Du YP. [Effect of yangxue qingnao granule on microcirculation and cerebral blood flow in patients with migraine]. *Zhongguo Zhong Xi Yi Jie He Xue Hui, Zhongguo Zhong Yi Yan Jiu Yuan Zhu Ban* [*Chinese Journal of Integrated Traditional & Western Medicine*] 2004;24:357–358.

Flower A, Liu JP, Chen S, et al. Chinese herbal medicine for endometriosis. *Cochrane Database Syst Rev* 2009;3:CD006568.

Fu QZ, Wang ZJ, Luo Y, et al. Effects of compound Guixin granule on hemorheology and serum Ca, Mg in migraineurs. *Chinese J Clin Rehabil* 2003a;7:3098–3099.

Fu QZ, Wang ZJ, Luo Y, You GX. Emotional disturbance of migraine and therapeutical effect of Chinese herb mixture granule guixin. *Chinese J Clin Rehabil* 2003b;7:2712–2713.

Gabriel C. Diagnosis and therapy of headaches and migraine in respect of traditional Chinese medicine (TCM). *Gynakologe* 2004;37:1110–1114.

Gaul C, Eismann R, Schmidt T, et al. Use of complementary and alternative medicine in patients suffering from primary headache disorders. *Cephalalgia* 2009;29:1069–1078.

Goldbach-Mansky R, Wilson M, Fleischmann R, et al. Chinese herb appears better than standard treatment for rheumatoid arthritis. *Ann Intern Med* 2009;151:229–240.

Gottschling S, Meyer S, Gribova I, et al. Laser acupuncture in children with headache: a double-blind, bi-center, placebo-controlled trial. *Pain* 2008;137:405–412.

Guo J. Tactics of acupuncture for migraine prophylaxis. *J Chin Integrated Med* 2010;8:210–214.

Guo L, Shi X. [The intervention effect of traditional Chinese medicine on meningeal nuclear factor expression of rats suffering from migraine]. *Shengwu Yixue Gongchengxue Zazhi* [*Journal of Biomedical Engineering*] 2007;24:646–649.

Harris RE, Zubieta JK, Scott DJ, et al. Traditional Chinese acupuncture and placebo (sham) acupuncture are differentiated by their effects on mu-opioid receptors (MORs). *Neuroimage* 2009;47:1077–1085.

He QY, Liang J, Zhang Y, Zhang J. Thirty-two cases of vascular headache treated by acupuncture combined with Chinese herbal decoction. *J Trad Chin Med* 2009;29:253–257.

Hibino T, Yuzurihara M, Terawaki K, et al. Goshuyuto inhibits platelet aggregation in guinea-pig whole blood. *J Pharmacol Sci* 2008;108:89–94.

Hoizey D, Hoizey M. *A History of Chinese Medicine.* Edinburgh: University Press; 1988.

Hu HQ, Zhou YH, Wang XL. Clinical study on effect of Xiaoyao nose drops in stopping episode of migraine. *Chin J Integrative Med* 2006;12:112–117.

Hu J, Chen Z, Zhong G, et al. Proteomic analysis of effects of Chinese herbs to calm the liver and suppress hyperactive yang in a rat migraine model. *Neural Regeneration Res* 2008;3:494–497.

Hu J, Wu ZC, Wang JJ, Jiao Y. [Comparison between modern and ancient thoughts about acupuncture treatment of migraine]. *Zhen Ci Yan Jiu* 2009;34:276–278.

Hu ZQ, Song LG, Mei T. [Clinical and experimental study on treatment of migraine with Shutianning granule]. *Zhongguo Zhong Xi Yi Jie He Xue Hui, Zhongguo Zhong Yi Yan Jiu Yuan Zhu Ban* [*Chinese Journal of Integrated Traditional & Western Medicine*] 2002;22:581–583.

Hui KK, Marina O, Liu J, Rosen BR, Kwong KK. Acupuncture, the limbic system, and the anticorrelated networks of the brain. *Auton Neurosci* 2010;157:81–90.

Huang JJ, Pang J, Lei LM, et al. [Observation on therapeutic effect of Jingjin therapy on migraine]. *Zhongguo Zhen Jiu* 2006;26:322–324.

Hunt KJ, Coelho HF, Wider B, Perry R, Hung SK, Terry R, Ernst E. Complementary and alternative medicine use in England: results from a national survey. *Int J Clin Pract* 2010;64:1496–1502.

Institute for Integrative Health. Comparative effectiveness research & integrative medicine. Stakeholder symposium. Baltimore; November 2009. Available at: http://tiih.org /cer-the-online-symposium-april-may-2010#cervideo. Accessed October 22, 2010.

Ishida K, Sato H. Kampo medicines as alternatives for treatment of migraine: six case studies. *Compl Ther Clin Practice* 2006;12:276–280.

Jena S, Witt CM, Brinkhaus B, et al. Acupuncture in patients with headache. *Cephalalgia* 2008;28:969–979.

Jia CS, Ma XS, Shi J, et al. Electroacupuncture at Qiuxu (GB 40) for treatment of migraine: a clinical multicentral random controlled study. *J Trad Chin Med* 2009; 29:43–49.

Jiang D. Management of migraine using traditional Chinese medicine. *J Chin Med* 2004;76:40–44.

Kozak S, Gantenbein AR, Isler H, et al. Nosology and treatment of primary headache in a Swiss headache clinic. *J Headache Pain* 2005;6:121–127.

Lao L, Hamilton GR, Fu J, Berman BM. Is acupuncture safe? A systematic review of case reports. *Altern Ther Health Med* 2003;9:72–83.

Lefaki T, Frantzeskos G, Zaimi D, Aspraki G. 431 headaches: the importance of number of sessions on the action of acupuncture. *Eur J Pain* 2009;13:S130.

Li XZ, Liu XG, Song WZ, et al. [Effect of acupuncture at acupoints of the Shaoyang meridian on cerebral glucose metabolism in the patient of chronic migraine]. *Zhongguo Zhen Jiu* 2008;28:854–859.

Li Y, Liang F, Yu S, et al. Randomized controlled trial to treat migraine with acupuncture: design and protocol. *Trials* 2008;9:57.

Li Y, Liang F, Yang X, et al. Acupuncture for treating acute attacks of migraine: A randomized controlled trial. *Headache* 2009;49:805–816.

Li Z, Li W, Chen ZQ, et al. Effect of Tianma Gouteng Yin on proteins in hypothalamus of migraine rats with hyperactivity of liver-yang. *Chin J Clin Rehabil* 2006;10:45–48.

Linde K, Streng A, Jürgens S, et al. Acupuncture for patients with migraine: a randomized controlled trial. *JAMA* 2005;293:2118–2125.

Linde K, Streng A, Hoppe A, et al. Randomized trial vs. observational study of acupuncture for migraine found that patient characteristics differed but outcomes were similar. *J Clin Epidemiol* 2007;60:280–287.

Linde K, Allais G, Brinkhaus B, et al. Acupuncture for migraine prophylaxis. *Cochrane Database Syst Rev* 2009a;1:CD001218.

Linde K, Allais G, Brinkhaus B, et al. Acupuncture for tension-type headache. *Cochrane Database Syst Rev* 2009b;1:CD007587.

Lipton RB, Göbel H, Einhäupl KM, et al. *Petasites hybridus* root (butterbur) is an effective preventive treatment for migraine. *Neurology* 2004;63:2240–2244.

Lundeberg T, Lund I, Sing A, Näslund J. Is placebo acupuncture what it is intended to be? [Electronic publication ahead of print.] *Evid Based Complement Alternat Med* 2011. Article ID 932407, 5 pages. doi:10.1093/ecam/nep049.

Luo S, Wang X, Kuang P. A clinical study of Yangxueqingnaokeli in preventive treatment of migraine. *Chin J Neurol* 2001;34:291–294.

Maciocia G. *The Foundations of Chinese Medicine.* London: Churchill Livingstone; 1989.

Maciocia G. *The Practice of Chinese Medicine* (2nd ed.). London: Elsevier; 2008.

Maclean W, Lyttleton J. *Handbook of Internal Medicine, Vol. 1.* Washington DC: Macarthur; 1998.

Maclean W, Lyttleton J. *Handbook of Internal Medicine, Vol. 3.* London: Pangolin Press; 2010.

MacPherson H, Liu B. The safety of Chinese herbal medicine: a pilot study for a national survey. *J Altern Complement Med* 2005;11:617–626.

MacPherson H, Thomas K, Walters S, Fitter M. The York acupuncture safety study: prospective survey of 34000 treatments by traditional acupuncturists. *BMJ* 2001;323:486–487.

MacPherson H, Scullion A, Thomas KJ, Walters S. Patient reports of adverse events associated with acupuncture treatment: a prospective national survey. *Qual Saf Health Care* 2004a;13:349–355.

MacPherson H, Sinclair-Lian N, Thomas K. Patients seeking care from acupuncture practitioners in the UK: a national survey. *J Public Health* 2004b;26:152–157.

Melchart D, Thormaehlen J, Hager S, et al. Acupuncture versus placebo versus sumatriptan for early treatment of migraine attacks: a randomized controlled trial. *J Intern Med* 2003;253:181–188.

Melchart D, Hagerc S, Hagerc U, et al. Treatment of patients with chronic headaches in a hospital for traditional Chinese medicine in Germany: a randomized, waiting list controlled trial. *Complem Ther Med* 2004;12:71–78.

Melchart D, Weidenhammer W, Streng A, et al. Acupuncture for chronic headaches: an epidemiological study. *Headache* 2006;46:632–641.

Metcalfe A, Williams J, McChesney J, et al. Use of complementary and alternative medicine by those with a chronic disease and the general population: results of a national population based survey. *BMC Complement Alt Med* 2010;10:58.

Molsberger AF, Boewing G, Diener HC, et al. Designing an acupuncture study: the nationwide, randomized, controlled, German acupuncture trials on migraine and tension-type headache. *J Altern Complement Med* 2006;12:237–245.

Moss CA. Five element acupuncture: treating body, mind, and spirit. *Altern Ther Health Med* 1999;5:52–61.

Napadow V, Dhond R, Park K, et al. Time-variant fMRI activity in the brainstem and higher structures in response to acupuncture. *Neuroimage* 2009;47:289–301.

Ni H, Simile C, Hardy AM. Utilization of complementary and alternative medicine by United States adults: results from the 1999 national health interview survey. *Med Care* 2002;40:353–358.

Odaguchi H, Wakasugi A, Ito H, et al. The efficacy of Goshuyuto in preventing episodes of headache. *Curr Med Res Opin* 2006;22:1587–1597.

Park K-H, Kim H-J, Baek S-Y, et al. Effect of acupuncture on blood flow velocity and volume in common carotid and vertebral arteries in migraine patients. *Med Acupuncture* 2009;21:47–54.

Paterson C, Zheng Z, Xue C, Wang Y. "Playing their parts": the experiences of participants in a randomized sham-controlled acupuncture trial. *J Altern Complement Med* 2008;14:199–208.

Peng C, Xie X, Wang L, et al. Pharmacodynamic action and mechanism of volatile oil from Rhizoma Ligustici Chuanxiong Hort. on treating headache. *Phytomedicine* 2009;16:25–34.

Pickett H, Blackwell JC. FPIN's clinical inquiries: acupuncture for migraine headaches. *Am Fam Physician* 2010;81:1036–1037.

Qin L, Gu S. Treatment of 60 migraine sufferers with penetration needling of points and point selection based on following the corresponding meridians. *Intl J Clin Acupunct* 2006;15:163–167.

Ramos-Font C, Vas J, Rebollo-Aguirre AC, et al. Preliminary results of a pragmatic randomised controlled trial in general practice investigating the effectiveness of acupuncture against migraine: qualitative analysis of brain perfusion SPECT. *Eur J Integrative Med* 2009;1:208–209.

Rossi P, Di Lorenzo G, Faroni J, et al. Use of complementary and alternative medicine by patients with chronic tension-type headache: results of a headache clinic survey. *Headache* 2006;46:622–631.

Rutberg S, Ohrling K. Experiences of acupuncture among women with migraine. *Adv Physiother* 2009;11:130–136.

Scheid, V. *Chinese Medicine in Contemporary China*. Durham, NC: Duke University Press; 2002.

Scott SW, Deare JC. Acupuncture for migraine. *Australian J Acupunct Chin Med* 2006;1:1–14.

Scottish Intercollegiate Guidelines Network. Diagnosis and management of headache in adults. 2008. Available at: http://www.sign.ac.uk/guidelines/fulltext/107/index.html. Accessed October 20, 2010.

Sheehan MP, Atherton DJ. A controlled trial of traditional Chinese medicinal plants in widespread non-exudative atopic eczema. *Br J Dermatology* 1992;126:179–184.

Shen Nong Ben Cao Jing [*The Divine Farmer's Materia Medica*]. Circa 300 BC. [Today it is hypothesized that it is a compilation of oral traditions written between about 300 BC and 200 AD.]

Sherman KJ, Coeytaux RR. Acupuncture for improving chronic back pain, osteoarthritis and headache. *J Clin Outcomes Manage* 2009;16:224–230.

Shi H, Li JH, Ji CF, et al. [Effect of electroacupuncture on cortical spreading depression and plasma CGRP and substance P contents in migraine rats]. *Zhen Ci Yan Jiu* 2010;35:17–21.

Srivastava KC. Aqueous extracts of onion, garlic and ginger inhibit platelet aggregation and alter arachidonic acid metabolism. *Biomed Biochim Acta* 1984;43:S335–S346.

Streng A, Linde K, Hoppe A, et al. Effectiveness and tolerability of acupuncture compared with metoprolol in migraine prophylaxis. *Headache* 2006;46:1492–1502.

Su HR, Su RP, Shao LY, Su B. Comparison of three-year relapse rate of chronic headache treated by combination of traditional Chinese medicine and Western medicine. *Chin J Clin Rehabil* 2005;9:43–45.

Sun Y, Gan TJ. Acupuncture for the management of chronic headache: a systematic review. *Anesth Analg* 2008;107:2038–2047.

Tao IF, Musial F, Dobos GJ. Acupuncture: what's the point? Why sham acupuncture doesn't exist. North American Research Conference on Complementary & Integrative Medicine; Minneapolis, MN; May 2009.

Thomas K, Coleman P. Use of complementary or alternative medicine in a general population in Great Britain: results from the National Omnibus survey. *J Public Health* 2004;26:152–157.

Thomas KJ, Nicholl JP, Coleman P. Use and expenditure on complementary medicine in England: a population based survey. *Complement Ther Med* 2001;9:2–11.

Thomas KJ, MacPherson H, Ratcliffe J, et al. Longer term clinical and economic benefits of offering acupuncture care to patients with chronic low back pain. *Health Technol Assess* 2005;9:1–109.

Tindle HA, Davis RB, Phillips RS, Eisenberg DM. Trends in use of complementary and alternative medicine by US adults: 1997–2002. *Complement Ther Med* 2006;14:20–30.

Tu JR. [Reasons for publication bias in acupuncture RCTs]. *Zhongguo Zhen Jiu* 2010;30:601–608.

Unschuld P. *Medicine in China: A History of Ideas*. Los Angeles: University of California Press; 1985.

U.S. Headache Consortium. U.S. Headache Consortium guidelines. April 25, 2000. Available at: https://www.americanheadachesociety.org/professionalresources/USHeadacheConsortiumGuidelines.asp. Accessed October 20, 2010.

Vanderheyden LC, Verhoef MJ, Hilsden RJ. The role of scientific evidence in decision to use complementary and alternative medicine. *Evid Based Integr Med* 2005;2:19–20.

VanderPloeg K, Yi X. Acupuncture in modern society. *J Acupunct Meridian Stud* 2009;2:26–33.

Van Kleef M, Mekhail N, van Zundert J. Evidence-based guidelines for interventional pain medicine according to clinical diagnoses. *Pain Pract* 2009;9:247–251.

Vickers A, Goyal N, Harland R, Rees R. Do certain countries produce only positive results? A systematic review of controlled trials. *Control Clin Trials* 1998;19:159–166.

Vickers AJ, Rees RW, Zollman CE, et al. Acupuncture for chronic headache in primary care: large, pragmatic, randomised trial. *BMJ* 2004;328:744.

Wakasugi A, Odaguchi H, Oikawa T, Hanawa T. Effects of goshuyuto on lateralization of pupillary dynamics in headache. *Autonomic Neuroscience-Basic & Clinical* 2008;139:9–14.

Walkey M. Abbreviated courses in acupuncture for physicians pose a serious problem. Available at: http://www.medicalacupuncturefacts.com/2010/03/24/abbreviated-courses-in-acupuncture-for-physicians-pose-a-serious-problem/. Accessed December 3, 2010.

Wang DN, Chen BT, Zhou YL. [Effect of new zhengtian pill on 5-hydroxytryptamine content in platelet and plasma of migraine patients]. *Zhongguo Zhong Xi Yi Jie He Xue Hui, Zhongguo Zhong Yi Yan Jiu Yuan Zhu Ban [Chinese Journal of Integrated Traditional & Western Medicine]* 1996;16:280–282.

Wang J, van der Heijden R, Spruit S, et al. Quality and safety of Chinese herbal medicines guided by a systems biology perspective. *J Ethnopharmacol* 2009;126:31–41.

Wang S, Cai Y, Zhou Z, Hu C. [Effect of Chuanjuzhitong capsule on the level of plasma endothelin in patient with migraine]. *Chin J Traditional Med Science Technology* 2002;9(4).

Wang S, Li W, Zhong G, et al. Acupuncture at the San Jiao meridian affects brain stem tissue G protein content in a rat migraine model. *Neural Regeneration Res* 2008;3:958–961.

Wang YY, Zheng Z, Xue CCL. Acupuncture for migraine. *Austral J Acupunct Chin Med* 2008;3:1–16.

Wayne PM, Hammerschlag R, Langevin HM, et al. Resolving paradoxes in acupuncture research: a roundtable discussion. *J Altern Complement Med* 2009;15:1039–1044.

Weidenhammer W, Streng A, Linde K, et al. Acupuncture for chronic pain within the research program of 10 German Health Insurance Funds: basic results from an observational study. *Complement Ther Med* 2007;15:238–246.

White A, Hayhoe S, Hart A, Ernst E. Adverse events following acupuncture: prospective survey of 32 000 consultations with doctors and physiotherapists. *BMJ* 2001;323:485–486.

White A, Cummings M, Barlas P, et al. Defining an adequate dose of acupuncture using a neurophysiological approach: a narrative review of the literature. *Acupunct Med* 2008;26:111–120.

Wing TA, Sedlmeier ES. Measuring the effectiveness of Chinese herbal medicine in improving female infertility. *J Chin Med* 2006;80:26–32.

Witt CM, Reinhold T, Jena S, et al. Cost-effectiveness of acupuncture treatment in patients with headache. *Cephalalgia* 2008;28:334–345.

Witt CM, Pach D, Brinkhaus B, et al. Safety of acupuncture: results of a prospective observational study with 229,230 patients and introduction of a medical information and consent form. *Forsch Komplementmed* 2009;16:91–97.

Wonderling D, Vickers AJ, Grieve R, McCarney R. Cost effectiveness analysis of a randomised trial of acupuncture for chronic headache in primary care. *BMJ* 2004;328(7442):747.

Xue CC, Zhang AL, Lin V, et al. Acupuncture, chiropractic and osteopathy use in Australia: a national population survey. *J Altern Complement Med* 2006;12:639–648.

Xue CC, Zhang AL, Lin V, et al. Acupuncture, chiropractic and osteopathy use in Australia: a national population survey. *BMC Public Health* 2008;8:105.

Xue CC, Zhang AL, Greenwood KM, et al. Traditional Chinese medicine: an update on clinical evidence. World Health Organization (WHO) Collaborating Centre for Traditional Medicine, Discipline of Chinese Medicine, School of Health Sciences, RMIT University, Bundoora, Victoria, Australia. *J Altern Complement Med* 2010;16:301–312.

Yamashita H, Tsukayama H, Sugishita C. Popularity of complementary and alternative medicine in Japan: a telephone survey. *Complement Ther Med* 2002;10:84–93.

Yarnell E, Abascal K. Botanical medicines for headache. *Altern Complement Ther* 2007;13:148–152.

Zhang W, Leonard T, Bath-Hextall FJ, et al. Chinese herbal medicine for atopic eczema. *Cochrane Database Syst Rev* 2004;4:CD002291.

Zhang Y, Liu HL, Wang LP. Evaluation of the quality of reports on acupuncture for migraine prophylaxis. *Chin J Evidence-Based Med* 2008;8:461–465.

Zhang Y, Zhang L, Li B, Wang LP. [Effects of acupuncture preventive treatment on the quality of life in patients of no-aura migraine]. *Zhongguo Zhen Jiu* 2009a;29:431–435.

Zhang Y, Wang L, Liu H, et al. The design and protocol of acupuncture for migraine prophylaxis: a multicenter randomized controlled trial. *Trials* 2009b;10:25.

Zhao CH, Stillman MJ, Rozen TD. Traditional and evidence-based acupuncture in headache management: theory, mechanism, and practice. *Headache* 2005;45:716–730.

Zhao FH, Ma B, Yi K, et al. Yangxue Qingnao grain for migraine. *Chin J Evidence-Based Med* 2008;8:887–891.

Zhao L, Ren YL, Liang FR. [Analysis of characteristics of meridians and acupoints selected for treating migraine in past dynasties based on data excavation]. *Zhongguo Zhen Jiu* 2009;29:467–472.

Zheng H, Chen M, Wu X, et al. Manage migraine with acupuncture: a review of acupuncture protocols in randomized controlled trials. *Am J Chin Med* 2010;38:639–650.

Zhong GW, Li W. Effects of acupuncture on 5-hydroxytryptamine1F and inducible nitric oxide synthase gene expression in the brain of migraine rats. *J Clin Rehabil Tissue Engineering Res* 2007;11:5761–5764.

Zhong GW, Li W, Luo YH, Chen GL, et al. Herbs for calming liver and suppressing liver-yang in treatment of migraine with hyperactive liver-yang syndrome and its effects on lymphocyte protein expression. *J Chin Integrative Med* 2009a;7:25–33.

Zhong GW, Li W, Luo YH, Wang SE, et al. [Acupuncture at points of the liver and gallbladder meridians for treatment of migraine: a multi-center randomized and controlled study]. *Zhongguo Zhen Jiu* 2009b;29:259–263.

Zhou JW, Li J, Li N, et al. [Transient analgesic effect of electro-acupuncture at Taiyang (EX-HN 5) for treatment of migraine with hyperactivity of the liver-yang]. *Zhongguo Zhen Jiu* 2007;27:159–163.

Zhu CQ, Xie W, Chan BT. [Effect of new zhengtian pill on expression of whole blood platelet membrane adhesion molecules in patients of migraine]. *Zhongguo Zhong Xi Yi Jie He Xue Hui, Zhongguo Zhong Yi Yan Jiu Yuan Zhu Ban [Chinese Journal of Integrated Traditional & Western Medicine]* 2001;21:822–824.

Naturopathy: Including Nutritional Considerations

Joseph Pizzorno, ND

INTRODUCTION

Migraine is a complex neurologic syndrome, with a pathophysiology that has not yet been clearly defined. It may be more accurate to say that the pathophysiology is not identical among all migraineurs, and the diversity in symptoms reflects this diversity in physiological dysfunction. Migraine is not due to any one specific cause, such as infection, inflammation, or tumor, although in most individuals it is thought to have a trigger, including both endogenous and exogenous factors (Levy et al., 2009), and there may be some shared degree of cortical hyperexcitability. Also, because migraine does not appear to have a uniform etiology or physiology, it is a disease defined by symptoms agreed upon by convention, and not necessarily reflective of the primary dysfunction. This chapter highlights the diverse biochemistry of migraineurs and reviews nutritional therapies that address the most likely underlying dysfunction.

BACKGROUND

The International Headache Society has defined migraines as headaches that last 4 to 72 hours, are typically unilateral, are pulsating, are associated with moderate to severe pain intensity, worsen with exertion, and are often accompanied by nausea and/or vomiting, and phonophobia and/or photophobia (Mueller, 2007). None of these symptoms is specific to migraine; indeed, all of them may occur in other types of headache. Also, approximately one-fourth of all migraineurs experience aura—a combination of positive and negative visual, sensory, and speech symptoms that lasts less than 1 hour and often precedes the headache. The presence of aura also adds significant morbidity and mortality risk; an increase in both all-cause and cardiovascular mortality has been found with this condition, as well as preeclampsia and both hemorrhagic and ischemic stroke (Schürks et al., 2009; Gudmundsson et al., 2010; Kurth et al., 2010).

The etiology of migraines was initially thought to be vascular in origin, although this hypothesis has since been largely replaced by a neuronal theory (Goadsby, 2009). Nevertheless, neither concept completely explains the diverse physiology of these headaches. At present, perhaps the most widely accepted theory is that a primary neurologic event occurs, which then initiates downstream events, including vascular changes. A maladaptive and recurrent activation of the peripheral trigeminocervical pain apparatus appears to play a critical role in this cascade of events (Cutrer, 2010), leading to activation of meningeal nociceptors and release of vasoactive peptides (e.g., substance P, neurokinin A, and calcitonin gene–related peptide [CGRP]) into the arteries they innervate, causing dilatation of meningeal arteries (as well as perivascular inflammation and extravasation of plasma proteins). Also, what begins as peripheral nociceptor activation ultimately projects to higher cortical centers in the brain (Loder, 2010).

What predisposes an individual to that initial neuronal event remains very much in question, and the significant diversity in migraine triggers makes any explanation quite complex. For example, stress, anxiety, insomnia, dietary factors, and hormonal changes are all known to be capable of producing a migraine. Thus either the various triggers must all be capable of initiating one specific process, such as the activation of meningeal nociceptors, or else a number of distinct pathways are capable of activating meningeal nociceptors (Levy et al., 2009). Although the precise mechanisms are unknown, a number of nutritional factors are thought to be involved in determining individual sensitivity to migraine, at least in part through mechanisms related to this underlying predisposition, including abnormal histamine metabolism, food allergies, dysfunctional neuronal mitochondrial function, methylenetetrahydrofolate reductase (MTHFR) gene polymorphisms, nitric oxide activity, and imbalances in neurotransmitter activity or neuromodulation. Additionally, telomeres of migraineurs were also recently shown to be shorter than controls, with the age of migraine onset being associated with the loss in relative telomere length (Ren et al., 2010)—likely a sign of increased oxidative stress and inflammation.

The following discussion of the pathophysiology highlights those causes most amenable to natural interventions.

IMMUNOGLOBULIN E, MAST CELLS, AND HISTAMINE: BUTTERBUR AND FOOD ALLERGIES

That at least some migraineurs demonstrate abnormal histamine release has been suspected for quite some time, at least partly because of the increased comorbidities of migraine and other allergic conditions. For example, a recent study found that the incidence of migraines in a population with allergic rhinitis was more than 14 times greater than the corresponding incidence in a control population (Ku et al., 2006). Similar studies found an increased risk of migraine among individuals with asthma, asthma-related symptoms, and other respiratory disorders, as well as among children with atopic disease (Mortimer et al., 1993; Aamodt et al., 2007). Indeed, one study of children with migraine found 40% to have positive allergy tests (IgE mediated), such that their migraines responded to either pharmacological or dietary treatment of the allergy (Wendorff et al., 1999). An increase in total IgE and histamine levels among adults with migraine has been also documented (Gazerani et al., 2003). The common element among those persons with various atopic diseases is likely the IgE-triggered mast cell release of histamine and other vasoactive substances.

Histamine is well known to cause vasodilation via the H_1 and H_2 receptors. Additionally, the increased vascular permeability caused by histamine may contribute to local neurogenic inflammation, which is suspected to be a key component of migraine pathology. Finally, histamine is thought to increase the release of nitric oxide (NO), which has also been implicated in migraine pathogenesis (discussed further later in this chapter) (Ku et al., 2006). The apparent role of histamine in migraine is also consistent with earlier studies that found elevated histamine levels in migraineurs, onset of symptoms after histamine administration, and alleviation of headache with an H_1-receptor blocking agent. However, histamine receptor antagonists have not always shown benefit for treating migraine, likely because they do little to modify the vascular effects of histamine.

The relationship between histamine, IgE, and migraine has translated into a therapeutic potential from dietary changes. An approach of identifying IgE antibodies and eliminating those foods that produce an immune response would be expected to lessen migraine frequency, and it may be particularly useful in an atopic patient. Previous trials of food elimination based on IgE testing have generally found positive effects from this strategy (Mansfield et al., 1985). Similarly, treatments that prevent mast cell degranulation and histamine release would also be expected to have therapeutic value, as has been demonstrated with the herb butterbur.

Butterbur

Components of butterbur have been found to be mast cell stabilizers, which prevent the release of histamine (Agosti et al., 2006) as well as prostaglandins. For this reason, initial clinical trials with a butterbur extract were done with patients suffering from allergic rhinitis, with results demonstrating comparable efficacy to standard antiallergy medications (Schapowal et al., 2004, 2005). The first clinical trial of butterbur use for migraine prophylaxis was published in 2000 and involved a population of 60 adults; a subsequent analysis of this trial's data found that the treatment significantly reduced migraine frequency compared to placebo, and possibly lessened the intensity of the headaches experienced. This analysis deemed 45% of patients receiving butterbur to be responders (defined as those patients experiencing a 50% or greater reduction in migraine frequency—a standard term used in most trials), compared with only 15% of patients receiving placebo (Diener et al., 2004).

Subsequent trials in both adults and children have generally found benefits from butterbur in migraine as well (Agosti et al., 2006). It seems noteworthy that the percentage of patients responding to butterbur (approximately 45%) is roughly equal to the percentage of children with migraines who had elevated IgE antibodies (discussed previously). Although butterbur has other mechanisms of action that may explain its benefit for migraine prophylaxis (it is an anti-inflammatory agent and a calcium-channel antagonist per Horak et al., 2009), the shared pathophysiology and efficacy between migraine and allergic rhinitis suggests that mast cell stabilization may be its primary effect in these two conditions.

Interestingly, in one study children who were able to reduce their migraine frequency through relaxation techniques were found to have a lower level of urine tryptase, an indicator of mast cell activation (Olness et al., 1999). In addition to highlighting the efficacy of stress reduction techniques, this small study suggested that histamine release is a possible mechanism by which stress

or anxiety may trigger migraines, or at least showed that mast cell stability may be a marker for migraines, if not part of a more active contributor.

Evidence: Butterbur, 1B+; IgE-based food elimination, 1B+.

Immunoglobulin G and Food Allergy

Although IgE activation of mast cells may have a more clearly defined mechanism in migraine physiology, the role of food is not likely to be limited to only this pathway. In addition to IgE, IgG antibodies appear to play a role in migraine development. In 2007, researchers measured the levels of IgG antibodies produced in response to more than 100 food antigens, and found not only a significant difference in the number of positive antibodies among those persons with migraine compared to controls, but also that elimination of these foods reduced the migraine burden (Arroyave Hernández et al., 2007).

Perhaps even more convincing was a double-blind, cross-over study published in 2010 (Alpay et al., 2010). In this study, 30 patients with migraine without aura had IgG levels measured against more than 250 foods, and were randomized to either a provocative diet for 6 weeks, rich in foods to which they were producing IgG antibodies, or an elimination diet, which was devoid of those foods. After a 2-week diet-free period, participants then were put on the alternative diet for 6 additional weeks (i.e., cross-over to either provocation or elimination diet). Both patients and their physicians were blinded to the results of the IgG tests, and any reduction in migraine attacks could be attributed directly to the consumption of specific foods to which IgG antibodies were produced. Analysis of these data found a significant reduction in both attack frequency and the number of days with headache when compared to the baseline data as well as the provocative dietary period (although attack severity and duration did not change). Specifically, more than 50% of patients had at least a 30% reduction in the number of attacks compared to baseline, and 20% had at least a 50% reduction in attack frequency.

The question that remains unanswered by these studies is by which mechanism of action IgG antibodies contribute to migraine initiation. It is likely that foods can induce or prevent migraines through several pathways, as indicated by the clinical success many physicians report anecdotally when using various elimination diets. For example, studies published in the 1980s reported tremendous clinical success by having patients avoid certain foods, and even developed a fairly consistent list of which foods most commonly produced migraines, such as cow's milk, eggs, chocolate, and wheat (Egger et al., 1983; Hughes et al., 1985; see Pizzorno & Murray, 2006, for complete list). Additionally, adoption of a low-fat diet has been shown to reduce headache frequency, duration, intensity, and medication use among patients with migraine (Bic et al., 1999).

The authors of the most recent study that measured IgG suggest that perhaps the inflammation produced by IgG antibody formation or activation is a key factor, as documented in a study published in 2008 that followed children with obesity (Wilders-Truschnig et al., 2008). In this study, obese children were found to have higher IgG production against specific foods than normal-weight children, and IgG levels were associated with both low-grade systemic inflammation (measured by CRP) and intimal media thickness of the common carotid arteries. Given the likely role of neurogenic inflammation in migraine, this theory seems plausible.

Evidence: IgG-based food elimination, 1B + ; oligoantigenic diet, 1B + .

MITOCHONDRIAL DYSFUNCTION: RIBOFLAVIN AND COENZYME Q10

One of the contributing factors to migraines, affecting perhaps as many as 40% of patients, appears to be mitochondrial dysfunction, which fortunately may be modified by nutritional interventions. Mitochondrial involvement has been postulated for some time, largely due to direct evidence from morphological, biochemical, and neuro-radiological studies (reviewed in Sparaco et al., 2006). The pertinent factors include documented lactic acidosis in the cerebrospinal fluid and reduced activity of specific enzymes involved in oxidative phosphorylation (e.g., succinate dehydrogenase, NADH–cytochrome-c–reductase) among migraine patients. Evidence in the same vein also includes phosphorus magnetic resonance spectroscopy analyses (P-MRS, a noninvasive test that can monitor ATP production and in vivo brain energy metabolism) indicative of an "unstable metabolic state of the brain and a decreased ability to cope with further energy demand" among migraineurs (Sparaco et al., 2006), pointing to either a primary or secondary mitochondrial dysfunction. Moreover, at least some migraineurs have been shown to have a carnitine palmityltransferase II deficiency, which responds to carnitine supplementation (Kabbouche et al., 2003).

Although genetic evidence for mitochondrial dysfunction in migraine has not identified any common mutations among migraineurs, a recent study does provide support for this theory. In patients with cyclic vomiting syndrome (CVS; considered a migraine-like condition or migraine equivalent) as well as in individuals with migraine without aura, the entire mitochondrial genome was sequenced and compared to controls (Zaki et al., 2009). In this study, the authors found a very high rate of two specific polymorphisms among those persons with CVS and migraine. First, a 16519C→T polymorphism was found in 70% of CVS patients (odds ratio [OR]: 6.2) and in 52% of migraineurs (OR: 3.6), compared to only 27% of controls. Second, the 3010G→A polymorphism was found in 29% of CVS patients (OR: 17.0) and 26% of migraineurs (OR: 15.0) compared to only 1.6% of controls. The findings from this study certainly lend credence to the idea that alterations in mitochondrial energy production predispose individuals toward migraine. (It should be noted that this study was restricted to patients with haplogroup H, with the term "haplogroup" indicating a common ancestor marked by some shared mtDNA mutations. Haplogroup H is more common among persons of European ancestry, and may actually correspond to greater metabolic activity than is found in other haplogroups.)

In addition to direct evidence, a considerable amount of indirect data points to a role of mitochondrial dysfunction. Specifically, the use of enhancers of oxidative phosphorylation has shown considerable benefits in migraine prevention, including the use of riboflavin and coenzyme Q10 (CoQ10). It also appears that the benefit of these nutrients may be influenced by mitochondrial polymorphisms.

Riboflavin

The use of riboflavin by patients with migraine was first published in 1994, and has since shown effectiveness for migraine prophylaxis in both adults and children at a dose of 200–400mg per day (Schoenen et al., 1994). For example, in a recent study nearly 70% of children and adolescents had a 50% or greater reduction in migraine frequency (responders) as well as a decrease in migraine intensity (Condò et al., 2009). In a 3-month randomized trial comparing riboflavin to placebo, 59% of those taking riboflavin were considered responders, compared to 15% of those taking placebo (Schoenen et al., 1998). Riboflavin is likely to be effective because it is the precursor of flavin mononucleotide and flavin adenine dinucleotide, both of which are required by enzymes in the electron transport chain, particularly complex I in this chain (Scholte et al., 1995).

Two additional studies with riboflavin are worth mentioning. The first compared the effect of both riboflavin

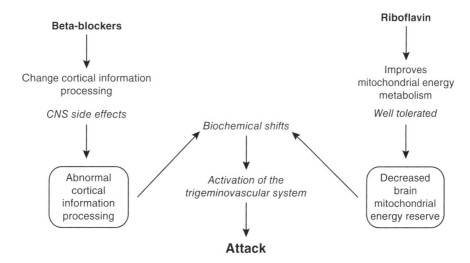

Figure 29.1 Probable Mechanisms of Action for Beta-Blocker and Riboflavin Prophylaxis in Migraine Pathophysiology. The distinct mechanisms for these two treatments suggest that they might potentially be effective in nonresponders to the alternate therapy; they also emphasize the lack of adverse effects seen with riboflavin treatment.

From Gentile G, et al. Frequencies of genetic polymorphisms related to triptans metabolism in chronic migraine. *J Headache Pain* 2010;11:151–156.

(400 mg per day) and beta-blockers (metoprolol 200 mg per day, bisoprolol 10 mg per day) on clinical responses as well as on the intensity dependence of auditory-invoked cortical potentials (migraineurs tend to have increased cortical activity in response to stimuli, a phenomenon confirmed in this study). Beta-blockers are known to be effective agents for migraine prophylaxis, but are suspected to work by a different mechanism than riboflavin, possibly by changing neuronal excitability or neurotransmitter activity. The first finding of this study was that the percentages of "responders" in both groups were statistically equivalent (53% and 55% had a reduction of more than 50% in pain attack frequency). The second finding, however, was that although riboflavin did not reduce the intensity dependence of cortical potentials, the beta-blocker treatment resulted in significant reduction, with clinical response directly associated with the reduction *in the beta-blocker group only*. The authors point out that the lack of reduction in intensity dependence in the riboflavin group does not point to any difference in clinical efficacy, as the two treatments were equally effective. Rather, it demonstrates the presence of two different mechanisms by which these treatments are thought to act, and possibly the diversity in migraine physiology. Perhaps most importantly, it suggests that if either treatment alone is ineffective (or if beta-blocker therapy is intolerable due to adverse effects), either changing treatments or combining treatments may be the most clinically effective intervention (Sándor et al., 2000). A follow-up clinical

trial examining the efficacy of combined therapy would be very interesting **(Figure. 29.1)**.

The second study involved the use of riboflavin in an experiment to see if a patient's haplogroup influences clinical improvement. The authors speculated that because no classic mtDNA mutations were found in common forms of migraine, more subtle mutations in the mitochondrial genome—as captured by haplogroup—might explain the apparent involvement of mitochondrial pathology (Di Lorenzo et al., 2009). Their speculation turned out to be accurate, as the "responder" rate in patients with haplogroup H was 44.8% compared to 77% in non-H haplogroups; the overall responder rate was 62.5%, a rate comparable to that obtained in previous controlled trials.

This study suggests several possibilities. Perhaps non-H haplogroups may be more responsive to riboflavin treatment because of impaired complex I activity in these haplogroups (which riboflavin would be expected to address), a relationship supported by previous studies (Ruiz-Pesini et al., 2000). Perhaps haplogroup H is protective for migraine due to a more functional complex I or, alternatively, perhaps it is less responsive to treatment because either a non-mitochondrial pathology is present, a component of the electron transport chain other than complex I is affected, or a distinct dysfunction is present in complex I that is not modifiable by increasing riboflavin levels. It appears that haplogroup H is decidedly not protective for migraine, being found at approximately the same frequency in persons with and without migraine. Indeed, it may actually increase the risk for other conditions with suspected mitochondrial involvement, including Alzheimer's disease and Parkinson disease (Pyle et al., 2005; Fesahat et al., 2007). The most likely hypothesis is that inefficiencies in other mitochondrial complexes (i.e., II, III, IV) are present in haplogroup H, which might respond to treatments that target those specific complexes.

Thus, although the responder rate seems high enough in all haplogroups to justify riboflavin as a prophylactic treatment, those persons with a non-H haplogroup are more likely to benefit (i.e., those with non-European ancestry have a greater likelihood of success). Exploration of the pathology associated with haplogroup H seems indicated to better address the underlying dysfunction.

Evidence: Riboflavin, 1A + .

Coenzyme Q10

Coenzyme Q10 was first used as a potential headache therapy in an open-label trial of adults with migraine, in whom it resulted in a mean reduction in migraine frequency of 13% at 1 month and 55% at 3 months (Rozen et al., 2002). CoQ10 has since been found to be significantly superior to placebo, delivering a nearly 50% response rate compared to a response rate of almost 15% for placebo in a randomized trial (Sàndor et al., 2005). Like riboflavin, this therapy's full benefit was not seen for at least 3 months, indicating that it may take time to increase mitochondrial function. Additionally, it had the greatest effect on reducing headache frequency and nausea, with no apparent effect on headache severity or duration.

In a more recent study, the serum CoQ10 levels of more than 1,500 children and adolescents with migraine were measured (Hershey et al., 2007). The researchers found that 32.9% of participants had a level of total CoQ10 below the reference range (less than 0.5 μg/mL), and a total of 74.6% had suboptimal levels (less than 0.7 μg/mL). When patients with a deficiency were then given supplemental CoQ10 (1–3 mg/kg/day), a response rate of nearly 50% was observed.

The high rate of CoQ10 deficiency observed likely reflects increased consumption of CoQ10 (versus inadequate production or absorption), perhaps due to increased oxidative or mitochondrial stress. Vascular inflammation may also play a role in generating reactive oxygen species, which in turn consume CoQ10. CoQ10 is known to transport electrons between complex I and complex II, as well as to function as a cellular antioxidant; thus it serves as a regenerator of vitamins C and E.

A trial designed to measure the impact of both riboflavin and CoQ10 when used together might prove very informative, and identifying specific mitochondrial pathologies in migraineurs should also help to predict the most effective treatment.

Evidence: CoQ10, 1B + .

MTHFR AND HOMOCYSTEINE: FOLATE, VITAMIN B$_{12}$, AND VITAMIN B$_6$

Although current thinking leans heavily toward migraine as having a neurologic origin, considerable evidence continues to support roles for a vascular component as well as abnormalities in platelet aggregation. A number of fascinating studies have examined the relationship between polymorphisms of the MTHFR gene, homocysteine elevations, and migraine. MTHFR catalyzes the conversion of 5,10-methylenetetrafirsthydrofolate into 5-methylenetetrahydrofolate, a cofactor for the remethylation of homocysteine to methionine, and the main circulating form of folate. The C677T polymorphism is a common variant of the MTHFR gene, and has been shown to have decreased enzymatic activity, leading to increased levels of the amino acid homocysteine. Hyperhomocysteinemia is an important risk factor for both peripheral and central cardiovascular disease, with researchers having identified a direct association between the TT genotype and such increased risk (Durga et al., 2004; Khandanpour et al., 2009). Homocysteine itself is likely to have direct vascular toxicity, at least in part through oxidative stress.

It appears that the C677T polymorphism and hyperhomocysteinemia are also associated with increased risk for migraine with aura in some populations (Pizza et al., 2010; Schürks et al., 2010). For example, a recent analysis of more than 400 migraineurs found that homocysteine levels exceeding 12.0 μM had an OR of 2.145 for migraine with aura, while levels greater than 15.0 μM carried a nearly sixfold increase in risk; the number of T alleles was found to be the greatest predictor of homocysteine status (Oterino et al., 2010).

A recent study also documented an increase in the total homocysteine concentration in the cerebrospinal fluid of 41% of migraineurs without aura compared to controls, and a surprising 376% increase in those migraineurs who also had aura (Isobe et al., 2010). It is suspected that the increase in homocysteine concentrations associated with the T allele may largely explain the increased risk for atherosclerotic conditions associated with migraine, which is significantly greater if aura is present.

Unfortunately, the results of this study do not help in determining whether migraine may have more of a vascular than a neurologic origin. In a recent review published in *Cephalalgia*, the authors concluded that endothelial dysfunction is not just more prevalent in migraineurs, but "may be the underlying patho-physiological process underlying this widespread vasculopathy" (Tietjen, 2009). Homocysteine may potentially contribute to a systemic vasculopathy by generating cerebral microvascular changes. However, as Isobe (2010) points out, homocysteine can also be metabolized into homocysteic acid (HCA), which closely resembles the excitatory neurotransmitter glutamate. HCA may generate excitotoxicity via activation of the *N*-methyl-D-aspartate receptor, as well as induce neuronal apoptosis, increase oxidative stress, and lead to a reduction in intracellular glutathione levels (Ratan et al., 1994a, 1994b). All of these effects point to the role of neuronal dysfunction as the root of migraine pathology.

Regardless of the mechanism by which impaired homocysteine metabolism leads to an increase in migraines, treatments that address this dysfunction have shown impressive clinical benefits. In a recent randomized, double-blind, placebo-controlled trial published in *Pharmacogenetics and Genomics*, a combination of folic acid, vitamin B_6, and vitamin B_{12} were given to 52 patients diagnosed with migraine with aura. Researchers found that vitamin supplementation not only reduced homocysteine levels by 39%, but also decreased the prevalence of migraine disability (based on the Migraine Disability Assessment [MIDAS] score) from 60% at baseline to 30% after 6 months, with no corresponding reduction seen in the placebo group. Unlike most prophylactic treatments, the vitamin combination also significantly reduced the pain severity of the participants' migraines (no change in this variable was noted in the placebo group). Somewhat unexpectedly, carriers of the C allele for the MTHFRC677T polymorphism experienced a greater response. The authors suggested quite astutely that this variation may reflect a need for a larger dose of B vitamins for those persons with the T allele if the therapy is to have a comparable effect (Lea et al., 2009).

In a smaller trial, the use of folic acid alone was evaluated among children presenting with hyperhomocysteinemia, migraine without aura, and at least one T allele (often both) or a second MTHFR polymorphism that also impairs enzyme activity (1298AC). Although this investigation was an open-label trial, the authors reported that not only did plasma homocysteine levels normalize in 100% of patients, but a complete resolution in migraines was also experienced in 62% of the

participants, a 75% reduction in an additional 31%, and a 50% reduction in the remaining population. Thus 100% of the patients experienced at least a 50% reduction in migraines, with the majority having complete resolution (Di Rosa et al., 2007). Note that the dose of folic acid was 5 mg per day in this study, compared to only 2 mg in the larger placebo-controlled trial.

Lastly, an interesting analysis found that the MTHFR genotype was associated not just with migraine diagnosis, but also with specific migraine phenotypes. Researchers analyzed the specific symptoms, triggers, and treatments for more than 250 migraineurs genotyped for the MTHFR C677T variant (Liu et al., 2010). They found the TT genotype to be significantly associated with migraine with aura diagnosis and unilateral head pain, whereas the CT genotype was associated with physical activity discomfort as well as stress as a migraine trigger. Additionally, the TT genotype was present in the highest percentage of participants suffering from unilateral head pain, the CC genotype was present in the lowest percentage of these individuals, and the CT genotype was linked to an intermediate value. This line of research may represent a step toward differentiating the various migraine symptoms as keys to specific pathology, instead of the amorphous classification of migraine based on a checklist of criteria, not underlying physiology.

Evidence: Folic acid with vitamin B_{12} and vitamin B_6, 1B + for migraine with aura; folic acid alone for migraine without aura, 2C +.

NITRIC OXIDE HYPOTHESIS OF MIGRAINE: VITAMIN B_{12}

Another component of migraine as well as other primary headaches is nitric oxide (NO). NO is involved in regulation of cranial blood flow; plays a role in nociceptor processing, particularly in the central nervous system; and has been shown to initiate migraines as well as to be involved during the entire duration of an attack (Olesen et al., 1994; Olesen, 2008). It appears to be linked to a number of important mediators of migraine, including serotonin, estrogen, and possibly CGRP, and its actions are likely mediated via cGMP. NO also seems to be closely tied to cortical spreading depression (CSD), the phenomenon that is thought to explain the aura of migraine.

Although nonselective nitric oxide synthase (NOS) inhibitors (i.e., L-NMMA) have been shown to reduce migraine frequency, the adverse effects associated with these drugs prevent their use, and as of yet no data for selective NOS inhibitors have been published. However, compounds that scavenge NO may be therapeutically effective for migraine, although at this point few data on their use for this indication have been published. For example, the superoxide radical is known to scavenge NO. During conditions of hypoxia, such as at high altitudes, there is less superoxide available and therefore more NO, possibly accounting for the increase in headaches at these elevations. It has also been shown that L-arginine supplementation increases both exhaled NO and headache frequency at high altitude, and may be expected to increase symptoms in some patients with migraine (Mansoor et al., 2005). Similarly, triptan overuse in migraine has been shown to increase headache frequency in some patients. An animal study recently found that this effect may be due to an induction of neuronal NOS and, therefore, elevated NO levels (De Felice et al., 2010).

A natural nitric oxide scavenger is vitamin B_{12}. After an initial in vitro study found that cobalamins could quench NO (Brouwer et al., 1996), a small open-label trial was done using intranasal hydroxocobalamin (1 mg) in migraineurs (Van der Kuy et al., 2002). Using a cut-off of 50% or more reduction in migraine attack frequency, 53% were found to be responders, while 63% had 30% or greater reductions in migraine frequency. Although a placebo effect is very unlikely to have been this effective, a follow-up controlled trial has not yet been done.

Evidence: Vitamin B_{12}, 2C + .

GLUTAMATE, DOPAMINE, AND TRACE AMINE RECEPTORS: MELATONIN, MAGNESIUM, AND DIET

One of the most accepted components of migraine is cortical synaptic hyperexcitability, and glutamate (along with aspartate)—the major excitatory neurotransmitter in the central nervous system—is thought to be one of the principal factors involved in this abnormality (Ramadan, 2003). Indeed, the balance between glutamate activity and gamma-aminobutyric acid (GABA), the major inhibitory neurotransmitter, regulates many functions of the brain and may be impaired in migraineurs. There may also be a role for glutamate receptors, as a study published in June 2010 in *BMC Medical Genetics* documented the first genetic evidence for an association between glutamate receptors and both migraine with and without aura (different polymorphisms were associated with each migraine type) (Formicola et al., 2010).

For many years, there has been a suspicion that trace amines, such as tyramine, octopamine, and synephrine,

may somehow contribute to migraine pathogenesis, either by influencing the action of glutamate to induce cortical hyperexcitability or by acting as "false neurotransmitters" (i.e., displacing biogenic amines from their storage vesicles). Not only have elevated levels of these trace amines recently been documented in primary headaches (D'Andrea et al., 2004), but the profile of these amines also appears to be different (albeit abnormal) between migraine with and without aura (D'Andrea et al., 2006). Additionally, the abnormalities in trace amine levels and metabolism may explain some of the autonomic disturbances, behavioral changes, and premonitory symptoms of migraine, as well as related symptoms in cluster headache (D'Andrea et al., 2007).

Nevertheless, despite these proven abnormalities, this theory of migraine development had not gained very much traction until recently, in part because the detection of these amines in human samples has been very difficult. There now appears to be renewed interest in pursuing this line of investigation, mostly due to the discovery of a new class of G-protein–coupled receptors with high affinity for these amines, known as trace amine receptors (TAARs). These trace amines are suspected to act as neurotransmitters at these receptors and as neuromodulators (i.e., influencing the effect of other neurotransmitters) at dopamine and norepinephrine synaptic clefts (Berry, 2004).

Both sympathetic and dopaminergic activity have long been suspected to play roles in migraine physiology, and the discovery of TAARs may provide insight into at least part of the mechanism involved. To briefly review dopaminergic involvement, dopamine appears to be responsible to some extent for some of the non-headache symptoms of migraine, such as nausea, vomiting, and hypotension. Moreover, migraineurs are known to be hypersensitive to dopamine agonists. For example, dopamine agonists have been shown to increase the number of yawns over time in migraineurs compared to controls (Blin et al., 1991). Dopamine is a derivative of the trace amine tyrosine, with the conversion of tyrosine to L-dopa occurring through the action of tyrosine hydroxylase (the rate-limiting step in production of dopamine), as well as norepinephrine and epinephrine. Thus an increase in trace amines may contribute to increased dopaminergic activity, explaining a number of migraine-related symptoms. Additionally, the first genetic evidence for an involvement of the dopaminergic system in migraine with aura was presented only in 2009—specifically, polymorphisms in dopamine-beta hydroxylase (which converts dopamine to norepinpehrine) and dopamine transporter genes (Todt et al., 2009).

Melatonin

Two potential therapeutic agents that address some of the underlying mechanisms related to altered neurotransmitter activity and neuromodulation in migraine are the hormone melatonin and the mineral magnesium. Animal studies have shown that melatonin can reduce the sensitivity of central dopamine receptors—the very type of hypersensitivity documented in individuals with migraine (Abílio et al., 2003). Melatonin also inhibits the release of dopamine, indicating it works via multiple pathways in reducing dopaminergic activity (Zisapel, 2001). Furthermore, a recent study found that levels of a urinary metabolite of melatonin, 6-sulfatoxymelatonin, were decreased in patients with chronic migraine (Masruha et al., 2010). Perhaps coincidentally, the production of melatonin in women with migraine was found to be "supersensitive to light"; that is, the production of melatonin was more markedly suppressed by the same intensity of light in migraineurs compared to controls (Claustrat et al., 2004). Given that the production of melatonin peaks during darkness, perhaps this relationship explains part of the photophobia experienced by some individuals with migraine. In any event, it appears that the very hormone that may prevent the excess dopaminergic activity found in migraine appears to be deficient in migraineurs compared to controls.

Only two clinical trials have been published in which melatonin was used as a migraine prophylactic, although unfortunately a control group was not included in either study. The first trial produced very impressive results, with a dose of 3 mg bringing about at least a 50% reduction in headaches in nearly 80% of patients, and a 100% response in 25% after 3 months of therapy (Peres et al., 2004). The second trial was done in children with either migraine or tension-type headache, and again was an open-label trial. In this study, 61% of participants were classified as responders, with nearly 20% reporting complete resolution of headaches (Miano et al., 2008). Given these impressive results in open-label trials, it is astonishing that randomized and blinded trials have not been done to further evaluate the efficacy of melatonin.

Evidence: Melatonin, 2C+.

Magnesium

Magnesium has a long history of use in migraine. It is known to have an effect on serotonin receptors, nitric oxide synthesis and release, and NMDA receptors; it may be the only compound known to block glutamate-dependent spreading depression; and its levels have been shown to be reduced in the brains of migraine patients, especially during a painful attack (Mauskop & Altura,,1998; D'Andrea & Leon, 2010). Although clinical trials have yielded mixed results over the years (most likely due to a variety of forms of magnesium used and the mode of administration), in general a therapeutic effect seems quite likely to exist. For example, in a recent placebo-controlled trial, 30 patients with migraine without aura were given 600 mg magnesium citrate per day over a 3-month period. Not only did the researchers observe a reduction in attack frequency and severity compared to placebo, but they also used computed tomography to document changes in cortical blood flow and other signs of therapeutic benefit compared to placebo (Köseoglu et al., 2008).

Although most of the migraine treatments discussed so far in this chapter are primarily used for prophylactic treatment of migraine, magnesium may be one with the potential to be a prophylactic treatment as well as to be used in acute migraine, when given intravenously. In a trial in which 1,000 mg magnesium sulfate IV was compared to placebo, magnesium was found to significantly reduce pain and other migraine symptoms in patients with migraine with aura. Although it did not provide pain relief in those migraineurs without aura, it did relieve other related symptoms, such as phonophobia and photophobia (Bigal et al., 2002).

Magnesium may also have an important role in menstrually related migraines. Serum ionized levels of magnesium were found to be deficient most of the time (approximately 15%) in women in a prospective evaluation of more than 250 women seen at a headache clinic, but during a menstrually related migraine the percentage of women with reduced ionized magnesium rose dramatically, to 45% (Mauskop & Altura, 2002). Serum ionized magnesium may be a better predictor of which patients might benefit from magnesium than total magnesium levels, which were found to be consistently normal in a previous study (which also found benefit of magnesium, particularly in those patients with a reduced ionized level) (Mauskop et al., 1996).

Evidence: Magnesium, 2B+.

Diet

Lastly, the role of dietary amines in migraine remains an open question. As discussed earlier, biogenic and trace amines do appear to affect migraine pathology, and their levels seem to be elevated in patients with migraine. However, increased production of these trace amines alone may be sufficient to explain this abnormality. For example, in the trial mentioned previously that found elevated plasma levels of trace amines in migraineurs, the participants were asked to rigorously avoid foods that contained relevant amounts of these compounds, making a dietary contribution seem much less likely (D'Andrea et al., 2004). In fact, a recent review of dietary amines and any related intolerance concluded that there was no association. However, this review disregarded several positive studies with which the authors found problems, making them ineligible for consideration. Somewhat troubling was the fairly high rate of headache cited in some of the placebo groups, which the author cited as "negative" evidence for any effect of dietary amines. For example, 19 out of 27 individuals given tyramine reported a headache, while 14 out of 27 given placebo did (Ryan, 1974). When a placebo causes a headache in more than 50% of patients, this finding suggests perhaps the placebo itself was not benign. Indeed, more recently the ingredients in placebo have come into question as being triggers of migraine themselves (Strong, 2000). Also, a study of red wine as a trigger suggests that an unknown component of red wine (not the alcohol or tyramine content) may be able to trigger migraines (Littlewood et al., 1988). Thus the "conclusive" evidence reported in Jansen et al. (2003) seems questionable.

Biogenic amines are found in the highest amounts in "yeast extracts, fish, chocolate, alcoholic drinks, and fermented products, such as cheese, soy products, sauerkraut, and processed meat" (Jansen et al., 2003). It may be worth considering these foods as potential migraine triggers, although this link has not been definitively proved. Interestingly, a recent analysis of the effects of a cocoa-rich diet in rats found that this diet altered expression of several key inflammatory proteins in trigeminal ganglion neurons, reduced neuronal expression of CGRP, and suppressed stimulation of nitric oxide synthase—all effects that would suggest the diet might have a benefit for migraineurs, despite chocolate-containing foods having a reputation as a frequent migraine trigger (Marcus et al., 1997; Cady & Durham, 2010).

Evidence: Dietary restriction of biogenic amines, 2C+.

ADDITIONAL NUTRITIONAL ASSOCIATIONS/THERAPIES

Vitamin D

Although the nutritional interventions mentioned earlier have at least plausible mechanisms of action given our current understanding of migraine pathophysiology, a number of other factors related to diet and nutrition have been associated with migraine, albeit without a solid basis for their connections. For example, in recent years the high prevalence of vitamin D insufficiency, along with the spectrum of conditions affected by low levels of this hormone, has garnered tremendous attention. Migraine may be one of these effects of vitamin D deficiency. Although no studies have been done to evaluate the vitamin D levels of patients with migraine or to examine the therapeutic use of vitamin D in these patients, a study published in August 2010 in *The Journal of Headache and Pain* found a significant correlation between increasing latitude and the prevalence of both tension-type headache and migraine, a relationship that would correspond well with the incidence of vitamin D deficiency (Prakash et al., 2010). Although several mechanisms might be responsible for this effect, including increased neuronal inflammation with deficiency, the role in migraine is not yet established. However, given the important role of vitamin D in many body systems, screening for insufficiency should be routine.

Evidence: Vitamin D, 0.

Body Mass Index

Obesity has also recently been shown to be associated with migraine, and weight loss may yield therapeutic benefit for reducing headaches in these patients (Bond et al., 2011). Interestingly, obesity does not seem to be associated with migraine prevalence, but rather with migraine frequency. In a population-based telephone interview of more than 30,000 participants, body mass index (BMI) was not associated with prevalence, but 20.7% of morbidly obese participants had 10 to 15 headache days per month, compared to only 4.4% of the normal-weight group, with intermediate values in the overweight and obese groups (Bigal et al., 2006). Additionally, BMI was associated with headache severity as well as migraine symptoms such as photophobia and phonophobia. A number of possibilities exist for this connection, including elevated CGRP levels in obese individuals that increase with fat intake, and elevated levels of several inflammatory cytokines, and markers, including substance P, tumor necrosis factor alpha and interleukin-6, and C-reactive protein (CRP). The hormones leptin and adiponectin may also play a role in the connection between obesity and migraine (Bond et al., 2011).

Evidence: Weight loss in overweight individuals, 0.

Thioctic Acid (Alpha Lipoic Acid)

Thioctic acid also has therapeutic potential for migraineurs, likely related to its effect on mitochondrial function, but possibly due to its antioxidant effects. In a randomized, single-blind trial, 600 mg thioctic acid or placebo was given to 44 participants with migraine with or without aura. Although no difference in the number of 50% responders was found between groups, those receiving thioctic acid experienced a reduction in frequency, headache days, and severity (Magis et al., 2007).

Evidence: Thioctic acid, 2B +.

Menstrual Migraines

At least half of women with migraines report some association with their menstrual cycles and headaches, experiencing either "pure menstrual" or "menstrually related" migraines (Gupta et al., 2007). This high rate of menstrual migraines is almost certainly due to changes in plasma levels of sex hormones, possibly via several mechanisms, including increased CGRP levels, enhanced cortical hyperexcitability owing to altered norepinephrine levels and adrenergic receptor sensitivity, decreased magnesium levels, and modulation of the synthesis of serotonin as well as several other mediators of migraine discussed previously (Gupta et al., 2007; **Figure 29.2**). Recent research has also noted the presence of several polymorphisms related to estrogen metabolism in female migraineurs (Oterino et al., 2008).

Given that changes in estrogenic fluctuations before menses are likely to be directly involved in migraine development, researchers gave a combination of phytoestrogens to 49 women with menstrual migraine in a placebo-controlled trial. The therapy consisted of 60 mg soy isoflavones, 100 mg dong quai, and 50 mg black cohosh given daily for 6 months. Evaluation of the results found an average frequency of migraine attack of 4.7 in the phytoestrogen group versus 10.3 in the placebo group (Burke et al., 2002). A second but very small study found improvement when patients were given soy isoflavones only, but no placebo was used to evaluate the effectiveness (Ferrante et al., 2004).

Evidence: Phytoestrogens for menstrual migraine, 2B +.

As mentioned previously, magnesium levels are known to be at their lowest during menstrually related attacks, and this decline may play a role in migraine initiation (Mauskop & Altura, 2002). When a double-blind, placebo-controlled trial was performed in 20 women with menstrually related migraines, the researchers found that not only did magnesium reduce the number of days with headache, but it also improved premenstrual complaints (Facchinetti et al., 1991).

Evidence: Magnesium for menstrual migraine, 2B +.

In a double-blind, controlled trial, 72 women with menstrual migraine received placebo for 5 days (2 days before menstruation and 3 days after menstruation) for 2 months, followed by a 1-month washout period, and then 400 IU vitamin E on the same 5-day schedule for the next two cycles (Ziaei et al., 2009). Although the authors' reason for choosing vitamin E does not seem consistent with current understanding (Wu et al., 2004), they found that this therapy reduced headache pain severity, functional disability, and the need for pain medications. Unfortunately, the authors did not report much of their data, including any change to the number of headaches in either period.

Evidence: Vitamin E for menstrual migraines, 2B +.

Omega-3 Fatty Acids

The role of inflammation in migraine suggests that omega-3 fatty acids such as eicosapentaenoic acid (EPA) and docosahexaenoic acid (DHA) would prove to have therapeutic value for reducing migraine attacks. Unfortunately, only two placebo-controlled studies have been done, with both finding no benefit from such therapy compared to placebo. This result may not necessarily indicate a lack of benefit of omega-3 fatty acids, however. In the more recent study, researchers found that such treatment produced a marked improvement in migraine frequency compared to baseline, but not compared to placebo, leading the authors to conclude that both the treatment arm (fish oil) and the placebo (olive oil) may have had clinical benefit (Harel et al., 2002). The second study also reported a high placebo effect, with olive oil used as placebo (Pradalier et al., 2001). Rather than rule out a potential benefit of omega-3 fatty acids, a more appropriately designed trial seems indicated.

Evidence: Omega-3 fatty acids, 2B +.

Feverfew

An extract of the herb feverfew has yielded mixed results in trials evaluating its efficacy for migraine prophylaxis. In one double-blind, randomized trial, this treatment

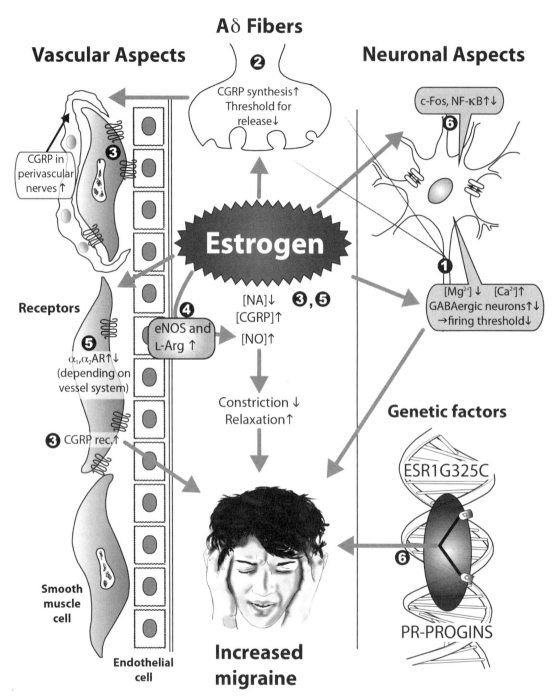

Figure 29.2 Schematic Representation of the Main Mechanisms by Which Estrogens May Increase the Incidence of Migraine. 1. Estrogens enhance neuronal excitability by decreasing the levels of Mg^{2+} and increasing Ca^{2+} concentrations. 2. Estrogens up-regulate the synthesis of CGRP in and its subsequent release from Aδ fibers. 3. At the vascular level, this increased CGRP release enhances vasodilatation, which acts in tandem with increased expression of CGRP receptors and inhibition of the sympathetic nervous system. 4. Estrogens enhance the production of NO via endothelial NO synthase (eNOS) from L-arginine (L-arg) by the endothelium. 5. The GABAergic and noradrenergic (α1- and α2-AR [adrenoceptors], as well as plasma concentrations of NA [noradrenaline]) systems may display both enhanced and attenuated effects in response to estrogens. 6. Estrogens also modulate the molecular markers c-fos and NF-κB, while mutations in both estrogen receptors (ESR1G325C) and progesterone receptors (PR-PROGINS) increase the risk for migraine.

Source: Gupta S, Mehrotra S, Villalón CM, et al. Potential role of female sex hormones in the pathophysiology of migraine. *Pharmacol Ther* 2007;113:321–340.

was found to be effective in only a small subset of migraineurs—namely, those with four or more attacks within the 28-day baseline period; its greatest efficacy was noted to occur at a dose of 6.25 mg three times per day (Pfaffenrath et al., 2002). A more recent study of this extract at the same dose found a reduction in migraine frequency by 1.9 attacks per month (from an initial rate of 4.76 attacks per month) in the feverfew group compared to a reduction of 1.3 attacks in the placebo group (Diener et al., 2005). Although the mechanism of action is not well understood, this herb is assumed to act by inhibiting prostaglandin production, affecting blood vessel vasoreactivity, and reducing the platelet secretion of serotonin.

Evidence: Feverfew, 1B + .

CONCLUSIONS

One goal of migraine therapy is to reduce the pain and other symptoms associated with these debilitating headaches, and many nutritional therapies have been shown to provide clinically meaningful benefits toward that purpose. As we gain a better understanding of migraine etiology, and recognize that each patient has unique triggers and a unique physiology (despite meeting the broader criteria of migraine headaches), however, a second—and perhaps more important—goal is the selection of therapies that address these root causes. Such an approach could lead to not only symptom reduction, but also a correction of the pathology behind migraine associated comorbidities. Avoiding foods to which antibodies are being produced may reduce both migraine symptoms and symptoms of allergic rhinitis or irritable bowel syndrome, for example. Similarly, identifying those persons with a genetic predisposition requiring greater levels of folic acid may not only prevent migraines, but also lead to a reduction in stroke risk owing to this shared pathology. The diagnosis of migraine may be best used as a starting point for assessment, not as a springboard directly into therapy. Thus it represents a clue to the specific abnormalities health-care providers might expect to find in their patients, which a more thorough assessment should reveal, allowing for much more specific therapies and broader benefit.

REFERENCES

Aamodt AH, Stovner LJ, Langhammer A, et al. Is headache related to asthma, hay fever, and chronic bronchitis? The Head-HUNT Study. *Headache* 2007;47:204–212.

Abílio VC, Vera JA Jr, Ferreira LS, et al. Effects of melatonin on behavioral dopaminergic supersensitivity. *Life Sci* 2003;72:3003–3015.

Agosti R, Duke RK, Chrubasik JE, et al. Effectiveness of *Petasites hybridus* preparations in the prophylaxis of migraine: a systematic review. *Phytomedicine* 2006;13:743–746.

Alpay K, Ertas M, Orhan EK, et al. Diet restriction in migraine, based on IgG against foods: a clinical double-blind, randomised, cross-over trial. *Cephalalgia* 2010;30:829–837.

Arroyave Hernández CM, Echavarría Pinto M, Hernández Montiel HL. Food allergy mediated by IgG antibodies associated with migraine in adults. *Rev Alerg Mex* 2007;54:162–168.

Berry MD. Mammalian central nervous system trace amines: pharmacologic amphetamines, physiologic neuromodulators. *J Neurochem* 2004;90:257–271.

Bic Z, Blix GG, Hopp HP, et al. The influence of a low-fat diet on incidence and severity of migraine headaches. *J Womens Health Gend Based Med* 1999;8:623–630.

Bigal ME, Bordini CA, Tepper SJ, et al. Intravenous magnesium sulphate in the acute treatment of migraine without aura and migraine with aura: a randomized, double-blind, placebo-controlled study. *Cephalalgia* 2002;22:345–353.

Bigal ME, Liberman JN, Lipton RB. Obesity and migraine: a population study. *Neurology* 2006;66:545–550.

Blin O, Azulay JP, Masson G, et al. Apomorphine-induced yawning in migraine patients: enhanced responsiveness. *Clin Neuropharmacol* 1991;14:91–95.

Bond DS, Roth J, Nash JM, et al. Migraine and obesity: epidemiology, possible mechanisms and the potential role of weight loss treatment. *Obes Rev* 2011;5:e362–371.

Brouwer M, Chamulitrat W, Ferruzzi G, et al. Nitric oxide interactions with cobalamins: biochemical and functional consequences. *Blood* 1996;88:1857–1864.

Burke BE, Olson RD, Cusack BJ. Randomized, controlled trial of phytoestrogen in the prophylactic treatment of menstrual migraine. *Biomed Pharmacother* 2002;56:283–288.

Cady RJ, Durham PL. Cocoa-enriched diets enhance expression of phosphatases and decrease expression of inflammatory molecules in trigeminal ganglion neurons. *Brain Res* 2010;1323:18–32.

Claustrat B, Brun J, Chiquet C, et al. Melatonin secretion is supersensitive to light in migraine. *Cephalalgia* 2004;24:128–133.

Condò M, Posar A, Arbizzani A, et al. Riboflavin prophylaxis in pediatric and adolescent migraine. *J Headache Pain* 2009;10:361–365.

Cutrer FM. Pathophysiology of migraine. *Semin Neurol* 2010;30:120–130.

D'Andrea G, Leon A. Pathogenesis of migraine: from neurotransmitters to neuromodulators and beyond. *Neurol Sci* 2010;31(suppl 1):S1–S7.

D'Andrea G, Terrazzino S, Leon A, et al. Elevated levels of circulating trace amines in primary headaches. *Neurology* 2004;62:1701–1705.

D'Andrea G, Granella F, Leone M, et al. Abnormal platelet trace amine profiles in migraine with and without aura. *Cephalalgia* 2006;26:968–972.

D'Andrea G, Nordera GP, Perini F, et al. Biochemistry of neuromodulation in primary headaches: focus on anomalies of tyrosine metabolism. *Neurol Sci* 2007;28(suppl 2):S94–S96.

De Felice M, Ossipov MH, Wang R, et al. Triptan-induced enhancement of neuronal nitric oxide synthase in trigeminal ganglion dural afferents underlies increased responsiveness to potential migraine triggers. *Brain* 2010;133:2475–2488.

Diener HC, Pfaffenrath V, Schnitker J, et al. The first placebo-controlled trial of a special butterbur root extract for the prevention of migraine: reanalysis of efficacy criteria. *Eur Neurol* 2004;51:89–97.

Diener HC, Pfaffenrath V, Schnitker J, et al. Efficacy and safety of 6.25 mg t.i.d. feverfew CO2-extract (MIG-99) in migraine prevention: a randomized, double-blind, multicentre, placebo-controlled study. *Cephalalgia* 2005;25:1031–1041.

Di Lorenzo C, Pierelli F, Coppola G, et al. Mitochondrial DNA haplogroups influence the therapeutic response to riboflavin in migraineurs. *Neurology* 2009;72:1588–1594.

Di Rosa G, Attinà S, Spanò M, et al. Efficacy of folic acid in children with migraine, hyperhomocysteinemia and MTHFR polymorphisms. *Headache* 2007;47:1342–1344.

Durga J, Verhoef P, Bots ML, et al. Homocysteine and carotid intima-media thickness: a critical appraisal of the evidence. *Atherosclerosis* 2004;176:1–19.

Egger J, Carter CM, Wilson J, et al. Is migraine food allergy? A double-blind controlled trial of oligoantigenic diet treatment. *Lancet* 1983;2:865–869.

Facchinetti F, Sances G, Borella P, et al. Magnesium prophylaxis of menstrual migraine: effects on intracellular magnesium. *Headache* 1991;31:298–301.

Ferrante F, Fusco E, Calabresi P, et al. Phyto-oestrogens in the prophylaxis of menstrual migraine. *Clin Neuropharmacol* 2004;27:137–140.

Fesahat F, Houshmand M, Panahi MS, et al. Do haplogroups H and U act to increase the penetrance of Alzheimer's disease? *Cell Mol Neurobiol* 2007;27:329–334.

Formicola D, Aloia A, Sampaolo S, et al. Common variants in the regulative regions of GRIA1 and GRIA3 receptor genes are associated with migraine susceptibility. *BMC Med Genet* 2010;11:103.

Gazerani P, Pourpak Z, Ahmadiani A, et al. A correlation between migraine, histamine and immunoglobulin E. *Scand J Immunol* 2003;57:286–290.

Goadsby PJ. The vascular theory of migraine: a great story wrecked by the facts. *Brain* 2009;132:6–7.

Gudmundsson LS, Scher AI, Aspelund T, et al. Migraine with aura and risk of cardiovascular and all cause mortality in men and women: prospective cohort study. *BMJ* 2010;341:c3966.

Gupta S, Mehrotra S, Villalón CM, et al. Potential role of female sex hormones in the pathophysiology of migraine. *Pharmacol Ther* 2007;113:321–340.

Harel Z, Gascon G, Riggs S, et al. Supplementation with omega-3 polyunsaturated fatty acids in the management of recurrent migraines in adolescents. *J Adolesc Health* 2002;31:154–161.

Hershey AD, Powers SW, Vockell AL, et al. Coenzyme Q10 deficiency and response to supplementation in pediatric and adolescent migraine. *Headache* 2007;47:73–80.

Horak S, Koschak A, Stuppner H, et al. Use-dependent block of voltage-gated Cav2.1 Ca^{2+} channels by petasins and eudesmol isomers. *J Pharmacol Exp Ther* 2009;330:220–226.

Hughes EC, Gott PS, Weinstein RC, et al. Migraine: a diagnostic test for etiology of food sensitivity by a nutritionally supported fast and confirmed by long-term report. *Ann Allergy* 1985;55:28–32.

Isobe C, Terayama Y. A Remarkable increase in total homocysteine concentrations in the CSF of migraine patients with aura. *Headache* 2010;50:1561–1569.

Jansen SC, van Dusseldorp M, Bottema KC, et al. Intolerance to dietary biogenic amines: a review. *Ann Allergy Asthma Immunol* 2003;91:233–240.

Kabbouche MA, Powers SW, Vockell AL, et al. Carnitine palmityltransferase II (CPT2) deficiency and migraine headache: two case reports. *Headache* 2003;43:490–495.

Khandanpour N, Willis G, Meyer FJ, et al. Peripheral arterial disease and methylenetetrahydrofolate reductase (MTHFR) C677T mutations: a case-control study and meta-analysis. *J Vasc Surg* 2009;49:711–718.

Köseoglu E, Talaslioglu A, Gönül AS, et al. The effects of magnesium prophylaxis in migraine without aura. *Magnes Res* 2008;21:101–108.

Ku M, Silverman B, Prifti N, et al. Prevalence of migraine headaches in patients with allergic rhinitis. *Ann Allergy Asthma Immunol* 2006;97:226–230.

Kurth T, Kase CS, Schürks M, et al. Migraine and risk of haemorrhagic stroke in women: prospective cohort study. *BMJ* 2010;341:c3659.

Lea R, Colson N, Quinlan S, et al. The effects of vitamin supplementation and MTHFR (C677T) genotype on homocysteine-lowering and migraine disability. *Pharmacogenet Genomics* 2009;19:422–428.

Levy D, Strassman AM, Burstein R. A critical view on the role of migraine triggers in the genesis of migraine pain. *Headache* 2009;49:953–957.

Littlewood JT, Gibb C, Glover V, et al. Red wine as a cause of migraine. *Lancet* 1988;1:558–559.

Liu A, Menon S, Colson NJ, et al. Analysis of the MTHFR C677T variant with migraine phenotypes. *BMC Res Notes* 2010;3:213.

Loder E. Triptan therapy in migraine. *N Engl J Med* 2010;363:63–70.

Magis D, Ambrosini A, Sándor P, et al. A randomized double-blind placebo-controlled trial of thioctic acid in migraine prophylaxis. *Headache* 2007;47:52–57.

Mansfield LE, Vaughan TR, Waller SF, et al. Food allergy and adult migraine: double-blind and mediator confirmation of an allergic etiology. *Ann Allergy* 1985;55:126–129.

Mansoor JK, Morrissey BM, Walby WF, et al. l-Arginine supplementation enhances exhaled NO, breath condensate VEGF, and headache at 4,342 m. *High Alt Med Biol* 2005;6:289–300.

Marcus DA, Scharff L, Turk D, et al. A double-blind provocative study of chocolate as a trigger of headache. *Cephalalgia* 1997;17:855–862.

Masruha MR, Lin J, de Souza Vieira DS, et al. Urinary 6-sulphatoxymelatonin levels are depressed in chronic migraine and several comorbidities. *Headache* 2010;50:413–419.

Mauskop A, Altura BM. Role of magnesium in the pathogenesis and treatment of migraines. *Clin Neurosci* 1998;5:24–27.

Mauskop A, Altura BM. Serum ionized magnesium levels and serum ionized calcium/ionized magnesium ratios in women with menstrual migraine. *Headache* 2002;42:242–248.

Mauskop A, Altura BT, Cracco RQ, et al. Intravenous magnesium sulfate rapidly alleviates headaches of various types. *Headache* 1996;36:154–160.

Miano S, Parisi P, Pelliccia A, et al. Melatonin to prevent migraine or tension-type headache in children. *Neurol Sci* 2008;29:285–287.

Mortimer MJ, Kay J, Gawkrodger DJ, et al. The prevalence of headache and migraine in atopic children: an epidemiological study in general practice. *Headache* 1993;33:427–431.

Mueller LL. Diagnosing and managing migraine headache. *J Am Osteopath Assoc* 2007;107:ES10–ES16.

Olesen J. The role of nitric oxide (NO) in migraine, tension-type headache and cluster headache. *Pharmacol Ther* 2008;120:157–171.

Olesen J, Thomsen LL, Iversen H. Nitric oxide is a key molecule in migraine and other vascular headaches. *Trends Pharmacol Sci* 1994;15:149–153.

Olness K, Hall H, Rozniecki JJ, et al. Mast cell activation in children with migraine before and after training in self-regulation. *Headache* 1999;39:101–107.

Oterino A, Toriello M, Cayón A, et al. Multilocus analyses reveal involvement of the ESR1, ESR2, and FSHR genes in migraine. *Headache* 2008;48:1438–1450.

Oterino A, Toriello M, Valle N, et al. The relationship between homocysteine and genes of folate-related enzymes in migraine patients. *Headache* 2010;50:99–168.

Peres MF, Zukerman E, da Cunha Tanuri F, et al. Melatonin, 3 mg, is effective for migraine prevention. *Neurology* 2004;63:757.

Pfaffenrath V, Diener HC, Fischer M, et al. The efficacy and safety of *Tanacetum parthenium* (feverfew) in migraine prophylaxis: a double-blind, multicentre, randomized placebo-controlled dose-response study. *Cephalalgia* 2002;22:523–532.

Pizza V, Bisogno A, Lamaida E, et al. Migraine and coronary artery disease: an open study on the genetic polymorphism of the 5, 10 methylenetetrahydrofolate (MTHFR) and angiotensin I-converting enzyme (ACE) genes. *Cent Nerv Syst Agents Med Chem* 2010;10:91–96.

Pizzorno J, Murray M. *Textbook of Natural Medicine* (3rd ed.). London: Elsevier; 2006.

Pradalier A, Bakouche P, Baudesson G, et al. Failure of omega-3 polyunsaturated fatty acids in prevention of migraine: a double-blind study versus placebo. *Cephalalgia* 2001;21:818–822.

Prakash S, Mehta NC, Dabhi AS, et al. The prevalence of headache may be related with the latitude: a possible role of vitamin D insufficiency? *J Headache Pain* 2010;11:301–307.

Pyle A, Foltynie T, Tiangyou W, et al. Mitochondrial DNA haplogroup cluster UKJT reduces the risk of PD. *Ann Neurol* 2005;57:564–567.

Ramadan NM. The link between glutamate and migraine. *CNS Spectr* 2003;8:446–449.

Ratan RR, Murphy TH, Baraban JM. Macromolecular synthesis inhibitors prevent oxidative stress-induced apoptosis in embryonic cortical neurons by shunting cysteine from protein synthesis to glutathione. *J Neurosci* 1994a;14:4385–4392.

Ratan RR, Murphy TH, Baraban JM. Oxidative stress induces apoptosis in embryonic cortical neurons. *J Neurochem* 1994b;62:376–379.

Ren H, Collins V, Fernandez F, et al. Shorter telomere length in peripheral blood cells associated with migraine in women. *Headache* 2010;50:965–972.

Rozen TD, Oshinsky ML, Gebeline CA, et al. Open label trial of coenzyme Q10 as a migraine preventive. *Cephalalgia* 2002;22:137–141.

Ruiz-Pesini E, Lapeña AC, Díez-Sánchez C, et al. Human mtDNA haplogroups associated with high or reduced spermatozoa motility. *Am J Hum Genet* 2000;67:682–696.

Ryan RE Jr. A clinical study of tyramine as an etiological factor in migraine. *Headache* 1974;14:43–48.

Sándor PS, Afra J, Ambrosini A, et al. Prophylactic treatment of migraine with beta-blockers and riboflavin: differential effects on the intensity dependence of auditory evoked cortical potentials. *Headache* 2000;40:30–35.

Sándor PS, Di Clemente L, Coppola G, et al. Efficacy of coenzyme Q10 in migraine prophylaxis: a randomized controlled trial. *Neurology* 2005;64:713–715.

Schapowal A, Petasites Study Group. Butterbur Ze339 for the treatment of intermittent allergic rhinitis: dose-dependent efficacy in a prospective, randomized, double-blind, placebo-controlled study. *Arch Otolaryngol Head Neck Surg* 2004;130:1381–1386.

Schapowal A, Study Group. Treating intermittent allergic rhinitis: a prospective, randomized, placebo and antihistamine-controlled study of Butterbur extract Ze 339. *Phytother Res* 2005;19:530–537.

Schoenen J, Lenaerts M, Bastings E. High-dose riboflavin as a prophylactic treatment of migraine: results of an open pilot study. *Cephalalgia* 1994;14:328–329.

Schoenen J, Jacquy J, Lenaerts M. Effectiveness of high-dose riboflavin in migraine prophylaxis: a randomized controlled trial. *Neurology* 1998;50:466–470.

Scholte HR, Busch HF, Bakker HD, et al. Riboflavin-responsive complex I deficiency. *Biochim Biophys Acta* 1995;1271:75–83.

Schürks M, Rist PM, Bigal ME, et al. Migraine and cardiovascular disease: systematic review and meta-analysis. *BMJ* 2009;339:b3914.

Schürks M, Rist PM, Kurth T. MTHFR 677C > T and ACE D/I polymorphisms in migraine: a systematic review and meta-analysis. *Headache* 2010;50:588–599.

Sparaco M, Feleppa M, Lipton RB, et al. Mitochondrial dysfunction and migraine: evidence and hypotheses. *Cephalalgia* 2006;26:361–372.

Strong FC 3rd. Why do some dietary migraine patients claim they get headaches from placebos? *Clin Exp Allergy* 2000;30:739–743.

Tietjen GE. Migraine as a systemic vasculopathy. *Cephalalgia* 2009;29:987–996.

Todt U, Netzer C, Toliat M, et al. New genetic evidence for involvement of the dopamine system in migraine with aura. *Hum Genet* 2009;125:265–279.

van der Kuy PH, Merkus FW, Lohman JJ, et al. Hydroxocobalamin, a nitric oxide scavenger, in the prophylaxis of migraine: an open, pilot study. *Cephalalgia* 2002;22:513–519.

Wendorff J, Kamer B, Zielińska W, et al. [Allergy effect on migraine course in older children and adolescents]. *Neurol Neurochir Pol* 1999;33(suppl 5):55–65.

Wilders-Truschnig M, Mangge H, Lieners C, et al. IgG antibodies against food antigens are correlated with inflammation and intima media thickness in obese juveniles. *Exp Clin Endocrinol Diabetes* 2008;116:241–245.

Wu D, Liu L, Meydani M, et al. Effect of vitamin E on prostacyclin (PGI2) and prostaglandin (PG) E2 production by human aorta endothelial cells: mechanism of action. *Ann NY Acad Sci* 2004;1031:425–427.

Zaki EA, Freilinger T, Klopstock T, et al. Two common mitochondrial DNA polymorphisms are highly associated with migraine headache and cyclic vomiting syndrome. *Cephalalgia* 2009;29:719–728.

Ziaei S, Kazemnejad A, Sedighi A. The effect of vitamin E on the treatment of menstrual migraine. *Med Sci Monit* 2009;15:CR16–CR19.

Zisapel N. Melatonin–dopamine interactions: from basic neurochemistry to a clinical setting. *Cell Mol Neurobiol* 2001;21:605–616.

Dietary Approaches

Damien Downing, MBBS, MSB

INTRODUCTION: A CASE HISTORY

A case history will illustrate the complexity that can occur in diet-related migraine. A man, age 40, consulted this chapter's author about migraines that always seemed to occur on weekends. As a fairly high-powered executive, he experienced work-related stress, and was clearly a Type A personality. He was normotensive and not overweight, and a physical examination revealed nothing relevant. The patient's diet contained no obvious sources of tyramine or other chemical triggers (this was some years ago, when the biogenic amine hypothesis for migraine was still popular); nevertheless, he had avoided red wine and cheese for several weeks without benefit.

The next working hypothesis was that the migraines were triggered by hypoglycemia due to caffeine and/or adrenaline withdrawal—that is, that he ran on adrenaline during the week, then slept in and relaxed on the weekends, probably becoming hypoglycemic in the process. However, elimination of caffeine, adjustment of diurnal pattern, and general destressing all made no difference.

Food intolerance seemed to be an unlikely mechanism underlying the patient's migraines, but was investigated anyway. The patient lived in Yorkshire and had a normative but high-protein diet, eating bacon for breakfast most days. On Saturdays, however, he often had a pork chop. To cut a long story short, we eventually established, by elimination and challenge dieting, that the pork chop was the trigger. The patient was intolerant to pork, but the process of curing altered the protein in bacon sufficiently that he tolerated it. After he eliminated both pork and bacon from his diet, his migraines cleared.

The lesson from this case history is summarized well in a recent review (Wöber & Wöber-Bingöl, 2010): "Taken together, virtually all aspects of life

413

have been suspected to trigger migraine or tension-type headache, but scientific evidence for many of these triggers is poor." This contention is confirmed by the reasonably large survey (n = 1,207) conducted by the Headache Center of Atlanta (Kelman, 2007), which reported the following self-identified frequencies for triggers: stress (80%), female cycle (65%), hunger (57%), weather (53%), insomnia (50%), odors (44%), light (38%), alcohol (38%), smoke (36%), food (27%), exercise (22%), sex (5%).

DIETARY TRIGGERS

Biogenic Amines

Tyramine is an amino compound that is present in matured and fermented foods. It is produced from the amino acid tyrosine in a slow process during fermentation and, therefore, is rarely present in any fresh food. In contrast, food that has spent time being fermented, matured, or cured may contain it. Foods known to contain tyramine include matured cheeses, cured meats, hung game, non-fresh fish, over-ripe fruits, fermented vegetable products (e.g., sauerkraut), and fermented soya products.

Tyramine's physiological effect appears to be mediated by its replacement of noradrenaline (norepinephrine) in presynaptic vesicles of nerves. Normally, this substitution has little effect, but as it is metabolized by the enzyme monoamine oxidase A (MAO), in persons taking monoamine oxidase inhibitors (MAOIs) tyramine may not be cleared and may accumulate in higher concentrations. The effect is, by action on peripheral (autonomic) nerve endings, to cause hypertension, tachycardia, and severe headache. If severe, this problem can amount to hypertensive crisis. Chocolate contains another amino compound, phenylethylamine, which has been postulated to have similar effects. Several other such compounds—most notably octopamine—also occur naturally.

The tyramine hypothesis for migraine arose when Hannington (1967) noted that the list of foods causing severe headaches in patients on MAOIs was similar to that reported as suspected dietary triggers by some migraine sufferers. In a pilot study, capsules of 100 mg tyramine were given to four migraineurs with a definite dietary history and provoked migraines in all cases; placebo capsules of 100 mg lactose did not. In four migraineurs with no known or suspected dietary triggers, neither the tyramine nor the lactose provoked symptoms.

Since that time, the amine hypothesis has been repeatedly studied clinically, and the results have disappointed. In 2003, a systematic review (Jansen et al., 2003) of randomized, controlled trials (RCTs) of biogenic amines'

effects identified 13 oral challenge studies, of which only 5 were positive in outcome. Of the 13 total studies, 3 were deemed ineligible for the meta-analysis and 6 yielded inconclusive findings. The remaining 4 conclusive studies (2 on tyramine and migraine, 1 on phenylethylamine from chocolate and headaches, and 1 on amines in red wine and symptoms) all reported no effect.

Moreover, in the open study of elimination diets conducted by Grant (1979), while 85% of subjects became migraine free on the allergen elimination diet, only 13% did so on the amine-free diet.

This overall negative finding has been countered by the speculation that only a subgroup of migraineurs are susceptible to tyramine's effects. Some scientists have estimated that these individuals represent 10% of the total migraine-affected population (unconfirmed news report). Moreover, the scientific plausibility of the amine hypothesis remains unrefuted, given the MAOI experience in particular.

Current findings in genomics do raise the possibility that a subgroup susceptible to this mechanism exists. Sulfotransferases are a large family of enzymes that add a sulfate group to a range of molecules. This addition has a predominantly inactivating effect, albeit not always a permanent one. Steroid hormones, for example, are mainly transported in the inactive, sulfated form, but can then be reactivated by sulfatase enzymes on cell surfaces.

The sulfotransferase enzymes coded for by the two genes SULT1A1 and SULT1A3 are mainly present in platelets; both are able to sulfate phenolic compounds—which the "biogenic amines" all are. SULT1A1 enzyme activity has been found to be reduced by approximately 50% in migraineurs compared to patients with tension headache or controls (Alam et al., 1997) and SULT1A3 has also been found to be lowered in at least one study (Marazzitti et al., 1994).

In common with several other enzyme genes, the SULT genes are inhibited (in some cases by 100%) by sulforaphane, which is present in most vegetables, but is found in significant quantities only in the cruciferi—that is, broccoli, cabbage, and cauliflower. The result of inhibiting the SULT gene is less production of the enzyme that it encodes and, therefore, less enzyme activity. This epigenetic effect may mean that foods can alter an individual's predisposition to migraine by altering the amine pathway, either instead of or as well as by triggering intolerance reactions. Our current understanding of genomics suggests that polymorphisms of these two genes might alter the response to inhibitors, such as assulforaphane, and inducers, thereby explaining the observed link between migraine and reduced enzyme activity. At the time of writing, this finding has not been reported in the published literature, but it is a fast-moving field.

Caffeine

Caffeine is a vasopressor and stimulant found in coffee, tea, cocoa, mate, and guarana, and is the most widely used psychoactive agent worldwide. The caffeine withdrawal syndrome is consequently well recognized and described. It involves some or all of the following symptoms, the overlap of which with migraine is evident (Griffiths et al., 2003): headache, fatigue, drowsiness, loss of concentration, irritability, anxiety, depression, nausea and vomiting, and motor performance impairment.

Although the typical headache of caffeine withdrawal is described as diffuse and not hemicranial, it is associated with considerable comorbidity of different types of headache including migraines, and many migraineurs report both caffeine consumption and caffeine avoidance/cessation as risk factors. One case-control study (n = 713) found caffeine consumption to be a modest risk factor for headaches regardless of type (Scher et al., 2004). Caffeine is also widely used as an adjuvant in analgesic medications for headache, even though a non-systematic review did not find a significant adjuvant effect with its inclusion (Gray et al., 1999).

The CYP1A2 gene codes for a major cytochrome P450 enzyme of the same name, which is responsible for 90% of caffeine metabolism—specifically, converting it into other dimethylxanthines. Known polymorphisms in this enzyme could well account for substantial variability in caffeine sensitivity. One of the most common of these polymorphisms, CYP1A2*1F, also known more simply as F allele (nucleotide change 164A → C, U.K. prevalence of the allele approximately 33%), is a highly inducible variant; inducers include cruciferous vegetables, chargrilled meat, and insulin (in diabetics). Exposure to these products can increase enzyme activity much more in persons with the variant form of the gene.

One population study (Gentile et al., 2010) found that the CC genotype (i.e., homozygous for the F allele) was significantly more common in migraineurs (**Table 30.1**). No

Table 30.1 Distribution of Genotype in Patients with Migraine and Healthy Controls

Genotype	Migraine Patients (%) [n = 104]	Healthy Controls (%) [n = 495]	P
CC	26.9	8.9	< 0.001
CA	40.4	45.9	
AA	32.7	45.2	

Source: Gentile G, Missori S, Borro M, et al. Frequencies of genetic polymorphisms related to triptans metabolism in chronic migraine. *J Headache Pain* 2010;11:151–156.

subtype analysis for caffeine sensitivity was performed, so this association is merely suggestive at present.

Alcohol

Hannington (1967) observed that alcohol was often reported as a trigger for migraines, and this finding has been confirmed by most surveys since then. For example, Hauge et al. (2011) noted that 22 of 126 questionnaire responders (17%) found alcohol to be a trigger; none of them said alcohol triggered 50% or more of their attacks. Kelman (2007) found that 37.8% of 1,307 migraineurs, and Garcia-Martín et al. (2010) 32% of 197 migraineurs, reported alcohol as a trigger.

Garcia-Martín et al. (2010) went on to examine polymorphisms of the genes for the enzyme alcohol dehydrogenase, in particular ADH2. One polymorphism of this gene, rs1229984, causes the substitution of the amino acid histidine for arginine at location 48 (i.e., Arg48His). Having the ADH2 His allele appears to protect against alcohol abuse and alcoholism (Eriksson et al., 2001). The same study revealed that the ADH2 His allele was significantly more common in migraineurs who reported alcohol as a trigger than in those who did not. However, the allele frequency was 7.1% versus 2.4%, respectively, while the frequency of the same allele in non-migraineurs was 7.6%, so it is difficult to see what this proves.

Food Intolerances

In 1930, Albert Rowe, a physician in Oakland, California, described a case series of 86 patients with migraine "due, in my opinion, to food allergy"—that is, shown to be triggered by the ingestion of specific foods. Rowe reported comorbidity of migraines with allergic toxemia (a term no longer in common medical use), which encompasses drowsiness, confusion, slowness of thought, mood changes, and fatigue (no statistics given), together with gastrointestinal symptoms such as bloating, discomfort, and change of bowel habit (occurring in 64% of the migraine group), as well as skin reactions (43%).

In 1979, an open study provided "proof of concept" for food intolerance as a cause of migraine (Grant, 1979). In this study, 126 patients attending a London hospital migraine clinic undertook elimination diets. For the first 5 days they ate only two foods considered to be low risks for triggering intolerances, and drank only bottled spring water; during this period, most had migraines or headaches in the first 3 days, but were free of them by the fifth day. The participants were then instructed to introduce common foods into their diet singly, to record their reactions, and thereafter to avoid any foods to which they did react. Ninety-one patients completed the process and continued afterward to avoid identified triggers. The first 60 consecutive patients to complete the trial were included in the analysis (52 were females). All patients improved; of the 60, only 9 (15%) still had headaches or migraines at follow-up. The foods most commonly identified as causing symptoms are summarized in **Table 30.2**.

The following year, another group of researchers (Monro et al., 1980) drew a similar conclusion—namely, that two-thirds of severe migraineurs are allergic to foods. Both this and a subsequent small ($n = 9$) study (Monro et al., 1984) used positive therapeutic response to cromoglycate to argue that the mechanism in migraine is allergic.

RCTs are scarce in this area, unfortunately. However, an elegant study in children, part of a series conducted at Great Ormond St. Children's Hospital in London, was a RCT (Egger et al., 1983). In this investigation, 88 children with severe frequent migraines underwent oligoantigenic diets; 78 of them (88%) recovered completely. In a second phase, 40 of the patients then underwent further double-blinded, placebo-controlled challenge testing to confirm the triggering foods. Twenty-six (65%) developed headaches after active challenge, but not after placebo challenge.

An especially noteworthy finding in the London study, in light of the Rowe (1930) case series cited earlier, is that the children's comorbidities that also improved with changes in diet included abdominal and central nervous symptoms, together with known allergic disorders such as asthma and eczema. Moreover, nonspecific and nondietary triggers such as stroboscopic effects and exertion no longer caused migraine when the children were on the diet. These findings were broadly confirmed in a subsequent RCT of an oligoantigenic diet in hyperkinesis; headaches including migraines also improved when patients were on the diet (Egger et al., 1985).

Use of allergy tests—whether skin tests or laboratory tests—to select foods to be eliminated introduces another set of variables into such studies, as opposed to selection by response to elimination and challenge dieting. It is perhaps not surprising, therefore, if the resulting response rates are lower.

One study (Mansfield et al., 1985)—the first ever to use double-blind, placebo-controlled food challenges in migraine—based individual diets on skin-prick testing; 43 adult subjects with migraine were instructed to avoid foods for which their prick tests were positive, as well as milk, eggs, wheat, and corn, for 1 month. Thirteen of them (31%) reported at least a 66% improvement in migraine frequency. These individuals then underwent active and placebo double-blind testing, and 6 (14%) developed migraines in response to the active challenge (none to placebo challenge).

The same research team performed a larger study on 104 adults using a similar experimental model. This investigation is described in a review article by the chapter's principal author (Vaughan, 1994), but the original article is not indexed. The 40 (38%) subjects with confirmed migraine who experienced a 50% or greater improvement on skin-prick–based diet underwent blinded challenges. Seventeen (16%) had migraines in response to active but not to placebo challenges.

A prospective audit (i.e., no controls, no blinding) using enzyme-linked immunosorbent assay (ELISA) IgG antibody testing (Rees et al., 2005) on migraine patients was conducted in 6 U.K. general practices. Sixty-one subjects started the trial, and 39 completed 2 months of diet change based on the IgG findings. On a scale of 0 (no benefit) to 5 (high benefit), 38.2% of these individuals reported considerable benefit (4 or 5), 29.4% some benefit (2 or 3), and 32.4% little or no benefit (0 or 1).

Most recently, a Turkish cross-over RCT also based individual diets on IgG antibody findings (Alpay et al., 2010). Thirty subjects with non-aura migraine underwent ELISA testing to identify food antigens, and were put on diets that either excluded identified foods or included them for a 6-week period, followed by a 2-week washout

Table 30.2 Foods Most Commonly Identified as Causing Migraine Symptoms

Food	Percentage of Subjects Reporting the Food as a Migraine Trigger
Wheat	78
Orange	39
Egg	45
Tea	40
Coffee	40
Chocolate	37
Milk	37
Beef	35
Corn	33
Cane sugar	33
Yeast	33
Mushrooms	30
Peas	28

Source: Grant EC. Food allergies and migraine. *Lancet* 1979; 1(8123):966–969.

and then the reverse diet. When patients were on the excluding diet, they experienced a 32% reduction in number of migraines (from 9.0 ± 4.4 to 6.2 ± 3.8; $P < 0.001$) and a 29% reduction in "headache days."

The less impressive outcome in these four trials suggests that neither skin-prick testing nor IgG antibody testing may be the optimal means to identify food triggers in patients with migraine. The results should be compared with the resolution in headaches found by Grant (85%) and by Egger (93%)—both uncontrolled and unblinded—and the 65% positive responses on blinded controlled challenge also found by Egger. Both studies based the interventional diets on the "real life" response to diet alone.

CONCLUSIONS

The studies by Grant and by Egger demonstrate that a majority—at least two-thirds—of migraineurs in well-conducted studies respond to elimination of food allergens. The mechanisms underlying this effect have not been elucidated, but the phenomenon can no longer be said to lack scientific plausibility. In contrast, response to biogenic amines as a mechanism for migraines is clearly plausible, but the evidence for it remains weak. It remains possible, however, that a genomic variation could account for a small subgroup of patients having migraines triggered in this manner.

Both caffeine and alcohol are other plausible migraine triggers, and in both cases known genomic variations could potentially explain a subgroup of patients responding in this way. Even so, the evidence suggests that neither substance is likely to be the sole or major trigger in any individuals. We are just at the start of our journey of discovery in genomic medicine, however, and are entitled to anticipate much greater understanding in the years to come, of migraine as of most diseases.

REFERENCES

Alam Z, Coombes N, Waring RH, et al. Platelet sulphotransferase activity, plasma sulphate levels and sulphation capacity in patients with migraine and tension headache. *Cephalalgia* 1997;17:761–764.

Alpay K, Ertas M, Orhan EK, et al. Diet restriction in migraine, based on IgG against foods: a clinical double-blind, randomised, cross-over trial. *Cephalalgia* 2010;30:829–837.

Egger J, Carter CM, Wilson J, et al. Is migraine food allergy? A double-blind controlled trial of oligoantigenic diet treatment. *Lancet* 1983;2(8355):865–869.

Egger J, Carter CM, Graham PJ, et al. Controlled trial of oligoantigenic treatment in the hyperkinetic syndrome. *Lancet* 1985;1(8428):540–545.

Eriksson CJ, Fukunaga T, Sarkola T, et al. Functional relevance of human ADH polymorphism. *Alcohol Clin Exp Res* 2001;25:157S–163S.

García-Martín E, Martínez C, Serrador M, et al. Alcohol dehydrogenase 2 genotype and risk for migraine. *Headache* 2010;50:85–91.

Gentile G, Missori S, Borro M, et al. Frequencies of genetic polymorphisms related to triptans metabolism in chronic migraine. *J Headache Pain* 2010;11:151–156.

Grant EC. Food allergies and migraine. *Lancet* 1979;1(8123):966–969.

Gray RN, McCrory DC, Eberlein K, et al. *Self-Administered Drug Treatments for Acute Migraine Headache. AHRQ Technical Reviews and Summaries.* Rockville, MD: Agency for Health Care Policy and Research; 1999.

Griffiths RR, Juliano LM, Chausmer AL. Caffeine pharmacology and clinical effects. In: Graham AW, Schultz TK, Mayo-Smith MF, et al., eds. *Principles of Addiction Medicine* (3rd ed.). Chevy Chase, MD: American Society of Addiction; 2003.

Hannington E. Preliminary report on tyramine headache. *Brit Med J* 1967;2:550–551.

Hauge AW, Kirchmann M, Olesen J. Characterization of consistent triggers of migraine with aura. *Cephalalgia* 2011;31:416–438.

Jansen SC, van Dusseldorp M, Bottema KC, Dubois AE. Intolerance to dietary biogenic amines: a review. *Ann Allergy Asthma Immunol* 2003;91:233–240.

Kelman L. The triggers or precipitants of the acute migraine attack. *Cephalalgia* 2007;27:394–402.

Mansfield LE, Vaughan TR, Waller SF., et al. Food allergy and adult migraine: double-blind and mediator confirmation of an allergic etiology. *Ann Allergy* 1985;55:126–129.

Marazzitti D, Bonuccelli U, Nuti A, et al. Platelet 3H-imipramine binding and sulphotransferase activity in primary headache. *Cephalalgia* 1994;14:210–214.

Monro J, Brostoff J, Carini C, Zilkha K. Food allergy in migraine: study of dietary exclusion and RAST. *Lancet* 1980;2(8184):1–4.

Monro J, Carini C, Brostoff J. Migraine is a food-allergic disease. *Lancet* 1984;2(8405):719–721.

Rees T, Watson D, Lipscombe S, et al. A prospective audit of food intolerance among migraine patients in primary care clinical practice. *Headache Care* 2005;2:105–110.

Rowe AH. Allergic toxaemia and migraine due to food allergy. *Calif West Med* 1930;33:785.

Scher AI, Stewart WF, Lipton RB. Caffeine as a risk factor for chronic daily headache: a population-based study. *Neurology* 2004;63:2022–2027.

Vaughan TR. The role of food in the pathogenesis of migraine headache. *Clin Rev Allergy* 1994;12:167–180.

Wöber C, Wöber-Bingöl C. Triggers of migraine and tension-type headache. *Handb Clin Neurol* 2010;97:161–172.

Normobaric and Hyperbaric Oxygen Therapy

Michael H. Bennett, MBBS, MD, FANZCA, CertDHM

INTRODUCTION

This chapter considers the evidence for the effectiveness and safety of oxygen administration for migraine. It includes both the use of oxygen at a high percentage of normal atmospheric pressure (normobaric oxygen therapy [NBOT]) and the use of 100% oxygen at pressures greater than 1 atmosphere (hyperbaric oxygen therapy [HBOT]). It also considers oxygen as an acute therapy for terminating individual attacks and as a preventive therapy for reducing the frequency of headache episodes.

Included in this chapter is a summary of the systematic review and meta-analysis of randomized controlled trials published through the Cochrane Collaboration (Bennett et al., 2008). Interested readers are referred to that regularly updated analysis for further details. The author is grateful to the staff and reviewers in the Cochrane Pain, Palliative, and Supportive Care review group for their assistance with that review.

THE GOAL OF OXYGEN THERAPY

Acute therapy for migraine aims to provide symptomatic treatment of the head pain and other symptoms associated with an acute attack. By comparison, the goal of preventive therapy is to reduce the frequency and/or intensity of attacks, thereby inducing an improvement in functional ability and quality of life. Preventive therapy is especially well suited to patients with very frequent or severe attacks, significant headache-related disability, or resistance to acute therapy. Oxygen administration over a wide dose range may potentially be of benefit in all these situations.

Therapeutic Approach to Migraine

Many accepted drug therapies for acute migraine exist, including nonspecific analgesics such as nonsteroidal anti-inflammatory drugs, and specific agents such as sumatriptan, ergotamine, and dihydroergotamine (DHE). A recent survey suggested that fewer than 20% of migraineurs regularly use migraine-specific agents, with triptans the class of drugs most commonly being prescribed for this indication (Bigal et al., 2009). Ergots are used by fewer than 1% of patients, while 68% rely on over-the-counter agents for headache relief. This pattern suggests there may be an unmet need for effective treatment strategies, and indeed novel delivery systems are being developed, including needle-free injectable triptans and inhalable dihydroergotamine (Silberstein, 2010).

Both drug and physical therapies have been thoroughly reviewed in previous chapters in this text. Drugs are effective in the majority of cases, although it is not uncommon for headache to recur within 48 hours (Bateman, 1993). Most people with migraine are able to manage even these recurrent headaches successfully at home with self-administered medication. Thus, while migraine is a problem, the number of individuals who fail to respond to accepted therapeutic approaches may be small. It is these patients who may benefit from a therapy delivered at a health facility, such as intravenous DHE, parenteral analgesics or antinauseants, or

(potentially) HBOT. In addition, refractory patients may be offered preventive drug treatments with potentially serious toxicities, such as methysergide. These individuals may also be candidates for other resource-intensive treatments such as HBOT.

NBOT, in contrast, is readily available, cheap, easy to administer, and safe. If it were shown to be an effective treatment strategy for migraine for some patients, it would be adopted for routine use by those individuals.

What Is Hyperbaric Oxygen Therapy?

Hyperbaric medicine is the treatment of health disorders using whole-body exposure to pressures greater than 1 atmosphere (760 mm Hg or 1 ATA). In practice, this therapy almost always entails the administration of oxygen at high inspired concentration (HBOT). The Undersea and Hyperbaric Medical Society (UHMS) defines HBOT as "a treatment in which a patient breathes 100% oxygen... while inside a treatment chamber at a pressure higher than sea level pressure (i.e. >1 atmosphere absolute or ATA)" (Gesell, 2008). Most treatments are delivered at between 1.5 and 3.0 ATA for 1 and 2 hours. For many indications, treatment is repeated on a daily or twice-daily basis for 20 to 40 total treatment sessions, although for migraine most authors have studied a single treatment aimed at relieving an acute headache.

The treatment chamber is an airtight vessel variously called a hyperbaric chamber, recompression chamber, or decompression chamber, depending on the clinical and historical context. Such chambers may be capable of accommodating a single patient (a mono-place chamber)

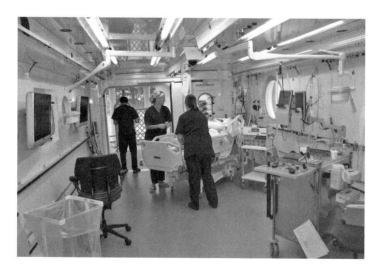

Figure 31.1 A Hyperbaric Oxygen Therapy Chamber Designed to Treat Multiple Patients at the Karolinska Institute, Stockholm Picture: Peter Kronlund.

or multiple patients and attendants as required (a multiplace chamber). A compartment within a large multiplace chamber is shown in **Figure 31.1**.

OXYGEN THERAPY IN HEADACHE

The Therapeutic Use of Oxygen

Supplemental oxygen breathing has a dose-dependent effect on oxygen transport, ranging from an improvement in hemoglobin oxygen saturation when a few liters per minute is delivered by simple mask at 1 ATA (NBOT), to an increase in the dissolved plasma oxygen sufficient

to sustain life without the need for hemoglobin at all when 100% oxygen is breathed at 3 ATA. Most HBOT regimens involve breathing oxygen at pressures between 2.0 and 2.8 ATA, and the resultant increase in arterial oxygen tensions to greater than 1,000 mm Hg has widespread physiological and pharmacological consequences. **Figure 31.2** summarizes the potential therapeutic mechanisms associated with oxygen therapy.

One direct consequence of high intravascular tension is to greatly increase the effective capillary–tissue diffusion distance for oxygen such that oxygen-dependent cellular processes can resume in hypoxic tissues. Important as this effect may be, the mechanism of action is not

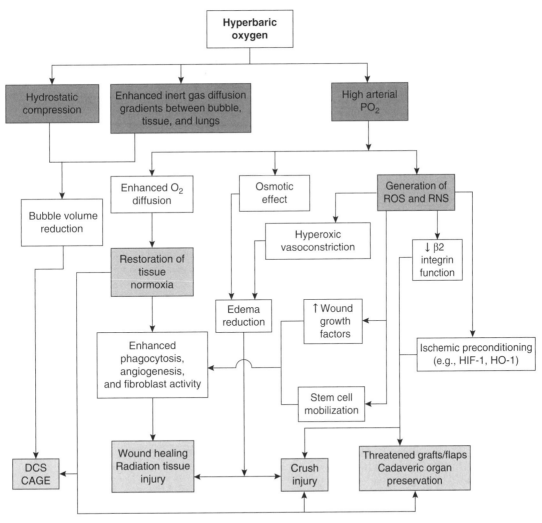

Figure 31.2 Summary of Mechanisms of Hyperbaric Oxygen. There are many consequences of compression and oxygen breathing. The cell signaling effects of HBOT are the least understood but potentially the most important. The relevance of these mechanisms is shown for several example indications (gray boxes). HBOT may provide a benefit in migraine through vasoconstriction with preservation of high tissue oxygen tension. ROS, reactive oxygen species; RNS, reactive nitrogen species; HIF-1, hypoxia inducible factor 1; HO-1, hemoxygenase 1; DCS, decompression sickness; CAGE, cerebral arterial gas embolism.

limited to the restoration of oxygenation in hypoxic tissue. Indeed, the pharmacological effects from such treatment are both profound and long-lasting. While removal from the hyperbaric chamber results in a rapid return of poorly vascularized tissues to their hypoxic state, even a single dose of HBOT produces changes on fibroblast, leukocyte, and angiogenic functions and antioxidant defenses that persist many hours after oxygen tensions are returned to pretreatment levels.

For the treatment of migraine, the most likely mechanism of action has been postulated as the reversal of vasodilatation through high intravascular oxygen tension in the intracranial arterial tree (Fife et al., 1994). Nevertheless, a number of alternative mechanisms are possible, as discussed later in this chapter.

It is widely accepted that oxygen in high doses produces adverse effects due to the production of reactive oxygen species (ROS) such as superoxide ($O_2^{.2-}$) and hydrogen peroxide (H_2O_2). It has become increasingly clear over the last decade that both ROS and reactive nitrogen species (RNS) such as nitric oxide (NO) participate in a wide range of intracellular signaling pathways involved in the production of a range of cytokines, growth factors, and other inflammatory and repair modulators. These reactive species can produce both beneficial and deleterious effects (Allen et al., 2008; Thom, 2009). NO is almost certainly the cell signal pathway responsible for vasoconstriction, for example.

Such mechanisms are complex and at times operate in an apparently paradoxical manner. For example, in the treatment of chronic hypoxic wounds, some effects of HBOT are to enhance the clearance of cellular debris and bacteria by providing the substrate for macrophage phagocytosis; to stimulate growth factor synthesis through increased production and stabilization of hypoxia inducible factor 1 (HIF-1); to inhibit leukocyte activation and adherence to damaged endothelium; and, through the induction of nitric oxide synthetase 3 (NOS-3 or eNOS), to mobilize bone marrow stem cells that will enable vasculogenesis (Milovanova et al., 2009; Thom, 2009). The interactions between these mechanisms remain the subject of very active investigation. One exciting development in our emerging understanding is the concept of *hyperoxic preconditioning,* in which a short exposure to HBO_2 can induce tissue protection against future hypoxic/ischemic insult. One clinical randomized trial has been completed that suggests HBOT delivered prior to coronary artery bypass grafting reduces biochemical markers of ischemic stress and improves neurocognitive outcome (Yogaratnam et al., 2010).

Mechanism of Oxygen Therapy for Headache

NBOT has been used with some success to treat both migraine and cluster headaches for many years (Alvarez, 1939; Kudrow, 1981) based on the ability of oxygen to constrict distal cerebral resistance vessels (Drummond & Anthony, 1985; Iversen et al., 1990). The observation that oxygen administered at higher pressures produces even further vasoconstriction (with preservation of tissue oxygenation) led directly to the suggestion that HBOT might favorably influence vascular headache that is resistant to conventional drug therapy (Fife et al., 1994).

More recently, some sources have suggested that HBOT may exert therapeutic effects through the action of oxygen as a serotonergic agonist and an immunomodulator of response to substance P (a short-chain neuropeptide involved in pain signal transmission). In a clinical study of the role of HBOT in cluster headache, Di Sabato et al. (1996) estimated the immunoreactivity of substance P in the nasal mucosa of patients treated with HBOT versus a sham exposure in a hyperbaric chamber. These authors found a significant reduction in the activity of substance P in the group exposed to HBO_2 and concluded that HBOT modulated the content of substance P by a mechanism as yet unknown. In a follow-up study in 1997, the same group was able to demonstrate that exposure to HBO_2 was associated with the reestablishment of a normal plateau effect on the binding of serotonin to mononuclear cells in 9 of 14 cluster headache patients following treatment with HBOT (Di Sabato et al., 1997). Both studies demonstrated a clinical response to HBOT.

Indeed, while acknowledging that vascular mechanisms are involved, some authors have suggested that inflammation plays a critical role in the genesis of a migraine episode (Goadsby, 1997; Hamel, 1999). If this view is correct, then the well-described moderation of inflammatory pathways by HBOT may influence acute attacks and provide a useful means of prophylaxis (Slotman, 1998; Sumen et al., 2001; Thom, 2009). Figure 31.2 summarizes some of these potential mechanisms.

Toxicity and Adverse Effects

Clinically, HBOT has been reported as a successful treatment for headache since at least 1972 (Wolff, 1972; Fife & Fife, 1989; Weiss et al., 1989), and sporadic reports have followed, including some comparative trials. Conversely, oxygen in high doses may increase oxidative stress through the production of oxygen-free radical species and is potentially toxic (Yusa et al., 1987; Thom, 2009). Indeed, the brain is particularly at risk, with acute oxygen toxicity often manifested by generalized seizures very similar to grand mal epileptic events. For this reason, it is appropriate to postulate that in some migraine patients, HBOT may do more harm than good.

While precautions against fire are required and standard practice in all areas where oxygen is in use, NBOT is generally considered safe in the absence of severe respiratory disease where spontaneous ventilation is dependent on the hypoxic drive. HBOT, in contrast, is associated with some risk of adverse effects, including damage to the ears, sinuses, and lungs from the effects of pressure; temporary worsening of short-sightedness; claustrophobia; and oxygen poisoning. Although serious adverse effects are rare, HBOT cannot be regarded as an entirely benign intervention. Consequently, any demonstrated benefit needs to be assessed with full knowledge of the potential adverse effects.

CLINICAL EVIDENCE FOR THE USE OF OXYGEN

Searching Strategy

To locate all the relevant evidence, a structured search was made over a wide range of resources from their inception to September 2010. While some modifications were required for individual databases, the general search criteria are given in **Table 31.1**. Those interested in the methodology employed for locating, selecting, and analyzing the clinical evidence are referred to the full Cochrane systematic review published in 2008 (Bennett et al., 2008).

In our meta-analysis, we included patients of any age and either gender with an acute episode or history of migraine (with or without aura) and followed the diagnostic guidelines established by the International Headache Society where possible (IHS, 2004).

Analytical Approach

In presenting outcome data, this chapter quotes individual studies where appropriate and utilizes a meta-analytical approach with data from several randomized trials combined using standard statistical techniques where possible (Bennett et al., 2008). Careful consideration was given to the appropriateness of meta-analysis in the presence of significant clinical or statistical variability among studies (heterogeneity).

Table 31.1 Indicative Search Strategy Used to Locate the Clinical Evidence Referred to in This Chapter

Example Search Strategy (MEDLINE)

1. Headache/
2. exp Headache Disorders/
3. (headache$ OR migrain$ OR cephalgi$ OR cephalalgi$).tw.
4. or/1-3
5. Hyperbaric Oxygenation/
6. Oxygen Inhalation Therapy/
7. Oxygen/ae, tu, to [Adverse Effects, Therapeutic Use, Toxicity]
8. Hyperoxia/
9. Atmosphere Exposure Chambers/
10. (hyperbar$ or HBO$).tw.
11. (high pressure oxygen or 100% oxygen).tw.
12. ((monoplace or multiplace) adj5 chamber$).tw.
13. or/5-12
14. 4 and 13
15. limit 14 to human

For the purposes of the meta-analysis, a fixed-effect model was used where there was no evidence of significant heterogeneity between studies, and a random-effects model when such heterogeneity was likely. Statistical heterogeneity was assessed using the I^2 statistic, and consideration was given to the appropriateness of pooling and meta-analysis if the proportion of variability likely due to differences between trials exceeded 40% ($I^2 > 40\%$).

For proportions (dichotomous outcomes), relative risk (RR) was used as an analytical technique. When data from cross-over trials contributed to an analysis, the intention was to use the Peto method for taking joint conditional probabilities into account, as described in Curtin et al. (2002). This approach proved infeasible with the data available, however, so the trials were instead analyzed as if they were parallel group in design. This generally conservative approach ignores the reduction in interpatient variability in cross-over studies.

Continuous data were converted to the mean difference (MD) using the inverse variance method, and an overall MD calculated. Testing for publication bias was not appropriate for the data available.

Subgroup analysis was considered where appropriate by calculation of RR or MD in each subgroup and examination of the 95% confidence intervals (CIs). Non-overlap in intervals was taken to indicate a statistically significant difference between subgroups. All analyses were made on an intention-to-treat basis where possible.

Clinical Reports Identified

The clinical outcomes considered relevant are listed in **Table 31.2**. In their meta-analysis, Bennett et al. (2008) identified 11 publications dealing specifically with the clinical use of oxygen for the treatment of migraine; in a repeat search carried out in September 2010, 3 additional publications were found (**Table 31.3**).

The first report of the administration of NBOT to patients with acute migraine seems to have been provided by Alvarez in 1939, with Wolff also reporting a small series in a textbook chapter in 1972. Although these reports suggested relief from pain in some individuals, the use of oxygen at 1 ATA by mask has not become widespread and is regarded generally as ineffective in reviews of the area (Nwosu & Khan, 2005; Sandor & Afra, 2005). There have been no reported comparative trials on the use of NBOT.

With regard to HBOT, three case series reported a total of 92 patients receiving oxygen at pressures between 2.0 ATA and 2.6 ATA (Fisher et al., 1988; Fife & Fife, 1989; Fife & Meyer, 1991). Although Fisher et al. reported only a 40% success rate, the two subsequent reports suggested a high success rate—approximately 90%—for termination of headache within 20 minutes in unselected subjects (Table 31.3). These encouraging reports led to the publication of five randomized controlled trials (RCTs) enrolling a modest total of 90 patients experiencing acute migraine; all of these studies employed HBOT in one arm (Fife et al., 1992; Hill, 1992; Myers & Myers, 1995; Wilson et al., 1998; Eftedal et al., 2004). Two utilized a crossover design (Hill, 1992; Wilson et al., 1998), and Fife and colleagues (Fife & Fife, 1989; Fife & Meyer, 1991) subsequently offered HBOT to those patients initially randomized to sham therapy. All trials gave HBOT at 2.0 ATA for 30 and 60 minutes, with the exception of the study conducted by Wilson et al. (1998), who used 2.4 ATA for 60 minutes. All of the studies provided patients with a single exposure to HBOT, except in the study carried out by Eftedal et al. (2004), who gave treatments over 3 consecutive days.

All trials provided a sham therapy and blinded both patients and assessors to the treatment received. The sham procedures varied, with air at 2 ATA being used by Hill (1992) and Eftedal et al. (2004), 10% oxygen at 2 ATA to maintain inspired oxygen tension near that of air at atmospheric pressure being used by Fife (Fife & Fife, 1989; Fife & Meyer, 1991), and 100% oxygen administration at or near atmospheric pressure being used by Myers and Myers (1995) and Wilson et al. (1998). Only Fife (Fife & Fife, 1989; Fife & Meyer, 1991), therefore, administered a true placebo therapy with no increased inspired oxygen tension in the sham therapy arm.

Table 31.2 Clinical Outcomes Considered Relevant for This Chapter

Purpose of Therapy	Outcomes Considered
Acute relief of headache	• Proportion of patients with pain-free response (complete resolution of headache pain) at 1, 2, and 4 hours. • Proportion of patients with headache pain reduction from moderate/severe to mild or none • Proportion of patients with sustained relief for 24 and 48 hours • Degree of headache relief or headache intensity • Functional status or disability • Proportion of patients requiring rescue medication • Proportion of patients with photophobia or phonophobia • Proportion of patients with nausea and/or vomiting
Prevention/amelioration of subsequent headache	• Frequency of attacks • Number of headache days • Days lost to work • Self-reported assessment of treatment success • Quality of life • Functional status or disability • Headache index
Adverse effects of therapy	• Adverse effects related to HBOT, such as the proportion of patients with visual disturbance (short and long term), barotrauma (aural, sinus, or pulmonary in the short and long term), and oxygen toxicity (short term) • Any other recorded adverse effects were reported and discussed

Table 31.3 Summary of Clinical Trials of Oxygen Therapy for Acute Migraine Headache

Publication Type	Author (Year)	Comments
Review (no primary data)	Nwosu and Khan (2005)	Qualitative review of HBOT for acute headaches.
	Sandor and Afra (2005)	Qualitative review of HBOT and NBOT for migraine.
	Bennett et al. (2008)	Cochrane systematic review with meta-analysis. HBOT effective for migraine relief (RR: 5.97; 95% CI: 1.46–24.38; $P = 0.01$) but not for prevention of future headaches.
Case series	Alvarez (1939)	Successful treatment of patients with acute migraine using NBOT (original data not accessed).
	Wolff (1972)	Patients received 90% oxygen and 10% carbon dioxide at 1 ATA. Outcome: relief of pain.
	Fisher et al. (1988)	15 patients with acute migraine receiving HBOT for other reasons. Outcome: 6 of 15 (40%) complete relief.
	Fife and Fife (1989)	26 patients with acute migraine given HBOT to maximum of 2.6 ATA up to 25 minutes. Outcome: 24 of 25 (92%) complete relief.
	Fife and Meyer (1991)	51 patients receiving 118 treatments with HBOT at 2 ATA. Outcome: 109 of 1,128 treatments resulted in relief (92%); 9% return of headache within 24 hours.
Randomized controlled trials (RCT)	Fife et al. (1992)	Acute therapy trial. Partial cross-over RCT (control to active after 30 minutes) with blinding of patients and investigators; 14 patients with migraine received 100% or 10% oxygen at 2.0 ATA. Outcome: significant pain relief.
	Hill (1992)	Acute therapy trial. Cross-over RCT with blinding of patients and investigators; 8 patients with migraine received 100% oxygen or air at 2.0 ATA. Outcome: pain relief.
	Myers and Myers (1995)	Acute therapy trial. RCT with assessor blinded; 20 patients with migraine received 100% oxygen at 1.0 ATA or 2.0 ATA. Outcome: significant headache relief.
	Wilson et al. (1998)	Acute therapy trial. Cross-over RCT with blinding of patients and investigators; 8 patients with migraine with aura received 100% oxygen at 1.1 ATA or 2.4 ATA. Outcome: headache severity, pericranial tenderness, and algometry.
	Eftedal et al. (2004)	Prophylaxis trial. RCT with blinding of patients and investigators; 40 patients with migraine with or without aura received 100% oxygen or air at 2.0 ATA for three consecutive days. Outcome: Hours of headache per week, number of days with headache per week, doses of attack terminating medication per week, and blood endothelin levels.

HBOT, hyperbaric oxygen therapy; NBOT, normobaric oxygen therapy; RR, relative risk.

Inclusion and exclusion criteria also varied across the trials. Three accepted patients with diagnoses confirmed by a neurologist or physician (Fife & Fife, 1989; Fife & Meyer, 1991; Myers & Myers, 1995; Wilson et al., 1998), whereas Eftedal et al. (2004) used the criteria of the International Headache Society (IHS, 1988) and Hill (1992) used the criteria of the Ad Hoc Committee of the National Institute of Neurological Diseases and Blindness (AHC, 1962). Most trials investigated the efficacy of oxygen for the termination of an acute headache attack, although the study conducted by Eftedal et al. (2004) was primarily designed to investigate prophylaxis. Consequently, only Eftedal et al. (2004) required a documented frequency of headaches over the previous 3 months of three to eight attacks per month. For most studies, the control arms used no specific anti-headache treatment; the exception occurred in the study carried out by Myers and Myers (1995), where NBOT was administered.

Table 31.4 Characteristics of Randomized Studies

Quality Dimension	Study Methodology	Comment
Adequate sequence generation	Fife et al., 1992: good	Used random draw of sealed envelopes
	Hill, 1992: unclear	Method unclear—only the first period before cross-over accepted for analysis because there was no cross-over if relief was obtained in the first period
	All others: unclear	No details of randomization given
Allocation concealment	Unclear in all studies	Generally no discussion of the method or temporal relationship between consent and randomization
Blinding	Fife et al., 1992; Hill, 1992; Wilson et al., 1998; Eftedal et al., 2004: good	Patients, investigators, and assessors blind
	Myers & Myers, 1995: fair	Assessor only blind
Incomplete outcome data addressed	Myers & Myers, 1995; Wilson et al., 1998: good	No losses to follow-up
	Eftedal et al., 2004: fair	Six patients enrolled but therapy not completed (5 HBOT, 1 sham); 1 patient lost to follow-up
	Hill, 1992: fair	One patient not treated
	Fife et al., 1992: fair	Some patients did not return for cross-over
Free of selective reporting	All trials: good	No evidence of a failure to report important outcomes

Only Eftedal et al. (2004) reported outcomes after the immediate therapy period, reflecting the focus on the prevention of headache in this trial. While the Cochrane review (Bennett et al., 2008) concentrated on clinical outcomes related to headache relief, other outcomes reported included the number of doses of attack-terminating medicine and plasma endothelin levels after therapy (Eftedal et al., 2004) and pericranial tenderness with algometry (Wilson et al., 1998).

Overall, these studies were judged to be of moderate to low methodological quality and, therefore, may be subject to bias. In particular, two of these reports were presented only as abstracts from meeting proceedings (Fife & Fife, 1989; Fife & Meyer, 1991; Hill, 1992). A summary of the Cochrane assessment of the quality is presented in **Table 31.4**.

SUMMARY OF THE RESULTS OF RANDOMIZED TRIALS

For many of the predetermined outcomes, there were no trials that reported comparative results of either HBOT or NBOT. This section summarizes those outcomes that were reported in randomized studies.

HBOT for an Acute Migraine Episode

Three trials reported the proportion of patients with resolution or significant relief of migraine within 40 to 45 minutes of the institution of HBOT (Hill, 1992; Fife et al., 1992; Myers & Myers, 1995), and there was a statistically significant increase in the proportion of patients with substantial relief of headache with HBOT. Overall, 29 of 40 patients (72.5%) obtained relief with HBOT, versus only 3 of 36 (8.3%) patients who received a sham therapy. The relative risk of obtaining relief was statistically significant (RR: 5.97; 95% CI: 1.46–24.38) and there was no indication of a difference when using either air or NBOT as a sham (**Figure 31.3**). The absolute risk difference of 64% between sham and HBOT suggests that the number needed to treat (NNT) to achieve one extra case of relieved headache is only two cases (95% CI: 1–2).

Wilson et al. (1998) reported on the related outcome of pain intensity immediately following therapy, enrolling eight patients in a cross-over study of NBOT versus HBOT. The cross-over was made when the individual patient presented for treatment of a second headache. Pain intensity on a visual analogue scale ranging from 0 (no pain) to 10 (worst pain) was lower following HBOT, but the difference was not statistically significant in this small trial (mean pain score: 3.5 [SD = 10.7] versus 6.3 [SD = 14]; mean difference: 2.80; 95% CI: 4.69 to 10.29; $P = 0.46$). When comparing each individual before and after each exposure, the reduction in intensity from pre-treatment to post-treatment was significantly greater in the HBOT arm than in the NBOT arm (HBOT 4.4 units reduction versus NBOT 0.2 reduction; $P = 0.03$).

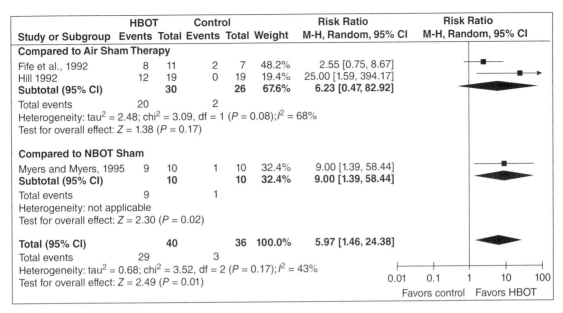

Figure 31.3 Forest Plot for the Resolution of an Acute Migraine Episode with Hyperbaric Oxygen Versus Sham. Relief is nearly six times more likely with HBOT (RR: 5.97).

NBOT for an Acute Migraine Episode

With respect to the use of NBOT, Myers and Myers (1995) used this therapy as the sham treatment for purposes of comparison to HBOT as described earlier. There was no indication that the administration of 100% oxygen was any more effective relative to HBOT than was air breathing (Figure 31.3). In this trial, only 1 of 10 patients (10%) obtained relief with NBOT versus 9 of 10 patients (90%) who received HBOT. In the two trials using air, the comparable figures were 2 of 26 patients (8%) and 20 of 30 patients (67%), suggesting little therapeutic benefit was derived from NBOT. Similarly, there was little indication of any benefit from NBOT in the study conducted by Wilson et al. (1998).

HBOT for the Prevention of Attacks

Eftedal et al. (2004) conducted the only trial that examined the ability of HBOT to prevent episodes of migraine, enrolling 40 patients (20 HBOT, 20 sham) in their investigation. There was no statistically significant difference in the mean number of days with headaches for the first week after therapy (HBOT 3.0 versus sham 2.87; MD: −0.13; 95% CI: −1.41 to 1.15; P = 0.84), nor during the fourth week (HBOT 2.52 versus sham 2.27; MD: −0.25; 95% CI: −1.52 to 1.02; P = 0.7) or the eighth week (HBOT 2.89 versus sham 2.14; MD: −0.75; 95% CI: −2.06 to 0.56;

P = 0.26). Likewise, there was not a significant reduction in the proportion of migraineurs requiring rescue medication (18 of 19 for the HBOT group versus 12 of 15 for the sham therapy; RR: 0.84; 95% CI: 0.64–1.11; P = 0.23). No trial has reported any data on the frequency of headaches, days off work, or other functional outcomes.

Eftedal et al. (2004) did not report the proportion of migraineurs experiencing nausea with or without vomiting in the week after therapy. There was no statistically significant difference between the groups (9 of 19 [47%] for the HBOT group versus 9 of 15 [60%] for the sham therapy; RR: 1.27; 95% CI: 0.68–2.38; P = 0.46).

NBOT for the Prevention of Attacks

The search revealed no series or comparative trials studying the use of NBOT for prevention of attacks. Thus there are no data on which to base any valuation of this therapy for that purpose.

ADVERSE EFFECTS AND CONTRAINDICATIONS TO HYPERBARIC OXYGEN

Adverse Effects of Therapy

The trials of HBOT for migraine made little effort to formally report any adverse effects of therapy. Myers and Myers (1995) noted that "no untoward effects were reported."

In contrast, Eftedal et al. (2004) reported that following enrollment, two patients refused to complete therapy due to claustrophobia, one developed an upper respiratory chest infection and was withdrawn by the investigators, and another patient was withdrawn following a pathological chest X-ray. Given that neither having a respiratory tract infection nor having a preexisting radiological abnormality on a chest radiograph can be described as an adverse effect of therapy, the two cases of claustrophobia were the only such events reported in these five trials. The other two cases do, however, suggest that not all patients will be suitable candidates for compression therapy.

It is not surprising that no serious complications were recorded in these small trials, as HBOT is generally well tolerated and safe in clinical practice. When adverse effects do occur, they may be associated with either increased pressure (barotrauma) or the administration of oxygen itself.

Barotrauma occurs when any noncompliant gas-filled space within the body does not equalize with environmental pressure during compression or decompression. Approximately 10% of patients complain of some difficulty equalizing middle ear pressure early in compression; while most of these problems are minor and can be overcome with training, 2% to 5% of conscious patients require middle ear ventilation tubes or formal grommets across the tympanic membrane (Lehm & Bennett, 2003; Ambiru et al., 2008). Other less common sites for barotrauma of compression include the respiratory sinuses and dental caries. The lungs are potentially vulnerable to barotrauma during decompression at the completion of each session, as expanding gas may be trapped behind blocked airways (e.g., in asthma) or abnormal lung tissue (e.g., in bullous disease). In practice, the rate of decompression following HBOT is so slow that pulmonary gas trapping is extremely rare in the absence of an undrained pneumothorax or lesions such as bullae.

The practical limiting factor for the dose of oxygen that can be delivered, either in a single treatment session or in a series of daily sessions, is oxygen toxicity. The most common acute manifestation is a seizure, which is often preceded by anxiety and agitation, during which time a switch from oxygen to air breathing may avoid the convulsion. Hyperoxic seizures typically consist of generalized tonic–clonic seizures followed by a variable post-ictal period. Such seizures arise when the antioxidant defense systems within the brain become overwhelmed. While clearly dose dependent, the onset of this effect is very variable, both between individuals and within the same individual on different days. In routine clinical hyperbaric practice, the incidence of hyperoxic

seizures is approximately 1 in 1,500 to 1 in 2,000 compressions. There are no known long-term consequences described following such seizures, and patients usually return to therapy the following day.

Chronic oxygen poisoning most commonly manifests as worsening myopia due to alterations in the refractive index of the lens following oxidative damage to lenticular proteins, similar to those associated with senescent cataract formation. As many as 75% of patients show deterioration in visual acuity after a course of 30 treatments at 2.0 ATA (Khan et al., 2003). Almost all return to pretreatment values 3 to 6 weeks after cessation of treatment. In any case, this adverse effect is not likely to be a problem after the single exposures used in most of these trials. A rapid maturation of preexisting cataracts has occasionally been associated with HBOT. Although a theoretical problem, the development of pulmonary oxygen toxicity over time does not seem to be problematic in practice—probably due to the intermittent nature of the exposure.

Contraindications to Hyperbaric Oxygen

There are few absolute contraindications to HBOT. The most commonly encountered conditions ruling out such therapy are untreated pneumothorax and a history of bleomycin administration. A pneumothorax may expand rapidly on decompression and come under tension. Prior to any compression, patients with a pneumothorax should have a patent chest drain put in place. The presence of other obvious risk factors for pulmonary gas trapping, such as bullae, should trigger a very cautious analysis of the risks of treatment versus the potential benefit.

Bleomycin is associated with a partially dose-dependent pneumonitis in approximately 20% of patients. This subgroup may be at particular risk of subsequent rapid deterioration in ventilatory function on exposure to high oxygen tensions. The relationship between pulmonary oxygen toxicity and bleomycin administration is not proven, particularly after long periods have elapsed between bleomycin and oxygen exposures. Nevertheless, any patient with a history of bleomycin administration should be carefully counseled prior to exposure to HBOT. For those recently exposed to doses greater than 200 mg and whose course was complicated by a respiratory reaction to bleomycin, compression should be avoided except in a life-threatening situation.

Practical Considerations

While HBOT administration may be an effective means for terminating migraine, there are problems of both cost and availability in applying this therapy in routine practice. For safe administration, HBOT requires relatively sophisticated equipment. For this reason, it is generally available only in specialist units, whether free-standing or hospital based. Many migraineurs do not have ready access to such facilities.

While the cost of hyperbaric therapy varies greatly around the world, one facility in Australia recently estimated the cost of a single session of treatment for an uncomplicated patient at $316 (Gomez-Castillo & Bennett, 2005). This strategy is not likely to be cost-effective compared to established therapeutic options for migraine. HBOT may be a useful option for patients who are refractory to other medications; however, this subgroup of patients has not been selected for study and the efficacy of HBOT in these patients is not known.

INTERPRETING THE CLINICAL EVIDENCE

Limitations of This Review

This review has included data from 11 trials, including 5 RCTs, and it is likely that these investigations represent all of the relevant clinical reports in this area. While every effort has been made to locate further unpublished data, it remains possible this review is subject to a positive publication bias, with results from generally favorable trials being more likely to achieve publication.

Generally, the methodological quality of the RCTs was assessed as moderate to low. Randomization was poorly described in all of the studies, and none appears to have been based on sound sample size calculations for expected differences. Other problems with synthesizing the results related to the failure to clearly report on important primary outcomes in many of the trials, poor reporting of means and standard deviations, and the variable methods used to report similar outcomes. Thus the results of this review must be interpreted with great caution.

Summary of Findings

We found evidence using pooled data from three trials that the administration of HBOT can substantially relieve an acute migraine attack (Fife et al., 1992; Hill, 1992; Myers & Myers, 1995). This analysis suggests more than 70% of patients will obtain relief within approximately 40 minutes (many within 15 or 20 minutes), with an NNT of 2 (95% CI: 1 to 2) compared to a sham therapy.

There was no evidence from a single trial that HBOT could prevent migraine episodes, reduce the incidence of nausea and vomiting, or reduce the requirement for rescue medication (Eftedal et al., 2004).

Only one small cross-over trial has reported pain intensity following HBOT (Wilson et al., 1998). While this small trial reported a significant reduction in pain intensity in the HBOT group (but not in the NBOT group), no statistically significant reduction in intensity was found when directly comparing HBOT and NBOT.

Planned subgroup analyses with respect to the dose of oxygen received (HBOT versus NBOT), session time, and length of treatment course were planned, but were not appropriate for the latter two variables. In terms of the oxygen dose used for the relief of migraine, HBOT appeared equally effective when compared to either air or NBOT, but no data were provided to suggest the minimum effective dose of HBOT. In most trials, patients underwent only a single therapeutic session at 2.0 ATA, with rapid relief of headache.

Overall, the level of evidence for the use of HBOT for the treatment of acute migraine is 2B+, while that for the prevention of migraine is 2B−. For the use of oxygen at 1 ATA, the evidence level for the treatment of acute migraine is 2B− and that for the prevention of migraine is 0.

CONCLUSIONS

The literature suggests that HBOT will effectively terminate migraine headache in the majority of patients in a general population of migraineurs. Nevertheless, the practical problems involved in the delivery of therapy suggest that HBOT should be reserved for those migraineurs who are resistant to standard pharmacological therapies. As there is no evidence available on the efficacy of HBOT in this subgroup of patients, a recommendation cannot be made that HBOT be used as a routine therapy. More research is required and should be specifically targeted at those individuals in whom standard pharmacological treatment has failed to control either the frequency or the severity of headache episodes.

HBOT cannot be recommended as a prophylactic therapy for migraine, and there is no evidence to support the practice of administering NBOT to patients with acute migrainous headache.

ACKNOWLEDGMENTS

Some of the material in this chapter has been reproduced from the following source: Bennett MH, French C, Schnabel A, et al. Normobaric and hyperbaric oxygen therapy for migraine and cluster headache. *Cochrane Database of Systematic Reviews* 2008;3:CD005219. Copyright Cochrane Collaboration, reproduced with permission of the first author.

REFERENCES

Ad Hoc Committee on the Classification of Headache of the National Institute of Neurological Diseases and Blindness. Classification of headache. *JAMA* 1962;179:717–718.

Allen BW, Demchencko IT, Piantadosi CA. Two faces of nitric oxide: implications for cellular mechanisms of oxygen toxicity. *J Appl Physiol* 2009;106:662–667.

Alvarez WC. The new oxygen treatment for migraine. *Am J Dig Dis* 1939;6:728.

Ambiru S, Furuyama N, Aono M, et al. Analysis of risk factors associated with complications of hyperbaric oxygen therapy. *J Critical Care* 2008;23:295–300.

Bateman DN. Sumatriptan. *Lancet* 1993;341:221–224.

Bennett MH, French C, Schnabel A, et al. Normobaric and hyperbaric oxygen therapy for migraine and cluster headache. *Cochrane Database Syst Rev* 2008;3:CD005219.

Bigal M, Borucho S, Serrano D, Lipton RB. The acute treatment of episodic and chronic migraine in the USA. *Cephalalgia* 2009;29:891–897.

Curtin F, Elbourne D, Altman DG. Meta-analysis combining parallel and cross-over clinical trials. *Statistics Med* 2002;21:2145–2159.

Di Sabato F, Giacovazzo M, Cristalli G, et al. Effect of hyperbaric oxygen on the immunoreactivity to substance P in the nasal mucosa of cluster headache patients. *Headache* 1996;36:221–223.

Di Sabato F, Rocco M, Martelletti P, Giacovazzo M. Hyperbaric oxygen in chronic cluster headaches: influence on serotonergic pathways. *Undersea Hyperbaric Med* 1997;24:117–122.

Drummond PD, Anthony M. Extracranial vascular responses to sublingual nitroglycerine and oxygen inhalation in cluster headache patients. *Headache* 1985;25:70–74.

Eftedal OS, Lydersen S, Helde G, et al. A randomised, double blind study of the prophylactic effect of hyperbaric oxygen therapy on migraine. *Cephalalgia* 2004;24: 639–644.

Fife CE, Meyer JS. Hyperbaric oxygen treatment of acute migraine headache. *Headache Quarterly* 1991;2:301–306.

Fife CE, Meyer JS, Berry JM, Sutton TE. Hyperbaric oxygen and acute migraine pain: preliminary results of a randomised blinded trial. *Undersea Biomed Res* 1992;19:106–107.

Fife CE, Powell MG, Sutton TE, Meyer JS. Transcranial Doppler evaluation of the middle cerebral artery from 1ATA to 3ATA PO2. *Undersea Hyperbaric Med* 1994;21(suppl):77.

Fife WP, Fife CE. Treatment of migraine with hyperbaric oxygen. *J Hyperbaric Med* 1989;4:7–15.

Fisher B, Jain KK, Braun E, Lehrl S. *Handbook of Hyperbaric Oxygen Therapy.* Amsterdam: Springer-Verlag; 1988.

Gesell L, ed. *Hyperbaric Oxygen Therapy Indications* (12th ed.). Durham: Undersea and Hyperbaric Medical Society Publications; 2008.

Goadsby PJ. Current concepts of the pathophysiology of migraine. *Neurol Clinics* 1997;15:27–42.

Gomez-Castillo JD, Bennett MH. The cost of hyperbaric therapy at the Prince of Wales Hospital, Sydney. *South Pacific Underwater Med J* 2005;35:194–198.

Hamel E. Current concepts of migraine pathophysiology. *Can J Clin Pharm* 1999;6(suppl A):9A–14A.

Hill RK. A blinded, crossover controlled study of the use of hyperbaric oxygen in the treatment of migraine headache. *Undersea Biomed Res* 1992;19(suppl):106.

International Headache Society. Classification and diagnostic criteria for headache disorders, cranial neuralgias and facial pain: 1st edition. *Cephalalgia* 1988;8 (suppl 7):29–34.

International Headache Society. Headache Classification Subcommittee of the International Headache Society. The International Classification of Headache Disorders: 2nd edition. *Cephalalgia* 2004;24(suppl 1):1–160.

Iversen HK, Nielsen TH, Olesen J, Tfelt-Hansen P. Arterial responses during migraine headache. *Lancet* 1990;336:837–839.

Khan B, Evans AW, Easterbrook M. Refractive changes in patients undergoing hyperbaric oxygen therapy: a prospective study. *Undersea Hyperbaric Med* 2003;24(suppl):9.

Kudrow L. Response of cluster headache attacks to oxygen inhalation. *Headache* 1981;21:1–4.

Lehm JP, Bennett MH. Predictors of middle ear barotrauma associated with hyperbaric oxygen therapy. *South Pacific Underwater Med Soc J* 2003;33:127–133.

Milovanova TN, Bhopale VM, Sorokina EM, et al. Hyperbaric oxygen stimulates vasculogenic stem cell growth and differentiation in vivo. *J Appl Physiol* 2009;106:711–728.

Myers DE, Myers RA. A preliminary report on hyperbaric oxygen in the relief of migraine headache. *Headache* 1995;35:197–199.

Nwosu IA, Khan AA. Hyperbaric oxygen therapy in primary headache: a research review. *Biom Research* 2005;16:143–160.

Sandor PS, Afra J. Nonpharmacologic treatment of migraine. *Curr Pain Headache Reports* 2005;9:202–205.

Silberstein SD. Meeting acute migraine treatment needs through novel treatment formulations. *Neurotherapeutics* 2010;7:153–158.

Slotman GJ. Hyperbaric oxygen in systemic inflammation: HBO is not just a movie channel anymore. *Crit Care Med* 1998;26:1932–1933.

Sumen G, Cimsit M, Eroglu L. Hyperbaric oxygen treatment reduces carrageenan-induced acute inflammation in rats. *Eur J Pharmacol* 2001;431:265–268.

Thom SJ. Oxidative stress is fundamental to hyperbaric oxygen therapy. *J Appl Physiol* 2009;106:988–995.

Weiss LD, Ramasastry SS, Eidelman BH. Treatment of a cluster headache patient in a hyperbaric chamber. *Headache* 1989;29:109–110.

Wilson JR, Foresman GH, Gamber RG, Wright T. Hyperbaric oxygen in the treatment of migraine with aura. *Headache* 1998;38:112–115.

Wolff HG. *Wolff's Headache and Other Head Pain* (3rd ed.). New York: Oxford University Press; 1972.

Yogaratnam JZ, Laden G, Guvendik L, et al. Hyperbaric oxygen preconditioning improves myocardial function, reduces length of intensive care stay, and limits complications post coronary artery bypass graft surgery. *Cardiovasc Revasc Med* 2010;11:8–19.

Yusa T, Beckman JS, Crapo JD, Freeman BA. Hyperoxia increases H_2O_2 production by brain in vivo. *J Appl Physiol* 1987;63:353–358.

Index